369 0246402

KU-067-224

Imaging in Oncological Urology

Jean J.M.C.H. de la Rosette
Michael J. Manyak
Mukesh G. Harisinghani
Hessel Wijkstra
Editors

Imaging in Oncological Urology

Forewords by:
Peter L. Choyke, M.D.
and
John M. Fitzpatrick MCh, FRCSI, FC Urol (SA), FRCSGlas, FRCS

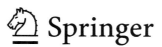 Springer

Editors
Jean J.M.C.H. de la Rosette
Department of Urology
Academic Medical Center
Amsterdam
The Netherlands
j.j.delarosette@amc.uva.nl

Michael J. Manyak
Department of Urology
The George Washington University
Washington
USA
mmanyak@mfa.gwu.edu

Mukesh G. Harisinghani
Department of Radiology
Massachusetts General Hospital
Boston
USA
mukesh@massmed.org

Hessel Wijkstra
Department of Urology
Academic Medical Center
Amsterdam
The Netherlands
h.wijkstra@amc.uva.nl

ISBN: 978-1-84628-514-1   e-ISBN: 978-1-84628-759-6
DOI 10.1007/978-1-84628-759-6

British Library Cataloguing in Publication Data
A catalogue record for this book is available from the British Library

Library of Congress Control Number: 2008938964

Springer Science+Business Media
springer.com

Foreword

The past decade has seen dramatic advances in urology and imaging. These changes are evident in improvements in laparoscopic surgery as well as in the emergence of multidetector CT, with multiplanar reformatting and FDG-PET-CT as routine imaging methods. The new minimally invasive procedures often require more exacting imaging as the surgeon does not have the same visual field of view as was possible with open procedures. Thus, it is appropriate now to provide an update on imaging advances for the benefit of urologists and radiologists alike. The increasing number of innovative imaging approaches to urologic tumors including CT, MRI, PET, SPECT, and endoscopic imaging can be perplexing and lead to over- and underestimations of the capabilities of modern imaging on the part of those who interpret them and those who use the information they provide for patient management. There is a growing "expectations gap" between what is expected and what is possible that needs to be closed. While previous books have focused on the more common urologic tumors such as bladder, prostate, and kidney cancer, none has attempted a comprehensive review of the state of the art of imaging in most of the tumors involved in urologic oncology. *Imaging in Urologic Oncology* addresses these challenges.

In the modern imaging department it is easy to forget how useful conventional plain radiography can be in urologic diagnosis. Much of our current understanding of urologic disease is based on the "classic appearance" on intravenous urograms, cystograms, or retrograde pyelograms. Therefore, conventional imaging provides the first "layer" in our understanding of urologic tumors. The next layer is cross-sectional imaging. The impact of cross-sectional imaging on the detection of renal and adrenal tumors can be seen from the steady decrease in the average size of renal tumors detected today in comparison to 10 years ago. Today subcentimeter tumors can be routinely identified and characterized. This has had important implications for the management of these lesions and the need to biopsy or observe them. Perhaps more profoundly it has shaken the concept of what tumors are, how often they occur, and how often they are occult. For the urothelial tract, CT and MR urography have become the new gold standard for diagnosis. The use of virtual endoscopy—based on CT or MRI data—is opening up new opportunities for early diagnosis with more complete characterization tumor invasion and staging of urothelial tract tumors. The use of MRI for prostate cancer detection continues to evolve with improvements in sensitivity and specificity as new techniques such as spectroscopy, diffusion weighted imaging, and dynamic contrast enhancement are employed. These subjects are reviewed in depth in this book.

The final layer in each section is radionuclide and PET imaging. Although these fields have played a minor role to date in urologic oncology, this situation is changing fast. The potential of these methods is obvious to anyone who experiences the dramatic diagnostic power of an FDG-PET-CT scan when detecting a metastatic lesion that, even in retrospect, was nearly invisible on the CT. Although the role of PET-CT is evolving in urologic oncology, it clearly has a promising future.

The final chapters of this book are appropriately devoted to the future. The editors had to make some difficult decisions about what to cover and they chose well. The insights of the contributing authors, all of whom are thought leaders in their areas, provide tantalizing insights into what is "around the corner." Image-guided therapeutic interventions have the potential to improve patient outcome, decrease morbidity, and speed procedure time while reducing costs. New contrast media will provide highly targeted and specific information on the biology of tumors without the need for biopsy. Optical contrast agents may dramatically improve the diagnostic capabilities of "white light" endoscopy, as it is currently performed, as targeted fluorescent conjugates are used to highlight tiny tumor clusters, while they are still completely curable. And finally, in a "back to the future" chapter, elasticity imaging may allow us to not only see cancers more easily but "feel" them as well.

Thus, *Imaging in Urologic Oncology* provides a needed resource to health care providers who are concerned with the diagnosis and management of urologic tumors in patients who suffer from them. It is this last group that stands to benefit most from this work.

Bethesda, MD, USA   Peter L. Choyke, M.D.

Foreword

The advances in urological imaging in the past decade have been considerable. The improvement in existing technology and the introduction of new methods of imaging have helped the clinician in urological oncology. For example, it is now much easier to be certain of the volume of disease and also its whereabouts; biopsy techniques have now become more reliable; interventional procedures to relieve ureteric obstruction have become more routine and certainly less traumatic for the patient. Innovation has been prevalent in the field of imaging in urological oncology and it is essential for urologists to maintain their knowledge of a fast-growing field.

It is often the case that radiologists send their descriptions of new techniques preferentially to their own specialist journals. I know that very frequently now imaging papers are being sent to urological journals, a practice I would thoroughly endorse speaking as editor-in-chief of such a journal. It is a pleasure therefore to introduce a book in which radiologists and urologists, whose main interests lie in urological oncology, have collaborated to produce an excellent textbook of imaging in urological oncology.

Each of the urological cancers is covered using a similar format in every case. The introduction is by a urologist, and the three sections on imaging for each cancer have been written by radiologists (although in some cases they are written by urologists). At the end of each cancer topic the urologists have written a section entitled "Considerations." In this they discuss the impact of imaging technology on the practice of urological oncology. It is a rather novel and in my opinion successful way of covering the subject and I feel that it should be required reading for urologists. Given the excellence of the writers and their high academic standing, I feel that it will be read by radiologists also. With the emphasis nowadays in cancer management on multi-disciplinary approaches, this book embodies that principle and will be a superb addition to the literature.

John M. Fitzpatrick MCh, FRCSI, FC Urol (SA), FRCSGlas, FRCS
Professor and Chairman Department of Surgery
Consultant Urologist Mater Misericordiae

Preface

Novel and significant changes in the area of oncologic imaging have had a positive impact on the ability to non-invasively stage bladder, prostate, penile, testicular, adrenal, and renal tumors. Most of these imaging enhancements are closely related and parallel the clinical impact of these tumors: for example as prostate cancer becomes the most common malignancy in men, there is a push to use imaging for both accurate staging prior to therapy and also as a means to follow patients after therapy. Most of the novel and cutting-edge therapeutic techniques being developed to treat these genitourinary tumors are increasingly more dependent on imaging for better tumor delineation and evaluation. The mainstay for imaging used to be conventional imaging techniques with transrectal and transabdominal ultrasound, angiography, and intravenous contrast studies. Significant improvements in image processing and resolution in cross-sectional imaging with computed tomography, magnetic resonance imaging, and now single photon emission computed tomography have brought dramatic changes in our ability to assess genitourinary malignancies of all types. Improvements in contrast agents and superimposition of functional studies with anatomical studies have now made molecular imaging with radionuclides part of our armamentarium for these neoplasms.

What can the expected impact of imaging be on the future of uro-oncology? Although the current orientation for imaging has been anatomic and organ specific, the striking improvements in imaging related to functional activity are now being combined with the anatomic data to give a more complete assessment of the disease process in all stages. The development of new molecular markers and the incorporation of virtual technology will provide a true fusion of technology that is bound to have an impact on our management of oncological problems. We are currently limited by our inability to detect disease at its earliest stages, follow it closely through a course of therapy, and monitor it after treatment. Imaging is a major key to improvements that may make management of cancer similar to that of other chronic diseases such as diabetes or hypertension. This text presents the state of the art for imaging in urological oncology and gives a glimpse of future directions for research in this exciting field.

Jean de la Rosette
Michael Manyak
Mukesh Harisinghani
Hessel Wijkstra

Contents

Contributors

Maurice C. Aalders, Msc, PhD Academic Medical Center, University of Amsterdam, Amsterdam, The Netherlands

Peter Albers, MD Department of Urology, Klinikum Kassel GmbH, Kassel, Hesse, Germany

Steve D. Allen, BSc (Hons), MBBS, MRCS, FRCR. Department of Imaging, Royal Marsden Hospital, Sutton, Surrey, UK

Gerasimos Alivizatos, MD. PhD, FEBU Second Urology Department, Athens Medical School, Kolonaki, Athens, Greece

Michalakis A. Averkiou, PhD Marie Curie Chair of Excellence, Biomedical Engineering Program Department of Mechanical Engineering, University of Cyprus

Rajinikanth Ayyathurai, MD, MS, MRCS (Ed) Department of Urology, University of Miami Miller School of Medicine, Miami, Florida, USA

Mark Bachner, MD 3rd Medical Department – Center for Oncology and Hematology, Ludwig Boltzmann-Institute for Applied Cancer Research Vienna (LBI-ACR VIEnna), Kaiser Franz Josef – Spital der Stadt Wien and Applied Cancer Research Institution for Translational Research Vienna (ACR-ITR VIEnna), Kundratstrasse 3, A-1100 Vienna, Austria

Alexander Becherer, MD Department of Nuclear Medicine, Landeskrankenhaus Feldkirch, Feldkirch, Austria

Michael A. Blake, MB, BCh, BA0, BSc, MRCPI, FFR(RCSI), FRCR Department of Radiology, Massachusetts General Hospital, Boston, MN, USA

Michael L. Blute, MD Department of Urology, Mayo Clinic College of Medicine, Rochester, MN, USA

Damien M. Bolton, MB, BS, BA, MD, FRCS, FRACS Department of Surgery, University of Melbourne, Heidelberg, Victoria, Australia

Adrienne H. Brouwers, MD, PhD Department of Nuclear Medicine and Molecular Imaging, University Medical Center Groningen, Groningen, The Netherlands

Ignasi Carrió, MD Department of Nuclear Medicine, Hospital de Sant Pau, Barcelona, Spain

David Cosgrove, MA, MSc, FRCP, FRCR Department of Radiology, Hammersmith Hospital, London, UK

Peter Dawson, PhD, FInstP, FRCP, FRCR Department of Imaging, UCL Hospitals, London, UK

Ferdinand Frauscher, MD   Department of Radiology II, Medical University Innsbruck, Innsbruck, Tyrol, Austria

Matthijs C.M. Grimbergen, BSc   Department of Medical Physics, University Medical Centre Utrecht, Utrecht, The Netherlands

Sigurdur Gudjonsson, MD   Department of Urology, Lund University Hospital, Lund, Sweden

James A. Guthrie, MRCP, FRCR, BA, MB, BChir   Department of Clinical Radiology, St James's University Hospital, Leeds, West Yorkshire, UK

Hamphrey R. Ham, MD, MSc, Phd   Department of Nuclear Medicine, Ghent University, Ghent, Belgium

Masoom A. Haider, MD, FRCP   Department of Medical Imaging, University of Toronto, Toronto, ON, Canada

Mukesh G. Harisinghani   Department of Radiology, White 270, Massachusetts General Hospital, Boston, USA

Robert P. Hartman, MD   Department of Diagnostic Radiology, Mayo Clinic College of Medicine, Rochester, MN, USA

Christopher James Harvey, BSc, MBBS, MRCP, FRCR   Department of Imaging, Hammersmith Hospital, London, UK

Axel Heidenreich, MD   Department of Urology, University of Cologne, Cologne, Germany

Hedvig Hricak, MD, PhD, Dr.hc   Department of Radiology, Memorial Sloan-Kettering Cancer Center, New York, USA

Cornelis A. Hoefnagel, MD, PhD   Department of Nuclear Medicine, Netherlands Cancer Institute, Amsterdam, The Netherlands

Simon Horenblas, MD, PhD, FEBU   Department of Urology, Netherlands Cancer Institute, Amsterdam, The Netherlands

Christian J. Ingui, MD   Department of Radiology, Boston Medical Centre, Boston, MA, USA

Brant A. Inman, MD, FRCSC   Assistant Professor of Urology, DUMC 2812, Duke University Medical Center, Durham, NC 27710

Audrey E.T. Jacques MBBS (BSc) MRCP FRCR   Department of Radiology, St Thomas Hospital, London, UK

Pieter L. Jager, MD, PhD   Department of Nuclear Medicine and Molecular Imaging, University Medical Center Groningen, Groningen, The Netherlands

Michael A.S. Jewett, MD, FRCSC   Department of Urology, University of Toronto, Toronto, Ontario, Canada

Kartik S. Jhaveri, MD   Department of Medical Imaging, University of Toronto, Toronto, Ontario, Canada

Adrian D. Joyce, MS, FRCS (Urol)   Department of Urology, St. James's University Hospital, Leeds, UK

Georgios Karanikas, MD   Department of Nuclear Medicine, Medical University of Vienna, Vienna, Austria

Louis R. Kavoussi, M.D   James Buchanan Brady Urological Institute, John Hopkins Medical Institutions, Baltimore, MD, USA

Eric A. Klein, MD Section of Urologic Oncology, Glickman Urologic and Kidney Institute, Cleveland, Ohio, USA

Bin K. Kroon, MD PhD Department of Urology, Leiden University Medical Center, Leiden, The Netherlands

M. Pilar Laguna, MD, PhD Department of Urology, Academic Medical Center, Amsterdam, The Netherlands

Nathan Lawrentschuk, MBBS Department of Surgery, University of Melbourne, Heidelberg, Victoria, Australia

Ton G. van Leeuwen Biophysical Engineering & Biomedical Technology Institute, University of Twente, AE Enschede, The Netherlands

Brian Lucey, MB, BCh, BAO, FFR (RCSI) Department of Radiology, Boston VA Healthcare System, West Roxbury, MA, USA

Agnieszka Maj-Hes, MD Department of Urology, Kaiser Franz Josef Hospital, Vienna, Austria

Murugesan Manoharan, MD, FRCS (Eng), FRACS (Urol) Department of Urology, University of Miami Miller School of Medicine, Miami, Florida, USA

Wiking Månsson, MD, PhD Department of Urology, Lund University Hospital, Lund, Sweden

Michael J. Manyak Department of Urology, The George Washington University, Washington, USA

Walter Scott McDougal, MD Department of Urology, Harvard Medical School, Boston, MA, USA

Michael Mitterberger, MD Department of Urology, Medical University of Innsbruck, Innsbruck, Austria

Markus Mitterhauser, PhD Department of Nuclear Medicine, Medical University of Vienna, Vienna, Austria

Michael Muntener, MD The Department of Urology, Johns Hopkins Hospital, Baltimore, MD, USA

Chung Yung Nio, MD Radiology Department, University of Amsterdam, Amsterdam, The Netherlands

Patrick O'Keeffe, M.B., B.Ch., M.R.C.P.I, F.F.R.R.C.S.I, F.R.C.R. Consultant Radiologist, Letterkenny General Hospital, Ireland

Martin O'Malley Department of Medical Imaging, University of Toronto, Toronto, ON, Canada

Juan Palou Department of Urology, Fundació Puigvert, Cartagena, Barcelona, Spain

Leo Pallwein, MD Department of Radiology II, University Hospital Innsbruck, Innsbruck, Austria

Alexandru Patriciu PhD, B.Sc, M.Sc.CompSci, M.Sc. MechEng, Ph.D Department of Electrical and Computer Engineering, McMaster University, Hamilton, ON, Canada

Doru Petrisor, PhD Department of Urology, John Hopkins University, Baltimore, MD, USA

Hendrik van Poppel, MD, PhD Department of Urology, University Hospital of KULeuven, Leuven, Belgium

Jens Rassweiler, MD Department of Urology, SLK Kliniken Heilbronn, Heilbronn, Baden-Württemberg, Germany

Gundula Rendl, MD Department of Nuclear Medicine, Medical University of Vienna, Vienna, Austria

Rodney Reznek, FRCP, FRCR Centre for Molecular Oncology and Imaging, London School of Medicine and Dentistry, London, UK

Theo M. de Reijke MD PhD FEBU Department of Urology, Academic Medical Center, Amsterdam, The Netherlands

David M. Rodin, MD Indian River Urology Association, Vero Beach, Florida, USA

Jean J.M.C.H. de la Rosette Department of Urology, Academic Medical Center, Amsterdam, The Netherlands

Mansi A. Saksena, MB, BS Department of Radiology, Massachusetts General Hospital, Boston, MA, USA

Evis Sala, MD, PhD, FRCR Department of Radiology, University of Cambridge and Addenbrookes Hospital, Hills Road, Cambridge, UK

Maria de Santis, MD 3rd Medical Department – Center for Oncology and Hematology, Ludwig Boltzmann-Institute for Applied Cancer Research Vienna (LBI-ACR VIEnna), Kaiser Franz Josef – Spital der Stadt Wien and Applied Cancer Research Institution for Translational Research Vienna (ACR-ITR VIEnna)/CEADDP, Kundratstrasse 3, A-1100 Vienna, Austria

Gary Schwartz, BS, BA Research and Development, Philips Ultrasound, Bothell, WA, USA

Andrew M. Scott MBBS (Hons) MD FRACP DDU Ludwig Institute for Cancer Research, Melbourne Centre for Clinical Sciences, Heidelberg, Victoria, Australia

Shomik Sengupta, MB, MS, FRACS Suite 103, Freemason's Medical Centre, East Melbourne, Victoria, Australia

Bindu N. Setty, MD, DNB Department of Radiology, Massachusetts General Hospital, Boston, MN, USA

Mark S. Soloway, MD Department of Urology, University of Miami Miller School of Medicine, Miami, Florida, USA

Rémi Souchon, PhD INSERM, U556, Lyon, France

Dan Stoianovici, PhD Department of Urology, John Hopkins University, Baltimore, MD, USA

Michael J. Stone, MD Department of Diagnostic Radiology, National Institutes of Health, Bethesda, Maryland, USA

Günther Strau, MD Department of Radiology, Kaiser Franz Josef – Spital der Stadt Wein, Kundrastrasse 3, A-1100 Vienna, Austria

Shahin Tabatabaei, MD Department of Urology, Harvard Medical School, Boston, MA, USA

Dogu Teber, MD, F.E.B.U Department of Urology, University of Heidelberg, SLK Kliniken, Heilbronn, Germany

David Thüer, MD Department of Urology, University of Cologne, Cologne, Germany

Renato A. Valdés Olmos, MD, PhD Department of Nuclear Medicine, Netherlands Cancer Institute, Amsterdam, The Netherlands

Christophe Vandewiele, MD, PhD   Department of Nuclear Medicine, Ghent University, Ghent, Belgium

Humberto Villavicencio, MD   Department of Urology, Fundació PuigvertC/Cartagena, Barcelona, Spain

Wolfgang Wadsak, PhD   Department of Nuclear Medicine, Medical University of Vienna, Vienna, Austria

Tze Min Wah, MBChB, FRCR   Department of Clinical Radiology, St James's University Hospital, Leeds, West Yorkshire, UK

Hessel Wijkstra   Department of Urology, Academic Medical Center, Amsterdam, The Netherlands

Bradford J. Wood, MD   Diagnostic Radiology Department, National Institutes of Health, Bethesda, MD, USA

Georg Zettinig, MD   Department of Nuclear Medicine, Medical University of Vienna, Vienna, Austria

Part I
Adrenal Carcinoma

Chapter 1

Adrenal Carcinoma: Introduction

G. Alivizatos

Introduction

The widespread use of high-resolution anatomic imaging modalities such as ultrasound, computed tomography (CT), and magnetic resonance imaging (MRI) has led to the increased detection of clinically silent adrenal masses. Incidental adrenal masses (incidentalomas) is a serendipitous finding in 0.3–5% of those patients who undergo one of these imaging investigations and 70–94% of these lesions are biochemically inert and benign and are therefore named adrenal adenomas. This percentage could be even higher, as shown from autopsy studies that the prevalence of adrenal masses is about 7% in patients 70 years of age or older [1]. In those with an extra adrenal malignancy the risk that an adrenal mass represents a metastasis is 6–35% and the assessment of such a case is a difficult procedure. Until recently, surgical resection, adrenal biopsy, and clinical follow-up were used in order to distinguish benign from malignant lesions.

Today, management of these adrenal masses is based upon their size, upon their biochemical activity, upon the patient age, and finally upon the radiologic characteristics on CT, MRI, and PET scans [2]. First, patients with solid adrenal masses should undergo biochemical assessment. Adrenalectomy is considered when biochemical overactivity is identified, when the adrenal mass is bigger than 6 cm, when suspicious findings are identified with the imaging modalities, and finally when there is documentation of an increase in the size of the suspected lesion. Controversial issues arise in the management of solid adrenal masses between 4 and 6 cm, while those patients with lesions less than 4 cm are usually monitored [2].

Improvements of both CT and MRI techniques have increased the effectiveness of these imaging modalities in distinguishing benign from malignant adrenal tumors [3–5]. At the same time, nuclear medicine studies using specific radiotracers have the advantage of providing functional metabolic information and when the findings of these studies are correlated with the results of the CT and MRI scans, the correct characterization of an adrenal lesion becomes more specific [6].

Positron emission tomography (PET) CT with 18-F flourodeoxyglucose (18-FDG) allows adrenal malignant tumors to be recognized and offers detailed morphological information [7].

In this chapter, recent developments in conventional and cross-sectional imaging techniques and also scintigraphy and PET imaging innovations for the characterization of adrenal masses will be presented and analyzed.

References

1. Lau J, Balk E, Rothberg M et al. Management of clinically inapparent adrenal mass. Rockville, MD: Agency for Healthcare Research and Quality; 2002. AHRQ Publication No. 02-014. Evidence Report/Technology Assessment No. 56.
2. NIH state-of-the-science statement on management of the clinically inapparent adrenal mass (incidentaloma). NIH Consens State Sci Statements 2002;19(2):1–25.
3. Heinz-Peer G, Memarsadeghi M, Niederle B. Imaging of adrenal masses. Curr Opin Urol. 2007;17(1):32–8.
4. Bessel-Browne R, O'Malley ME. CT of pheochromocytoma and paraganglioma: risk of adverse events with i.v. administration of nonionic contrast material. AJR Am J Roentgenol. 2007;188(4):970–4.
5. Jhaveri KS, Wong F, Ghai S, Haider MA. Comparison of CT histogram analysis and chemical shift MRI in the characterization of indeterminate adrenal nodules. AJR Am J Roentgenol. 2006;187(5):1303–8.
6. Gross MD, Avram A, Fig LM, Rubello D. Contemporary adrenal scintigraphy. Eur J Nucl Med Mol Imaging. 2007;34(4):547–7.
7. Metser U, Miller E, Lerman H, Lievshitz G, et al. 18F-FDG PET/CT in the evaluation of adrenal masses. J Nucl Med. 2006;47(1): 32–7.

G. Alivizatos (✉)
Second Urology Department, Athens Medical School, Sismanoglio Hospital, Kolonaki, Athens, Greece

J.J.M.C.H. de la Rosette et al. (eds.), *Imaging in Oncological Urology*,
DOI 10.1007/978-1-84628-759-6_1, © Springer-Verlag London Limited 2009

Chapter 2

Cross-Sectional Imaging of Adrenal Masses

T.M. Wah, J.A. Guthrie, and A.D. Joyce

Masses encountered in the absence of hyperfunctioning syndromes will first be considered, and then the appearances of adrenal glands in the context of the syndromes of hormonal excess.

Non-functioning Adrenal Masses

Over the last two decades, with the increasing use of computed tomography (CT) and magnetic resonance imaging (MRI), there has been a rise in the detection of unsuspected adrenal masses when investigating unrelated diseases. These masses are frequently referred to as adrenal incidentalomas [1, 2], and such incidentalomas are usually, but not always, without clinical consequence. In autopsy series, the prevalence of incidental adrenal masses is about 2.1% which may range from 1.4% in the younger patients to 8.7% in the

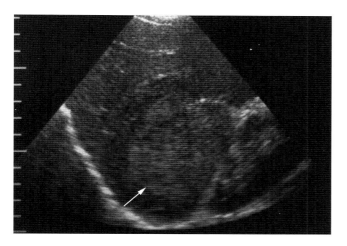

Fig. 2.1 Ultrasound showed a large mildly echogenic right adrenal mass situated in the hepato-renal space (*arrow*)

older patients [3–6], and in CT series adrenal nodules greater than 1 cm in diameter are detected in 0.35–5% of cases [7–10]. Most incidentalomas are benign, non-hormonally active, adrenal cortical adenomas; however, they may be hormonally active, but clinically unsuspected, in up to 10% of cases [11]. The other clinically significant conditions that need to be considered are pheochromocytomas, the rare adrenal cortical carcinoma, and in the cancer patient an adrenal metastasis.

Adrenal masses may occasionally be identified with conventional imaging techniques such as ultrasound (Fig. 2.1) or rarely indirectly through intravenous urography, but these techniques do not have a role in their characterization. It is through the use of CT or MRI that adrenal masses are most commonly identified, and these techniques have the crucial roles of assessing and characterizing both benign and malignant adrenal masses. The findings at CT and MR may allow a specific diagnosis or limit the differential diagnosis which may be further refined when clinical or biochemical information is taken into account.

Adenoma

Adenomas are the commonest adrenal tumors. Hormonally inactive adenomas are common in the general population with a prevalence of 3% [5] and adenomas greater than 1 cm are detected on abdominal CT in 0.35–5% of patients [7–10].The incidence is higher in patients with diabetes mellitus, hypertension, and in elderly females [3, 12]. In patients with adenomas they are bilateral in 9.5% [13].

On CT the normal adrenal gland appears as a chevron or Y-shaped structure with a smooth contour and a length of 2–4 cm [14]. The maximal width of the body of the normal gland is 1.2 cm and each limb 5 mm [15] (Fig. 2.2). Adenomas are usually round in shape, less than 3 cm in diameter, with a smooth outline, homogeneous internal architecture, and may have the same density as normal adrenal

T.M. Wah (✉)
Department of Radiology, St. James's University Hospital, Leeds LS9 7TF, United Kingdom, tze.wah@leedsth.nhs.uk

J.J.M.C.H. de la Rosette et al. (eds.), *Imaging in Oncological Urology*,
DOI 10.1007/978-1-84628-759-6_2, © Springer-Verlag London Limited 2009

(a)   (b)

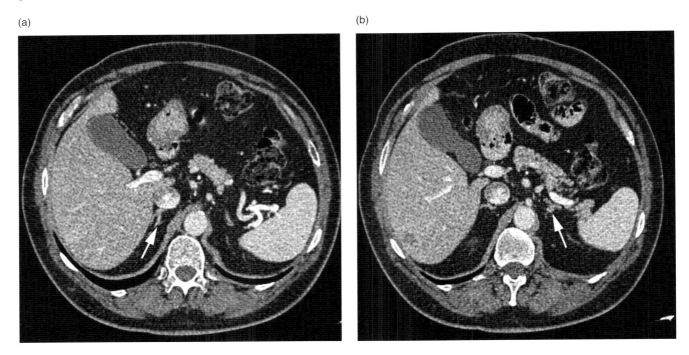

Fig. 2.2 Axial contrast enhanced CT shows a normal (**a**) right and (**b**) left adrenal glands (*arrows*)

tissue (Fig. 2.2). Most adenomas contain large amounts of intra-cytoplasmic fat, the precursor for hormone synthesis. The attenuation of adrenal adenomas varies according to the quantity of this intracellular fat with mean measurements ranging from −10 to 30 HU (Fig. 2.3a) [16]. Calcification, necrosis, and hemorrhage are extremely rare [17]. Adenomas enhance after IV contrast (Fig. 2.3b) and characteristically have a more rapid washout of contrast than adrenal

(a)   (b)

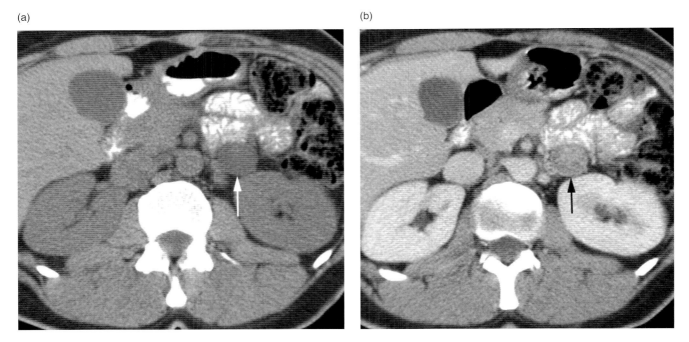

Fig. 2.3 Axial (**a**) unenhanced and (**b**) contrast enhanced CT shows a small left adrenal adenoma with a smooth outline, with a mean HU of eight and homogeneous enhancement following IV contrast (*arrow*)

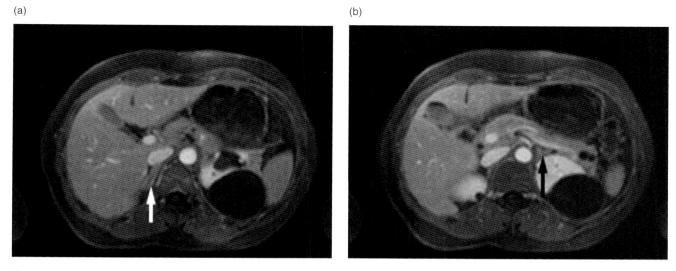

Fig. 2.4 Axial contrast enhanced MRI shows a normal (**a**) right and (**b**) left adrenal glands (*arrows*) (Reprinted with permission from Grainger, RG, Thomas, AMK, In: Dawson, P, Cosgrove, DO, Grainger, RG (eds) *Textbook of Contrast Media*, Oxford: ISIS Medical Media Ltd, 1999)

metastases, pheochromocytomas, and adrenal carcinomas [10, 18–20].

On MRI, the signal characteristics are similar to normal adrenal glandular tissue, i.e., typically hypo-intense on T1 and iso-intense or slightly hyper-intense on T2-weighted images (Fig. 2.4). These properties are not sufficiently useful to differentiate an adenoma from metastases as the range of signal intensity overlaps with that of metastases. However, chemical shift imaging is a useful means to identify the presence of intra-cytoplasmic fat and can distinguish adenomas from metastases (Fig. 2.5a and b) [21, 22]. A minority of adrenal adenomas have a relatively small proportion of intracellular fat. These lipid poor adenomas are more difficult to

differentiate from metastases as they have higher CT attenuation measurements (Fig. 2.6) and do not display loss of signal with chemical shift imaging (Fig. 2.7a and b).

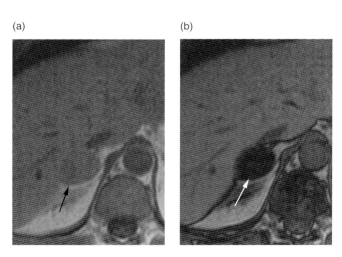

Fig. 2.5 Axial MRI using chemical shift imaging with T1-weighted gradient echo (GRE) MRI during (**a**) in-phase and (**b**) out-of phase images that demonstrate signal drop out in the left adrenal mass (*arrow*) typical of a benign adenoma

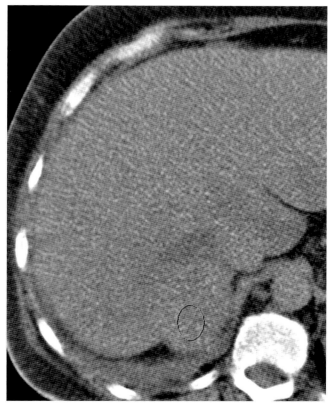

Fig. 2.6 Axial unenhanced CT shows a right adrenal metastasis which displays higher CT HU and has a mean of 44 HU

(a) (b)

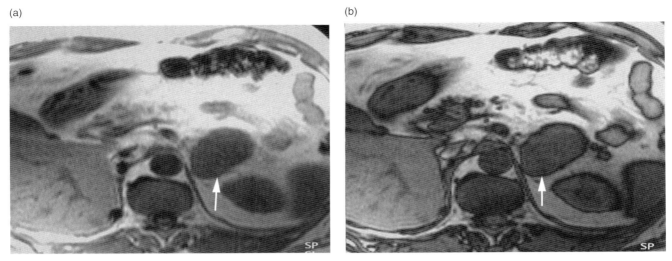

Fig. 2.7 Axial MRI showing a left adrenal metastasis (*arrow*) with no drop in signal between the in-phase GRE T1 sequence (**a**) and the out-of-phase GRE T1 sequence (**b**) as there is an absence of intracellular fat in most metastases

Metastases

Adrenal masses are frequently detected during the staging of oncology patients. The commoner primary tumors that metastasize to the adrenal gland are melanoma (50%), lung, breast, thyroid, and kidney [23, 24]. The prevalence of adrenal metastases is clearly likely to be higher in patients dying of cancer or in late stages of the disease than at presentation, but even in the presence of a primary neoplasm, only 27% of the cases of adrenal masses were due to metastatic disease in a postmortem series [23]. The prevalence of non-hyperfunctioning adenomas is such that at presentation even bilateral adrenal masses are almost as likely to be due to adenomas as metastases [25]. Patients with malignant disease may also develop mild diffuse enlargement of the adrenal glands in the absence of metastases; it is proposed that this is due to hyperplasia [26].

The significance of an adrenal metastasis to a patient's management is potentially profound. In the majority of cancers, an adrenal metastasis indicates systemic disease and that the disease is not likely to be cured by radical excision of a primary tumor and local nodal groups. The exception to this is ipsilateral adrenal involvement of a renal carcinoma. In the presence of widespread metastases, adrenal metastasis may not influence the overall management plan and therefore requires no further evaluation. If an adrenal mass is the only potential site of distant disease identified at presentation and this would make the morbidity of radical surgery unjustifiable, it is important to fully characterize the adrenal lesion. This most frequently occurs when staging bronchial carcinomas.

At presentation, adrenal metastases may be large or small, unilateral or bilateral in location. The CT and MR char-acteristics of adrenal metastases are non-specific. On CT and MRI, small metastases have homogeneous enhancement and larger metastases tend to have heterogeneous enhancement with areas of internal hemorrhage and necrosis and more complex contour (Fig. 2.8). Calcification is rarely seen in adrenal metastases. On MRI, they are typically hypo-intense when compared to liver on T1-weighted sequences (Fig. 2.7a) and mildly hyper-intense on T2-weighted sequences. These signal relationships are variable and metastases can also appear iso- or hypo-intense to liver on

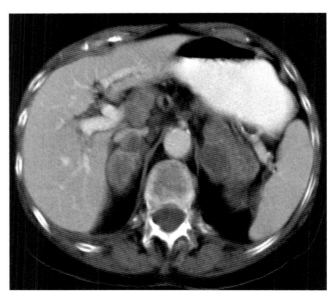

Fig. 2.8 Axial contrast enhanced CT of bilateral colorectal cancer adrenal metastases with heterogeneous enhancement and irregular contours (Reprinted with permission from Grainger, RG, Thomas, AMK, In: Dawson, P, Cosgrove, DO, Grainger, RG (eds) *Textbook of Contrast Media*, Oxford: ISIS Medical Media Ltd, 1999)

T2-weighted sequences [21, 27]; some may even have a relatively long T2 that mimics pheochromocytoma.

Adenoma Versus Metastases

When characterizing an adrenal mass in a cancer patient the objective is primarily achieved by positively establishing an alternative diagnosis to metastasis, and this usually means an incidental adenoma. The properties exploited on both CT and MR to make the diagnosis of adenoma are the same; adenomas are diagnosed by the demonstration of high lipid content, in the absence of mature fatty elements, or by the rapid washout of intravenous (IV) contrast. These are independent properties. Positron emission tomography (PET) can also be used to exploit functional properties of adrenal masses to determine their nature. If the ultimate conclusion from non-invasive investigation of an adrenal mass is that it is a metastasis, in the context of a newly presenting neoplasm and the primary is otherwise operable with curative intent, many would still seek histological confirmation with a percutaneous biopsy. It is important not to deny a patient a potentially curative procedure and a high level of evidence is required to determine this.

Role of CT

CT-Unenhanced Attenuation

Most adrenal masses are detected on CT as the upper abdomen is examined during the hepatic portal venous phase at approximately 65 s following IV contrast injection. This timing is optimal to detect hypovascular liver metastases but a poor vascular phase to discriminate between adrenal adenomas and metastases, as there is considerable overlap in mean attenuation between these two conditions at this vascular phase [28]. It has been shown, however, that unenhanced CT can be used to accurately differentiate between adrenal adenomas and metastases [28–30]. Adenomas usually have lower mean Hounsfield units (HU) than metastases when a region of interest is placed over a representative area of the mass. The optimal threshold attenuation value on unenhanced CT for diagnosing adrenal adenomas is 10 HU, with the sensitivity and specificity for masses less than 10 HU are 71 and 98%, respectively [30]. If a higher attenuation threshold is adopted there is an increase in sensitivity but a reduction in specificity. There is limited body of evidence that analysis of histograms of the pixel HU values can discriminate adenomas from metastases [31] when a region of interest is drawn over an adrenal mass on portal venous phase acquisitions. In this study, the presence of negative HU values was found to be indicative of benign disease avoiding the need for further investigation or more elaborate analysis. While this finding is promising, this work needs to be confirmed by other groups prior to advocating the widespread adoption of this practice.

CT – Washout of Contrast

Adenomas have rapid loss of attenuation after the administration of contrast when compared with metastases. This reduction in attenuation is due to the rapid washout of contrast and may occur as early as 5 min. Measuring the HU in a region of interest at 10–15 min is a useful indicator to differentiate adenomas from metastases [32]. In most series, the delayed CT HU at 15 min of less than 30–40 HU is almost always adenoma (Fig. 2.9a and b). This can be refined by calculating the percentage of contrast washout giving a predictor that is independent of the type, amount, and injection rate of the contrast material.

The percentage of enhancement washout of an adrenal mass is calculated using the following equation:

$$\% \text{ of enhancement washout} = [(E - D)/(E - U)] \times 100$$

where E is the enhanced CT HU at 60 s, D the delayed CT HU at 15 min, and U the unenhanced CT HU.

Using the threshold value of 60% at 15 min, the sensitivity and specificity of the diagnosis of adrenal adenomas are 88 and 96%, respectively [19]. There is an apparent independence of this rapid HU washout from the lipid content of the adenoma, with lipid-poor adenomas of mean HU < 10 having similar washout patterns as lipid-rich adenomas [33]. In order to calculate the percentage washout of an adrenal mass a non-contrast acquisition needs to have been obtained; in practice this is not always available, particularly if the patient has not been scanned before. An alternative approach in this circumstance can be employed. If the adrenal mass is identified on the portal venous acquisition prior to the patient leaving the department, a delayed acquisition can be obtained and the percentage of relative enhancement washout can be calculated. This avoids the need to bring the patient back for an unenhanced acquisition or full tri-phasic study.

The percentage of relative enhancement washout = $[(E-D)/E] \times 100$

Using relative enhancement washout threshold of 40%, the sensitivity and specificity for the diagnosis of adrenal adenomas are 96 and 100%, respectively [33].

(a)   (b)

(c)

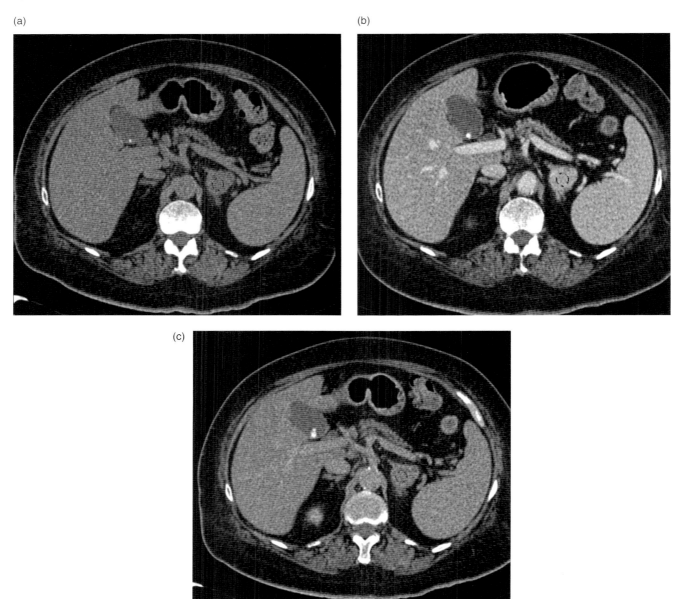

Fig. 2.9 (a), (b), (c) Axial CT washout series of a left adrenal adenoma which displays HU of 25, 102, and 51, respectively, on the unenhanced CT, portal venous phase, and 15 min delayed acquisitions following contrast enhancement, giving a value of 66% washout

Chemical Shift MRI

Chemical shift MRI imaging techniques exploit the different resonant frequencies for the hydrogen atom in water and triglyceride (lipid) molecules. This can be considered as two overlapping waves with different frequencies. The sampling for the in-phase images occurs when the peaks overlap causing the hydrogen atoms in both water and lipid to contribute to signal, whereas sampling when a peak and a trough overlap, the out-of phase images, results in a loss of signal. The magnitude of this loss of signal is dependent on the relative proportions of lipid and water occupying the same voxel.

As adrenal adenomas containing both intracellular fat and water chemical shift MRI imaging cause signal dropout in the out-of-phase when compared with the in-phase imaging (Fig. 2.10a and b). A lack of signal dropout indicates malignant adrenal mass [34] as metastases lack of intracellular fat (Fig. 2.7a and b).

The signal loss with chemical shift imaging can be assessed by a variety of ways, using both visual analysis and quantitative methods. The quick and simple visual assessment of the signal pattern on the in- and out-of-phase images has a sensitivity and specificity of 78 and 87%, respectively [22] and is adequate in most cases. When visually

(a)

(b)

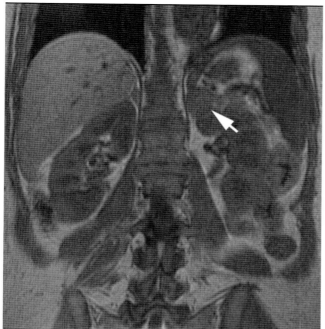
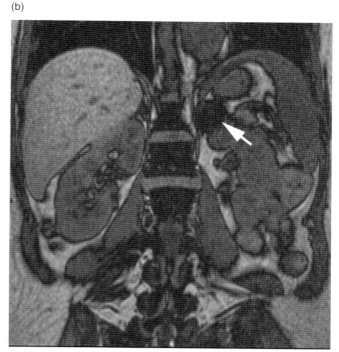

Fig. 2.10 Coronal MRI using chemical shift imaging with T1-weighted gradient echo MRI during (**a**) in-phase and (**b**) out-of-phase images that demonstrate signal dropout in the left adrenal mass (*arrow*) consistent with a benign adenoma

assessing the adrenal glands on in- and out-of-phase images, care should be taken to window the images so as to give the spleen a similar appearance on each set of images as the eye may be deceived particularly if the liver is fatty. Quantitative analysis may be helpful in equivocal cases, and ratios of signal loss in the adrenal gland alone or against that of liver, spleen, or paraspinal muscle on the in- and out-of-phase images have been suggested [35]. However, fatty infiltration of the liver makes it an unreliable organ as a standard (Fig. 2.11a and b). Spleen is the better reference organ although it may be affected by iron overload [36].

The adrenal to spleen ratio

$$(ASR) = \frac{[\text{Signal Intensity Opposed Phase (adrenal lesion/Spleen)}]}{[\text{Signal Intensity in Phase (adrenal lesion/Spleen)}]} \times 100.$$

The thresholds for MR-based ratios are less established than HU measurements in CT.

Using an ASR of ≤ 70% the diagnosis of benign adenoma has a sensitivity and specificity of 78 and 100%, respectively [16, 37]. Alternatively, a signal loss of adrenal lesion on the out-of-phase images of >20% is diagnostic of benign adenoma [16, 37].

Chemical shift imaging can be coupled with washout of gadolinium chelates to characterize adrenal masses. In a study of 114 patients with 134 adrenal masses and histolopathological specimens obtained in all, the sensitivity for adenoma characterization was 94% with a specificity of 95% [38]. Metastases were diagnosed with a sensitivity of 100%

and a specificity of 96%. The evaluation of contrast washout in this study was a qualitative visual assessment rather than a quantitative methodology. There is little comparative data between unenhanced CT and chemical shift MR; there is some evidence that chemical shift MR can confidently diagnose adenomas with mean HU > 10 on CT [39, 40].

Positron Emission Tomography (PET)

PET has an increasing role to play in the primary staging of many malignancies. The initial surgical staging for some cancers, such as bronchial carcinoma, is with CT and those in whom surgery is still an appropriate option undergoing whole body PET. Activity within an adrenal mass is an indicator of malignancy [41]. While there are false positives and negatives, as with any test series reporting on large numbers of adrenal masses, patterns are beginning to emerge. The largest experience published to date is with lung cancer where a sensitivity of 93% and a specificity of 90% for adrenal metastases were obtained using 18F-FDP PET in 113 adrenal masses in 94 patients [42]. The role of PET in this clinical setting will depend on the nature of the primary under consideration and will not completely remove the need to assess the CT images. Other PET tracers such as 11C-metomidate are currently under evaluation in the diagnosis of masses of adrenal origin [43]. The diagnostic value of PET will be discussed in detail in the next chapter.

(a)

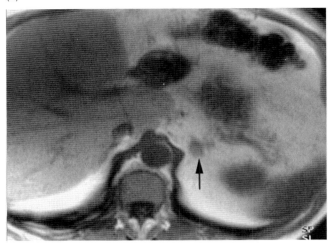

(b)

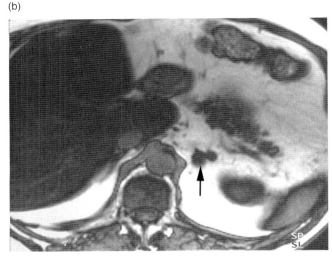

Fig. 2.11 Axial GRE MRI demonstrating the chemical shift effects of both a fatty liver and left adrenal adenoma (*arrow*) on an in-phase T1 sequence (**a**) and an out-of-phase T1 sequence (**b**) where both become dark due to signal dropout from the presence of intracellular fat. The liver is not a reliable internal visual reference for the assessment of adrenal masses due to its variable fat content

Percutaneous Biopsy

Percutaneous biopsy can be readily performed under CT or ultrasound guidance. The indication for biopsy has decreased now that the diagnosis of adenoma can be made with greater confidence through non-invasive means. If the adrenal is believed to be the only site of metastatic disease preventing radical treatment of a primary cancer with curative intent then it is the policy in our institution to obtain a biopsy. The accuracies from larger series are typically 90% plus [44, 45]. Complication rates are low but include hemorrhage, pneumothorax, pancreatitis, and needle track seeding of tumor.

Adrenal Carcinoma

Adrenal carcinomas are rare tumors, with a reported incidence of up to two cases per million [46] and a bimodal incidence with a childhood peak in the first decade and a second peak between 20 and 54 years [47]. There is a female predominance. Childhood tumors tend to present with virilization and have a less aggressive course than adult tumors which if functional tend to present with Cushing's syndrome (see below). Non-functioning tumors are more common in older patients and men [48] and often have a poor prognosis. Non-functioning tumors frequently produce hormones or their precursors but in insufficient quantity to cause a clinical syndrome; these tumors present with non-specific signs of abdominal pain, fever, weakness, and weight loss [49] or are discovered as an incidental adrenal mass. Asymptomatic masses comprise up to 12% of cases in surgical series of

adrenal carcinomas [50]. Childhood tumors are associated with hemihypertrophy and the Beckwith–Wiedemann syndrome [48].

Adrenal carcinomas are usually large masses greater than 6 cm in diameter with central necrosis and calcification is seen on CT in 20–30% of the cases [51, 52] (Fig. 2.12). Enhancement is often heterogeneous reflecting the presence of necrosis and significantly less washout of contrast is found at 10 min than with adenomas [20]. Tumors have a propensity to invade large draining adrenal veins and tumor thrombus extending into the left renal vein or inferior vena cava is common [46]. It is important to define the proximal extent of the

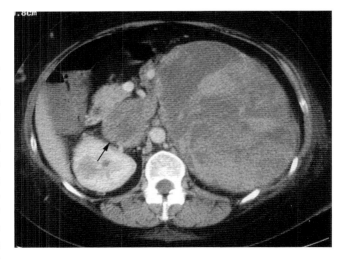

Fig. 2.12 Contrast enhanced CT shows a large heterogeneous enhancing left adrenal carcinoma with extension into the inferior vena cava (*arrow*) via the left renal vein invasion

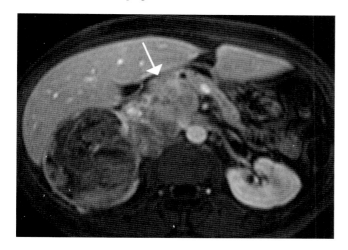

Fig. 2.13 Contrast enhanced MRI shows a large heterogeneous enhancing right adrenal carcinoma with adjacent bulky lymph node (arrow) metastasis effacing the inferior vena cava

tumor to provide information for surgical planning regarding vascular control [53]. This can be assessed using CT with coronal reconstructions but if contrast mixing artifacts are problematic color flow Doppler or MRI may be used. Common sites of dissemination are lymph nodes (Fig. 2.13), lung, and liver [49]. A minority of adrenal carcinomas are more homogeneous and resemble adenomas; it is however exceptionally uncommon for tumors smaller than 3 cm to be adenocarcinomas. With increasing size the risk of carcinoma also increases and for this reason many advocate the resection of tumors over 5 cm [54].

The MRI features of adrenal carcinomas reflect the morphological diversity described above. The majority are large complex masses with non-specific appearances and they are often hyper-intense on both T1- and T2-weighted sequences as a result of central necrosis and internal hemorrhage [55] (Fig. 2.14 a, b, and c). Other carcinomas are more homogeneous and chemical shift effects due to intracellular fat

(a)   (b)

(c)

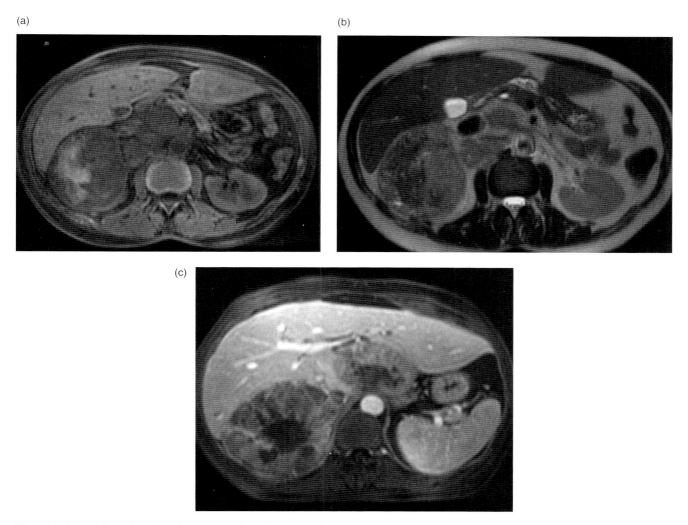

Fig. 2.14 A large right adrenal carcinoma with enlarged para-caval lymph nodes: (**a**) the high signal represents internal hemorrhage fat-suppressed T1-weighted, (b) T2-weighted, and (c) gadolinium-enhanced MRI

may be observed in a minority [56, 57]. As with CT they often demonstrate heterogeneous enhancement with avascular areas due to the presence of necrosis. The components that do enhance typically show marked enhancement with slow washout [38]. Venous extension especially into the inferior vena cava is well seen on coronal or sagital acquisitions [56, 58].

The prognosis of adrenal carcinoma is poor with 5-year survival 20–45% [59]. The mainstay of treatment is complete surgical excision and the role of imaging in addition to establishing the diagnosis is to provide a pre-surgical map of the anatomic extent of the tumor. There have been few chemotherapeutic advances in recent years and mitotane remains the agent of choice for residual or recurrent disease although only has a limited effect [59].

Pheochromocytoma

It is important to consider pheochromocytoma within the differential diagnosis of the incidentally discovered adrenal mass. Pheochromocytoma is derived from chromaffin cells and is the commonest tumor of the adrenal medulla. These tumors secrete an excess of catecholamines and most patients present with symptoms resulting from these hormones with episodic hypertension, flushing, and palpitations. The hypertension and cardiac arrhythmias may be life threatening. In 10% of cases these tumors are clinically silent and detected on imaging as an incidental mass [60, 61]. The diagnosis is usually made by biochemical findings of elevated catecholamines or their metabolites in blood or urine. The role of imaging is usually to locate the tumors.

Pheochromocytomas can occur anywhere in the autonomic system from the base of the skull to bladder although 90% occur within the adrenal medulla [62] and 98% within the abdomen [63]. Most extra-adrenal pheochromocytomas are within the paravertebral sympathetic ganglia, the organ of Zuckerkandl (Fig. 2.15), or rarely the urinary bladder. The incidence of extra-adrenal tumors is higher in the sporadic group than those associated with the multiple endocrine neoplasia syndromes (MEN 2a or 2b), neurofibromatosis, or von Hippel–Lindau disease [64]. Tumors are multiple in 10% of the sporadic cases and 30% of the cases when associated with systemic disease [65, 66]. Approximately 10% of pheochromocytomas are malignant, with the incidence higher in extra-adrenal masses and when the tumors are greater than 6 cm in size [67, 68].

The typical pheochromocytoma on CT is a well-defined oval mass with a density similar to liver or muscle on the unenhanced acquisition (i.e., a mean HU of greater than 10). Following contrast the tumor displays avid enhancement, which reflects the vascular nature of the tumor, although washout of contrast is, however, typically less than that of

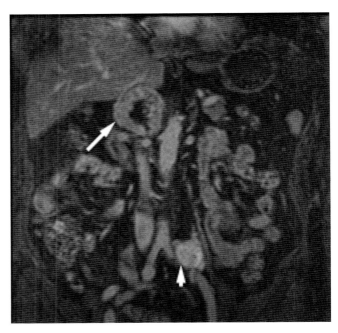

Fig. 2.15 Coronal gadolinium-enhanced MRI demonstrating two extra-adrenal pheochromocytomas (*arrows*)

adrenal adenomas [20]. Suspected pheochromocytoma was traditionally a contraindication to the use of iodinated contrast agents in the absence of α and β blockade, and while some authorities would still urge caution in the use of IV contrast there is some evidence that the use of low osmolar non-ionic contrast agents is safe [69, 70]. It should be appreciated that pheochromocytomas have a very wide spectrum of radiological appearances. The larger masses often have heterogeneous attenuation and enhancement secondary to internal hemorrhage or central necrosis (Fig. 2.16). Tumors

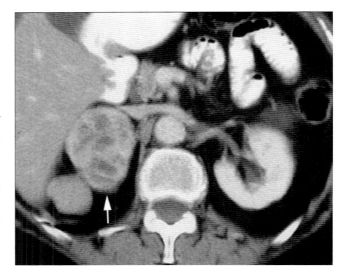

Fig. 2.16 Axial contrast-enhanced CT shows a large right adrenal pheochromocytoma with heterogeneous enhancement (*arrow*)

(a)

(b)

(c)

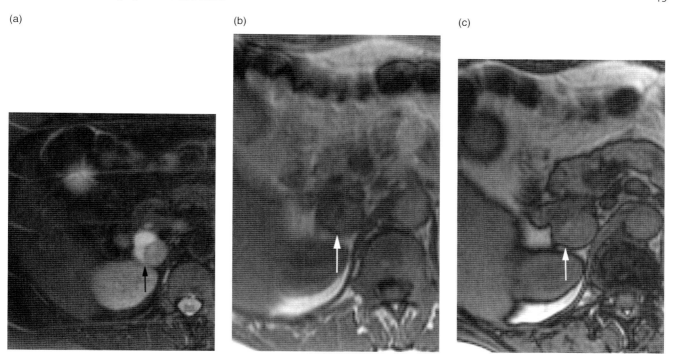

Fig. 2.17 Axial MRI illustrating a complex right adrenal pheochromocytoma (*arrow*) with high signal on FSE fat-suppressed T2 (**a**) and intermediate signal on in-phase GRE T1 (**b**) and no loss of signal on the out-of-phase GRE T1-weighted sequence (**c**)

may be almost entirely cystic or contain sufficient fat to lower the attenuation below 10 HU and rarely contain macroscopic fatty elements [63]. In a CT series of 33 patients with pheochromocytomas there was very little difference in size and other imaging characteristics between incidental and symptomatic tumors although calcification was a commoner finding in the symptomatic group [71] and non-hormonally active tumors are usually larger than hormonally active tumors[9].

On MRI pheochromocytomas are typically of low signal on T1 and high signal on T2-weighted sequences [72] (Fig. 2.17a, b, and c). While typical, these characteristics are not specific as they overlap with adrenal metastases [73]. The high signal on T2 imaging is useful to help locate extra-adrenal tumors and aids in the differentiation from an adrenal adenoma. In 35% of the cases, they may not have long T2, therefore display atypical signal intensity on T2-weighted sequences [58]. Necrosis, hemorrhage, and cystic degeneration all contribute to the complexity of appearances on MR on T1 and T2. Pheochromocytoma enhances avidly following gadolinium injection although this is rarely necessary for its characterization (Fig. 2.18) [74]. Radionucleotide imaging is of value in locating pheochromocytomas, with radio-iodine-labeled meta-iodobenzylguanidine (MIBG) having a specificity approaching 100% [75] and a sensitivity of 84% [76].

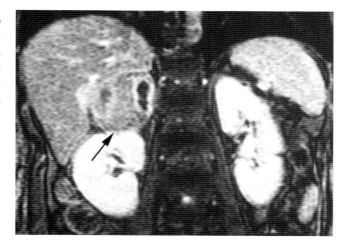

Fig. 2.18 Coronal MRI following gadolinium enhancement shows a large right adrenal pheochromocytoma with avidly heterogeneous enhancement (*arrow*)

Myelolipoma

A myelolipoma is a benign tumor that is composed of bone marrow elements such as mature fat and hemopoietic tissue. In one pathology series of 418 adrenal tumors derived from postmortem and surgical cases, myelolipomas accounted for 2.6% of primary adrenal tumors [77]; similar incidences are

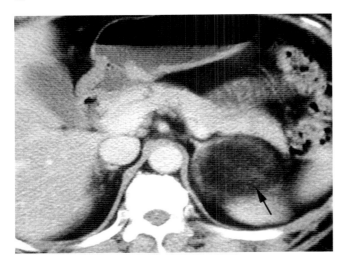

Fig. 2.19 Axial contrast-enhanced CT shows a large left adrenal myelolipoma (*arrow*) which is predominantly of fatty attenuation.

have also been reported [80, 81] and apart from a few isolated cases [82, 83] are usually hormonally inactive.

On CT, myelolipomas are characterized by the presence of a mass with areas of fatty differentiation and these appear as low-density zones with negative value Hounsfield units (HU) ranging from −30 to −100 HU [84, 85] (Fig. 2.19). Radiologically these tumors may seem to be composed almost entirely of fat but varying amounts of soft tissue elements are seen and calcification is present in up to 20% of cases. In a small proportion of cases no fatty elements are identified and the diagnosis cannot be made radiologically. On MRI the appearances are reflected by the amount of mature fat and bone marrow elements in the tumor. The fatty content is usually high signal on T1 and intermediate signal on T2-weighted sequences with loss of the high signal from fat when fat suppression techniques are used (Fig. 2.20a and b). The bone marrow content is usually low signal on T1 and moderate signal on T2-weighted sequences [86, 87]. The differential diagnosis for fat containing adrenal tumors includes lipomas, angiomyolipomas, teratomas, and liposarcomas; all are very uncommon and only the latter malignant [77]. Myelolipomas diagnosed on CT or MRI are treated conservatively, except in a few cases, where a large myelolipoma cannot be distinguished from a retroperitoneal sarcoma. Surgery or biopsy may then be indicated for definitive diagnosis.

observed in large radiological series [38]. These tumors are usually asymptomatic although occasionally larger tumors may cause flank pain particularly when undergoing necrosis or spontaneous hemorrhage [79, 80]. Myelolipomas are usually found in adrenal glands but extra-adrenal locations

(a)   (b)

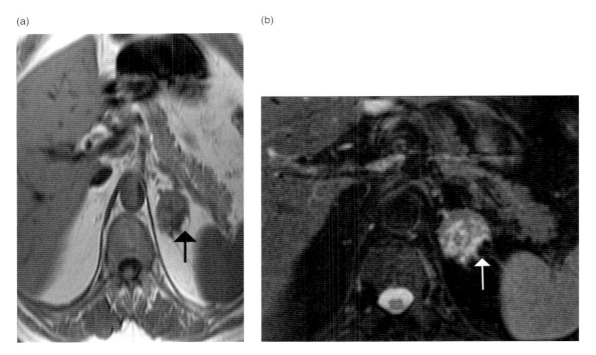

Fig. 2.20 Axial MRI showing a left adrenal myelolipoma which displays mixed signal with only a small focal fatty component of high signal (*arrow*) on the GRE T1-weighted sequence (**a**) and focal loss of signal (*arrow*) on the fat-suppressed T2-weighted sequence (**b**)

Adrenal Hemorrhage

Adrenal hemorrhage can be unilateral or bilateral, and may be spontaneous, traumatic, or related to anticoagulation. Blunt abdominal trauma usually results in unilateral adrenal hemorrhage, affecting the right adrenal gland more frequently than the left [88, 89]. The presence of bilateral adrenal hemorrhage is usually due to anticoagulation therapy or blood dyscrasias; other less common causes are stress related to surgery, sepsis, and hypotension and, rarely, trauma [90]. Adrenal hemorrhage may also be caused by adrenal vein thrombosis secondary to venous catheterization [91] and the presence of preexisting neoplasia, particularly lung metastasis, although this is very uncommon [92]. Bilateral adrenal hemorrhage may result in functional insufficiency [93].

On CT, the acute or subacute adrenal hemorrhage usually has an unenhanced attenuation value of 50–90 HU. This can be followed by serial CTs, with diminishing size and HU of the adrenal mass as a result of re-absorption of the hemorrhage. In the chronic phase, calcification of the adrenal hematoma may be seen (Fig. 2.21). However, acute adrenal hemorrhage can mimic an enhanced adrenal mass on a post-contrast CT and unenhanced images may be of value in establishing the diagnosis [94]. In the context of trauma stranding in the adjacent fat is often seen, and patients usually have severe injuries with other organ injury evident and a poorer prognosis [88, 89]. Conversely with relatively minor blunt trauma or the absence of other organ

injury, another cause for an adrenal mass should be considered. On MRI, the appearances depend on the evolution of the adrenal hemorrhage that varies from acute to chronic stages with the hemoglobin breakdown. In the acute phase, deoxyhemoglobin causes signal loss on T1- and T2-weighted sequence. In the subacute phase, the presence of methemoglobin leads to high signal on T1-weighted sequences and in the chronic phase, it has low signal on both T1- and T2-weighted sequences due to hemosiderin deposition [95].

Adrenal Cysts

Adrenal cysts are uncommon and usually unilateral with a female preponderance. There are four types of cysts based on histological findings: endothelial (commonest), epithelial, parasitic, and post-traumatic pseudocysts as a result of adrenal hemorrhage [96]. On CT, cysts range from simple to complex. The simple cyst is characterized by a smooth, round, non-enhancing, and near-water density mass with a thin wall (less than or equal to 3 mm) and are usually benign. The more complex cysts may contain soft tissue nodules, septa, calcification, and blood [97] and should be evaluated with caution as there is overlap with malignant adrenal masses, including adrenal carcinoma [97]. Surgery may be required to obtain the diagnosis of a complex adrenal cyst. Pheochromocytomas may be cystic and should be considered within the differential diagnosis of a complex cyst (see above); therefore hormonal hyperfunction should be sought before contemplating surgery or biopsy of these masses. Occasionally adenomas may be cystic with subclinical hyperfunctioning adenomas may also be found as cystic adrenal lesions [98]. On MRI, a simple cyst is low signal on T1 and high signal on T2-weighted sequences (Fig. 2.22a and b) and complex cysts will contain soft tissue components, septa, and blood.

Lymphoma

Involvement of the adrenal glands with lymphoma is commoner with diffuse disease from non-Hodgkin's lymphoma than Hodgkin's disease and occurs in approximately 4% of cases [99]. In the majority of such cases involvement is bilateral. Primary adrenal lymphoma is extremely rare and usually occurs in the absence of other sites of retroperitoneal lymphoma in elderly males [100, 101]. Primary or secondary involvement of the adrenal glands with lymphoma will occasionally cause adrenal failure [99, 102].

On CT, lymphoma is usually a solid homogeneous mass that exhibits minimal post-contrast enhancement [103];

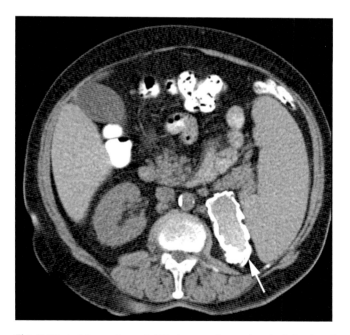

Fig. 2.21 Axial unenhanced CT shows a large chronic left adrenal hematoma with peripheral calcification (*arrow*)

(a)

(b)

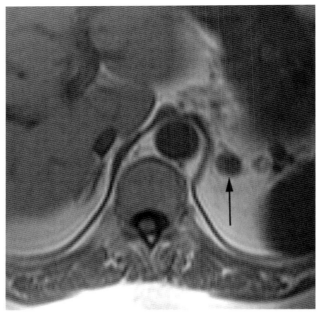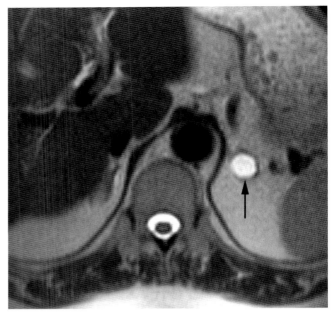

Fig. 2.22 Axial-unenhanced MRI shows a simple left adrenal cyst (*arrow*) with (**a**) low signal on T1-weighted and (**b**) high signal on T2-weighted images

occasionally the morphology of the gland is preserved but it is diffusely enlarged. Calcification is unusual without previous radiotherapy. On MRI, lymphoma cannot be differentiated from other malignant adrenal masses, as it has homogeneous low signal on T1 and moderate high signal on T2-weighted sequences [55]. However, due to the absence of intracellular fat, lymphoma can be differentiated from adenoma using chemical shift imaging [104].

Hemangioma

Adrenal hemangioma is rare benign tumor that is composed of vascular channels lined by a single layer of endothelium [105]; radiological descriptions are of case reports with no large series. They are usually large (>10 cm) presenting as an incidental finding, being hormonally inactive. Malignant hemangiosarcoma does occur within the adrenal gland but is even rarer [106].

The imaging features of adrenal hemangiomas may resemble those in other organs or be non-specific, appearing as a large well-defined mass of soft tissue density on unenhanced CT with inhomogeneous contrast enhancement. Most contain foci of calcification either from pheboliths within the vascular channels of the tumor or from previous hemorrhage [107]. If peripheral nodular enhancement with progressive filling in is observed, the diagnosis can be made radiologically, but this is not always present with other patterns of

enhancement such as thin peripheral rim enhancement, and in these circumstances the diagnosis cannot be made preoperatively [108–110]. On MRI, adrenal hemangiomas are low in signal on T1 when compared to liver [55] and extremely high signal on T2-weighted images. Occasionally, there is central high signal on T1 from internal hemorrhage. Following gadolinium, there is persistent peripheral enhancement on delayed images. These tumors are usually removed because of the risk of bleeding or uncertainty in diagnosis with a large complex adrenal mass.

Neuroblastoma

This is the commonest extracranial solid tumor of childhood [111] and may occur anywhere along the parasympathetic plexus. Tumors (50–80%) arise within the adrenal medulla and the chest is another common site. Eighty-five percent of the cases occur in children less than 5 years, with a peak at 2 years. Neuroblastoma is an extremely rare cause of an adrenal mass in adults and not addressed in detail in this review; a detailed account is provided by Ng et al. [112]. When the tumor is present in adults and adolescents it has a worse prognosis with metastases occurring in the bones, lymph nodes, liver, pleura, and dura [113, 114]. The imaging findings are similar for both adults and children. CT and MRI can be used to stage the tumors as both provide good anatomical delineation although MR is the preferred imaging

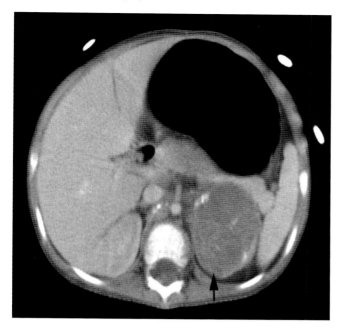

Fig. 2.23 Axial contrast-enhanced CT in a 3-year-old boy showing a large low-attenuation adrenal neuroblastoma with peripheral calcification (*arrow*)

technique in children so as to avoid ionizing radiation. Neuroblastoma tends to encase the aorta and inferior vena cava. Calcification occurs in up to 85% of the tumors (Fig. 2.23), which may be difficult to appreciate on MRI but it is usually unimportant for staging.

Ganglioneuroma

Ganglioneuromas are another rare tumor that may arise within the adrenal gland. These tumors are formed of Schwann and ganglion cells derived from cells of neural crest origin and may occur in any age group. Ganglioneuromas may be found anywhere along the paravertebral sympathetic plexus, with approximately 50% occurring within the abdomen and 40% of these arising within the adrenal medulla [115]. The tumors are usually hormonally inactive and discovered as an incidental mass, but they may occasionally secrete vasoactive intestinal peptide and catecholamines, and composite tumors with pheochromocytomas are also reported [116].

Ganglioneuromas are usually large, with sizes ranging from 4 to 22 cm in Radin's series and extra-adrenal retroperitoneal tumors may be even larger. On CT the tumors are typically non-specific homogeneous masses of lower attenuation than the muscle on pre- and post-contrast images and relatively uniform enhancement in small tumors and mild heterogeneity in larger tumors. Small calcific foci may be present.

On MRI, ganglioneuromas have lower signal than liver on T1 and higher signal than liver on T2 with greater heterogeneity than on T1 or CT [116, 117]. Extra-adrenal tumors may encase the major retroperitoneal vessels without causing occlusion.

Granulomatous Disease

The adrenal glands may become involved with the granulomatous diseases such as tuberculosis, histoplasmosis, and blastomycosis. Both adrenal glands are usually involved but this may be asymmetrical. Imaging features are usually non-specific and also depend on the stage of presentation. Early in the disease there is typically bilateral enlargement with preservation of the adrenal chevron or inverted Y shape; this is followed by progressive loss of volume and calcification [118, 119]. The glands may loose their shape to become more mass-like and of heterogeneous density with central low attenuation from caseous necrosis and ring enhancement [119, 120]. Granulomatous disease should be considered within the differential diagnosis of bilateral adrenal enlargement along with lymphoma and hemorrhage particularly if there is adrenal hypo-function and no history of malignancy. Percutaneous adrenal biopsy is required to confirm the diagnosis and organism in the absence of more accessible sites.

Incidental Adrenal Mass: Imaging and Treatment Algorithm

Having discovered an adrenal mass a diagnosis needs to be established. Any patient presenting with a clinically inapparent adrenal masses requires a complete history and physical examination, biochemical evaluation for hormone excess, and imaging evaluation for characterization of the adrenal mass. In patients with widespread metastases, unless the clinical management is influenced, further characterization with radiology is not indicated. In the absence of a recent presentation of malignancy, the biochemical evaluation, based on the guidance from the NIH Conference [4], is outlined in Table 2.1. Either CT or MRI can be used to locate and characterize the adrenal tumor. An imaging pathway for the evaluation of a non-functional mass is outlined in the flow chart in the chapter 4 (see below). Not all steps need to be taken; some may prefer to go straight to MR rather than recall the patient for a characterization CT study, and in the context of malignancy some cancers will be routinely staged by PET.

Most complex adrenal masses, not believed to represent a metastasis, require surgical excision if the patient

Table 2.1 Hormonal evaluation of incidental adrenal masses (NIH Conference, 2002) [4] (Reprinted with permission from Grainger, RG, Thomas, AMK, In: Dawson, P, Cosgrove, DO, Grainger, RG (eds) *Textbook of contrast Media*, Oxford: ISIS Medical Media Ltd, 1999)

Hormonal state	Screening test
Excess glucocorticoid	Overnight 1 mg dexamethasone suppression test
Hyperaldosteronism	Serum potassium
	Plasma aldosterone-to-plasma rennin activity ratio (abnormal if > 30)
Pheochromocytoma	24-h urinary catecholamines or plasma-free metanephrines

is fit and the tumor can be completely excised. Complex tumors in which macroscopic clearance is unlikely require a percutaneous biopsy. In patients with hormonally inactive adrenal masses with features of an adenoma, size is an important determining factor in the patient's management. Most adrenal masses less than 3 cm are adrenal adenomas, whereas greater than 6 cm, a mass has an increasing likelihood of being an adrenal carcinoma. Resection is recommended for all tumors with the characteristics of an adenoma if above 6 cm in diameter because of this risk of malignancy. Adrenalectomy can be performed as an open or laparoscopic procedure, with some preferring an open resection for tumors believed to represent carcinomas [4, 121, 122]. Surgery should also be considered in all patients with hormonally active adrenal cortical tumors that are clinically symptomatic. However, for sub-clinical hormonally active adrenal cortical tumors less than 6 cm in diameter there is lack of evidence to support either surgery or non-surgical approach.

To date the number of such longitudinal studies of patients with incidental non-function adenomas is small. There is some evidence that up to 22% of tumors with the characteristics of adenomas will increase in size over 10 years (some decreasing in size), with up to 10% developing sub-clinical hormonal hypersecretion (usually hypercortisolism) and a small number developing overt clinical syndromes when followed up [123, 124]. The development of carcinoma is an extremely rare event. In patients with tumors less than 4 cm the NIH consensus group advocated follow-up imaging after 6–12 months with longer hormonal follow-up. If there is no increase in size and no evidence of excess hormonal production, they recommend no further follow-up. The decision to operate or monitor adrenal masses 4–6 cm in size is also difficult and the approach should depend on factors other than size.

Adrenal Hyperfunction

Adrenal masses may present as the result of excessive hormone elaboration. Hormonally active adrenal tumors may occur in either the adrenal cortex or medulla. The hormones that are produced determine the clinical and biochemical presentations. Imaging is primarily used to locate the adrenal source of the hormone, differentiating adenomas or other functioning masses from hyperplastic conditions in order to assist with patient management. Hormonal evaluation should also be part of the assessment of any incidental detected adrenal mass and should aim to determine whether the patient has a pheochromocytoma, primary aldosteronism (Conns syndrome), glucocorticoid excess (Cushing's syndrome), or virilizing or feminizing tumors (Table 2.1).

Adrenal Cortex

Primary Hyperaldosteronism (Conn's Syndrome)

Primary hyperaldosteronism is characterized by hypertension, hypokalemia, and metabolic alkalosis. The condition is rare and accounts for less than 0.5% of patients with hypertension. The causes are adrenal adenoma (79%), bilateral adrenal hyperplasia (20%), and extremely rarely adrenal carcinoma (less than 1%) [125–127]. The diagnosis should first be established biochemically by demonstrating aldosterone excess with suppressed renin prior to contemplating radiological investigation. Imaging plays an important role in differentiating between these causes as bilateral adrenal hyperplasia is treated medically and adrenal adenomas (or carcinomas) are optimally treated with surgical excision.

Adrenocortical adenomas are usually small with a mean size of 1.8 cm [51] and up to 20% less than 1 cm in diameter [128]. Detection of the adrenal adenomas is related to size, and the ease of detection increases with increasing size. Observers using CT typically have sensitivities of approximately 85–90% in detecting adenomas (Fig. 2.24a and b) [51, 129, 130] and are able to resolve nodules less than 1 cm [131]. The MR features of Conn's adenomas are similar to those of non-hyperfunctioning adenomas and the performance in detecting adenomas and differentiating from hyperplasia is similar to that of CT [132–135].

The traditional approach in differentiating between adenoma and hyperplasia has been to attempt to make a positive diagnosis of an adenoma and in the absence of such a tumor assumes the diagnosis of bilateral hyperplasia. This approach was in part born of necessity as there was neither the imaging capability nor the established criteria to positively diagnose hyperplasia. Problems arise when an incidental non-functioning adenoma co-exists with a contra-lateral hyperfunctioning adenoma, which can result in misinterpretation of bilateral adrenal hyperplasia. Similarly, a macron-

(a)   (b)

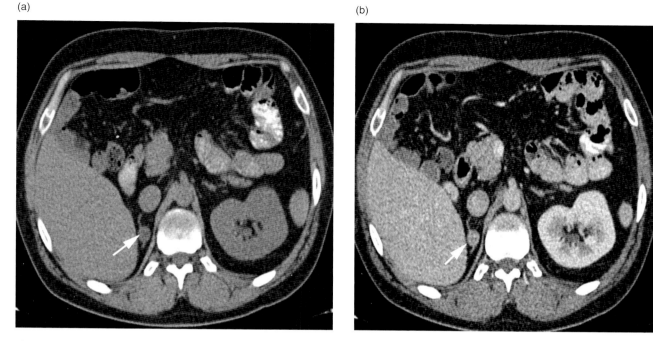

Fig. 2.24 Axial CT shows a small, well-defined and round right adrenal (Conn's) adenoma (*arrow*) on the (**a**) unenhanced and (**b**) contrast-enhanced CT

odule in nodular hyperplasia may be diagnosed as a solitary adenoma. However, the spatial resolution of both CT and MR continues to improve and data is emerging to allow the positive diagnosis of hyperplasia. When Conn's syndrome is secondary to hyperplasia, the limbs but not the bodies of the adrenal glands become enlarged on CT [134]. In this series a mean limb thickness of 3 mm excluded hyperplasia, a mean limb thickness greater than 3 mm gave a sensitivity of 100% and a specificity of 54% for hyperplasia, and a mean limb thickness greater than 5 mm gave a specificity of 100% and a sensitivity of 47% for hyperplasia. In standard clinical practice, in the presence of a solitary adenoma with a normal contra-lateral adrenal gland as detected on cross-sectional imaging, further imaging is not required before surgery [133, 136, 137]. Patients in whom surgery is contemplated but where the diagnosis is not clearcut require venous sampling to establish the source of aldosterone production. Patients with bilateral normal adrenal glands, bilateral nodules, or a unilateral nodule with contra-lateral enlargement of the adrenal gland should have venous sampling to distinguish between hyperplasia and an adenoma which would influence their management [137–139]. Lingham et al. suggest modifying this approach on the basis of adrenal limb size; if a nodule is seen and the mean limb thickness is less than 3 mm the diagnosis of a functioning adenoma is established, if the limb thickness is >5 mm then hyperplasia is established, however, venous sampling being required if the mean limb thickness is <3 mm with no nodules identified or 3–5 mm with or with-

out a nodule. While this protocol seems attractive it has yet to be tested prospectively [134].

Cushing's Syndrome

Cushing's syndrome is the result of an excess of glucocorticoids and causes characteristic clinical and biochemical features. The commonest cause of Cushing's syndrome is iatrogenic through the therapeutic administration of corticosteroids. Endogeneous causes can be broadly divided into ACTH-dependent and ACTH-independent disease. ACTH-independent disease is always adrenal in origin whereas ACTH-dependent Cushing's syndrome is caused by excess production of ACTH by a pituitary tumor (Cushing's disease) or less frequently an ectopic ACTH source. The biochemical diagnosis of Cushing's syndrome is made on the basis of a raised serum cortisol with loss of the usual diurnal rhythm and incomplete suppression of cortisol production after 2 mg of oral dexamethasone. Adrenal Cushing's syndrome is indicated by failure to suppress cortisol production with a high dose of dexamethasone, and failure of cortisol and ACTH to respond to corticotropin-releasing hormone stimulation.

Radiology has an important role in both ACTH-dependent and ACTH-independent Cushing's syndrome. In ACTH-dependent disease the underlying pituitary adenoma needs to be identified or an ectopic source sought. Invasive venous sampling methods may be needed to supplement anatomic investigation. With ACTH-independent disease it is important to differentiate between a unilateral adrenal cause which occurs in 92% of cases [140] and bilateral disease. Cushing's syndrome is associated with considerable morbidity and treated with surgery whenever possible. In addition to identifying the side and unilateral nature of the underlying cause imaging can help to plan the surgical approach; large potentially malignant tumors may require an open operation whereas those with smaller tumors and benign features generally can be undertaken with a laparoscopic approach [141].

The Imaging Features of Adrenal Glands in Cushing's Syndrome

ACTH-Dependent Cushing's Disease

In 80–85% of cases of Cushing's syndrome the cause is due to excess ACTH production from either a pituitary or an ectopic source [142]. The adrenal glands may appear normal or hyperplastic on CT or MRI. Hyperplasia is usually bilateral and may be smooth when the gland appears thickened or elongated (Fig. 2.25); alternatively the hyperplasia may appear nodular which can be mistaken for rare forms of primary adrenal disease. Marked hyperplasia suggests the presence of an ectopic ACTH source and could be related to the time period of ACTH stimulation [131]. Fifteen percent of the ACTH-dependent Cushing's syndrome is related to non-pituitary ectopic ACTH production [143]. Overt ectopic ACTH secretion is usually from small cell carcinoma and is usually clinically apparent with lack of the clinical features of Cushing's syndrome and has a relatively

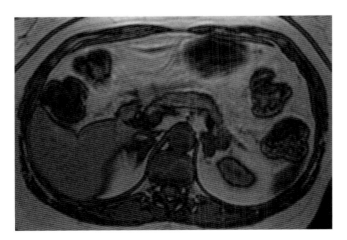

Fig. 2.25 Axial-unenhanced out-of-phase GRE T1-weighted MRI showing bilateral thickening of the limbs of the adrenal glands typical of adrenal hyperplasia

short clinical history. Conversely, "occult" ectopic ACTH secretion presents as more indolent clinical course and simulates Cushing's syndrome secondary to pituitary or adrenal adenoma [143]. Bronchial carcinoid tumors are the commonest cause for the occult presentation and account up to 79% of cases [131, 144]. These tumors are small (0.4–2 cm) and thin section CT is therefore required to locate these tumors and they typically enhance with contrast administration. Other ectopic ACTH sources include small islet cell of the pancreas, pheochromocytoma, medullary thyroid carcinomas, and thymic carcinoids [143].

Adrenocortical Adenoma

Adrenal adenomas account for 10–20% of Cushing's syndrome cases, with the average tumor size typically ranging from 2 to 3.5 cm [51, 140, 142] but can be much larger. The contra-lateral adrenal gland may be atrophic due to diminished ACTH stimulation. With CT and MRI functional adenomas have similar characteristics to non-hyperfunctioning adenomas (see above). Functioning adenomas causing Cushing's syndrome may also occur within myelolipomas [140, 145]; in these rare cases the imaging findings are dominated by the myelolipoma component.

Adrenal Carcinoma

Adrenal carcinomas account for up to 15% of the cases of Cushing's syndrome [146]. The radiological features of adrenal carcinomas are discussed above. In 90% of cases they produce an excess of steroids and this results in Cushing's syndrome in 50–60% [147, 148]. Virilization syndromes secondary to carcinomas are less frequent and oestrogen secretion syndromes and primary aldosteronism are very rare [47].

Primary Pigmented Nodular Adrenocortical Disease (PPNAD)

PPNAD occurs in infant and young adults and is a rare cause of Cushing's syndrome [149]. The symptoms are usually mild and the diagnosis is usually delayed with severe osteoporosis [131]. The condition gains its name from the presence of lipofuscin, a brown pigment, that is evident at histology. PPNAD may be part of the Carney complex with cardiac myxomas, spotty skin pigmentation, testicular tumors, or a growth hormone secreting pituitary adenoma [150]. Treatment for PPNAD is by bilateral adrenalectomy, and family screening is recommended due to the autosomal dominant transmission, and given the association with the Carney complex, a cardiac echo undertaken.

In this condition the findings within the adrenal glands are of multiple bilateral nodules; these are usually small and less than 5 mm in size but nodules of 1–2 cm may be seen in older patients. For children less than 10 years, the nodules are usually less than 3 mm and may not be detected by either CT or MRI. In older patients they may be detected with CT/MRI. On MRI, the nodules are low signal when compared with the adjacent "atrophic" cortical tissue on T1- and T2-weighted images [151] and demonstrate chemical shift signal loss [140]. The radiological appearances overlap with pituitary-dependent hyperplasia but can clearly be differentiated by the presence of a low ACTH.

ACTH-Independent Macronodular Hyperplasia (AIMAH)

This is the rarest cause of Cushing's syndrome first described in 1964 [152]. The adrenal glands are replaced by multiple large (>4 cm) nodules with obliteration of the normal adrenal outline. The nodules of AIMAH are hyper signal on T2 than pituitary-induced hyperplasia and appear hyperintense to the liver. On T1-weighted images the nodules are iso-intense with muscle and also demonstrate chemical shift signal loss and peripheral enhancement following contrast [140]. The pituitary glands appear normal on CT and MR.

Adrenogenital Syndrome

In children, congenital adrenal hyperplasia is the commonest cause of virilization. This is due to inborn error in the enzyme 11b- or 22-hydroxylase which is important in the production of cortisol and aldosterone. This leads to excess ACTH with chronic adrenocortical stimulation causing gross enlargement of the adrenal glands; they are easily detected by US, CT, or MRI. There is a risk of malignant transformation into adenoma or carcinoma as a result of long-term stimulation [153]. Androgen-secreting tumors are rare and include both carcinomas and adenomas, with carcinomas being commoner of the two. They are usually large and can easily be detected with CT/MRI.

Adrenal Medulla

Pheochromocytoma

This is the commonest tumor of the adrenal medulla. They arise from chromaffin cells and secrete catecholamines. Patients frequently present with a variety of symptoms including episodic hypertension, flushing, and palpitations. The diagnosis is usually established with biochemical evaluation with 24-h urinary catecholamines or plasma-free metanephrines. Imaging is primarily used to localize the tumor and is described above.

Neuroblastoma and Ganglioneuroblastoma

Neuroblastoma is the commonest extracranial solid tumor of childhood [111]. It usually originates from the neural cells of the sympathetic nervous system. The majority occur in children less than 5 years and have a peak incidence of 2 years. Ganglioneuroblastoma are found in older children and have more benign behavior. The radiological characteristics are described above.

Conclusion

The incidental adrenal mass and the search for the source of an excess of adrenal hormones both represent frequent challenges for cross-sectional radiologists. There has been considerable progress in the understanding of the imaging characteristics of these adrenal masses and conditions so as to enable reliable therapeutic decisions to be made, in the majority of cases through non-invasive means. There are still gaps in our knowledge particularly in the optimal follow-up of non-hormonally active adenomas, and imaging techniques continue to evolve.

References

1. Geelhoed GW, Druy EM. Management of the adrenal 'incidentaloma'. Surgery 1982;92:866–74.
2. Prinz RA, Brooks MH, Churchill R, Graner JL, Lawrence AM, Paloyan E, et al. Incidental asymptomatic adrenal masses detected by computed tomographic scanning. Is operation required? JAMA. 1982;248:701–4.
3. Kokko JP, Brown TC, Berman MM. Adrenal adenoma and hypertension. Lancet. 1967;1:468.
4. MG Melvin, MKB Beverly, DB Glenn, KK Campbell, JA Carney, PA Godley, et al. Management of the clinically inapparent adrenal mass ('Incidentaloma'). NIH Conference. Ann Interm Med. 2003;138:424–29.

5. Commons RR, Callaway CP. Adenomas of theadrenal cortex. Archiv Intern Med. 1948;81:37–41.

6. Hedeland H, Ostberg G, Hokfelt B. On the prevalence of adrenocortical adenomas in an autopsy material in relation to hypertension and diabetes. Acta Med Scand. 1968;184:211–4.

7. Kloos RT, Gross MD, Francis IR, Korobkin M, Shapiro B. Incidentally discovered adrenal masses. Endocr Rev. 1995;16:460–84.

8. Glazer HS, Weyman PJ, Sagel SS, Levitt RG, McClennan BL. Nonfunctioning adrenal masses: incidental discovery on computed tomography. Am J Roentgenol. 1982;139:81–5.

9. Aso Y, Homma Y. A survey on incidental adrenal tumours in Japan. J Urol. 1992;147:1478–81.

10. Dunnick NR, Korobkin M, Francis I. Adrenal radiology: distinguishing benign from malignant adrenal masses. Am J Roentgenol. 1996;167:861–7.

11. Mantero F, Masini AM, Opocher G, Giovagnetti M, Arnaldi G. Adrenal incidentaloma: an overview of hormonal data from the National Italian Study Group. Horm Res. 1997;47:284–9.

12. Dunnick R. Adrenal imaging: current status. Am J Roentgenol. 1990;154:927–36.

13. Caoili EM, Korobkin M, Francis IR, Cohan RH, Platt JF, Dunnick R, et al. Adrenal masses: characterization with combined unenhanced and delayed enhanced CT. Radiology. 2002;222:629–33.

14. Montagne J-P, Kressel HY, Korobkin M, Moss AA. Computed tomography of the normal adrenal glands. Am J Roentgenol. 1978;130:963–66.

15. Vincent JM, Morrison ID, Armstrong P, Reznek RH. The size of normal adrenal glands on computed tomography. Clin Rad. 1994;49:453–5.

16. Korobkin M, Giordano TJ, Brodeur FJ, Francis IR, Siegelman ES, Quint LE, et al. Adrenal adenomas: relationship between histologic lipid and CT and MR findings. Radiology. 1996;200:743–7.

17. Francis IR, Gross MD, Shapiro B, Korobkin M, Quint LE. Integrated imaging of adrenal disease. Radiology. 1992;184:1–13.

18. Krestin GP, Friedmann G, Fischbach R, Neufang KFR, Allolio B. Evaluation of adrenal masses in oncologic patients: dynamic contrast enhanced MR vs. CT. J Comput Assist Tomogr. 1991;15:104–10.

19. Korobkin M, Bordeur FJ, Francis IR, Quint LE, Dunnick NR, Londy F. CT time-attenuation washout curves of adrenal adenomas and nonadenomas. Am J Roentgenol. 1998;170:747–52.

20. Szolar DH, Korobkin M, Reittner P, Berghold A, Bauernhofer T, Trummer H, et al.. Adrenocortical carcinomas and adrenal pheochromocytomas: mass and enhancement loss evaluation at delayed contrast-enhanced CT. Radiology. 2005;234:479–85.

21. Reinig JW, Doppman JL, Dwyer AJ, Johnson AR, Knop RH. Adrenal masses differentiated by MR. Radiology. 1986;158:81–4.

22. Outwater EK, Siegelman ES, Radecki PD, Picoli CW, Mitchell DG. Distinction between benign and malignant adrenal masses: value of T1-weighted chemical shift MR imaging. Am J Roentgenol. 1995;165:579–83.

23. Abrams HL, Spiro R, Goldstein N. Metastases in carcinoma: analysis of 1000 autopsied cases. Cancer. 1950;3:74–85.

24. Zornova J, Bracken R, Wallace S. Radiologic features of adrenal metastases. Urology. 1976;8:295–9.

25. Katz RL, Shirkhoda A. Diagnostic approach to incidental adrenal nodules in the cancer patient. Results of a clinical, radiologic and fine-needle aspiration study. Cancer. 1985;55:1995–2000.

26. Vincent JM, Morrison ID, Armstrong P, Reznek RH. Computed tomography of diffuse, non-metastatic enlargement of the adrenal glands in patients with malignant disease. Clin Rad. 1994;49:456–60.

27. Kier R, McCarthy S. MR characterisation of the adrenal masses: field strength and pulse sequence considerations. Radiology. 1989;171:671–4.

28. Korobkin M, Brodeur FJ, Yutzy GG, et al. Differentiation of adrenal adenomas from nonadenomas using CT attenuation values. Am J Roentgenol. 1996;166:531–6.

29. Lee MJ, Hahn PF, Papanicolau N, Schoellnast H, Preidler KW, Samonigg H. Benign and malignant adrenal masses: CT distinction with attenuation coefficients, size and observer analysis. Radiology. 1991;179:415–8.

30. Boland GW, Lee MJ, Gazelle GS, Halpern EF, McNicholas MM, Mueller PR. Characterization of adrenal masses using unenhanced CT: an analysis of the CT literature. Am J Roentgenol. 1998;171:201–4.

31. Bae KT, Fuangtharnthip P, Prasad SR, Joe BN, Heiken JP. Adrenal masses: CT characterization with histogram analysis method. Radiology. 2003;228:735–42.

32. Szolar DH, Kammerhuber F. Quantitative CT evaluation of adrenal gland masses: a step forward in the differentiation between adenomas and nonadenomas? Radiology. 1997;202:517–21.

33. Caoili EM, Korobkin M, Francis IR, Cohan RH, Dunnick NR. Delayed enhanced CT of lipid-poor adrenal adenomas. Am J Roentgenol. 2000;175:1411–5.

34. Mitchell DG, Crovello M, Matteucci T, Petersen RO, Miettinen MM. Benign adrenocortical masses: diagnosis with chemical shift MR imaging. Radiology. 1992;185:345–51.

35. Fujiyoshi F, Nakajo M, Fukukura Y, Tsuchimochi S. Characterization of adrenal tumours by chemical shift fast low-angle shot MR imaging: comparison of four methods of quantitative evaluation. Am J Roentgenol. 2003;180:1649–57.

36. Mayo-Smith WW, Lee LJ, McNicholas MM, Hahn PF, Boland GW, Saini S. Characterization of adrenal masses (<5 cm) by use of chemical shift MR imaging: observer performance verses quantitative measures. Am J Roentgenol. 1995;165:1651–91.

37. McNicholas MM, Lee MJ, Mayo-Smith WW, Hahn PF, Boland GW, Mueller PR. An imaging algorithm for the differential diagnosis of adrenal adenomas and metastases. Am J Roentgenol. 1995;165:1453–9.

38. Heinz-Peer G, Hönigschnabl S, Schneider B, Niederle B, Kaserer K, Lechner G. Characterization of adrenal masses MR Imaging with Histopathologic correlation. Am J Roentgenol. 1999;173:15–22.

39. Israel GM, Korobkin M, Wang C, Hecht EN, Krinsky GA. Comparison of Unenhanced ct and chemical shift MRI in evaluating lipid-rich adrenal adenomas. Am J Roentgenol. 2004;183:215–9.

40. Outwater EK, Siegelman ES, Huang AB, Birnbaum BA. Adrenal masses: correlation between CT attenuation value and chemical shift ratio at MR imaging with in-phase and opposed-phase sequences. Radiology. 1996;200:749–52. Erratum in: Radiology. 1996;201:880.

41. Maurea S, Mainolfi C, BazzicaloL, Panico MR, Imparato C, Alfano B, et al. Imaging of adrenal tumours using FDG PET: comparison of benign and malignant lesions. Am J Roentgenol. 1999;173:25–9.

42. Kumar R, Xui Y, Yu JQ, Takalkar A, El-Haddad G, Potenta S, et al. 18F-FDG PET in evaluation of adrenal lesions in patients with lung cancer. J Nucl Med. 2004;45:2058–62.

43. Minn H, Salonen A, Friberg J, Roivainen A, Viljanen T, Langsjo J, et al. Imaging of eadrenal incidentalomas with PET using (11)C-metomidate and (18)F-FDG. J Nucl Med. 2004;45:972–9.

44. Silverman SG, Mueller PR, Pinkney LP, Koenker RM, Selter SE. Predictive value of image-guided adrenal biopsy: analysis of results of 101 biopsies. Radiology. 1993;187:715–8.

45. Welch TJ, Sheedy PF II, Stephens DH, Johnson CM, Swensen SJ. Percutaneous adrenal biopsy: review of a 10 year experience. Radiology. 1994;193:341–4.

46. Hedican SP, Marshall FF. Adrenocortical carcinoma with intracaval extension. J Urol. 1997;158:2056–61.

47. Wajchenberg BL, Albergaria Pereira MA, Medonca BB, Latronica AC, Campos Carneiro P, Alves VA, et al. Adrenocortical carcinoma: clinical and laboratory observations. Cancer. 2000;88:711–36.

48. Dunnick NR. Adrenal carcinoma. Radiol Clin North Am. 1994;32:99–108.

49. Boscaro M, Fallo F, Barzon L, Daniele O, Sonino N. Adrenocortical carcinoma: epidemiology and natural history. Minerva Endocrinol. 1995;20:89–94.

50. Gomez-Rivera F, Medina-Franco H, Arch-Ferrer JE, Heslin MJ. Adrenocortical carcinoma: a single institution experience. Am Surg. 2005;71:90–4.

51. Dunnick NR, Doppman JL, Gill JR Jr, Strott CA, Keiser HR, Brennan MF. Localization of adrenal tumours by computed tomography and venous sampling. Radiology. 1982;142:429–33.

52. Fishman EK, Deutch BM, Hartman DS, Goldman SM, Zerhouni EA, Seigelman SS. Primary adrenocortical carcinoma: CT evaluation with clinical correlation. Am J Roentgenol. 1987;148;431–5.

53. Dunnick NR, Doppman JL, Geelhoed GW. Intavenous extension of endocrine tumours. Am J Roentgenol. 1980;135:471–6.

54. Terzolo M, Ali A, Osella G, Mazza E. Prevalence of adrenal carcinoma among incidentally discovered adrenal masses. A retrospective study from 1989 to 1994. Gruppo Piemontese Incidentalomi Surrenalici. Arch Surg. 1997;132:914–9.

55. Krebs TL, Wagner BJ. MR imaging of the adrenal gland: radiologic-pathologic correlation. Radiographics. 1998;18:1425–40.

56. Schlund JF, Kenney PJ, Brown ED, Egglin TK, Saini S, Mueller PR, et al. Adrenocortical carcinoma: MR imaging appearance with current techniques. J Magn Reson Imaging. 1995;5:171–74.

57. Yamada T, Saito H, Moriya T, Tsuboi M, Ishibashi T, Sato A, et al. Adrenal carcinoma with a signal loss on chemical shift magnetic resonance imaging. J Comput Assist Tomogr. 2003;27:606–8.

58. Lee MJ, Mayo-Smith WW, Hahn PF, Ascher SM, Brown JJ, Semelka RC. Sate-of-the-art MR imaging of the adrenal gland. Radiograhics 1994;14:1015–29.

59. Roman S. Adrenocortical carcinoma. Curr Opin Oncol. 2006;18:36–42.

60. Sutton MG, Sheps SG, Lie JT. Prevalence of clinically unsuspected pheochromoctoma: review of a 50-year autopsy series. Mayo Clin Proc. 1981;56:354–60.

61. Lucon AM, Pereira MAA, Mendonca BB, Goldberg MA, Boland GW, Saini S, et al. Pheochromocytoma: study of 50 cases. J Urol. 1997;157:1208–12.

62. Radin DR, Ralls PW, Boswell WD Jr, Colletti PM, Lapin SA, Halls JM. Phaechromocytoma detection by unenhanced CT. Am J Roentgenol. 1986,46:741–4.

63. Blake MA, Kalra MK, Maher MM, Sahani DV, Sweeney AT, Mueller PR, et al. Pheochromocytoma: an imaging chameleon. Radiographics. 2004;24 Suppl 1:S87–99.

64. Whalen RK, Althausen AF, Daniels GH. Extra-adrenal pheochromocytoma. J Urol. 1992;147:1–10.

65. Atuk NO, McDonald T, Wood T, Carpenter JT, Walzak MP, Donaldson M, et al. Familial pheochromocytoma, hypercalcemia and von Hippel Lindau disease: a ten year study of a large family. Medicine (Baltimore). 1979;58:209–18.

66. Horton WA, Wing V, Eldridge R. Von Hippel-Lindau disease: clinical and pathological manifestations in nine families with 50 affected members. Arch Intern Med. 1976;136:769–77.

67. van Heerden JA, Sheps SG, Hamberger B, Sheedy PF II, Poston JG, ReMine WH. Pheochromocytoma: current status and changing trends. Surgery. 1982;91:367–73.

68. Proye C, Fossati P, Fontaine P, Lefebvre, Decoulx M, Wemeau JL, et al. Dopamine-secreting pheochromocytoma: an unrecognised entity? Classification of pheochromocytomas according to their type of secretion. Surgery. 1986:100;1154–62.

69. Raisanen J, Shapiro B, Glazer GM, Desai S, Sisson JC. Plasma catecholamines in pheochromocytoma: effect of urographic contrast media. Am J Roentgenol. 1984;143:43–6.

70. Mukherjee JJ, Peppercorn PD, Reznek RH, Patel V, Kaltsas G, Besser M, et al. Pheochromocytoma: effect of non-ionic contrast medium in CT on circulating catecholamine levels. Radiology. 1997;202:227–31.

71. Motta-Ramirez GA, Remer EM, Herts BR, Gill IS, Hamrahian AH. Comparison of CT findings in symptomatic and incidentally discovered pheochromocytomas. Am J Roentgenol. 2005;185:684–8.

72. Cirillo RL Jr, Bennett WF, Vitellas KM, Poulos AG, Bova JG. Pathology of the adrenal gland: imaging features. Am J Roentgenol. 1998;170:429–35.

73. Varghese JC, Hahn PF, Papanicolaou N, Mayo-Smith WW, Gaa JA, Lee MJ. MR differentiation of phaeochromocytoma from other adrenal lesions based on qualitative analysis of T2 relaxation times. Clin Rad. 1997;52:603–6.

74. van Gils APG, Falke THM, van Erkel AR, Arndt JW, Sandler MP, van der Mey AG, et al. MR imaging and MIBG scintigraphy of pheochromocytomas and extra-adrenal functioning paragangliomas. Radiographics. 1991;11:37–57.

75. Tenenbaum F, Lumbroso J, Schlumberger M, Mure A, Plouin PF, Caillou B, et al. Comparison of radiolabeled octreotide and meta-iodobenzylguanidine (MIBG) scintigraphy in malignant pheochromocytoma. J Nucl Med. 1995;36:1–6.

76. Guller U, Turek J, Eubanks S, Delong ER, Oertli D, Feldman JM. Detecting pheochromocytoma: defining the most sensitive test. Ann Surg. 2006;243:102–7.

77. Lam KY, Lo CY. Adrenal lipomatous tumours: a 30 year clinicopathological experience at a single institution. J Clin Pathol. 2001;54:707–12.

78. Goldman HB, Howard RC, Patterson AL. Spontaneous retroperitoneal haemorrhage from a giant myelolipoma. J Urol. 1996;155:639.

79. Russell C, Goodacre BW, vanSonnenberg E, Orihuela E. Spontaneous rupture of adrenal myelolipoma: spiral CT appearance. Abdom Imaging. 2000;25:431–4.

80. Sneiders A, Zhang G, Gordon BE. Extra-adrenal perirenal myelolipoma. J Urol. 1993;150:1496–7.

81. Kammen BF, Elder DE, Fraker DL, Siegelman ES. Extra-adrenal myelolipoma: MR imaging findings. Am J Roentgenol. 1998;171:721–3.

82. WeinerSN, Weiner SN, Bernstein RG, Lowy S, Karp H. Combined adrenal adenoma and myelolipoma. J Comput Assist Tomogr. 1981;5:440.

83. Whaley D, Becker S, Presbrey T, Shaff M. Adrenal myelolipoma associated with Conn syndrome: CT evaluation. J Comput Assist Tomogr. 1985;9:959.

84. Musante Musante F, Derchi LE, Zappasodi F, Bazzocchi M, Riviezzo GC, Banderali A, et al. Myelolipoma of the adrenal gland: sonographic and CT features. Am J Roentgenol. 1988;151:961.

85. Palmer WE, Gerard-McFarland EL, Chew FS. Adrenal myelolipoma. Am J Roentgenol. 1991;156:724.

86. Cyran KM, Kenney PJ, Memel DS, Yacoub I. Adrenal myelolipoma. Am J Roentgenol. 1996;166:395–400.

87. Rao P, Kenney PJ, Wagner BJ, Davidson AJ. Imaging and pathologic features of myelolipoma. Radiographics. 1997;17:1373–85.

88. Rana AI, Kenney PJ, Lockhart ME, McGwin G Jr, Morgan DE, Windham ST III, et al. Adrenal gland hematomas in trauma patients. Radiology. 2004;230:669–75.

89. Burks DW, Mirvis SE, Shanmuganathan K. Acute adrenal injury after blunt abdominal trauma: CT findings. Am J Roentgenol. 1992;158:503–7.

90. Xarli VP, Steale AA, Davis PJ, Buescher ES, Rios CN, Garcia-Bunnel R. Adrenal haemorrhage in the adult. Medicine (Baltimore). 1978;57:211–21.

91. Bayliss RIS, Edwards OM, Starer F. Complications of adrenal venography. BJR. 1970;43:531–3.

92. Outwater E, Bankoff MS. Clinically significant adrenal hemorrhage secondary to metastases. Computed tomography observations. Clin Imaging. 1989;13:195–200.

93. Wolverson MK, Kannegiesser H. CT of bilateral adrenal hemorrhage with acute adrenal insufficiency in the adult. Am J Roentgenol. 1984;142:311–4.

94. Ling D, Korobkin M, Silverman PM, Dunnick NR. CT demonstration of bilateral adrenal haemorrhage. Am J Roentgenol. 1983;141:307–8.

95. Boland GW, Lee MJ. Magnetic resonance imaging of the adrenal gland. Crit Rev Diagn Imaging. 1995;36:115–74.

96. Cheema P, Cartegena R, Staubitz W. Adrenal cysts: diagnosis and treatment. J Urol. 1981;126:396–9.

97. Rozenblit A, Morehouse HT, Amis SE Jr. Cystic adrenal lesions: CT features. Radiology. 1996;201:541–8.

98. Bellantone R, Ferrante A, Raffaelli M, Boscherini M, Lombardi CP, Crucitti F. Adrenal cystic lesions: report of 12 surgically treated cases and review of the literature. J Endocrinol Invest. 1998;21:109–14.

99. Paling MR, Williamson BRJ. Adrenal involvement in non-Hodgkin lymphoma. Am J Roentgenol. 1983;141:303–5.

100. Salvatore JR, Ross RS. Primary bilateral adrenal lymphoma. Leuk lymphoma. 1999;34:111–7.

101. Kumar R, Xui Y, Mavi A, El-Haddad G, Zhuang H, Alavi A. FDG-PET imaging in primary bilateral adrenal lymphoma: a case report and review of the literature. Clin Nucl Med. 2005;30:222–30.

102. Pimental M, Johnston JB, Allan DR, Greenberg H, Bernstein CN. Primary adrenal lymphoma associated with adrenal insufficiency: a distinct clinical entity. Leuk lymphoma. 1997;24:363–7.

103. Moulton JS. CT of the adrenal gland. Semin Roentgenol. 1988;13:288–303.

104. Reinig JW, Stutley JE, Leonhardt CM, Spicer KM, Margolis M, Caldwell CB. Differentiation of adrenal masses with MR imaging: comparison of techniques. Radiology. 1994; 192:41–6.

105. Honig SC, Klavans MS, Hyde C, Siroky MB. Adrenal haemangioma: an unusual adrenal mass delineated with magnetic resonance imaging. J Urol. 1991;146:400–2.

106. Ferrozzi F, Tognini G, Bova D, Zuccoli G, Pavone P. Haemangiosarcoma of the adrenal glands: CT findings in two cases. Abdom Imaging. 2001;26:336–9.

107. Kawashima A, Sandler CM, Fishman EK, Charnsangavej C, Yasumori K, Honda H, et al. Spectrum of CT findings in non-malignant disease of the adrenal gland. Radiographics. 1998;18:393–412.

108. Rieber A, Brambs HJ. CT and MR imaging of adrenal hemangioma. A case repot. Acta Radiol. 1995;36:659–61.

109. Yamada T, Ishibashi T, Saito H, Majima K, Takahashi S, Moriya T. Two cases of adrenal hemangioma: CT and MRI findings with pathological correlations. Radiat Med. 2002;20:51–6.

110. Marotti M, Sucic Z, Krolo I, Dimanovski J, Klaric R, Ferencic Z, et al. Adrenal cavernous hemangioma: MRI, CT and US appearance. Eur Radiol. 1997;7:691–4.

111. Young JL Jr, Miller RW. Incidence of malignant tumours in US children. J Paediatr. 1975;86:245–58.

112. Ng YY, Kingston JE. The role of radiology in the staging of neuroblastoma. Clin Rad. 1993;47:226–35.

113. Franks LM, Bollen A, Seeger RC, Stram DO, Matthay KK. Neuroblastoma in adults and adolescents: an indolent course with poor survival. Cancer. 1997;79:2028–35.

114. Feinstein RS, Gatewood OM, Fishman EK, Goldman SM, Siegelman SS. Computed tomography of adult neuroblastoma. J Comput Assist Tomogr. 1984;8:720–26.

115. Enzinger FM, Weiss SW. Soft tissue tumours. 3rd ed. St. Louis, Mo: Mosby-Year Book; 1995. 929–64.

116. Radin R, David CL, Goldfarb H, Francis IR. Adrenal and extra-adrenal retroperitoneal ganglioneuroma: imaging findings in 13 adults. Radiology 1997;202:703–7.

117. Johnson GL, Hruban RH, Marshall FF, Fishman EK. Primary adrenal ganglioneuroma: CT findings in four patients. Am J Roentgenol. 1997;169:169–171.

118. Buxi TB, Vohra RB, Sujatha, Byotra SP, Mukherji S, Danial M. CT in adrenal enlargement due to tuberculosis: a review of literature with five new cases. Clin Imaging. 1992;16:102–8.

119. Doppman JL, Gill JR Jr, Nienhuis AW, Earll JM, Long JA Jr. CT findings in Addison's disease. J Comput Assist Tomogr. 1982;6:757–61.

120. Wang YX, Chen CR, He GX, Tang AR. CT findings of adrenal glands in patients with tuberculous Addison's disease. J Belge Radiol. 1998;81:226–8.

121. Vaughan ED Jr. Surgery of the adrenals. Scientific World Journal. 2004;28-4 Suppl 1:400–26.

122. Micali S, Peluso G, De Stefani S, Celia A, Sighinofi MC, Grande M, et al. Laparoscopic adrenal surgery: new frontiers. J Endourology 2005;19(3):272–8.

123. Barzon L, Scaroni C, Sonino N, Fallo F, Paoletta A, Boscaro M. Risk factors and long-term follow-up of adrenal incidentalomas. J Clin Endocrinol Metab. 1999;84(2):520–6.

124. Bülow B, Jansson S, Juhlin C, Steen L, Wahrenberg H, Valdmarsson S, et al. Adrenal incidentaloma – follow-up results from a Swedish prospective study. Eur J Endocrinol. 2006; 154:419–23.

125. Weinberger MH, Grim CE, Hollifield JW, Kem DC, Ganguly A, Kramer NJ, et al. Primary aldosteronism: diagnosis, localization and treatment. Ann Intern Med. 1979;90:386–95.

126. Ferris JB, Bevers DG, Brown JJ, et al. Clinical, biochemical and pathological features of low rennin ('primary') hyperaldosteronism. Am Heart J. 1978;95:375–88.

127. Greathouse DJ, McDermott MT, Kidd GS, et al. Pure primary hyperaldesteronism due to adrenal cortical carcinoma. Am J Med. 1984;76:1132–7.

128. Dunnick NR, Leight GS, Roubidoux MA, Leder RA, Paulson E, Kurylo L. CT in the diagnosis of primary aldosteronism: sensitivity in 29 patients. Am J Roentgenol. 1993;160:321–4.

129. Lumachi F, Marzola MC, Zucchetta P, Tregnaghi A, Cecchin D, Favia G, et al. Non-invasive adrenal imaging in primary aldosteronism. Sensitivity and positive predictive value of radiocholesterol scintigraphy, CT scan and MRI. Nucl Med Commun. 2003;24:683–8.

130. Lingam RK, Sohaib SA, Rockall AG, Isidori AM, Chew S, Monson JP, et al. Diagnostic performance of CT versus MR in detecting aldosterone-producing adenoma in primary hyperaldosteronism (Conn's syndrome). Eur Radiol. 2004;14: 1787–92.

131. Doppman JL, Travis WD, Nieman L, Miller DL, Chrousos GP, Gomez MT, et al. Cushing syndrome due to primary pigmented nodular adrenocortical disease: findings at CT and MR imaging. Radiology. 1989;172:415–20.

132. Rossi GP, Chiesura-Corona M, Tregnaghi A, Zanin L, Perale R, Soattin S, et al. Imaging of aldosterone-secreting adenomas: a prospective comparison of computed tomography and magnetic resonance imaging in 27 patients with suspected primary aldosteronism. J Hum Hypertens. 1993;7:357–63.

133. Sohaib SA, Peppercorn PD, Allan C, Monson JP, Grossman AB, Besser GM, et al. Primary hyperaldosteronism (Conn's syndrome): MR imaging findings. Radiology. 2000;214:527–31.

134. Lingam RK, Sohaib SA, Vlahos I, Rockall AG, Isidori AM, Monson JP, et al. CT of primary hyperaldosteronism (Conn's syndrome): the value of measuring the adrenal gland. Am J Roentgenol. 2003;181:843–9.

135. Lumachi F, Marzola MC, Zucchetta P, Tregnaghi A, Cecchin D, Favia G, et al. Non-invasive adrenal imaging in primary aldosteronism. Sensitivity and positive predictive value of radiocholesterol scintigraphy, CT scan and MRI. Nucl Med Commun. 2003;24:683–8.

136. Gross MD, Falke THM, Shapiro B, Sandler MP. Adrenal glands. In: Sandler MP, Patton JA, Gross MD, Shapiro B, Falke THM, editors. Endocrine imaging. Norwalk, CT: Appleton and Lange; 1992. pp. 271–349.

137. Sheaves R, Goldin J, Reznek RH, Chew SL, Dacie JE, Lowe DG, et al. Relative value of computed tomography scanning and venous sampling in establishing the cause of primary hyperaldosteronism. Eur J Endocrinol. 1996;134:308–13.

138. Doppman JL, Gill JR. Hyperaldosteronism: sampling the adrenal veins. Radiology. 1996;198:309–12.

139. Blevins LS Jr, Wand WS. Primary aldosteronism: an endocrine perspective. Radiology. 1992;184:599–600.

140. Rockall AG, Babar SA, Sohaib SA, Isidori AM, Diaz-Cano S, Monson JP, et al. CT and MR imaging of the adrenal glands in ACTH-independent cushing syndrome. Radiographics. 2004;24:435–52.

141. Prager G, Heinz-Peer G, Passler C, Kaczirek K, Schindl M, Scheuba C, et al. Surgical strategy in adrenal masses. Eur J Radiol. 2002;41:70–7.

142. Symington T. The adrenal cortex. In: Bloodworth JMB Jr, editor. Endocrine pathology: general and surgical, 2nd ed. Baltimore: William and Wilkins. pp 444–52, 483.

143. Howlett TA, Drury PL, Perry L, Doniach I, Rees LH, Besser GM. Diagnosis and management of ACTH-dependent Cushing's syndrome: comparison of the features in ectopic and pituitary ACTH production. Clin Endocrinol. 1986;24:699–713.

144. Vincent JM, Trainer PJ, Reznek RH, Marcus AJ, Dacie JE, Armstrong P, et al. The radiological investigation of occult ectopic ACTH-dependent Cushing's syndrome. Clin Radiol. 1993;48:11–7.

145. Matsuda T, Abe H, Takase M, Arakawa A, Matsumoto T, Fujime M, et al. Case of combined adrenal cortical adenoma and myelolipoma. Pathol Int. 2004;54:725–9.

146. Hutter AM, Kayhoe DE. Adrenal cortical carcinoma. Am J Med. 1966;41:572–80.

147. Bodie B, Novick AC, Pontes JE, Straffon RA, Montie JE, Babiak T, et al. The Cleveland Clinic experience with adrenal cortical carcinoma. J Urol. 1989;141:257–60.

148. Tauchmanovà L, Colao A, Marzano LA, Sparano L, Camera L, Rossi A, et al. Adrenocortical carcinomas: twelve-year prospective experience. World J Surg. 2004;28:896–903.

149. Grant CS, Carney JA, Carpenter PC, van Heerden JA. Primary pigmented nodular adrenocortical disease: diagnosis and management. Surgery. 1986;100:1178–83.

150. Bain J. Carney's complex (letter). Mayo Clin Proc. 1986;61:508.

151. Peppercorn PD, Reznek RH. State-of-the-art CT and MRI of the adrenal gland. Eur Radiol. 1997;7:822–36.

152. Kirschner MA, Powell RD Jr, Lipsett MB. Cushing's syndrome: nodular cortical hyperplasia of adrenal glands with clinical and pathological features suggesting adrenocortical tumor. J Clin Endocrinol Metab. 1964;24:947–55.

153. Falke THM, van Seters AP, Schaberg A, Moolenaar AJ. Computed tomography in untreated adults with virilizing congenital adrenal cortical hyperplasia. Clin Radiol. 1986; 37:155–60.

Chapter 3

Adrenal Carcinoma – Radionuclide Imaging

A. Becherer, G. Karanikas, M. Mitterhauser, W. Wadsak, G. Zettinig, and G. Rendl

Introduction

The adrenal glands are small organs situated in the retroperitoneum, slightly superior and medial to the upper kidney poles, the right somewhat higher and more dorsal than the left. Their size is variable in adults with a weight from 4 to 6 g. The adrenals consist of two entirely different tissue types, the cortex and the medulla.

In fact, regarding their function, cortex and medulla can be considered as two different endocrine organs. Embryologically, the cortex is of mesodermal origin whereas the medulla derives from the neuroectoderm. Histologically, the cortex is divided into the outer *zona glomerulosa*, responsible for mineralocorticoid synthesis, the intermediate broad *zona fasciculata* where primarily glucocorticoid hormones are produced and the inner *zona reticularis*, synthesizing androgenic steroid hormones. The cortex represents about 90% of the total adrenal volume. The medulla secretes the catecholamines epinephrine and norepinephrine.

The adrenal glands have been a target for functional imaging with radiolabeled tracers for more than 30 years because of the unique characteristics of their hormonal products. Using specific substrates of the adrenals, nuclear medicine is able to localize adrenal masses and to characterize them regarding their cortical or medullary origin. Most adrenal tumors are benign, thus this group represents the main indication for radionuclide adrenal imaging. Like their benign counterparts, the rare malignant adrenal tumors might arise from the adrenal cortex or from the medulla. The following chapter gives an overview over the current status of nuclear medicine for in vivo visualization of malignant adrenal lesions.

Radiotracers for Imaging of Adrenal Lesions

Adrenocortical Tumors

Adrenal tumors are principally frequent findings. It is estimated that approximately 8% of the population is bearing an adrenal nodule. Mostly an adrenal nodule is detected by chance on abdominal ultrasound, CT, or MRI.

Once detected, the question for the biological significance of the incidentaloma might be an important question. In patients with an extraadrenal malignant tumor it might represent an adrenal metastasis. Patients may even present with the adrenal lesion as the first sign of a malignant primary tumor. In other cases the incidentaloma is of primary adrenocortical or medullary origin.

The various kinds of adrenocortical neoplasms have different clinical features depending on their hormone products and/or their biological dignity. Many of them are diagnosed clinically by their characteristic symptoms like Cushing's syndrome, Conn's syndrome, feminization, or virilization. Some of them are found biochemically when an endocrine screening is started because of hypertension or electrolyte abnormalities.

Increasing numbers of asymptomatic adrenal tumors are detected incidentally on radiological imaging for other indications, referred to as incidentalomas. The incidence of incidentalomas has been increasing during recent years, reflecting the improvements in imaging technology. As much as 1% to almost 7% in patients over 70 years old will reveal an incidentaloma while incidentalomas are found on autopsy in about 6% [1–3].

Adrenocortical carcinoma (ACC) contributes only to a minor proportion of adrenal neoplasms. The annual incidence is 1–2 per million [4, 5]. However, the tumor is highly aggressive leading to 0.2% of cancer deaths in the USA [4, 6]. Surgery of the primary tumor as well as distant metastases is the only therapeutic modality with possible curative effect. Thus, accurate staging is crucial and any imaging

A. Becherer (✉)
Landeskrankenhaus Feldkirch, Department of Nuclear Medicine,
Carinagasse 47, A-6807 Feldkirch, Austria
alexander.becherer@lkhf.at

J.J.M.C.H. de la Rosette et al. (eds.), *Imaging in Oncological Urology*,
DOI 10.1007/978-1-84628-759-6_3, © Springer-Verlag London Limited 2009

procedure improving the detection of tumor lesions bears the potential of influencing survival positively.

Cholesterol Analogues

The backbone of all steroid hormones is cholesterol (Fig. 3.1). This chemical structure of steroid hormones led researchers to use radiolabeled cholesterol as an adrenal tracer. Beierwaltes et al. demonstrated the feasibility of in vivo visualization of adrenal function by 131Iodine-labeled 19-iodocholesterol [7–9]. The uptake ratios of the adrenals to the adjacent organs are increasing over several days to as high as 170 for adrenal/liver ratio and 300 for adrenal/kidney ratio, respectively [10]. A few years later, another tracer

with superior pharmacokinetics was identified which is in use till date as NP-59 (6β-[131I]iodomethyl-19-norcholest-5(10)-en-3β-ol) [11]. As an alternative, NP-59 with a 75Selenium label was used [12].

NP-59 is bound to plasma low-density lipoproteins (LDL) and internalized into the cell by the specific LDL receptor [13, 14]. Radiolabeled metabolic products are not recovered, probably because of the behavior of NP-59 as an enzyme inhibitor of hormone synthesis rather than as a metabolic precursor of steroid hormones [15].

NP-59 scanning has a higher radiation burden to the patient than other radionuclide or radiological imaging procedures established in daily practice because of the necessarily long half-life of the radiolabel. The low photon flux does not allow for tomographic SPECT imaging, only planar scintigraphy is possible (Figs. 3.2 and 3.3).

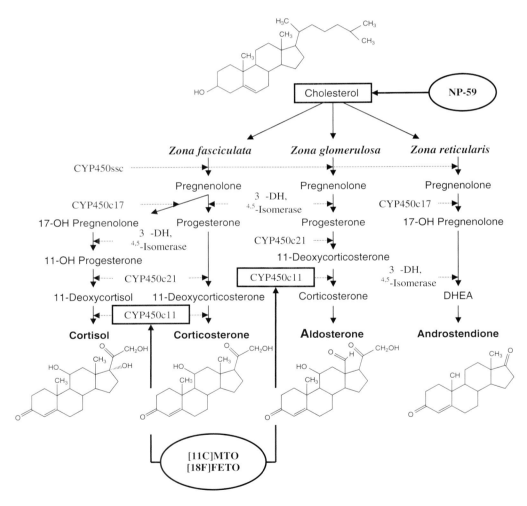

Fig. 3.1 Pathways of adrenocortical hormone synthesis. Targets for radionuclide tracers NP-59, [11C]MTO, and [18F]FETO are highlighted in bold boxes. Abbreviations: CYP450ssc=cytochrome p450-linked side-chain cleaving enzyme, desmolase; 3βDH = 3β-dehdrogenase; CYP450c21 = 21β-hydroxylase; CYP450c17 = 17α-hydroxylase; CYPc11 = 11β-hydroxylase; NP-59 = 6β-[131I]iodomethyl-19-norcholest-5(10)-en-3β-ol; [11C]MTO = [11C]metomidate; [18F] FETO = [18F]fluorethyl-etomidate

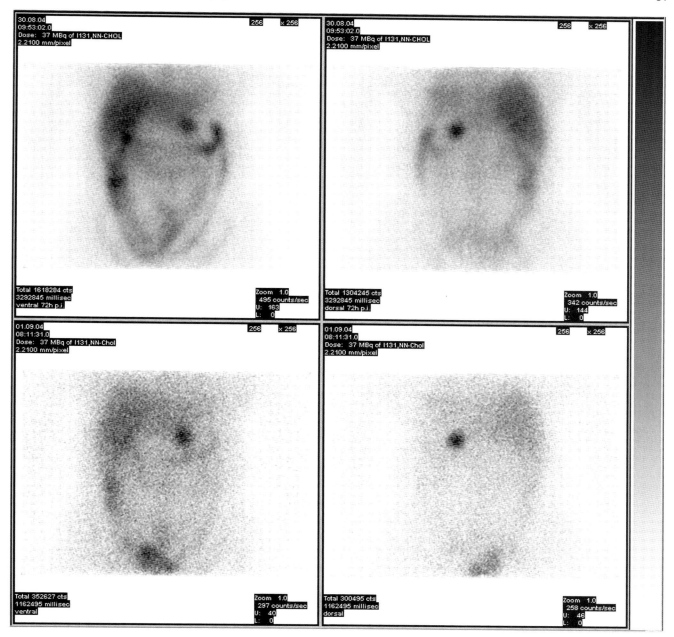

Fig. 3.2 NP-59, planar scans, upper row: 3 days p.i., lower row: 5 days p.i.; left column: anterior view, right column: posterior view. Clinically: Cushing's syndrome, caused by a left-sided benign adrenal adenoma

PET-Tracers

2[18F]Fluoro-2-deoxy-glucose ([18F]FDG)

Warburg has published the basic studies on tumor metabolism as early as in the 1930s [16]. He was able to show that cancer cells are mainly using glucose for their energy demands. This was the rationale for using the glucose derivative [18F]FDG for imaging malignant lesions, first in brain tumors [17], then in thyroid cancer and lymphoma [18, 19], and other malignant entities [20, 21]. In the following years, [18F]FDG was shown to be effective in the detection of a wide range of malignant tumors and clinical [18F]FDG-PET became a relevant imaging modality in oncology [22–24].

Most malignant adrenal lesions are metastatic lesions. Bronchial cancer, breast cancer, and sarcomas are the most common primaries that cause secondary tumors to the

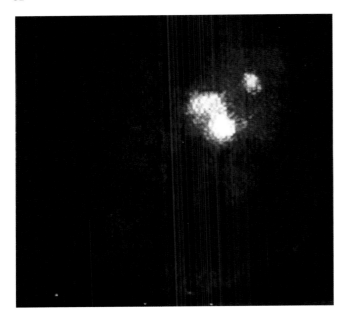

Fig. 3.3 NP-59, planar scan in posterior view 5 days p.i.: a large right-sided adrenocortical carcinoma with a pulmonary metastasis. Clinically: Cushing's syndrome

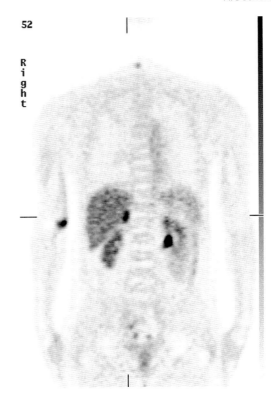

Fig. 3.4 [18F]FDG-PET, coronal slice. Metastasis in the right adrenal gland from a non-small cell bronchial carcinoma. The lesion shows up with high tracer uptake over the upper pole of the right kidney

adrenals (Fig. 3.4). The usefulness of [18F]FDG-PET for the evaluation of indeterminate adrenal masses in patients with various primary tumors is well documented [25–28]. Boland et al. scanned 20 patients with lung cancer, colorectal cancer, lymphoma, and other tumors with 24 adrenal lesions [29]. Fourteen lesions were malignant which were all diagnosed correctly by PET. Many data are available on adrenal metastases in lung cancer. Another report by Maurea et al. on unilateral adrenal lesions also included primary adrenal lesions in patients with no other malignancies and showed that PET permits non-invasive differentiation of malignant adrenal lesions from benign neoplastic ones [30]. The same group studied 30 patients with non-hypersecreting unilateral adrenal tumors [31]. Gadolinium-enhanced MR was compared to different modalities of adrenal scintigraphy. MR was performed using SE T1- (pre- and post-gadolinium DTPA) and T2-weighted images as well as in- and out-phase chemical-shift imaging (CSI). Radionuclide studies consisted of NP-59, [131I], and [18F]FDG-PET scans. Eight lesions were malignant (four adrenal carcinomas, one sarcoma, and three metastatic tumors) and all of them were imaged with [18F]FDG while NP-59 uptake was present only in adenomas. Gadolinium-enhanced MRI was less accurate than [18F]FDG in visualizing adrenal malignomas.

A study by our own group was focused on patients with proven adrenocortical carcinoma [32]. Ten patients were included, two in the primary staging setting, eight in the follow-up phase. All known sites of ACC lesions showed markedly increased [18F]FDG uptake. In three patients, previously unknown lesions were identified by PET in the lung

(one lesion), the abdomen (three lesions), and the skeleton (multiple), respectively. One false-positive liver focus was shown by PET aside from the true-positive lung metastases in the same patient. [18F]FDG-PET detected 23 lesions with a sensitivity and specificity of 100 and 95%, respectively. The tumor stage was modified in three patients, which resulted in a subsequent change in therapeutic management in two patients. In this study, several PET-positive patients were scanned under medication with 1,1-dichloro-2-(o-chlorophenyl)-2-(p-chlorophenyl)-ethane (o,p' DDD, mitotane) which did not hamper tracer uptake by the tumors and their metastases. However, the influence of medical treatment of adrenocortical carcinoma with mitotane or suramin on tracer uptake in radionuclide imaging remains an issue.

A case report demonstrated further the possible impact of [18F]FDG-PET in staging of juvenile adrenocortical carcinoma [33]. Only PET made it possible to detect an additional paravertebral metastasis, which was then resected. Given the adverse prognosis of the tumor in non-resectable or not resected tumors it can be assumed that PET has improved the survival of this patient.

Figures 3.5, 3.6, 3.9, and 3.10 show examples of [18F]FDG-PET scans of adrenocortical carcinomas.

The data on [18F]FDG in adrenocortical carcinoma are sparse, of course, but show a similar diagnostic accuracy as

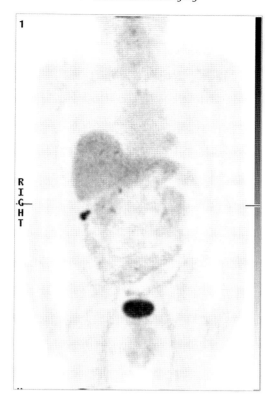

Fig. 3.5 [18F]FDG-PET, multiintensity projection (MIP). Local relapse (implantation metastasis) after resection of the primary tumor by right adrenalectomy

in other tumor entities where much more studies are available like cancers of the digestive tract or bronchial carcinoma. From those it can be derived that [18F]FDG-PET is of undoubtful value in re-staging and follow-up of adrenocortical carcinoma.

Specific Adrenocortical Tracers

Based on steroid hormone biosynthesis, there has been a search for tracers aside from labeled cholesterol derivatives with specific binding capability to the adrenal cortex. The synthesis of adrenocortical steroids proceeds from cholesterol through several enzymes and cytochrome P450 (Fig. 3.1).

Cholesterol is bound to the adrenals by LDL receptors and then stored in lipid droplets after esterification. LDL receptors are abundant in adrenocortical cells. Cholesterol ester hydrolase catalyzes the formation of free cholesterol in the lipid droplets, which are transported to the mitochondria by a sterol carrier protein. There it is converted to pregnenolone by cholesterol desmolase. Pregnenolone is the last common precursor of corticosteroids, mineralocorticoids, and adrenal androgens in all three zones. From there, the zones use dif-

ferent pathways to form their hormones, dependent on the specific enzymatic composition of the zones.

In *zona glomeruosa* cells the synthesis of glucocorticoids and androgens is blocked by a lack of 17α-hydroxylase (CYP450c17). Therefore pregnenolone is converted to progesterone by 3β-dehydrogenase (3β-DH) and progesterone to 11-deoxycorticosterone by 21β-hydroxylase (CYP450c21). The next step is the synthesis of corticosterone by 11β-hydroxylase (CYP450c11). Eventually the enzyme 18α-hydroxylase (CYPP450c18), which is only present in the *zona glomerulosa*, converts corticosterone to aldosterone.

In the *zona fasciculata*, the hormones cortisol and corticosterone are synthesized by the use of CYP450c17, 3β-DH, CYP450c21, and, finally, CYP450c11. In the *zona reticularis*, no CYP450c11 is present, thus the step of forming glucocorticoids is blocked.

It was again Beierwaltes et al. who developed agents for imaging of the adrenal cortex based on enzyme inhibition for conventional scintigraphy [34, 35]. CYP450c11 expression is increased in benign adenomas as well as in adrenocortical carcinomas, whereas it is not found in secondary adrenal lesions like metastatic bronchial carcinoma lesions and others [36]. Thus this enzyme can be used as a tracer target for labeling tissue specifically involved in glucocorticoid and mineralocorticoid incretion. Metyrapone has been synthesized as a potent inhibitor of P450c11, labeled with radioiodine and with carbon-11 for PET [37, 38]. Both tracers, however, did not fulfill the expectations for in vivo imaging.

[11C]Metomidate ([11C]MTO)

Other CYP450c11 inhibitors are etomidate and its derivatives. Etomidate is widely used for general anesthesia and has proven to be a safe drug in much higher amounts than required for radionuclide scans. Animal experiments with 11C-labeled metomidate (O-[11C]methyl-metomidate ([11C]MTO), and O-ethyl-1-[11C]-etomidate ([11C]ETO), and PET showed high uptake in the adrenal glands [36]. Because of shorter synthesis time, higher radiochemical yields and higher specific radioactivity, [11C]MTO was found to be more suitable for clinical purposes (Fig. 3.7).

Clinical studies with [11C]MTO showed promising results in imaging of adrenal cortex and adrenocortical lesions [39–42]. Adrenal lesions show impressive high uptake in comparison to lesions of other origin, as does the normal adrenal cortex. Another organ with rather high physiologic uptake is the stomach while liver, kidneys, and intestine have low uptake (Fig. 3.8). The tracer shows biliary excretion, which explains for the intestinal uptake. The gall bladder shows only moderate radioactivity concentration. Hence [11C]MTO is well suited for a non-invasive

(a)   (b)

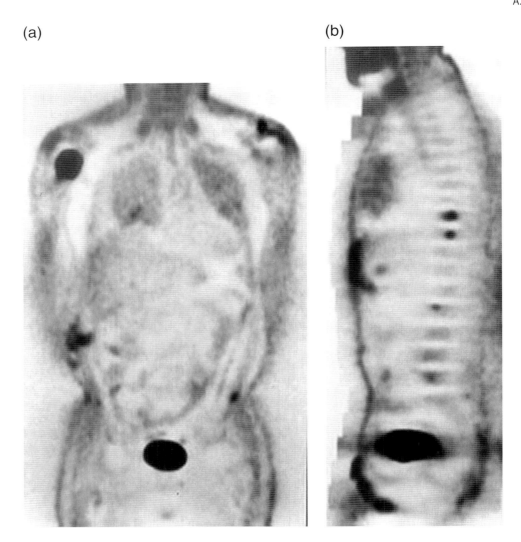

Fig. 3.6 [18F]FDG-PET, selected coronal (a) and sagittal (b) slices, scan without attenuation correction. One week after right adrenalectomy PET shows bone metastases, particularly in the right humerus and the left ilical bone (a) and the spine (b) and multiple small pulmonary hot spots consistent with lung metastases (a). Non-specific post-surgical uptake in the right flank

detection of adrenocortical tissue either if it is normal gland or neoplastic tissue. Zettinig et al. investigated 16 patients with various adrenal lesions, 13 of them having a benign lesion, 1 an adrenocortical carcinoma, 1 with a malignant pheochromocytoma, and 1 adrenal secondary malignancy [39–42]. All lesions of adrenal origin showed high [11C]MTO uptake although it was not possible to differentiate between the adrenocortical carcinoma and the benign lesions. The SUVs ranged from 11.5 to 32.2, the carcinoma was in the lower range with an SUV of 14.3. One drawback of this study was that only one patient with an adrenocortical carcinoma could be included because of the rareness of the disease and the prospective design. In this case [11C]MTO was superior in comparison to [18F]FDG in terms of visualization of lung metastasis (Fig. 3.9). There was further a clear distinction of adrenal and non-adrenal lesions, the latter having an SUV from 1.8 to 2.8. The absolute standardized uptake values of patients with Conn's syndrome were 10% higher than those of patients with Cushing's syndrome, albeit this difference was not significant; on the other hand, the lesion/normal adrenal gland ratio was higher in patients with Cushing's syndrome, which was interpreted as an indicator that [11C]MTO uptake is sensitive to suppression by the excessive hormone incretion of the contralateral lesion.

A more recent study from Hennings and co-workers retrospectively investigated 173 patients who had at least 1 out of 212 [11C]MTO-PET scans at their department [43]. This work confirmed the observation of Zettinig that aldosteronomas have higher uptake values than adenomas with glucocorticoid production but not the difference in the ratios of lesion to normal adrenals. This study comprised of ten patients with adrenocortical carcinoma whose SUVs were lower by

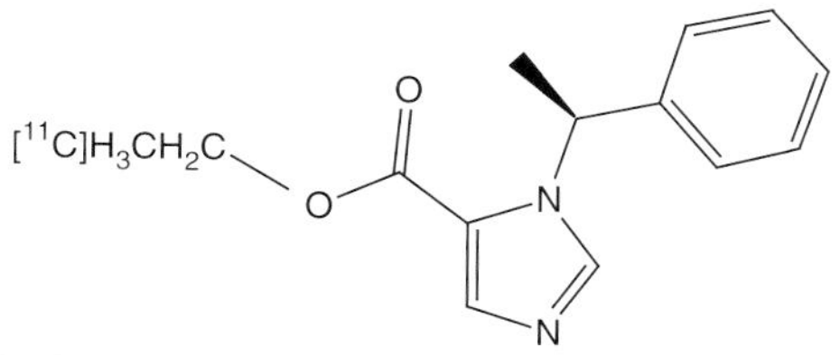

[¹¹C]H₃CH₂C

a) [11C]Etomidate (ETO)

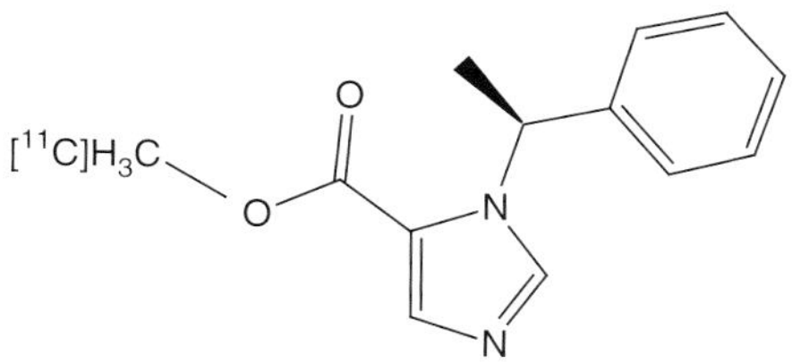

[¹¹C]H₃C

b) [11C]Metomidate (MTO)

¹⁸F

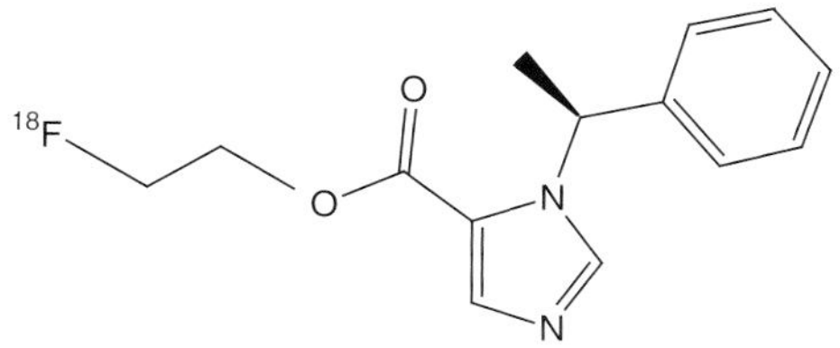

c) [18F]Fluorethyl-Desethyl-Etomidate (FETO)

Fig. 3.7 Chemical structures of [11C]ETO (a), [11C]MTO (b), and [18F]FETO (c)

50% than aldosteronomas and by 25% than glucocorticoid-producing lesions. An uptake ratio above 1.4 between the two adrenal glands was associated with a 99.5% risk of bearing an adrenal tumor, although it was not possible to identify a value predictive for an adrenocortical carcinoma.

It is not always the case that [11C]MTO is superior in imaging of adrenocortical carcinoma in comparison to [18F]FDG as is demonstrated in Figs. 3.10 and 3.11. Uptake properties might depend on tumor differentiation

with increasing glucose consumption and thus increasing [18F]FDG uptake when the tumor de-differentiates.

[18F]Fluorethyl-desethyl-etomidate ([18F]FETO)

A major drawback of [11C]MTO is the short half-life of the carbon-11 label of approximately 20 minutes, limiting its use to centers with its own cyclotron facility. To enable specific adrenal PET imaging remote from a cyclotron, a search for a fluorine-18-labeled etomidate analogue has been undertaken. Eventually, the fluorethyl-etomidate compound was found to be suited for this purpose (Fig. 3.7c). Wadsak and Mitterhauser developed a procedure in which [18F]FETO can be synthesized with reproducible acceptable radiochemical yields of almost 15% (decay corrected) within 80 minutes [44]. Therefore this tracer is a promising alternative to [11C]MTO for a wider use of adrenal PET imaging. Animal studies showed the high specific uptake in the adrenal glands at 30 minutes p.i. which was more than tenfold in relation to the next hottest organ, the lungs, expressed in % uptake per gram tissue [45]. The imaging potential of FETO was subsequently proven in healthy volunteers [46]. Figure 3.12 a demonstrates the increase of the adrenal-to-liver ratio over time, and Fig. 3.12b shows an example of a PET scan in a patient with an adenoma in the left adrenal gland and Cushing's syndrome with good contrast of the adrenals, the lesion-bearing as well as the contralateral normal one. As this tracer is the most recent development for adrenal imaging there are no clinical studies on its value in imaging of adrenocortical lesions to date. Its imaging properties correspond to those from [11C]MTO but it offers the physical possibility for broader distribution. Hence, these studies are likely to follow soon. First results show that FETO visualizes hormonally active and inactive benign and malignant lesions. Figures 3.13–3.15 give several examples of [18F]FETO scans of patients with various adrenocortical tumors. The examples highlight the high tracer affinity to adrenal cortex and its primary tumors (Fig. 3.14) and the high specificity (Fig. 3.15).

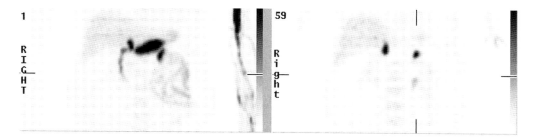

Fig. 3.8 [11C]MTO-PET, MIP (left frame), and coronal slice through the adrenals. Typical pattern with high adrenal and gastric uptake while the other organs display low uptake and are helpful for anatomic orientation. Characteristic visualization of the veins proximal to the injection site

(a)

(b)

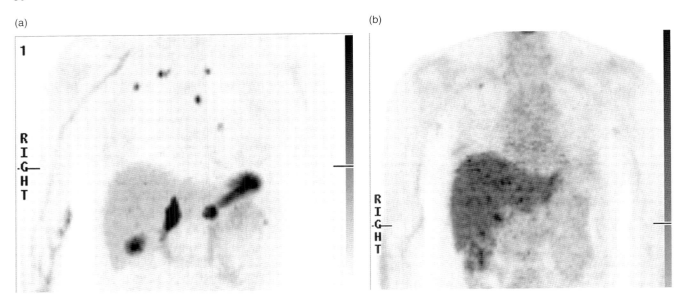

Fig. 3.9 (a) [11C]MTO-PET, MIP. Multiple small pulmonary metastases of a resected left-sided adrenocortical carcinoma, loco-regional relapse in the left diaphragmal crus. The right adrenal gland appears hypertrophic, non-specific gastric uptake. (b) [18F]FDG-PET, MIP. Only one lung lesion in the right apex shows tracer uptake, no visualization of the lesion in the left diaphragm

(a)

(b)

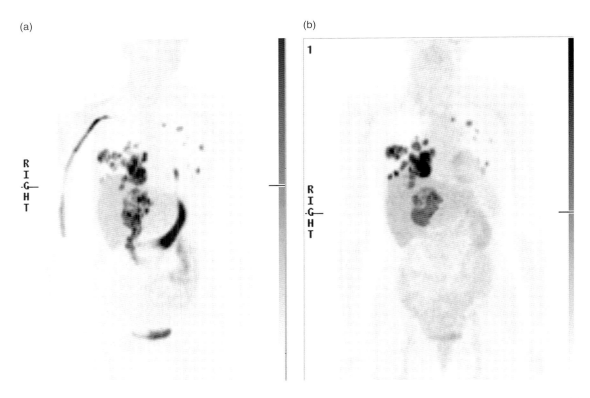

Fig. 3.10 (a) [11C]MTO-PET, (b) [18F]FDG-PET, MIPs of both scans. Large right-sided adrenocortical carcinoma with metastases in both lungs, predominantly in the right lung and the liver. Identical information by [11C]MTO and [18F]FDG regarding the extent and the number of lesions

(a)

(b)

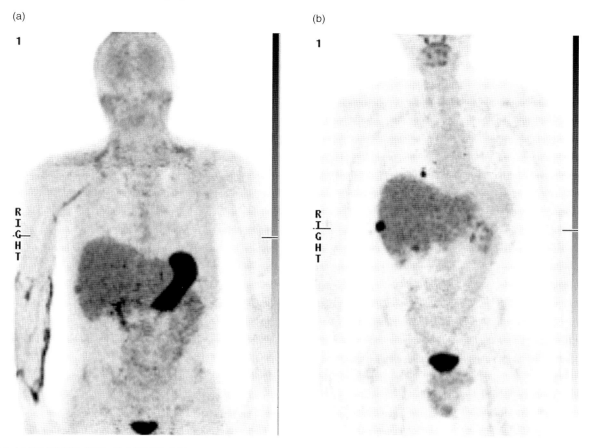

Fig. 3.11 (a) [11C]MTO-PET, (b) [18F]FDG-PET, MIPs. [18F]FDG has a much higher contrast in the subcapsular liver metastasis. The small lung lesion is even missed by [11C]MTO

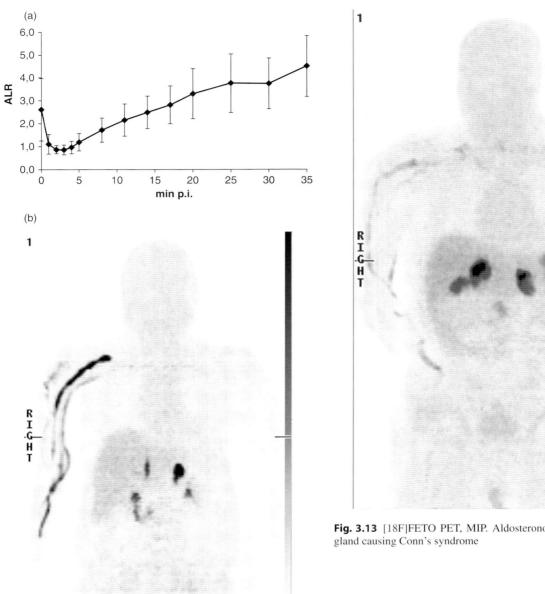

(a)

ALR

min p.i.

(b)

1

RIGHT

Fig. 3.13 [18F]FETO PET, MIP. Aldosteronoma in the right adrenal gland causing Conn's syndrome

Fig. 3.12 (a) Adrenal-to-liver ratios (ALRs). The ALR is a measure for the visual contrast between adrenals and the liver as reference region. All values represent arithmetic means; error bars indicate standard deviation. Image taken from [46] with kind permission of the publisher. (b) [18F]FETO distribution 30–40 minutes after injection in a patient with a cortisol-producing adenoma in the left adrenal (MIP): highest uptake in the adenoma, lower uptake in the right adrenal, low uptake in kidneys, liver, lungs, and soft tissue, low urinary excretion. Tracer uptake in the veins of the arm where the tracer has been injected is typical

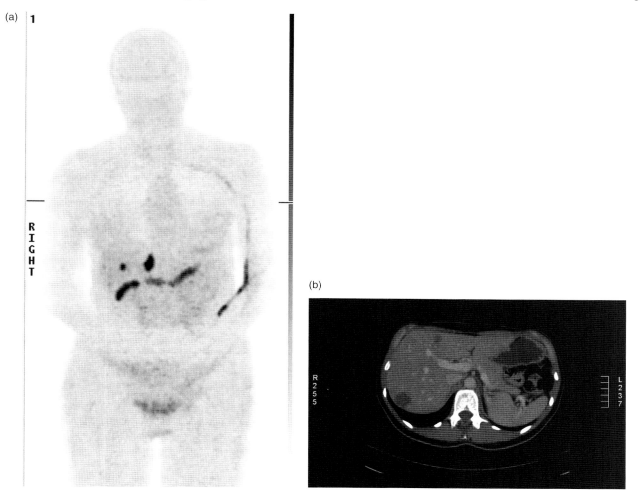

Fig. 3.14 (a) [18F]FETO PET, MIP. Adrenocortical carcinoma, Status post left adrenalectomy. A small hepatic metastasis is visualized with very high contrast despite a size of only 16 mm, normal right adrenal gland. (b) Oblique axial multiplanar MSCT image of the liver with venous phase contrast enhancement. Note two hypodense lesions, the ventral lesion is slightly hypodense (typical appearance for metastasis, corresponding to the PET-positive lesion) while the large dorsal lesion shows ring-like nodular enhancement, characteristic for a hemangioma, without any tracer uptake

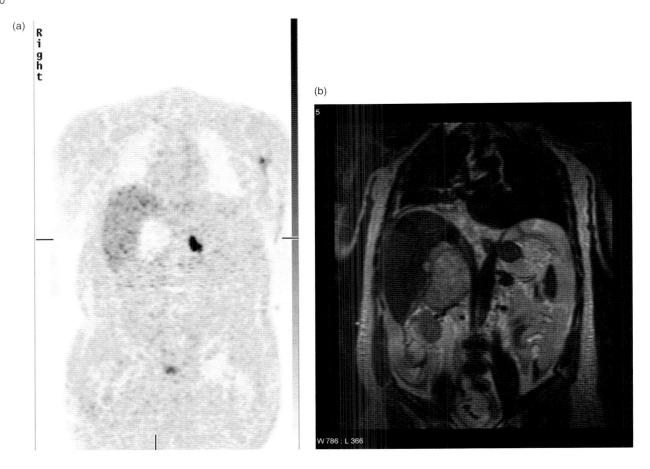

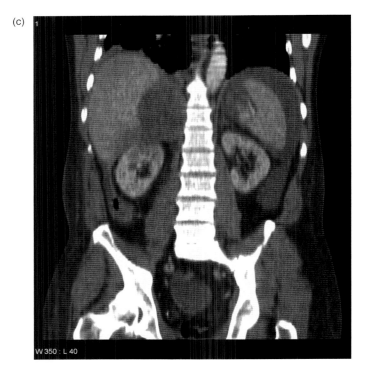

Fig. 3.15 (a) [18F]FETO PET, coronal slice. The patient showed up with a large right adrenal tumor and multiple lung metastases, highly suspicious for a primary adrenal carcinoma on CT with contrast media, venous phase (b) and even on MRI, turbo spin echo, without fat saturation (c). The tumor showed no tracer uptake in the PET scan, but appeared even photopenic. Histology revealed a rhabdomyosarcoma

Conclusions

Imaging of primary adrenocortical tumors consists of specific imaging of the adrenal cortex with labeled cholesterol and planar scintigraphy and inhibitors of 11β-hydroxylase and PET as well as non-specific imaging of glucose consumption and PET. For *in vivo* characterization of the histologic nature of an adrenal lesion specific tracers are mandatory. PET is the gold standard in this regard due to the by far better imaging properties. [18F]FETO and [11C]MTO both bind predominantly to 11β-hydroxylase and will visualize the lesions as long as they are not completely dedifferentiated. For the assessment of adrenal lesions whether they are malignant or non-malignant the first choice tracer is still [18F]FDG-PET. For the staging and follow-up of adrenocortical carcinomas not only is [18F]FDG highly useful but also [18F]FETO and [11C]MTO might be helpful as they can also visualize metastases of adrenocortical carcinomas. The new generation of integrated PET/CT scanners will further improve the diagnostic accuracy.

References

1. Kloos RT, Gross MD, Shapiro B, Francis IR, Korobkin M, Thompson NW. Diagnostic dilemma of small incidentally discovered adrenal masses: role for 131I-6beta-iodomethyl-norcholesterol scintigraphy. World J Surg. 1997;21(1):36–40.
2. Thompson GB, Young WF, Jr. Adrenal incidentaloma. Curr Opin Oncol. 2003;15(1):84–90.
3. Zarco-Gonzalez JA, Herrera MF. Adrenal incidentaloma. Scand J Surg. 2004;93(4):298–301.
4. Third nationalcancer survey: incidence data. *DHEW Publishers No (NIH) 75–787 NCI monograph*. Bethesda: National Cancer Institute; 1975. p. 41.
5. Dackiw AP, Lee, JE, Gagel RF, Evans DB. Adrenal Cortical Carcinoma. World J Surg 2001;25(7):914–926.
6. Wajchenberg BL, Albergaria Pereira MA, Medonca BB, et al. Adrenocortical carcinoma: clinical and laboratory observations. Cancer. 2000;88(4):711–36.
7. Beierwaltes WH, Lieberman LM, Ansari AN, Nishiyama H. 131 I-19-iodocholesterol in the diagnosis of adrenal disease. J Lab Clin Med. 1971;78(6):986–7.
8. Lieberman LM, Beierwaltes WH, Conn JW, Ansari AN, Nishiyama H. Diagnosis of adrenal disease by visualization of human adrenal glands with 131 I-19-iodocholesterol. N Engl J Med. 1971;285(25):1387–93.
9. Conn JW, Cohen EL, Lucas CP, et al. Visualization of aldosterone-producing tumors (APT) by scintillation scanning (SS) employing tracer amounts of 131 -iodocholesterol. J Lab Clin Med. 1971;78(5):814–5.
10. Counsell RE, Ranade VV, Blair RJ, Beierwaltes WH, Weinhold PA. Tumor localizing agents. IX. Radioiodinated cholesterol. Steroids. 1970;16(3):317–28.
11. Sarkar SD, Beierwaltes H, Ice RD, et al. A new and superior adrenal scanning agent, NP-59. J Nucl Med. 1975;16(11):1038–42.
12. Sarkar SD, Ice RD, Beierwaltes WH, Gill SP, Balachandran S, Basmadjian GP. Selenium-75-19-selenocholesterol-a new adrenal scanning agent with high concentration in the adrenal medulla. J Nucl Med. 1976;17(3):212–7.
13. Freeman DA, Counsell RE. Cellular internalization, transport, and esterification of iodine-125-NP59 by MA-10 Leydig tumor cells. J Nucl Med. 1991;32(3):495–9.
14. Rubello D, Bui C, Casara D, Gross MD, Fig LM, Shapiro B. Functional scintigraphy of the adrenal gland. Eur J Endocrinol. 2002;147(1):13–28.
15. Harbert JC. The adrenal glands and neural crest tumors. In: Harbert JC, Eckelman WC, Neumann RD, editors. Nuclear medicine: diagnosis and therapy. New York: Thieme Medical Publishers; 1996. pp. 745–58.
16. Warburg O. The metabolism of tumors. London: Constable Press; 1930.
17. Patronas NJ, Brooks RA, DeLaPaz RL, Smith BH, Kornblith PL, Di Chiro G. Glycolytic rate (PET) and contrast enhancement (CT) in human cerebral gliomas. AJNR Am J Neuroradiol. 1983;4(3):533–5.
18. Joensuu H, Ahonen A. Imaging of metastases of thyroid carcinoma with fluorine-18 fluorodeoxyglucose. J Nucl Med. 1987;28(5):910–4.
19. Paul R. Comparison of fluorine-18-2-fluorodeoxyglucose and gallium-67 citrate imaging for detection of lymphoma. J Nucl Med. 1987;28(3):288–92.
20. Strauss LG, Clorius JH, Schlag P, et al. Recurrence of colorectal tumors: PET evaluation. Radiology. 1989;170(2):329–32.
21. Minn H, Soini I. [18F]fluorodeoxyglucose scintigraphy in diagnosis and follow up of treatment in advanced breast cancer. Eur J Nucl Med. 1989;15(2):61–6.
22. Hoh CK, Schiepers C, Seltzer MA, et al. PET in oncology: will it replace the other modalities? Semin Nucl Med. 1997;27(2):94–106.
23. Delbeke D. Oncological applications of FDG PET imaging: brain tumors, colorectal cancer, lymphoma and melanoma. J Nucl Med. 1999;40(4):591–603.
24. Delbeke D. Oncological applications of FDG PET imaging. J Nucl Med. 1999;40(10):1706–15.
25. Erasmus JJ, Patz EF, Jr., McAdams HP, et al. Evaluation of adrenal masses in patients with bronchogenic carcinoma using 18F-fluorodeoxyglucose positron emission tomography. AJR Am J Roentgenol. 1997;168(5):1357–60.
26. Yun M, Kim W, Alnafisi N, Lacorte L, Jang S, Alavi A. 18F-FDG PET in characterizing adrenal lesions detected on CT or MRI. J Nucl Med. 2001;42(12):1795–9.
27. Kumar R, Xiu Y, Yu JQ, et al. 18F-FDG PET in evaluation of adrenal lesions in patients with lung cancer. J Nucl Med. 2004;45(12):2058–62.
28. Frilling A, Tecklenborg K, Weber F, et al. Importance of adrenal incidentaloma in patients with a history of malignancy. Surgery. 2004;136(6):1289–96.
29. Boland GW, Goldberg MA, Lee MJ, et al. Indeterminate adrenal mass in patients with cancer: evaluation at PET with 2-[F-18]-fluoro-2-deoxy-D-glucose. Radiology. 1995;194(1):131–4.
30. Maurea S, Mainolfi C, Bazzicalupo L, et al. Imaging of adrenal tumors using FDG PET: comparison of benign and malignant lesions. AJR Am J Roentgenol. 1999;173(1):25–9.
31. Maurea S, Caraco C, Klain M, Mainolfi C, Salvatore M. Imaging characterization of non-hypersecreting adrenal masses. Comparison between MR and radionuclide techniques. Q J Nucl Med Mol Imaging. 2004;48(3):188–97.
32. Becherer A, Vierhapper H, Potzi C, et al. FDG-PET in adrenocortical carcinoma. Cancer Biother Radiopharm. 2001;16(4):289–95.

33. Kreissig R, Amthauer H, Krude H, et al. The use of FDG-PET and CT for the staging of adrenocortical carcinoma in children. Pediatr Radiol. 2000;30(5):306.

34. Beierwaltes WH, Wieland DM, Ice RD, et al. Localization of radiolabeled enzyme inhibitors in the adrenal gland. J Nucl Med. 1976;17(11):998–1002.

35. Beierwaltes WH, Wieland DM, Mosley ST, et al. Imaging the adrenal glands with radiolabeled inhibitors of enzymes: concise communication. J Nucl Med. 1978;19(2):200–3.

36. Bergstrom M, Bonasera TA, Lu L, et al. In vitro and in vivo primate evaluation of carbon-11-etomidate and carbon-11-metomidate as potential tracers for PET imaging of the adrenal cortex and its tumors. J Nucl Med. 1998;39(6):982–9.

37. Robien W, Zolle I. Synthesis of radioiodinated metyrapone – a potential adrenal imaging agent. Int J Appl Radiat Isot. 1983;34(6):907–14.

38. Damani LA, Mitterhauser M, Zolle I, Lin G, Oehler E, Ho YP. Metabolic and pharmacokinetic considerations in the design of 2-phenyl substituted metyrapone derivatives: 2-methoxyphenylmetyrapone as a radioligand for functional diagnosis of adrenal pathology. Nucl Med Biol. 1995;22(8):1067–74.

39. Bergstrom M, Juhlin C, Bonasera TA, et al. PET imaging of adrenal cortical tumors with the 11beta-hydroxylase tracer 11C-metomidate. J Nucl Med. 2000;41(2):275–82.

40. Khan TS, Sundin A, Juhlin C, Langstrom B, Bergstrom M, Eriksson B. 11C-metomidate PET imaging of adrenocortical cancer. Eur J Nucl Med Mol Imaging. 2003;30(3):403–10.

41. Hennings J, Lindhe O, Bergstrom M, Langstrom B, Sundin A, Hellman P. 11C-metomidate positron emission tomography of adrenocortical tumours in correlation with histopathological findings. J Clin Endocrinol Metab. 2006;91(4):1410–1414.

42. Zettinig G, Mitterhauser M, Wadsak W, et al. Positron emission tomography imaging of adrenal masses: (18)F-fluorodeoxyglucose and the 11beta-hydroxylase tracer (11)C-metomidate. Eur J Nucl Med Mol Imaging. 2004;31(9):1224–30.

43. Hennings J, Lindhe O, Bergstrom M, Langstrom B, Sundin A, Hellman P. [11C]metomidate positron emission tomography of adrenocortical tumors in correlation with histopathological findings. J Clin Endocrinol Metab. 2006;91(4):1410–4.

44. Wadsak W, Mitterhauser M. Synthesis of [18F]FETO, a novel potential 11-beta hydroxylase inhibitor. J Labelled Comp Radiopharm. 2003;46(4):379–88.

45. Mitterhauser M, Wadsak W, Wabnegger L, et al. In vivo and in vitro evaluation of [18F]FETO with respect to the adrenocortical and GABAergic system in rats. Eur J Nucl Med Mol Imaging. 2003;30(10):1398–401.

46. Wadsak W, Mitterhauser M, Rendl G, et al. [(18)F]FETO for adrenocortical PET imaging: a pilot study in healthy volunteers. Eur J Nucl Med Mol Imaging. 2006;33(6):669–672.

Chapter 4

Considerations: Imaging in Adrenal Carcinoma

A.D. Joyce, J.A. Guthrie, and T.M. Wah

Adrenal masses will frequently be encountered by the radiologist and urologist. It is important to accurately characterize these lesions so that the patient can be managed appropriately. The diagnostic challenge arises from a small number of diagnoses which are of critical significance amongst a high prevalence of non-hyperfunctioning adrenal adenomas ("incidentalomas") and a number of other uncommon benign adrenal conditions which are usually without clinical consequence. Adrenal masses may be discovered incidentally during the investigation of unrelated symptoms, as part of a cancer staging investigation, or sought during the investigation of a biochemical or endocrine imbalance. Whilst there is a wide differential diagnosis for an adrenal mass a diagnosis can often be established when the morphological features are coupled with the clinical history and biochemical findings. In this chapter on considerations we aim to provide an algorithm on the use of diagnostic imaging of adrenal masses.

Imaging is becoming increasingly important in trying to assist the clinician in the determination of the significance of these lesions, the potential need for surgery, and the malignancy risk of these lesions if a conservative approach is under consideration. Most studies advise removal of an adrenal lesion >6 cm, whereas masses <3 cm can be observed. The question arises for those lesions between 3 and 6 cm, and some authors advocate the removal of all lesions in excess of 3 cm. Under these circumstances the need for an imaging algorithm is extremely useful and we advocate the following protocol to assist clinicians in their difficult deliberations (Fig. 4.1).

Adrenal surgery is very much a multidisciplinary effort with close co-operation between endocrinologists, surgeons, and anesthetists, to achieve a safe outcome.

Few urologists are active in adrenal surgery, predominantly due to the increasing role of laparoscopy in the surgical management of this condition and the fact that this option in some areas is offered on a wider scale by general surgeons rather than urologists.

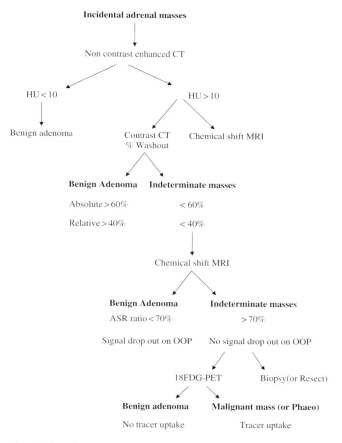

Fig. 4.1 Imaging algorithm for characterization of adrenal masses

T. Wah (✉)
Department of Radiology, St. James's University Hospital, Leeds, LS9 7TF, United Kingdom,tze.wah@leedsth.nhs.uk

J.J.M.C.H. de la Rosette et al. (eds.), *Imaging in Oncological Urology*,
DOI 10.1007/978-1-84628-759-6_4, © Springer-Verlag London Limited 2009

Chapter 5

Renal Cell Carcinoma: Introduction

H. Van Poppel and D. Thüer

Epidemiology

Primary malignant renal epithelial neoplasms account for 3% of adult malignancies [1]. The mean age at the time of diagnosis is about 70 years and, as shown in Fig. 5.1, there is a predominance of men over women in the range of 1.5–3.1. US, CT, and MRI all contribute to the increased detection of all types of renal parenchymal mass lesions, including those that require surgery and those where surgery has to be avoided. An increased incidence of renal cell carcinoma is reported while the incidence of the less common transitional cell carcinomas (TCC) of the renal pelvis is stable or decreasing (Fig. 5.2). Due to the systematic use of abdominal ultrasound and CT scan, a majority of tumors are now detected in an early stage. At present, 25–40% of clinically diagnosed RCC are found incidentally [2]. A total of 25–30% of patients with RCC have overt metastases at initial presentation and, in addition, a substantial fraction of patients have subclinical metastases at that time explaining the unsatisfactory outcome of treatment [3, 4].

Malignant tumors are detected at earlier stages. The mortality from RCC is increasing parallel to trends in incidence. Survival is closely related to initial stage; 5-year survival is 50–90% for localized disease, decreasing to 0–13% for metastatic disease [3]. Table 5.1 shows the relative 5-year survival percentage rate for RCC and TCC.

There are no generally accepted risk factors for RCC. There are some epidemiologic data indicating that a smoking habit, obesity, hypertension, or exposure to certain heavy metals such as cadmium may favor the development of RCCs.

Pathology

Understanding the underlying gross pathology and histological correlates provides an essential substrate for explaining the radiological characteristics of these masses. Many pathologists still rely on hematoxylin- and eosin-stained preparations of surgical specimens to achieve the histological diagnosis of renal cell carcinoma (RCC) [4, 5]. From clinicopathological observations, it has been observed that a neoplasm may change its pattern of differentiation in time and that it does not necessarily retain the phenotype of its presumed progenitor cell. Thus it can be explained that in the past, lectin and immunohistochemical studies using markers for different parts of the adult renal tubular system yielded conflicting results regarding the proximal versus distal tubular origin of renal cell tumors. Furthermore, renal cell carcinomas may be composed of mixtures of clear and granular cells or clear and chromophilic cells. Such observations would suggest that a transition between phenotypes occurs during progression.

During the last decades, it has become increasingly clear that the initiation and progression of solid tumors is governed by alterations of genes that control growth and differentiation. Tumor development is based on specific and separate molecular mechanisms in different cells, and therefore they are almost completely different. There is a specific combination of chromosomal and mitochondrial DNA alterations marking distinct types of tumor genes of putative tumor suppressor genes [6].

Classification

The morphological classification of renal cell neoplasm in adult relies on three essential criteria: first the aspect of the tumor cells (i.e., clear cells, chromophilic cells (basophilic or eosinophilic), chromophobic cells, oncocytes, collecting duct cells, and sarcomatoid or fusiform cells); second the

H.V. Poppel (✉)
University Hospital of KULeuven, UZ Gasthuisberg, Herestraat 49, B-3000 Leuven, Belgium, hendrik.vanpoppel@uz.kuleuven.ac.be

J.J.M.C.H. de la Rosette et al. (eds.), *Imaging in Oncological Urology*, DOI 10.1007/978-1-84628-759-6_5, © Springer-Verlag London Limited 2009

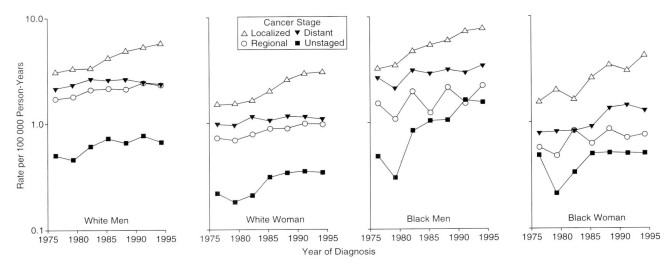

Fig. 5.1 Age-Adjusted (1970 US Standard) Incidence Rates Per 100,000 Person-Years for Renal Cell Carcinoma by Sex, Race, and Tumor Stage at Diagnosis–SEER, 1975–1977 to 1993–1995

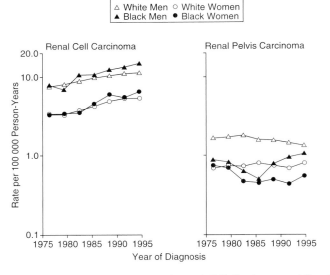

Fig. 5.2 Evolution of Incidence of Renal Cell Carcinoma and Renal Pelvis Carcinoma

Diagnosis

Clinical symptoms of RCC, such as hematuria, palpable tumor, and flank pain, are becoming less frequent. Asymptomatic tumors are more commonly diagnosed [11]. Clinical examination has a limited role in diagnosing RCC, but it may be valuable in assessing co-morbidity [12]. In case of hematuria, additional tumors of the genitourinary tract should be excluded [13]. The most commonly assessed laboratory parameters are

- Hemoglobin and erythrocyte sedimentation rate: prognosis
- Creatinine: overall kidney function
- Alkaline phosphatase: liver metastasis, bone metastasis
- Liver function tests: Stauffer syndrome

Serum calcium is frequently included in the preoperative assessment because of its association with paraneoplastic manifestation, which may have clinical implications [13].

The majority of tumors are diagnosed by abdominal ultrasound performed for various reasons. Standard radiological procedure is an abdominal CT scan with and without contrast medium. It serves to document the diagnosis of RCC and provides information on the function and morphology of the contralateral kidney [14]. Additional diagnostic procedures, such as magnetic resonance imaging, angiography, or fine needle biopsy, have a very limited role, but may be considered in selected cases [15].

Abdominal CT scan assesses primary tumor extension and provides information on venous involvement and on metastatic spread to locoregional lymph nodes, adrenals, contralateral kidney, liver, etc. [14]. Chest X-ray is

architecture (solid (acinar), tubulopapillary, tubular, tubulocystic); and third the nuclear grade, based on increasing numbers of nuclear and nucleolar atypia. Based on these morphological criteria, classification of the majority of renal cell neoplasms is feasible, with few exceptions only. This morphology-based classification is now supported by cytogenetic analysis. Five major groups of malignant renal epithelial neoplasms are distinguished [7–10] and are summarized in Table 5.2.

Table 5.1 Relative 5-Year Survival Percentage Rate for Patients With Renal Cell Carcinoma or Renal Pelvis Carcinoma by Sex, Race, and Time Period—SEER, 1975-1995

Cancer Stage	No. of Cases	5-Year Survival, %							
		White Men		White Women		Black Men		Black Women	
		1975-1985	1986-1995	1975-1985	1986-1995	1975-1985	1986-1995	1975-1985	1986-1995
		Renal Cell Carcinoma							
Total Invasive	31 105	50	61	49	59	50	51	55	58
Localized	14 605	82	89	82	86	82	75	83	84
Regional	6384	54	62	48	59	52	52	49	44
Distant	7890	7	9	5	7	10	7	6	8
Unstaged	2226	35	31	27	21	24	21	33	35
		Renal Pelvis Carcinoma							
Total Invasive	4985	64	58	58	50	57	70	51	48
Localized	2132	85	87	81	70	...	...	...	...
Regional	1907	52	48	48	49	...	...	...	...
Distant	608	10	4	1	4	...	...	...	...
Unstaged	338	49	46	30	43	...	...	...	...

*SEER indicates Surveillance, Epidemiology, and End Results program; ellipses, the number of cases and the number who died were too small for meaningful assessment of survival.

Table 5.2 Classification of renal epithelial neoplasms (Heidelberg classification)

Malignant renal epithelial neoplasms
    Renal carcinoma conventional (clear cell type)
    Papillary renal carcinoma (chromophobic type)
    Chromophobic carcinoma
    Collecting duct carcinoma
    Medullary carcinoma
    Unclassified renal carcinoma

Benign renal epithelial neoplasms
    Adenoma
    Metanephric adenoma
    Oncocytoma

performed to assess pulmonary spread. If indicated by signs and symptoms, other diagnostic procedures may be applied, such as bone scan, brain CT and chest CT [11].

Treatment

Radiological characterization of these tumors (differentiation from angiomyolipoma, oncocytoma, and complicated cysts) is a continuous challenge and an essential prerequisite for appropriate management [16]. The chances of cure by surgery most strongly depend on stage (primarily) and grade (secondarily) of the disease [17] and the presence or absence of micro-vascular invasion [18].

Since its introduction in 1963 by Charles Robson, radical nephrectomy including Gerota's fascia has been considered as the standard treatment for RCC, the objective of the procedure being to excise all tumor with an adequate margin, regardless of size. There is no evidence to favor a specific sur-

gical approach. In selected cases of small (< 4 cm) peripheral lesions, an organ-sparing approach is today advocated. Final evaluation of oncologic efficacy is pending [19, 20]. The number of imperative indications for kidney-sparing surgery has been rather constant during the last years, while the number of elective indications are steeply increasing. The complication rate of this type of surgery has recently become more than acceptable.

Alternative treatment strategies are available now, in particular for smaller tumors (<4 cm), and include open or laparoscopic tumorectomy, partial nephrectomy, radiofrequency ablation, and cryotherapy [21, 22]. The two latter minimally invasive procedures have a problem with the assessment of cure, and surgery has to deal with possible multifocality and local recurrence because of incomplete resection [23].

Since small adenocarcinomas of the kidney have the propensity to microscopic vascular invasion and thus metastatic potential, a watchful waiting policy [24] can only be proposed in a highly selected group of patients. Tumors of 3 cm in diameter or smaller can give rise to metastases [25]. On the other hand, a certain number of small solid tumors are benign. A small renal oncocytoma, angiomyolipoma, or metanephric adenoma can often not be recognized prior to surgery. If all suspicious solid tumors were to be treated by radical surgery, a significant number of kidneys without malignancy would be resected. This has been one of the factors in favor of conservative kidney surgery together with a significant increase of incidentally detected small tumors.

The survival of most patients who have progression after imperative conservative surgery is indeed determined by the presence of occult metastatic disease, not recognized at the time of surgery. A retrospective analysis showed a local recurrence rate of 0–10% after nephron-sparing surgery, 2.5–4% after thermoablative interventions, and 2–3% after (radical) nephrectomy [26]. Whether the local recurrences were due to incomplete resection or due to multifocality of the tumor is not clear, but often locally advanced tumors were operated for which a higher risk of local recurrence can be anticipated.

If surgery cannot eradicate all tumor deposits, tumor nephrectomy remains palliative therapy and should be considered in the context of multimodality treatment (e.g., in conjunction with immunotherapy or targeted therapies) [27, 28]. Certain cases, such as bilateral tumors, a solitary tumor-bearing kidney, multifocal lesions, renal insufficiency, or an occasional palliative situation, will require individual decisions.

Adrenalectomy is generally recommended. The sparing of the ipsilateral adrenal gland in the case of a smaller tumor of the lower half of the kidney is currently being evaluated [29]. A formal lymph node dissection is a valuable diagnostic tool (staging); however, therapeutic efficacy is unproven [30, 31]. Cytoreduction and immunotherapy was the treatment of choice for metastatic RCC. Radical nephrectomy and surgery of metastasis is an option in case of solitary metastasis or limited metastatic spread. With the advent of the targeted therapies the place and timing of surgery in metastatic patients needs to be further defined. In 2008 most patients are treated with targeted agents while immunotherapy is restricted to good risk metastatic patients.

Follow-up

Follow-up of patients with RCC after surgical treatment is recommended to detect local recurrence and distant metastases as early as possible to permit additional treatment when indicated and if possible. Such therapy may include resection of pulmonary metastasis or locoregional recurrences; certain cases may also be candidates for immunomodulating therapy. With this in mind, a regular postoperative follow-up of patients with RCC is proposed [32–34].

Prognostic factors and the type of surgical intervention (radical versus partial or nephron-sparing surgery) are relevant in determining the most efficient follow-up regimen. The only established prognostic factor is tumor stage according to the TNM system. After nephron-sparing tumor resection (elective or imperative indication), the possibility of local recurrence necessitates ultrasound or CT control of the remnant kidney.

Conclusion

The incidence of renal cell carcinoma is increasing, and imaging has a very important place in early detection, in diagnosis and staging, as well as in the follow-up. Expert ultrasonography can give a lot of information but still contrast-enhanced CT scan remains the diagnostic tool of choice. MRI will have a place in patients with renal failure, contrast allergy, and for the special indication of invasion of the inferior vena cava.

After nephron-sparing surgery, the follow-up of the ipsilateral and contralateral kidney should be done on a regular basis. Ultrasound would be very useful in these indications but again a contrast-enhanced CT scan at yearly or two-yearly intervals remains standard.

References

1. Murphy WM, Beckwith JB, Farrow GM. Tumors of the kidney. In: Murphy WM, Beckwith JB, Farrow GM, editors. Atlas of tumor pathology. Tumors of the kidney, bladder and related urinary structures. Washington DC: Armed Forces Institute of Pathology; 1994. p. 92–145.
2. McCredie M. Bladder and kidney cancers. Cancer Surv. 1994;19:343–68.
3. Motzer RJ, Matzumdar M, Bacik J, Russo P, Berg WJ, Metz EM. Effect of cytokine therapy on survival for patients with advanced renal cell carcinoma. J Clin Oncol. 2000;18:1928–35.
4. Weiss LM, Gelb AB, Medeiros LJ. Adult renal epithelial neoplasms. Am J Clin Pathol. 1995;103:624–35.
5. Cohen C, McCue PA, Derose PB. Histogenesis of renal cell carcinoma and oncocytoma. An immunohistochemical study. Cancer. 1988;62:1946–51.
6. Fleming S, O'Donnell M. Surgical pathology or renal epithelial neoplasms: recent advantages and current status. Histopathology. 2000;36:195–202.
7. Störkel S, van den Berg E. Morphological classification of renal cancer. World J Urol. 1995;13:153–8.
8. Kovacs G. Molecular differential pathology or renal cell tumors. Histopathology. 1993;22:1–8.
9. Dal Cin P, Polito P, Van den Berghe H. Genetics of renal tumors. Pathologica. 1998;90:101–107.
10. Hughson MD, Johnson LD, Silva FG, Kovacs G. Nonpapillary and papillary cell carcinoma: a cytogenetic and phenotypic study. Mod Pathol. 1993;6: 449–56.
11. Belldegrun A, deKernion JB. Renal tumours. In: Walsh PC, Retik AB, Vaughan ED, Wein AJ, editors. Campbell's urology. Philadelphia: W.B.Saunders. 1998; p. 2283–326.
12. Messing EM, Young TB, Hunt VB, Emoto SE, Wehbie JM. The significance of asymptomatic microhematuria in men 50 or more years old: Findings of a homescreening study using urinary dipsticks. J Urol. 1987;137:919–922.
13. Sufrin G, Chasan S, Golio A, Murphy GP. Paraneoplastic and serologic syndromes of renal adenocarcinoma. Semin Urol. 1989;7:158–171.
14. Bechtold RE, Zagoria RJ. Imaging approach to staging of renal cell carcinoma. Urol Clin N Am. 1997;24:507–22.

15. Newhouse JH. The radiologic evaluation of the patient with renal cancer. Urol Clin N Am. 1993;20:231–46.

16. Barbaric ZL. Imaging work-up: is it renal carcinoma and is it operable? Semin Urol Oncol. 1996;14:196–202.

17. Giberti C, Oneto F, Martorana G, Rovida S, Carmignani G. Radical nephrectomy for renal cell carcinoma: long-term results and prognostic factors on a series of 328 cases. Eur Urol. 1997;31:40–8.

18. Van Poppel H, Vandendriessche H, Boel K, Mertens V, Goethuys H, Haustermans K, et al. Microscopic vascular invasion is the most relevant prognosticator after radical nephrectomy for clinically nonmetastatic renal cell carcinoma. J Urol. 1997;158:45–9.

19. Novick AC. Nephron-sparing surgery for renal cell carcinoma. Br J Urol. 1998;82:321–4.

20. Van Poppel H, Bamelis B, Oyen R, Baert L. Partial nephrectomy for renal cell carcinoma can achieve long-term tumor control. J Urol. 1998;160:674–8.

21. Uzzo RG, Novick AC. Nephron-sparing surgery for renal tumors: indication, techniques and outcomes. J Urol. 2001;166: 6–11.

22. Pavlovich CP, Walther MM, Choyke PL, Pautler SE, Chang R, Linehan WM, et al. Percutaneous radio frequency ablation of small renal tumors: initial results. J Urol. 2002;167:10–5.

23. Mouraviev V, Joniau S, Polascik TJ, Van Poppel H. Current status of minimally invasive ablative techniques in the treatment of small renal tumours. Eur Urol. 2007;51:328–36.

24. Bosniak MA. Observation of small incidentally detected renal masses. Semin Urol Oncol. Nov 1995;13:267–72.

25. Bosniak MA. Radical nephrectomy for renal cell carcinoma 30mm. or less: long-term follow results. J Urol. 1996;155: 1196–9.

26. Lohr M, Rohde D. Recurrent disease in renal cell carcinoma. "Local recurrence" after kidney-sparing and radical resection. Urologe A. 2005;44(4):358–68.

27. Figlin RA. Renal cell carcinoma: management of advanced disease. J Urol. 1999;161:381–7.

28. Mickisch GH, Garin A, Van Poppel H, de Prijck L, Sylvester R. Radical nephrectomy plus interferon-alpha based immunotherapy compared with interferon-alpha alone in metastatic renal cell carcinoma: a randomized trial. Lancet. 2001;358: 966–70.

29. Wunderlich H, Schlichter A, Reichelt O, Zermann DH, Janitzky V, Kosmehl H, Schubert J. Real indications for adrenalectomy in renal cell carcinoma. Eur Urol. 1999; 35;272–6.

30. Schafhauser W, Ebert A, Brod J, Petsch S, Schrott KM. Lymph node involvement in renal cell carcinoma and survival chance by systematic lymphadenectomy. Anticancer Res. 1999;19: 1573–8.

31. Marshall FF, Steinberg GD, Pound CR, Partin AW. Radical surgery for renal-cell carcinoma: caval neoplastic excision, adrenalectomy, lymphadenectomy, adjacent organ resection. World J Urol. 1995;13:159–62.

32. Sandock DS, Seftel AD, Resnick MI. A new protocol for the follow up of renal cell carcinoma based on pathological stage. J Urol. 1994;154:28–31.

33. Hafez KS, Novick AC, Campbell SC. Patterns of tumour recurrence and guidelines for follow up after nephron sparing surgery for sporadic renal cell carcinoma. J Urol. 1997;157: 2067–70.

34. Levy DA, Slaton JW, Swanson DA, Dinney CP. Stage specific guidelines for surveillance after radical nephrectomy for local renal carcinoma. J Urol. 1998;159:1163–7.

Chapter 6

Renal Cell Carcinoma: Conventional Imaging Techniques

B.C. Lucey and C. Ingui

Introduction

The investigation of renal cell carcinoma (RCC) is best performed using cross-sectional imaging, either CT or MRI. Sonography has a role in the diagnosis, however, IVU and plain radiographs are of limited value in the investigation of RCC and the role of IVU is decreasing all the time.

Plain Radiography

A plain radiograph (or KUB) may be obtained in the evaluation of patients presenting with abdominal pain or hematuria. Plain radiographs have an extremely low sensitivity for detecting RCC and are useful in very few cases. Extremely large renal masses may escape detection until they cause symptoms related to compression on adjacent structures. In such cases, the mass may occasionally be identified as a soft tissue density on the plain radiograph. Alternatively, the mass may displace the bowel resulting in a paucity of bowel gas in the expected area of the bowel. Such a finding should prompt further evaluation with cross-sectional imaging. Calcification of a mass seen on a plain radiograph always warrants further evaluation. Although calcification occurs in only approximately 1% of renal cysts [1], renal cysts are so common that calcification is not uncommonly identified. The distinction is important as calcification may occur in 8–18% of RCC [1–4]. It can be difficult to differentiate benign from malignant calcification on plain radiographs alone. The morphology of the calcification does not help as calcification in a RCC may be linear, punctuate, or lobular. Calcification in renal cysts is most commonly linear, however, may also be punctuate or even appear as a conglomerate mass [1, 4]. The location of the calcification

within the mass is a better indicator as to the underlying pathology [1]. Calcification within cysts tends to be peripheral but central calcification within a mass is an indicator of malignancy, with approximately 85% of masses with central calcification seen on plain radiography proving to be malignant [1]. When peripheral calcification is detected, this poses a greater problem as up to 20% of masses with peripheral calcification may yet prove to be malignant [2, 4]. Therefore, given the degree of uncertainty surrounding the nature of calcification within a renal mass, cross-sectional imaging of most masses demonstrating calcification is advisable.

A plain radiograph may also show evidence of metastatic disease. By this time, the disease is by definition well advanced. Common locations for metastatic disease from RCC are the bones. The vertebrae, imaged ribs, and pelvis should be evaluated for evidence of usually expansile, lytic lesions. The lung bases are also imaged on a KUB and these should be evaluated for evidence of metastatic disease. RCC metastases to the lungs tend to be large well-defined masses. A pleural effusion may be the only clue to the presence of metastatic disease that is not on the imaged portion of the lung.

Intravenous Urogram

The IVU is rapidly fading out as an imaging modality for any indication. This is particularly so in the investigation of RCC. The abnormalities in an IVU caused by a RCC may be divided into contour abnormalities, contrast abnormalities, and collecting system abnormalities.

RCC may distort the renal outline. This is best seen on the nephrographic phase of the IVU. Such a contour deformity presents a diagnostic dilemma, however, as simple renal cysts may have a similar appearance. It is not possible to characterize the deforming lesion as solid or cystic without further imaging. To obtain maximum sensitivity to identify such contour-deforming masses, multiple tomograms should

B.C. Lucey (✉)
Boston Medical Center and Boston University, 88 East Newton Street, Atrium 2, Boston, MA 02118, USA, brian.lucey@bmc.org

J.J.M.C.H. de la Rosette et al. (eds.), *Imaging in Oncological Urology*,
DOI 10.1007/978-1-84628-759-6_6, © Springer-Verlag London Limited 2009

be obtained at different levels, as a conventional radiograph may not appreciate a mass projecting anterior or posterior to the kidney [5, 6]. A large renal mass may alter the axis of the kidney, however, there is such variety in the normal renal outline that this finding is of limited value.

A large RCC may result in occlusion of the renal vein. This may result from tumor growth into the vessel. This may be detected by a delayed nephrogram or even a lack of excretion of contrast from the kidney. Other causes of these findings should be excluded before attributing these to RCC; however, these findings should prompt further evaluation with cross-sectional imaging. A filling defect within the nephrogram may also be seen in RCC. This is seen in cases where the tumor is less vascular than the normal cortex. Occasionally, a defect in the nephrogram may be seen in large RCC with a necrotic center.

RCC may distort the collecting system on the excretory images of the IVU. Although transitional cell carcinoma more commonly produces filling defects within the collecting system itself, RCC produces distortion, stretching, and obstruction of the collecting system. These findings are more frequently seen in masses that are located centrally within the kidney rather than masses that cause renal outline distortion. Displacement and stretching of the calyces or infundibula may also be caused by cysts and as such, too much should not be read into this finding on IVU alone. Cysts, however, will not demonstrate local invasion, and the presence of irregularity within the calyceal wall or a filling defect within the calyx represents malignancy. Tumor may also result in obstruction of a calyx or infundibulum. Ureteric obstruction with hydronephrosis may also occur.

Sonography

Renal masses, as with masses elsewhere, may be either benign or malignant. The final diagnosis is made histologically; however, there are imaging features that can suggest the diagnosis on sonography. Benign solid renal tumors include oncocytoma and angiomyolipoma (AML). Multilocular cystic nephroma is a rare benign cystic tumor that often occurs in children. This consists of multiple cysts with fibrous septae surrounded by a dense capsule. This tumor is sonographically indistinguishable from a cystic renal cell carcinoma; however, multiloculated cystic nephroma has a tendency to protrude into the renal collecting system. This finding helps to give an increased pre-test probability that the mass is benign but is not specific enough to obviate surgical resection.

Oncocytoma is a benign tumor of the proximal collecting tubules. As it is benign, it may grow to a large size before coming to clinical attention. Oncocytoma may present with pain or hematuria and are often found incidentally on imaging performed for other purposes. The oncocytoma mass is usually a solid mass that appears homogenous on sonography. The echotexture is commonly hypoechoic compared to the normal renal parenchyma but smaller lesions may be almost isoechoic. The classic description of an oncocytoma contains a central scar that may be either hyperechoic or hypoechoic [7, 8], although identifying a scar is uncommon. The presence or absence of a central scar is insufficient evidence for not removing the mass. Calcification within an oncocytoma has been reported but this appearance is uncommon [9].

In contrast to an oncocytoma, the diagnosis of angiomyolipoma may often be made on sonography. AML is always a benign tumor of the kidney that contains elements of fat, muscle, and vessels in varying proportions. The sonographic appearances vary depending upon the proportions of each element in the mass. Fat-containing AMLs are echogenic on sonography [10]. When identified, the diagnosis may be made with a high degree of confidence. There are isolated reports of fat-containing renal cell carcinomas [11, 12], however, these are rare and AML is a frequent incidental finding. On occasion, the mass is of mixed echogenicity or even hypoechoic [13]. This makes the diagnosis a little less certain particularly if there has been hemorrhage into the mass. A renal mass protocol CT scan is often helpful in clarifying the diagnosis in cases of uncertainty. CT is highly sensitive at detecting fat within a mass [14].

Malignant tumors of the kidney are overwhelmingly renal cell adenocarcinomas. Other rare malignant tumors include sarcomas and Wilms' tumor. Lymphoma and metastases to the kidneys are more common than the latter two categories but are uncommon findings compared to RCC. A majority of renal cell carcinomas (RCC) are detected incidentally on imaging performed for other indications [15]. This includes renal or abdominal sonography or abdominal CT or MR examination.

On sonography, RCC may be hypoechoic (Fig. 6.1), isoechoic, or occasionally hyperechoic (Fig. 6.2) to normal renal parenchyma although the most common echotexture is isoechoic to renal cortex [16, 17]. Usually the mass appears as a well-defined, encapsulated lesion that may have either smooth or irregular margins. RCC may be identified by the contour deformity present when the mass is exophytic (Fig. 6.4). Despite being isoechoic, when the mass is located centrally, even small masses may be identified by interrupting the normal corticomedullary interface. RCC often contains areas of heterogeneity that are not seen in the relatively uniform echotexture of the normal kidney. In a small percentage ($<5\%$) of cases, RCC may be hyperechoic to the normal renal parenchyma. This may be confusing as a benign angiomyolipoma may also have this sonographic appearance

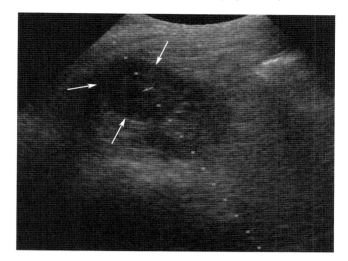

Fig. 6.1 Sonographic image showing large, solid hypoechoic mass on the superior pole of the kidney representing a renal cell carcinoma (*arrows*)

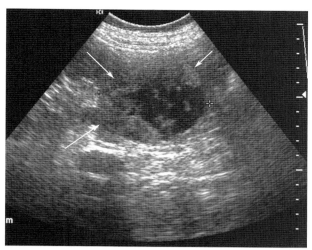

Fig. 6.3 Sonographic image showing large mass on the inferior pole of the left kidney. This mass is solid with large hypoechoic cystic areas within it representing a cystic renal cell carcinoma. Note the thickened irregular wall (*arrows*)

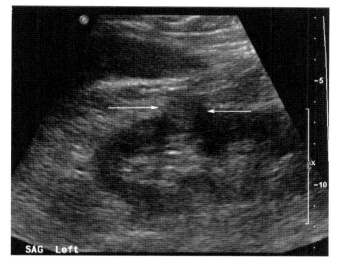

Fig. 6.2 Sonographic image showing small, solid hyperechoic mass on the lateral inter-polar area of the kidney representing a renal cell carcinoma (*arrows*)

the inability of the sound waves to penetrate the calcification. The presence of calcification within the central portion of the mass is of concern for malignancy. Peripheral calcification is less concerning but should always be followed with cross-sectional imaging. Occasionally, RCC may be extremely hypoechoic on sonographic evaluation. This usually indicates a cystic renal neoplasm (Fig. 6.3). Although these may initially be confused with renal cysts, these tumors will show evidence of a thickened nodular wall, often contain septae, and may contain debris. These findings help to distinguish cystic renal neoplasms from cysts. Large RCC may undergo extensive central necrosis and these tumors may also appear hypoechoic. There is seldom difficulty in identifying these masses as malignant as again these have thickened irregular walls. Another sonographic feature that separates benign from malignant masses is color flow within the mass. Cysts, either simple or complex, do not demonstrate flow when interrogated by color Doppler. RCC will demonstrate flow in almost all cases. In a vast majority of cases flow will be seen throughout the mass. In the small number of hypoechoic RCC masquerading as a cyst, flow will be identified in the thickened irregular wall. A renal mass that exhibits blood flow within it requires cross-sectional imaging for more complete evaluation.

A further use for color Doppler in the evaluation of RCC lies in the ability to interrogate the renal veins. Given the propensity for RCC to invade the ipsilateral renal vein, once an RCC is detected on sonography, an attempt should be made to identify tumor thrombus in the renal vein. The incidence of renal vein invasion is reported to be of the order of 5–33% and invasion of the IVC between 5 and 10% of patients with RCC [19] (Fig. 6.5). One study reports values

when the hyperechoic fat is identified. This sonographic appearance of increased reflectivity mimicking fat is more commonly found in smaller masses measuring less than 3 cm in diameter [18]. This is important given the trend toward early detection due to increased imaging for other purposes. The increased echogenicity may be caused by internal hemorrhage in various stages of degradation or alternatively may be caused by calcification within the tumor. Calcification occurs in approximately 10% of RCC [1] and is usually easily distinguished by posterior acoustic shadowing although the presence of extensive calcification may make further evaluation of the mass difficult by sonography given

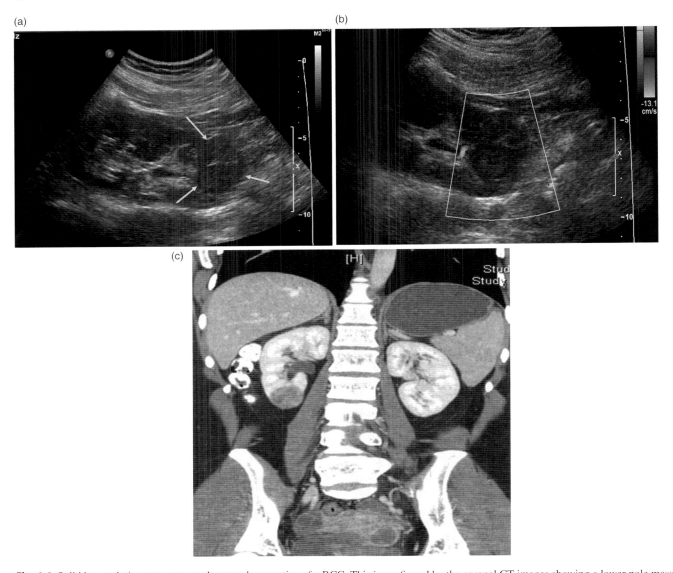

Fig. 6.4 Solid hypoechoic mass seen on ultrasound suggestive of a RCC. This is confirmed by the coronal CT images showing a lower pole mass

of renal vein involvement in 18% with caval extension in 11% [20]. Pathology studies report slightly different results. Hoehn reported renal vein invasion on histology in 46% and IVC invasion in only 4% of patients [21]. The figures for renal vein and IVC invasion are likely to be lower with the improved imaging available today. As RCC is detected earlier with increased and improved imaging, the size at which RCC is being detected is becoming smaller. Smaller RCC has decreased propensity for renal vein invasion. The difficulty with identifying renal vein or IVC invasion lies primarily in identifying the renal vessels themselves. The renal veins may be identified in approximately 81% of patients on the right but only 54% on the left [19]. This clearly tells us that sonography is limited in the evaluation of renal vein invasion.

The added value of color Doppler increases the accuracy of sonography to 87% with a sensitivity of 75%, a specificity of 96%, a positive predictive value of 92%, and a negative predictive value of 85% for detecting renal vein invasion [22]. In one study, color Doppler sonography was 100% accurate in assessing the presence and extent of inferior vena caval involvement by tumor thrombus [22]. The overall accuracy for detecting venous involvement for both the renal veins and the inferior vena cava was 93%, the sensitivity was 81%, and the specificity was 98% [22]. The primary difficulty, however, is identifying the vessel at all rather than identifying tumor within the vessel.

The sonographic appearance of tumor invasion in the renal veins is similar to that of intravenous thrombus

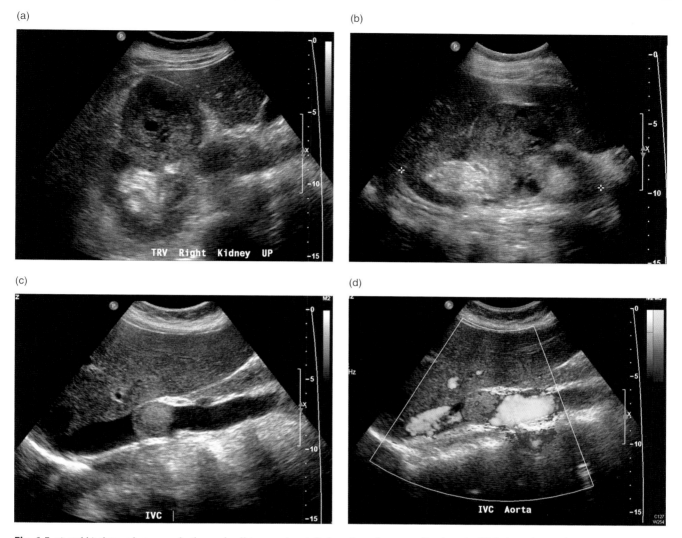

Fig. 6.5 a) and b) show a large exophytic renal cell tumor. c) and d) show thrombus extending into the IVC along the renal vein with an occlusion of the IVC. The flow seen on the power Doppler image suggests that this is tumor thrombus rather than bland thrombus

seen in other veins, most commonly the veins of the lower extremities. Intravenous thrombus may appear as a hyperechoic focus within the renal vein although this finding is not particularly sensitive. The other findings that may suggest thrombus in the lower extremities are not applicable to the renal veins. These include augmentation and compression techniques that increase the sensitivity for detecting thrombus. As the RCC spreads into the renal vein, it promotes intravascular coagulation that may in turn produce more thrombus within the renal vein. The use of color Doppler may be helpful in distinguishing this bland thrombus from tumor thrombus. Tumor thrombus may demonstrate color flow within the thrombus itself. Bland thrombus will not have flow within it. It is frequently extremely difficult to document color flow within tumor thrombus from RCC invasion into the renal vein. This is because not only may

the renal veins not be seen using sonography, but also the quantity of thrombus may be small and it may be difficult to appreciate true color flow separate from flow in the adjacent pulsating artery or surrounding vessels or even flow from patient related movement or respiration. At the point at which color flow may be clearly identified within the thrombus, it is almost always apparent that there is renal vein invasion from the RCC. Renal vein invasion may be clearly identified with a high degree of both sensitivity and specificity using either CT or MR technology. Therefore, even with color Doppler, sonography is less sensitive and less specific than either CT or MR and certainly takes longer to perform than CT and almost as long as MR. This raises another issue. Despite attempting to document renal vein invasion on imaging, it is far from clear if renal vein invasion by RCC is of any clinical significance. There have been multiple recent reports, mostly in the surgical or urological literature, that suggest that the presence or absence of renal vein or even IVC invasion does not significantly impact long-term survival in patients with RCC [23–25]. With the exception of IVC involvement above the level of the diaphragm, renal vein or IVC invasion by RCC is less important than the local staging of the tumor.

The sensitivity for sonography in detecting RCC varies widely depending on the size of the mass, the skills of the sonographer, and the quality of the technology used. The true sensitivity lies between that of IVP and CT [26, 27] or MRI. Sonography has been reported to identify 26% of masses <1 cm in size, 60% of masses between 1 and 2 cm in size, and 82% of masses between 2 and 3 cm in size [28–30]. The value of sonography in characterizing renal masses is the ability to differentiate between solid and cystic masses. This is useful for characterizing masses as simple or complex cysts but is poor at differentiating between various solid masses. In addition to the benign and malignant solid renal masses already discussed, other conditions may also appear as solid renal masses. These include inflammatory conditions such as focal pyelonephritis, abscess, xanthogranulomatous pyelonephritis, hematoma, renal infarct, and pseudotumor represented by a prominent column of Bertin. Given the poor specificity of sonography, CT or MR evaluation is required for characterization of renal masses identified on sonography.

Cystic renal cell carcinoma is more difficult to detect. A vast majority of cystic renal masses are benign cysts, either simple or complex and a majority of malignant renal masses are solid. This creates concern at the possibility of mis-characterizing a malignant cystic mass as benign. Most cystic RCC appear as complex cysts with thick septations, thick irregular walls, often heterogeneous, and may contain calcification. A majority of cystic RCC is a unilocular cystic mass but up to 30% may be multiloculated masses. In these cases, distinguishing the cystic RCC from multiloculated cystic nephroma is difficult and the mass needs to be surgically excised regardless. A solid vascular nodule in the wall of a cyst is a diagnostic feature of cystic RCC.

Sonography may be used for both the detection of RCC and occasionally for staging. As far as staging is concerned, if a renal mass suspicious for RCC is identified on sonography, an attempt should be made to stage the tumor as accurately as possible. The kidney should be evaluated to locate a possible second tumor. If found, this may indicate that the masses may represent renal metastases from an unknown primary tumor rather than represent a primary RCC although multiple RCC may occur particularly in patients with von Hippel–Lindau disease. Local extension into the perinephric fat is extremely difficult to identify with certainty on sonography unless gross. Tumor extension into the ipsilateral renal vein and inferior vena cava should be looked for and when present may be identified on sonography. Venous extension of RCC occurs in up to 30% of cases and extension into the inferior vena cava is reported in approximately 5% of cases [31, 32]. These figures are likely to decrease as more and more RCC are detected earlier as incidental masses. Local lymph node spread may occasionally be identified although this also may be difficult on sonography and not identifying lymphadenopathy does not in any way exclude the possibility and CT or MR is required for complete evaluation for lymphadenopathy, particularly in the retroperitoneum. Liver metastases may also be identified on sonography when present. Direct invasion of the liver by a right-sided RCC is uncommon.

Intraoperative Sonography

As we have seen, sonography is extremely limited in the evaluation of RCC. One area in which sonography may continue to be useful is in the intraoperative assessment of RCC. As nephrectomy becomes less common in the management of RCC, partial nephrectomy is becoming more so. Laparoscopic partial nephrectomy is now the management of choice for patients with RCC that does not involve both poles of the kidney or the renal sinus. For patients unfit for laparoscopic partial nephrectomy, radiofrequency ablation is an alternative. When performing laparoscopic surgery, identification of the branches of the renal arteries and veins is necessary and definition of the tumor margin is of paramount importance. The vessels require identification to avoid inadvertent transaction during laparoscopic procedures. This is best performed by preoperative CT or MR examination. Delineation of the tumor margin, however, is less exact by preoperative imaging modalities. At surgery, ideally a 5 mm rim of normal renal parenchyma is removed in an attempt to reduce the possibility of tumor recurrence. When performing laparoscopic partial nephrectomy, on occasion, it can be difficult to clearly identify the tumor margin and hence difficult to ensure a 5 mm margin of normal renal parenchyma. The use of sonography in the operating room is of value in identifying the tumor margins and this allows the surgeon to accurately perform a partial nephrectomy and ensuring an acceptable resection margin. In addition, intraoperative sonography (IOUS) may help to identify the relationship of the tumor to small vessels and the renal hilum when appropriate. IOUS requires special transducers developed specifically for the purpose. These transducers are small and may easily pass through the laparoscopy port sites. As the transducers are placed directly onto the kidney, high-frequency transducers are required. These are in the 10–13 mHz range.

Transabdominal sonographic transducers are generally in the 2–5 mHz range. By using such high-frequency transducers, the image quality and special resolution are excellent, and differentiation between tumor and normal renal parenchyma may be possible. No gel is required for IOUS as the tissue itself produces sufficient liquid to permit excellent contact. Normal saline may be used to create improved contact should this be required. IOUS is being used with increasing frequency for patients undergoing hand-assisted laparoscopic nephrectomy or partial nephrectomy [33]. It is also of benefit for the intraoperative identification of tumor thrombus extending into the renal vein or IVC [34, 35].

Sonographic Contrast Agents

There has been recent interest in the use of contrast agents for sonography. This is fundamentally an attempt to make up for the deficiencies of grey-scale sonography in general and in the kidney, used primarily for the detection of RCC. There is little doubt that the addition of sonographic contrast agents will improve detection and characterization of renal masses. RCC are, for the most part, vascular tumors and anything that increases the conspicuity of the supplying vessels should help with detection. One report comparing grey-scale sonography to contrast-enhanced sonography [36] found that anechoic areas within the tumor and a pseudo-capsule were seen in 87 and 77% of the RCC on the contrast-enhanced exam, whereas these features were seen in only 53 and 17% of the cases on the grey-scale sonography, respectively. The diagnostic sensitivity, specificity, and accuracy for RCC with contrast were 97, 93, and 95%, respectively. However, those for RCC using grey-scale sonography were 70, 86, and 78%, respectively. A similar study [37] identified the presence of a pseudo-capsule using grey-scale sonography in 3 of 14 RCC yielding a sensitivity of 21%. Sonographic contrast-enhanced harmonic imaging revealed the presence of a pseudo-capsule in 12 of 14 RCC yielding a sensitivity of 85.7%. Although these findings suggest that there is benefit to contrast-enhanced sonography for the detection and characterizing of RCC, to date, no large study has compared contrast-enhanced sonography to state-of-the-art CT or MR for the detection and characterizing of renal masses.

Summary

In summary, plain film has little value in the detection of RCC. The use of IVU has dramatically decreased and, in most major centers, is no longer performed for evaluation of hematuria. It is a limited method of investigation that will soon disappear altogether. Sonography will always have a role in the detection of incidental RCC despite having a limited role in characterizing renal masses. Although the use of color Doppler sonography and contrast-enhanced sonography does improve the detection and characterization of renal masses, at present, renal mass protocol CT or MR is required for complete evaluation of renal masses that are identified on sonography.

References

1. Daniel WW, Hartman GW, Witten DM, Farrow GM, Kelalis PP. Calcified renal masses: a review of 10 years experience at the Mayo Clinic. Radiology. 1972;103:503–8.
2. Kikkawa K, Lasser EC. "Ring-like" or "rim-like" calcification in renal cell carcinoma. AJR. 1969;107:737–42.
3. Phillips TL, Chin FG, Palubinskas AJ. Calcification in renal masses: an eleven-year survey. Radiology. 1963;80:786–94.
4. Sniderman KW, Krieger JN, Seligson GR, Sos TA. The radiologic and clinical aspects of calcified hypernephroma. Radiology. 1979;131:31–5.
5. Kass DA, Hricak H, Davidson AJ. Renal malignancies with normal excretory urograms. AJR. 1983;141:731–4.
6. Demos TC, Schiffer M, Love L, Waters WB, Moncada R. Normal excretory urograms in patients with primary kidney neoplasms. Urol Radiol. 1985;7:75–9.
7. Goiney RC, Goldenberg L, Cooperberg PL, Charboneau JW, Rosenfield AT, Russin LD, et al. Renal oncocytoma: sonographic analysis of 14 cases. AJR. 1984;143:1001–4.
8. Wasserman NF, Ewing SL. Calcified renal oncocytoma. AJR. 1983;141:747–9.
9. Williamson B. Benign neoplasms of the renal parenchyma. In: Pollack HM, editor. Clinical urography. Philadelphia: WB Saunders; 1990. p. 1199.
10. Hartman DS, Goldman SM, Friedman AC, Davis CJ, Madewell JE, Sherman JL. Angiomyolipoma: ultrasonic-pathologic correlation. Radiology. 1981;139:451–8.
11. Schuster TG, Ferguson MR, Baker DE, Schaldenbrand JD, Solomon MH. Papillary renal cell carcinoma containing fat without calcification mimicking angiomyolipoma on CT. AJR. 2004;183:1402–4.
12. Hammadeh MY, Thomas K, Philip T, Singh M. Renal cell carcinoma containing fat mimicking angiomyolipoma: demonstration with CT scan and histopathology. Eur Radiology. 1998;8:228–9.
13. Seigel CL, Middleton WM, Teefey SA, McClennan BL. Angiomyolipoma and renal cell carcinoma: US differentiation. Radiology. 1996;198:789–93.
14. Kurosaki Y, Tanaka Y, Kuramoto K, Itai Y. Improved CT fat detection in small kidney angiomyolipomas using thin sections and single voxel measurements. J Comput Assist Tomogr. 1993;17:745–8.
15. Lightfoot N, Conlon M, Kreiger N, Bissett R, Desai M, Warde P, et al. Impact of noninvasive imaging on increased incidental detection of renal cell carcinoma. Eur Urol. 2000;37:521–7.
16. Coleman BG, Arger PH, Mulhern CB, Pollack HM, Banner MP, Arenson RL. Grey-scale sonographic spectrum of hypernephromas. Radiology. 1980;137:757–65.
17. Charboneau JW, Hattery RR, Ernst EC, James EM, Williamson B, Hartman GW. Spectrum of sonographic findings in 125 renal masses other than benign simple cyst. AJR. 1983;140:87–94.

18. Forman HP, Middleton WM, Melson GL, McLennan BL. Hyperechoic renal cell carcinoma: increase in detection at US. Radiology. 1993;188:431–4.

19. Hofmann R, Schutz W, Leyh H, Braun J. Sonographic detection of thromboses of the renal veins and vena cava in adenocarcinoma of the kidney. Ultraschall Med. 1985;6:312–5.

20. Schwerk WB, Schwerk WN, Rodeck G. Venous renal tumor extension: a prospective US evaluation. Radiology. 1985;156:491–5.

21. Hoehn W, Hermanek P. Invasion of veins in renal cell carcinoma – frequency, correlation and prognosis. Eur Urol. 1983;9:276–80.

22. Habboub HK, Abu-Yousef MM, Williams RD, See WA, Schweiger GD. Accuracy of color Doppler sonography in assessing venous thrombus extension in renal cell carcinoma. AJR Am J Roentgenol. 1997;168(1):267–71.

23. Kim HL, Zisman A, Han KR, Figlin RA, Belldegrun AS. Prognostic significance of venous thrombus in renal cell carcinoma. Are renal vein and inferior vena cava involvement different? J Urol. 2004;171:596–7.

24. Ficarra V, Righetti R, D'Amico A, Rubilotta E, Novella G, Malossini G, et al. Renal vein and vena cava involvement does not affect prognosis in patients with renal cell carcinoma. Oncology. 2001;61:10–5.

25. Tongaonkar HB, Dandekar NP, Dalal AV, Kulkarni JN, Kamat MR. Renal cell carcinoma extending to the renal vein and inferior vena cava: results of surgical treatment and prognostic factors. J Surg Oncol. 1995;59:94–100.

26. Warshauer DM, McCarthy SM, Street L, Bookbinder MJ, Glickman MG, Richter J, et al. Detection of renal masses: sensitivities and specificities of excretory urography/linear tomography, US and CT. Radiology. 1988;169:363–5.

27. James-Dow CA, Choyke PL, Jennings SB, Linehan WM, Thakore KN, Walther MM. Small (<3 cm) renal masses: detection with CT versus US and pathologic correlation. Radiology. 1996;198:785–8.

28. Amendola MA, Bree RL, Pollack HM, Francis IR, Glazer GM, Jafri SZ, et al. Small renal carcinomas: resolving a diagnostic dilemma. Radiology. 1988;166:637–41.

29. Smith SJ, Bosniak MA, Megibow AJ, Hulnick DH, Horii SC, Raghavendra BN. Renal cell carcinomas: earlier discovery and increased detection. Radiology. 1989;170:699–703.

30. Curry NS, Schabel SI, Betsill WL. Small renal neoplasms: diagnostic imaging, pathologic features and clinical course. Radiology. 1986;158:113–7.

31. Goncharenko V, Gerlock AJ, Kadir S, Turner B. Incidence and distribution of venous extension in 70 hypernephromas. AJR. 1979;133:263–5.

32. Madayag MA, Ambos MA, Lefleur RS, Bosniak MA. Involvement of the inferior vena cava in patients with renal cell carcinoma. Radiology. 1979;133:321–6.

33. Tanaka K, Dobashi M, Yamada Y, Kawabata G, Kamidono S, Hara I. Hand-assisted laparoscopic radical nephrectomy using intraoperative ultrasonography for left renal cell carcinoma involving a level I renal vein tumor thrombus. Int J Urol. 2006;13(2):171–3.

34. Hsu TH, Jeffrey RB Jr, Chon C, Presti JC Jr. Laparoscopic radical nephrectomy incorporating intraoperative ultrasonography for renal cell carcinoma with renal vein tumor thrombus. Urology. 2003;61(6):1246–8.

35. Sundaram CP, Rehman J, Landman J, Oh J. Hand assisted laparoscopic radical nephrectomy for renal cell carcinoma with inferior vena caval thrombus. J Urol. 2002;168(1):176–9.

36. Park BK, Kim SH, Choi HJ. Characterization of renal cell carcinoma using agent detection imaging: comparison with gray-scale US. Korean J Radiol. 2005;6(3):173–8.

37. Ascenti G, Gaeta M, Magno C, Mazziotti S, Blandino A, Melloni D, et al.. Contrast-enhanced second-harmonic sonography in the detection of pseudocapsule in renal cell carcinoma. AJR Am J Roentgenol. 2004;182(6):1525–30.

Chapter 7

Cross-Sectional Imaging of Renal Cell Carcinoma

A.E.T. Jacques and R.H. Reznek

Introduction

Renal cell carcinoma accounts for approximately 3% of all cancer cases [1]. The stage of the disease at presentation is the single most important prognostic factor, as surgery remains the only curative treatment option. Cross-sectional imaging therefore has a vital role in early detection and accurate staging of renal cell carcinoma. A steady increase in the incidence of renal cell carcinoma since the 1970s has been observed [2], which is paralleled by an improved 5-year survival rate [3, 4]. This increase in survival can be attributed in part to the increased detection of small tumors resulting from the recent widespread use of cross-sectional imaging. Prior to the introduction of body computed tomography (CT) in the mid-1970s, 6–13% of renal cell carcinomas were detected incidentally in asymptomatic patients [5, 6], compared with up to 61% since [7, 8]. In addition the proportion of smaller and lower stage tumors at presentation has increased. Prior to 1980, fewer than 6% of renal cell carcinomas were 3 cm or less at diagnosis, compared with 25% currently [6]. This incidence now matches that of earlier autopsy series [9].

Diagnosis

Computed Tomography

In addition to the detection of renal mass lesions, CT plays a principle role in the characterization of these lesions. Space-occupying lesions of the kidney are extremely common in the adult population, the vast majority being simple benign cysts which generally do not pose a diagnostic problem to the radiologist. However, a majority of solid renal space occupying lesions are renal cell carcinomas. Because of this, percutaneous biopsy or needle aspiration of renal masses is not recommended as routine because of problems associated with tumor seeding and high false-negative rates [10–12]. Biopsy is reserved when tumors other than renal cell carcinoma are suspected (metastases, lymphoma). Lesion characterization with CT therefore forms an important role in directing appropriate patient management strategies. The typical appearance of renal cell carcinoma on CT is of a heterogeneous, predominately solid mass which enhances by more than 10 HU following contrast medium administration, and are often larger than 3 cm in diameter (Fig. 7.1). Thick or punctate calcification and areas of necrosis may be present. Renal cell carcinomas are typically hypervascular and prominent collateral vessels are often demonstrated (Fig. 7.2). Evidence of local or distant disease extension may help to confirm the

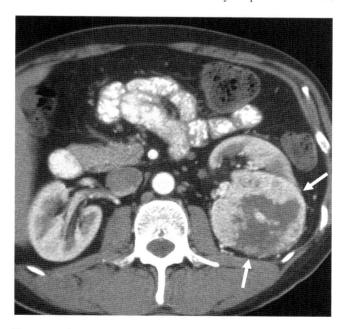

Fig. 7.1 Axial CT scan following administration of intravenous contrast medium showing a well-defined, avidly enhancing mass within the left kidney (*arrows*). There is central low attenuation due to necrosis. The appearances are typical for renal cell carcinoma

A.E.T. Jacques (✉)
Academic Department of Radiology, St Bartholomew's Hospital, West Smithfield, London EC1A 7BE, UK

J.J.M.C.H. de la Rosette et al. (eds.), *Imaging in Oncological Urology*,
DOI 10.1007/978-1-84628-759-6_7, © Springer-Verlag London Limited 2009

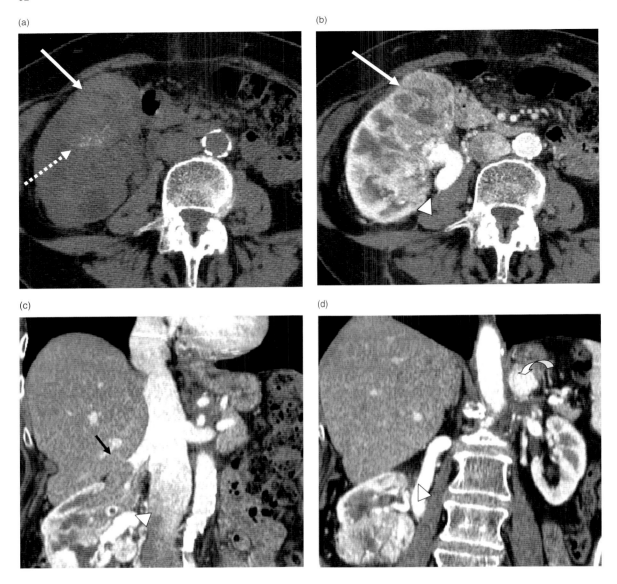

Fig. 7.2 Right renal cell carcinoma; stage T3b M1. (**a**) Axial unenhanced CT scan showing a large, heterogeneous soft tissue mass (*arrow*) arising from the right kidney with areas of calcification (*hashed arrow*) and necrosis. (**b–d**) axial and coronal reformatted images obtained after the administration of intravenous contrast medium showing avid and inhomogeneous enhancement of the tumor. (**c**) Non-enhancing thrombus (*black arrow*) is seen filling the right renal vein and an adjacent second renal vein (arrow head in **b–d**). (**d**) An enhancing mass is seen in the left suprarenal region in keeping with an adrenal metastasis (*curved arrow*)

diagnosis, in particular their propensity to invade the renal vein and inferior vena cava (IVC) (Fig. 7.2). Solid lesions particularly when small may be homogeneous and differentiation from solid benign lesions needs to be considered.

CT Characterization of the Small (<3 cm) Renal Mass

Much research has centered on characterizing the small (3 cm or less) renal mass, the detection of which has increased with the widespread use of CT and US. Most renal cell car-

cinomas of this size are predominately solid and homogeneous, measure greater than 20–25 HU, and enhance following contrast medium administration [13, 14]. Once detected, the recommended clinical management of small renal masses has been largely influenced by observations of their relatively slow growth rates and lower propensity to metastasize [3, 12, 13, 15]. Previously in fact, such lesions were labeled benign renal cortical adenomas by some pathologists and were detected incidentally at autopsy. These are in fact histologically indistinguishable from renal cell carcinomas but are of a lower grade and stage with variable patterns of growth [15]. The need to surgically resect all such lesions is debated particularly in the elderly and those with other co-morbid conditions from which the patient may succumb rather than the small renal cell carcinoma. A recognized management pathway has been accepted. First, the solid nature of an incidentally detected renal mass greater than 20–25 HU on CT needs to be confirmed as a significant proportion of these will represent cysts of increased density due to the presence of haemorrhage, debris, or pus within. If not confirmed as a simple cyst on ultrasound (US) repeated thin collimation contrast-enhanced CT is performed. Five millimeter collimation at least should be acquired, although 1.25 or 2.5 mm thin slices can be reconstructed using MDCT techniques. Images are acquired following intravenous administration of iodinated water-soluble contrast medium. Contrast enhancement is recognized as the most sensitive feature in the evaluation of the renal mass and enhancement is achieved when an increase in attenuation of more than 10 HU is observed [13, 14]. In assessing lesions enhancement, comparison must always be made to the unenhanced scan and care should be taken in the placement of the region of interest (ROI) marker. There is currently no agreed increase in Hounsfield unit measurement that can be reliably taken as evidence of enhancement. Previously, with non-helical CT scanners, an increase of 10 HU was taken as enhancement. However, it is currently felt that reconstruction algorithms and beam hardening may lead to greater variations in density measurements with the newer helical scanners [16]. Some authors now recommend the threshold should be increased to between 10 and 20 HU [16] and if a renal mass enhances by this degree, further evaluation should be considered for characterization. Attention should be made to apparent "pseudoenhancement" in renal cysts which may arise secondary to image reconstruction algorithms of modern scanners to adjust for beam hardening artifacts. It may also occur in small (<2 cm) cysts which are completely surrounded by enhancing renal tissue. It is suspected when a cyst appears simply on the unenhanced scan but increases in density by 10–15 HU following contrast administration. These lesions can often be characterized as simple cysts with US.

While most renal cell carcinomas will demonstrate enhancement, caution regarding some hypovascular tumors should be made. In particular, the papillary cell variant of renal cell carcinomas has been shown to demonstrate lower contrast medium enhancement in the corticomedullary phase, compared with conventional (clear cell) renal cell carcinomas [17–19]. In a recent study of 35 cases of papillary renal cell carcinoma, 36% showed no definite enhancement during the corticomedullary (30 s) phase but demonstrated delayed enhancement during the nephrographic (90 s) phase. No definite enhancement was shown by 34.2% in either phase of the scan [20].

The decision to remove those tumors between 2 and 3 cm in size will depend on the age and co-morbidity of the patient with resection reserved for those medically fit and

less than 75 years of age. Smaller lesions (<1.5 cm), which we are increasingly detecting, can be observed in younger patients. It may not always be possible to characterize such small lesions due to partial averaging effects and they are often labeled as "indeterminate." However a large proportion of these will be small simple cysts. Follow-up should be individualized, taking into account history of previous renal tumors, known primary malignancy, family history or predisposing familial syndrome, age, and surgical suitability [21]. Using current multislice CT techniques it may be possible to characterize some of these lesions based on contrast medium enhancement. As with larger lesions if enhancement is demonstrated the lesion may represent a small neoplasm. However, based on the observation of very slow growth rates of renal cell carcinomas of this size, surgical excision is not necessarily indicated and 6 month follow-up is generally advised. If there is no change is size after 1 year then follow-up can be yearly. If the mass increases in size to 2 cm and the patient is a surgical candidate, then resection could be considered [13].

Cystic Renal Mass Lesions

Particular attention always has to be paid to the cystic or partially cystic mass, with features not entirely consistent with a simple cyst. Such features include increased density, the presence of internal septations, wall thickening, nodular projections, calcification, and enhancement. These features make it difficult to exclude a malignant lesion and can be categorized according to the Bosniak cyst classification system [22–24] (Table 7.1). Category I lesions fulfill the criteria for benign simple cysts and need no further follow-up. Category II lesions are benign but have one or two more complex features and include septations (Fig. 7.3a), minimal benign calcification, and hyperdense cysts. Again they do not require further follow-up or imaging. These include hyperdense cysts exhibiting attenuation values greater than water (>20 HU) because of proteinaceous or hemorrhagic contents. They should be well defined, homogeneous, nonenhancing, with no irregularities and less than 3 cm to classify as a category II lesion. In addition at least a quarter of the lesion must extend outside of the kidney so the smoothness and thickness of some of its wall can be evaluated [23]. Hyperattenuating cysts are considered suspicious if they are irregular in contour, inhomogeneous, demonstrated enhancement, or appear solid on US [24]. These lesions may represent small cystic renal cell carcinomas and surgery should be considered. Category III and IV lesions (Fig. 7.3b–d) are those with malignant features and must be removed surgically. Category IV lesions are clearly malignant cystic renal cell carcinomas while category III lesions have some features by which they cannot be distinguished radiologically from

Table 7.1 Radiological features of cystic renal lesions (adapted from [22–24])

Radiological feature	Simple cyst	Benign pattern	Follow-up lesion	Indeterminate lesion with suspicious features	Malignant lesion
	Bosniak I	Bosniak II	Bosniak IIF	Bosniak III	Bosnick IV
Calcification	None	Small amount of thin, linear calcification in wall or septum. No associated soft tissue or enhancement	Thick and nodular calcification with no other suspicious features	Thick, irregular, or punctuate calcification plus any other suspicious features	As in III but with associated enhancing soft tissue, nodularity, or wall thickening
Septations	None	Thin (< 1 mm), smooth septae attached to wall with no thickened elements	Minimally thickened, only just >1 mm, but smooth and no other suspicious features	Thickened (>1 mm), irregular septae. Thickened at insertion point of wall. Associated with solid elements	As in III but also very irregular, numerous, and associated with solid enhancing soft tissue
Wall	Imperceptible. Smooth, well-defined contour	Thin (< 1 mm) with no associated soft tissue nodule or thickening	Smooth focal minimal thickening only	Thickened (>1 mm), irregular or associated with soft tissue nodules	As in III but more extensive
Nodules	None	None	None	Enhancing soft tissue nodules. Soft tissue mass abutting cyst wall	As in III but more extensive
Density of cyst contents	Density of contents <10 HU	Density of contents >20 HU but non-enhancing and <3 cm = benign hyperdense cyst	Hyperdense cyst >3 cm or <3 cm in a kidney with multiple complicated cystic lesions	Irregular contour, poorly defined margin. Inhomogeneous. Enhancing components	As in III

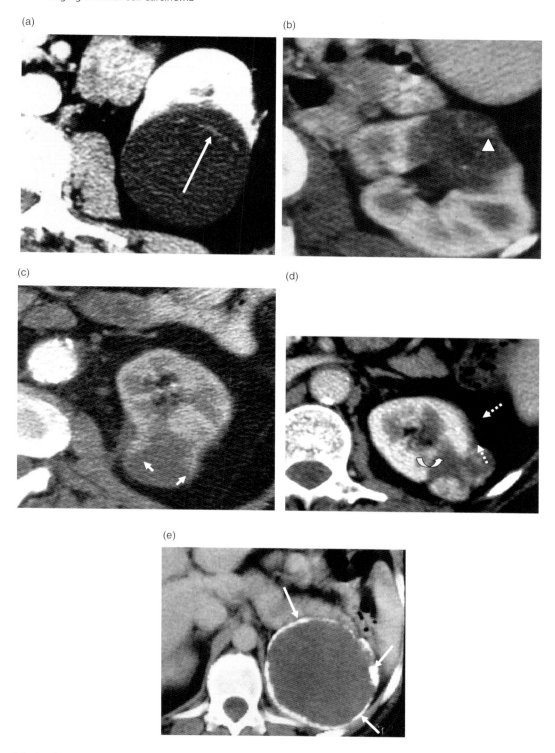

Fig. 7.3 Bosniak classification of cystic renal lesions. Axial CT scans following contrast medium administration in four different patients. (**a**) A well-defined homogeneous cystic lesion with an imperceptible wall is seen arising from the left kidney. It contains a thin (<1 mm) single septation (*long arrow*) with no thickening at its point of attachment, in keeping with a Bosniak II renal cyst. (**b**) A multi-septated cystic lesion is seen arising from the left kidney with septal thickening at the point of attachment to the cyst wall (*arrow head*). This lesion is categorized as a Bosniak III renal cyst and warrants further evaluation. This was a pathologically proven cystic renal cell carcinoma. (**c**) Cystic renal lesion with focal areas of wall thickening (*short arrows*) in keeping with a Bosniak III renal cyst. This lesion was proven to be a complicated benign cyst with hemorrhage. (**d**) Focal enhancing soft tissue nodule (*curved arrow*) within a renal cyst with multiple thickened septations and wall thickening seen also (*dashed arrows*) in keeping with a Bosniak IV cystic lesion. This was found to be a renal cell carcinoma. (**e**) Cystic renal lesion with heavy peripheral calcification (*arrows*). When there are no associated enhancing soft tissue components this lesion is classified as Bosniak IIF. Follow-up with repeat imaging in 3–6 months is recommended

malignant lesions. A proportion will be found to be benign and include multiloculated cysts and chronically infected or hemorrhagic cysts (Fig. 7.3c). More recently another category (IIF) has been added to this classification system and includes benign complicated cysts which require follow-up over time to confirm stability [23]. Features in this group include those with numerous but thin septa, septal, or wall enhancement but no soft tissue component or hyperdense category II lesions which are totally intrarenal or greater than 3 cm [23]. It also includes those with large amounts of calcification but no enhancing soft tissue components (Fig. 7.3e). The risk of malignancy in a Bosniak IIF lesion that is being followed up is approximately 5% [23] compared with 25–100% in a surgical lesion (Bosniak III) [25].It is important for radiologists to give some indication as to the significance of their findings when describing cystic renal lesions. Follow-up at 3–6 month interval for a Bosniak IIF lesion is often recommended in the first instance.

MRI

CT has been traditionally considered by radiologists to be the investigation of choice for the detection and characterization of focal renal lesions, with MRI being reserved for specific problem solving. However, MRI is considered the primary imaging modality in certain groups of patients particularly those with chronic renal insufficiency, those in whom contrast-enhanced CT is contraindicated, and those who require multiple follow-up imaging for surveillance to avoid the burden of repeated CT examinations. This becomes particularly pertinent in patients with known or family history of syndromes associated with renal cell carcinoma such as Von Hipple Lindau syndrome (VHL) and tuberous sclerosis (TS). Given its improved contrast resolution compared with CT, some authors find MRI better for the detection and characterization of the very small (less than 1.5 cm) renal lesions [26]. Again this is important for those with VHL or TS in whom renal cell carcinomas can arise within small simple cysts.

Although the original Bosniak classification of renal cysts is based on CT findings, the same approach can be used when characterizing lesions with MRI (see Table 7.1) [26]. Upgrading of lesions might occur, however, with MRI which may detect more or thicker septa or demonstrate subtle enhancement compared with CT in some cases. A disadvantage of MRI is its inability to depict calcification which is poorly visualized as a signal void. Proteinaceous or hemorrhagic contents of complex cysts are easily demonstrated on MRI, however, owing to their T1 shortening effect resulting in high signal intensity on T1-weighted imaging. Although hemorrhagic foci can be present in renal cell carcinomas,

lack of gadolinium enhancement must be observed to diagnose a hemorrhagic cyst [27].

Small solid renal cell carcinomas have similar signal intensity to surrounding renal parenchyma on T1- and T2-weighted imaging and are less well seen (Fig 7.9). However, they enhance differently to renal parenchyma following administration of gadolinium and become more conspicuous. Gadolinium enhancement of the wall of a necrotic renal cell carcinoma enables differentiation from a complex cyst where the wall does not enhance. MRI sequences combined with fat suppression techniques increase the contrast to noise ratio between tumor and surrounding fat on T2-weighted and gadolinium enhanced T1-weighted images and improves the conspicuity of small renal tumors [27]. Fat suppression also allows differentiation from fat containing benign renal angiomyolipomas.

Staging – CT and MRI

Accurate preoperative staging of renal cell carcinoma is vital, given that surgery is the only potentially curative treatment option. The Robson and TNM systems are commonly used for staging renal cell carcinoma and are summarized in Table 7.2. The presence of metastatic lymphadenopathy, extensive local organ invasion, and distant metastases determines operability. Previously all operable tumors were treated with radical nephrectomy plus ispsilateral adrenalectomy, and the distinction between Robson stages 1 and 2 tumors was less relevant. However, with the introduction of less aggressive treatment options such as nephron sparing surgery or radiofrequency ablation, this distinction is vital for appropriate surgical planning if local recurrence is to be avoided. This distinction is a challenge for the radiologist with increasing frequency of lower stage tumors at presentation.

Tumor extension into the renal vein and IVC is treated with thrombolectomy, but preoperative knowledge of the level of tumor extension will predict surgical approach. Extension of tumor thrombus above the level of the hepatic vein confluence will require a midline abdominal rather than flank incision, and for extension into the supradiaphragmatic IVC, the incision is extended caudally to a midline sternotomy and intraoperative cardiopulmonary bypass maybe required [28]. Direct tumor invasion of the IVC wall carries a worse prognosis which can be improved with caval wall resection and vascular reconstructive surgery [29].

Radiological staging can be achieved with a combination of ultrasound, CT, and magnetic resonance imaging (MRI). CT has been the imaging modality of choice for RCC staging, with the accuracy for each stage approaching 100% and overall accuracy of 91% [30]. Staging accuracies of between

Table 7.2 Renal cell carcinoma staging systems

Robson stage	Description	TNM stage
	Tumor contained within the renal capsule	
I	< 7 cm	T1
	> 7 cm	T2
II	Tumor spread to perinephric fat and/or ipsilateral adrenal gland	T3a
	Venous tumor thrombus	
III-A	Renal vein only	T3b
	Infradiaphragmatic IVC	T3c
	Supradiaphragmatic IVC	T4b
III-B	Regional lymph node metastases	N1–N3
III-C	Venous tumor thrombus and regional lymph node metastases	
IV-A	Direct invasion of adjacent organs outside Gerota's fascia	T4a
IV-B	Distant metastases	M1a–M1d, N4

74 and 96% have been reported with MRI [31–38]. In clinical practice, MRI is used for specific problem solving such as detecting early perinephric invasion and demonstrating venous, including IVC wall, invasion. However with recent advances in CT technology, multidetector row CT (MDCT) can now provide multiplanar imaging, three-dimensional volume-rendered imaging, and angiographic reconstructions of the renal vasculature (Figs. 7.4 and 7.5), thus increasing the staging accuracy of CT [37]. CT will continue to be the most widely used imaging modality of choice for the detection of distant metastases and for the overall staging of renal cell carcinoma. MRI may nevertheless still have an advantage in predicting direct invasion of the inferior caval wall [39].

Perinephric Invasion

The detection of tumor extension beyond the renal capsule and into the perinephric fat can be difficult with CT or MRI. The most reliable sign is the presence of a discrete soft tissue mass measuring at least 1 cm within the perinephric fat and is 98% specific for diagnosing stage 2 disease (Fig. 7.6). However, this sign will be absent in the majority of patients with stage 2 disease and the sensitivity of this finding on CT is only 46% [30]. Early signs on CT which may suggest perinephric extension include, indistinct tumor margin, blurring of the renal outline, thickening of the perirenal fascia and stranding of the perinephric fat (Fig. 7.6). Thickening of the perirenal fascia becomes a more sensitive indicator of extension when focal and contiguous with the tumor [40]. Perinephric fat stranding alone is a poor indicator of stage 2 disease and is seen in up to 50% of those with stage 1 tumor confined to the kidney [30] where it may be attributable to edema, inflammation, or fibrosis (Fig. 7.7). Staging can also be difficult in the presence of perirenal hemorrhage (Fig. 7.8). Using high-resolution MDCT to generate 1 mm reconstructed images in multiple planes, the diagnostic accuracy can be increased to 95% with high positive and negative predictive values of 100 and 93%, respectively [38].

On MRI, similar parameters for diagnosing perinephric fat infiltration exist and the presence of focal extension of tumor is the most reliable finding. Perinephric stranding extending from the renal capsule, of low signal on T1- and T2-weighted sequences, is in keeping with fibrosis rather than direct tumor extension [33]; however, thickened strands (>5 mm) or strands of similar signal intensity to the tumor are suggestive of tumor infiltration. The limitations of detecting extracapsular invasion exist on MRI as well as on CT. MRI, however, has a high negative predictive value for excluding extracapsular invasion of 97–100% [36, 41] which is as helpful for surgical planning (Fig. 7.9).

On MRI a low signal intensity pseudocapsule composing of fibrous tissue and compressed renal parenchyma can be seen surrounding the tumor in up to 59% of stage 1 renal cell carcinomas [41, 42]. T2-weighted imaging is more sensitive for detecting the pseudocapsule which is seen almost exclusively in renal cell carcinoma [42] (Figs. 7.9 and 7.10). It is seen more commonly in tumors less than 4 cm in size and is associated with lower tumor grades. Interruption of the pseudocapsule is suggestive of stage 2 disease while its preservation may help determine suitability for nephron sparing surgery, particularly enucleation.

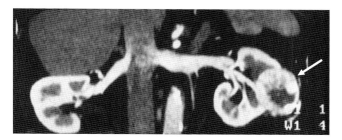

Fig. 7.4 Left renal cell carcinoma; Stage T1a. Coronal reformatted CT scan obtained after the administration of intravenous contrast medium showing a small, enhancing renal cell carcinoma, exophytic to the midpole of the left kidney (*arrow*). The relationship of the tumor to adjacent vessels is clearly demonstrated

(a)   (b)

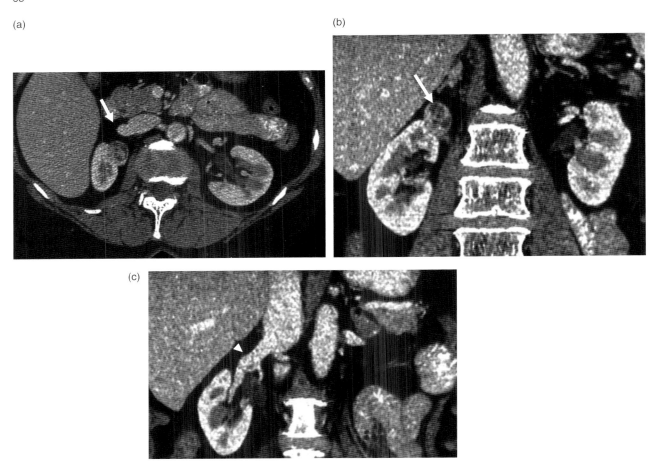

(c)

Fig. 7.5 Right renal cell carcinoma; Stage T1a. Axial (**a**) and (**b,c**) coronal reformatted image CT scans following administration of intravenous contrast medium showing a small, enhancing renal cell carci-noma exophytic to the upper pole of the right kidney (*arrow*). The relationship of the tumor to adjacent vessel (*arrow head*) is clearly demonstrated

(a)   (b)

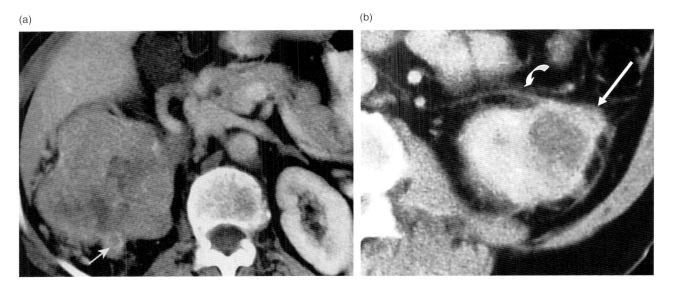

Fig. 7.6 Stage T3a renal cell carcinoma. Axial CT scans following intravenous contrast medium in two different patients (**a, b**) showing large focal renal cell carcinomas with bulging nodular tumor projec-tions (*arrows*) in keeping with perinephric invasion. In (**b**) there is focal thickening of the adjacent Gerota's fascia (*curved arrow*) in keeping with tumor extension

(a) (b)

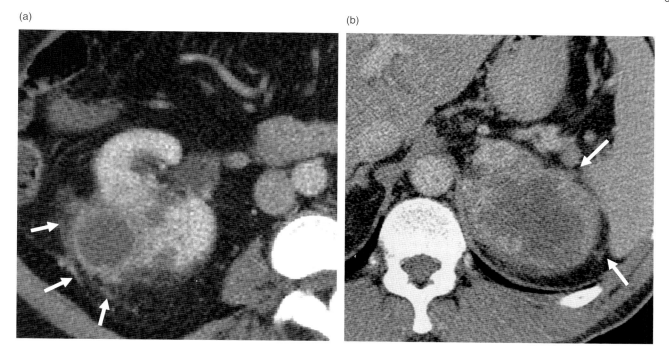

Fig. 7.7 Renal cell carcinoma staging; perinephric stranding versus edema. Axial CT scans following intravenous contrast medium administration in two different patients (**a, b**) showing focal renal cell carcinomas with prominent perinephric stranding (*arrows*). In both cases stage T1 was confirmed pathologically. The perinephric stranding was secondary to edema rather than tumor invasion

(a) (b)

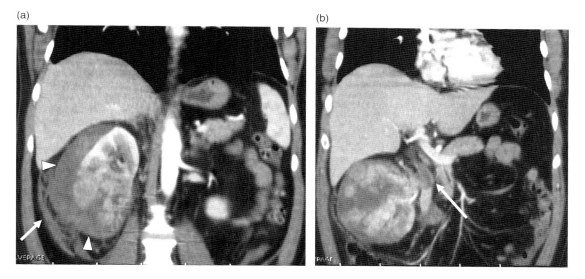

Fig. 7.8 Coronal reformatted CT scans following intravenous contrast medium administration. This patient presented with right flank pain. (**a**) CT scan revealed a large right renal cell carcinoma with extensive perirenal hematoma (*arrow heads*) extending along conal fascia (*arrow*). Local staging of this tumor was difficult in the presence of marked perirenal hematoma and edema. (**b**) Thrombus within the IVC seen as non-enhancing filling defect below the level of the hepatic veins

(a)   (b)

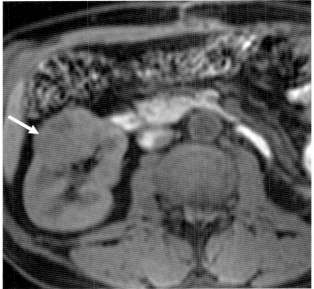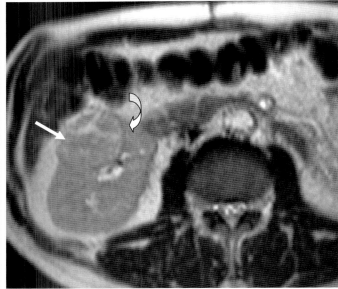

Fig. 7.9 Stage T1a right renal cell carcinoma. (**a**) T1-weighted fat-saturated and (**b**) T2-weighted MRI sequences showing focal renal cell carcinoma arising from the right kidney. No evidence of perinephric invasion and the surrounding fat plane is well visualized. An intact

low signal intensity pseudocapsule (*curved arrow*) is seen on the T2-weighted image (**b**) although it is partially obscured anteriorly by adjacent bowel

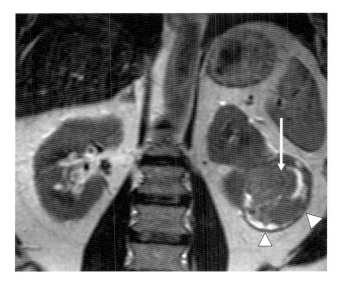

Fig. 7.10 Coronal T2-weighted MRI showing focal left-sided renal cell carcinoma (*arrow*) with an intact low signal intensity pseudocapsule (*arrow heads*) in keeping with stage T1 disease

Collecting System Invasion

Invasion of the collecting system by renal cell carcinoma is not included at present in the criteria for staging by either the Robson or the TNM systems but is important in assessing suitability for nephron sparing surgery. It is seen in up to 14% of cases [43], usually in larger tumors and in the presence

of hematuria. It is also associated with a worse prognosis with an overall 3-year survival rate of 39% reported in one recent study compared with 62% for those without collecting system involvement [43]. The difference in prognosis is more pronounced in those with lower stage tumors (Robson stages 1 and 2). Clearly, partial nephrectomy would not be appropriate for these patients. MRI has been shown to exclude collecting system invasion with a negative predictive value of 100% [41].

Vascular Invasion

Renal cell carcinoma extension has been reported into the renal vein in 10–23% and into the IVC in 5–7% of cases at surgery [28, 29, 44, 45] and is more common in tumors arising from the right kidney. Venous invasion was not seen in tumors <4.5 cm in size in one large series [45] and was seen more commonly in tumors >7 cm compared with those <5 cm in size (61 versus 12%) in another series [46]. The presence of tumor thrombus alone does not influence prognosis once completely resected; however accurate preoperative detection and prediction of the upper level of extension has an important role in surgical planning. Optimum detection of tumor invasion of the renal vein and IVC by CT requires acquisition of thin sections at 60 s after commencing injection of contrast medium, at which time peak opacification

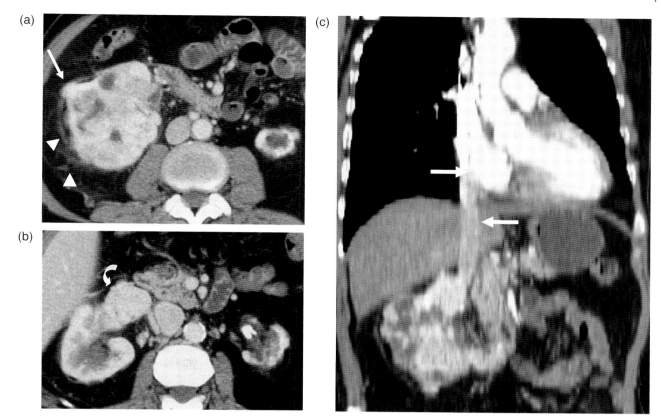

Fig. 7.11 Right renal cell carcinoma with renal vein and IVC thrombus. CT scan following intravenous contrast medium administration. (**a**) Large right renal cell carcinoma with perinephric stranding, thickening of Gerota's fascia (*arrow heads*), and bulging tumor contour (*arrow*) in keeping with perinephric invasion. (**b**) The renal vein (*curved arrow*) appears to be markedly distended and was initially thought to be patent although contained enhancing thrombus as confirmed following resection. (**c**) Coronal reformatted images show IVC thrombus as low density filling defect, extending above the hepatic vein confluence into the right atrium (*arrows*)

of the renal vein and IVC is achieved (Fig. 7.11). Detection of tumor thrombus depends on the presence of a persistent filling defect with or without a peripheral rim of contrast, and this sign is associated with a high positive predictive value [30, 47]. Indirect signs include vessel caliber enlargement and the presence of collateral vessels although both of these appearances can occur as a result of neovasularization and arteriovenous shunting in a hyperdynamic circulation induced by some renal cell carcinomas. The sensitivity and specificity of CT for the detection of venous invasion is approximately 79 and 97%, respectively [30, 45], with difficulties arising in determining the level of extension when near the hepatic vein confluence or in the region of the right atrium (Figs. 7.11c and 7.12).

Because of these limitations, MRI has found a place as the more reliable method with sensitivities and specificities ranging between 82–100 and 87–100%, respectively, for the detection and prediction of level of venous thrombus extension [33, 39, 45, 48–50] (Figs. 7.12–7.14). Thrombus is diagnosed as high to intermediate signal intensity with loss of the normal flow void within the vessel on T1 and T2

spin echo sequences (Figs. 7.13 and 7.14). Images acquired in the coronal plane are particularly useful for determining the upper level of extension (Figs. 7.13 and 7.14). Fast gradient echo sequences enable acquisition in a single breath hold with less motion artifact and can be combined with cardiac gating for detection of intracardiac extension. Flowing blood is fully magnetized throughout the gradient echo sequence and returns a high signal allowing differentiation between low signal bland thrombus or blood clot and intermediate signal tumor thrombus [49]. However, in practice the signal intensity may be variable and the use of intravenous gadolinium to demonstrate enhancement of tumor thrombus versus non-enhancing bland thrombus is more reliable [39] (Fig. 7.15). Tumor thrombus may directly invade the IVC in 25–64% of those with venous extension [29, 39, 49] and is associated with worse prognosis compared with bland thrombus. Hatcher et al. [29] reported 26% 5-year survival in a group with caval wall invasion compared with 69% in those with mobile thrombus, with improved survival rate of 57% following complete resection of the invaded segment of caval wall. Preoperative diagnosis of wall invasion is desirable for

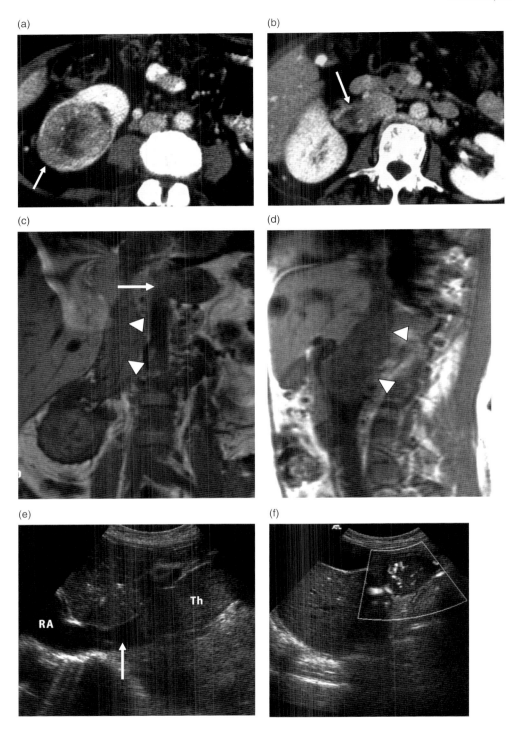

Fig. 7.12 Right renal cell carcinoma with renal vein and IVC invasion. (**a**, **b**) Contrast-enhanced CT scan showing (**a**) well-defined enhancing renal cell carcinoma in the right kidney with (**b**) tumor extension in the renal vein (*arrow*). (**c**) Coronal and (**d**) sagittal T1-weighted MRI images confirming the presence of thrombus extending into the intra-hepatic IVC. (**e**, **f**) Ultrasound images showing echogenic thrombus (Th) within the IVC but not extending into the right atrium (RA). (**f**) Vascularity is seen within the thrombus confirming tumor rather than bland thrombus

(a)

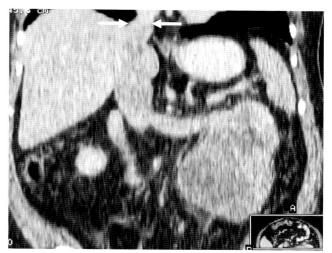

(b)

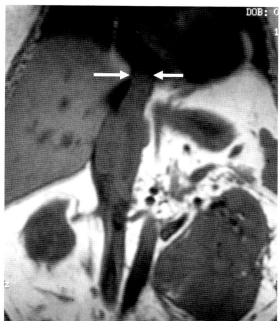

Fig. 7.13 Left renal cell carcinoma with tumor thrombus; CT and MRI correlation. (**a**) Coronal reformatted CT and (**b**) coronal T1-weighted MRI both show a large left renal cell carcinoma and tumor thrombus within the IVC. The upper level of extension of thrombus within the IVC is visualized (*arrows*) which is above the hepatic vein confluence but not into the right atrium

(a)

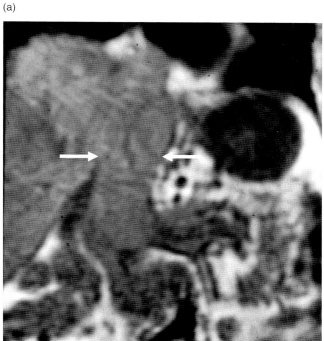

(b)

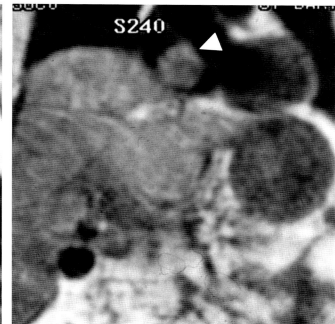

Fig. 7.14 IVC thrombus from renal cell carcinoma. (**a, b**) Coronal T1-weighted MRI showing the IVC expanded by intermediate signal intensity thrombus (*arrows*). The thrombus extends above the level of the hepatic vein confluence and is seen within the right atrium (*arrow head*)

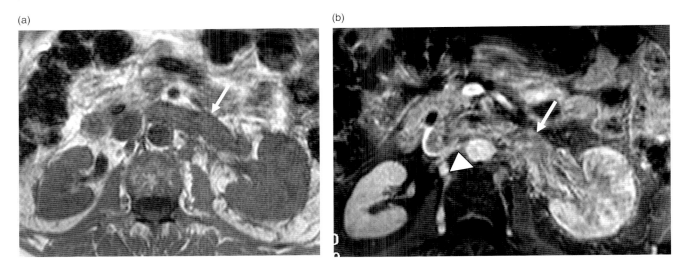

Fig. 7.15 Tumor thrombus. Axial (**a**) T1-weighted and (**b**) T1 fat-saturated images post-gadolinium administration. The left renal vein is expanded by thrombus (*arrows*) which extends into the IVC (*arrow*

head). The thrombus avidly enhances following contrast administration, confirming tumor rather than bland thrombus

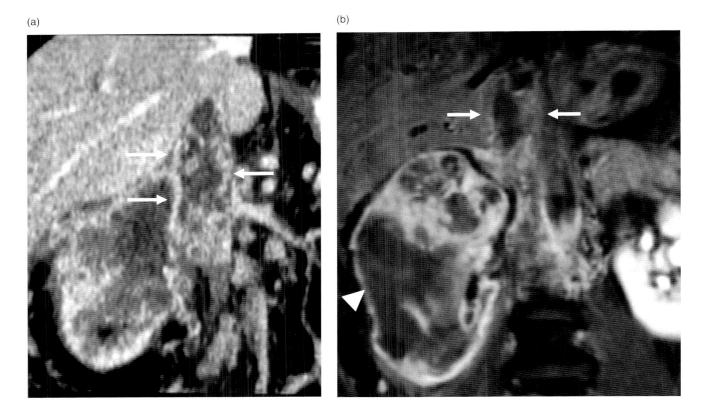

Fig. 7.16 IVC tumor thrombus (two different patients). (**a**) Coronal reformatted CT following intravenous contrast medium administration and (**b**) coronal post-contrast-enhanced T1-weighted fat-saturated MRI showing enhancing tumor thrombus within the IVC. Both CT and MRI

demonstrate enhancement of the IVC wall (*arrows*) in keeping with wall invasion by tumor thrombus. Large right renal cell carcinoma (*arrow head*) in (**b**)

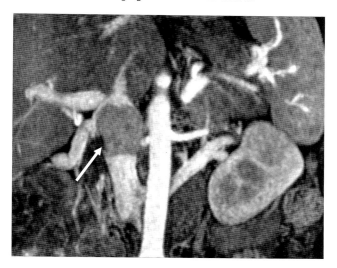

Fig. 7.17 Multidetector row CT images following intravenous contrast medium administration. Images are reformatted in a coronal plane to provide angiographic images. The arterial and venous anatomy is well demonstrated and there is non-enhancing thrombus within the IVC (*arrow*) at the level of the hepatic venous confluence

the surgeon as removal may require vascular reconstruction or be complicated by higher rates of bleeding (Fig. 7.16). Wall invasion is suggested on MRI where there is loss of clarity of the low signal intensity vessel wall, thickening, or altered signal intensity of the wall. It is more confidently diagnosed in the presence of a direct breach of the vessel wall with enhancing tumor seen on either side. Overall the accuracy for wall invasion reaches 92–94% [39, 49], with 100% sensitivity and 89% specificity reported in one study [39].

Using MDCT, 1 mm thin slices can be acquired and reformatted into maximum intensity projections allowing assessment of arterial and venous anatomy. Images can be reformatted longitudinally along the line of the vessel with improved depiction of vascular anatomy (Fig. 7.17). Using this technique, accuracy rates of up to 100% for the detection and localization of venous thrombus have been reported [51].

Lymph Nodes

Lymph node metastases in patients with renal cell carcinoma indicate worse prognosis and are associated with an increased incidence of distant metastases and local recurrence. At present size remains the main criterion for determining lymph node involvement, with short axis diameter of greater than 1 cm considered abnormal. CT is well placed to demonstrate local and distant nodal groups and contrast enhancement is advised to differentiate large collateral vessels from nodes. The limitations of using size criteria are well recognized, with nodes greater than 1 cm found to contain normal or hyperplastic lymphoid tissue in up to 43% of cases [29, 30, 32]. The incidence of enlarged reactive locoregional nodes is increased in the presence of tumor necrosis and venous invasion [52]. Conversely micrometastases within normal-sized lymph nodes will result in false-negative rates of about 4% [52]. Suspicious features of normal-sized nodes include a round rather than oval shape, loss of the normal fatty hilum, and contrast enhancement similar to the primary tumor. However, these features would be more likely in the presence of nearly or completely replaced nodes rather than micrometastases. Overall, using a size threshold of 1 cm, the sensitivity and specificity for diagnosing lymph node involvement have been reported as 83 and 88%, respectively [30].

The same limitations of using size criteria to define abnormality apply to MRI. However, recent developments in lymph node-specific contrast agents show promising results in differentiating metastatic nodes irrespective of size. Ultra-supramagnetic iron oxide particles (USPIOs) are administered intravenously as a suspension of tiny iron oxide nanoparticles which are taken up by normal reticuloendothelial tissue. They induce a magnetic susceptibility effect on MRI, most marked on T2* sequences and which results in signal dropout in tissues which have taken up the agent. On precontrast T2* sequences, normal or hyperplastic reactive nodes are of high signal intensity and subsequently lose signal as they take up the agent. Nodes in which the normal macrophages are replaced by tumor will remain of high signal intensity either uniformly if completely replaced or heterogeneously if partially involved. Data on the use of USPIOs for cancers elsewhere in the body have been reported [53, 54] and show significantly higher sensitivity for the detection of nodal metastases compared with conventional MRI.

Stage IV Disease

Local Organ Invasion

Detection of local and distant organ involvement (stage IV) is crucial to the staging of renal cell carcinoma and for treatment planning. The presence of extensive local organ invasion or widespread metastases will usually preclude surgery and other treatment options such as interferon or interleukin-2 therapies will be considered. Locally invasive stage IV disease represents direct tumor invasion through Gerota's fasica and into adjacent structures such as erector spinae and psoas muscles, liver, tail of pancreas, spleen, and diaphragm (Fig. 7.18). The most reliable signs of organ invasion are

(a)

(b)

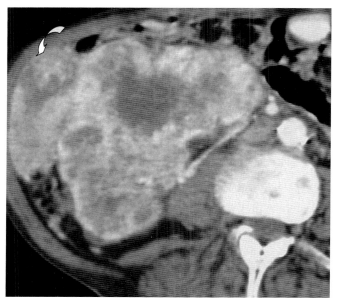
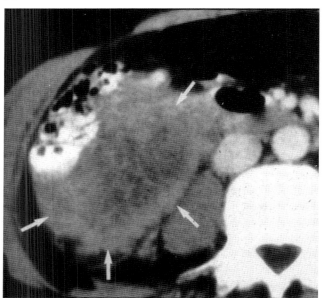

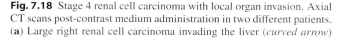

Fig. 7.18 Stage 4 renal cell carcinoma with local organ invasion. Axial CT scans post-contrast medium administration in two different patients. (**a**) Large right renal cell carcinoma invading the liver (*curved arrow*) and (**b**) local perinephric invasion and invasion of the serosal surface of adjacent bowel loops (*arrows*)

either enlargement or change in density of the affected organ or both. Obliteration of the fat plane between tumor and adjacent organ is not a reliable sign and is reported in 15% of those without invasion [30]. Multiplanar imaging with MDCT improves visualization of adjacent organ invasion, with accuracy up to 100% reported [51].

On MRI accuracy rates of 97–100% for detection of local organ invasion have been reported [33] although the validity of specific radiological signs is difficult to evaluate as these patients are usually excluded from surgery. As on CT, direct visualization of tumor within adjacent organs is the most reliable sign, and the excellent contrast resolution and multiplanar imaging capabilities of MRI make it useful for assessing local organ invasion.

Distant Metastases

Up to 30% of patients have distant metastases present at the time of diagnosis, the most frequent sites being lung, bone, liver, and brain [2]. Early detection of metastases is important for predicting prognosis, which remains poor with a 2-year survival rate of 10–20% for those presenting with metastatic disease. Regional lymph node involvement at presentation is a strong predictor of disease dissemination and when present, distant metastatic disease is present in up to 93% according to autopsy data [55]. In selected patients, chemoreductive nephrectomy and metastasectomy is being considered

for those with limited metastases and is being performed either alone or in conjunction with systemic immunotherapy. Survival rates improved by up to 50% have been reported [56, 57].

CT is the primary imaging tool for the detection of distant metastases and has the advantage over MRI of being able to image a large volume of the patient in a short time. It is therefore ideal for the detection of distant metastases particularly to the lungs, liver, and lymph nodes. MRI is usually reserved for specific problem solving such as adrenal and liver lesion characterization and spine and brain imaging as dictated by patient symptoms. The diagnosis of metastases at specific sites on CT and MRI will now be considered.

Lung

Pulmonary metastases are the most frequent site of distant disease seen in up to 61% of patients who subsequently develop metastases following nephrectomy for initially isolated renal cell carcinoma [58–60]. In an autopsy series of 554 patients with clinically unrecognized renal cell carcinoma, 21% had evidence of metastatic spread, with 74% of these having lung metastases [55]. Pulmonary and mediastinal metastases are frequently asymptomatic and detection is best achieved with CT. The lungs are the most frequent site of solitary metastases [55] and are the commonest site considered for metastasectomy. If complete metastasectomy is achieved, 5-year survival rates of 39–45% have been reported [61–63]. Improved survival following resection is associated with a fewer number of metastases and absence of mediastinal lymph node metastases. These features need to be considered on the preoperative CT if appropriate patient selection is to be achieved, although limitations of predicting lymph node involvement with cross-sectional imaging have already been discussed.

Liver

CT is the primary tool for initial staging of renal cell carcinoma, and the liver is often imaged during the portal venous phase of contrast enhancement as part of a standard "chest/abdomen/pelvis" staging CT protocol. However, as with the primary tumor, hepatic metastases from renal cell carcinoma are frequently hypervascular and will often enhance during the arterial phase of contrast infusion, becoming isointense with surrounding enhanced liver parenchyma on the portal venous phase. Indeed, they may be more conspicuous on the precontrast images or as they enhance early during the hepatic arterial phase of contrast infusion. For patients being considered for liver metastasectomy where precise knowledge of the number and distribution of liver metastases is required, repeat triple phase CT of the liver should be considered.

Liver MRI has a role in the characterization of focal liver lesions and can differentiate benign lesions such as cysts, hemangiomas, and focal nodular hyperplasia from metastases with a high degree of accuracy. Liver metastases from all primary tumors are most commonly mildly hypointense on T1-weighted MRI and moderately hyperintense on T2-weighted MRI [64]. Patterns of enhancement aid lesion characterization and this is commonly achieved following intravenous administration of gadolinium chelates. Serial imaging is obtained during arterial (18–30 s), portal venous (45–60 s), and delayed (90–120 s) phases post-injection. As described, liver metastases from renal cell carcinoma are typically hypervascular and enhancement during the arterial phase of gadolinium administration leads to signal intensity greater than that of surrounding liver parenchyma in 80% [64].

Other MRI contrast agents specific to liver parenchyma are being used for the detection and characterization of focal liver lesions. These include manganese-based compounds which are taken up by hepatocytes and supraparamagnetic iron oxide (SPIO) agents which target liver Kupffer cells. Both of these agents have been shown to improve lesion detection rate when compared with dynamic contrast-enhanced CT, and are of particular value in detecting small sub-centimeter lesions [65–68]. SPIO-enhanced MRI results in improved detection rates with sensitivity of

up to 97% [65], compared with around 73–85% for CT. Again, improved detection of liver metastases is important in patients being considered for metastasectomy.

Adrenal

Metastases to the adrenal gland are uncommon, 4.3% reported in one large series [69] (Fig. 7.19). The ipsilateral gland can become involved either by direct invasion from an upper pole tumor or by hematogenous or lymphatic extension. At present ipsilateral adrenal gland involvement is classified as stage T3a by the TNM staging system, which also includes invasion of the perinephric fat into this group (see Table 7.2). However, in reality, involvement of the ipsilateral adrenal gland confers a worse prognosis compared with perinephirc fat invasion, with higher lymph node involvement at presentation and lower 5-year survival rate reported [70, 71]. Indeed, disease to the ipsilateral adrenal gland confers a prognosis more similar to those with stage T4. Identification of adrenal gland involvement is important to plan surgery because currently adrenalectomy is not routinely performed. CT features suggesting involvement include adrenal gland enlargement, displacement, nodules, or irregularity and have been shown to be sensitive (100%) but less specific (76%) for the diagnosis [72, 73].

Incidentally detected adrenal masses are seen in up to 9% of the adult population on abdominal CT [74, 75]. The most frequent differential diagnosis to consider is that of a benign cortical adenoma. These are seen in 29–57% of patients with underlying malignancy [76–78]. Adrenal adenomas can be confidently diagnosed on CT by virtue of their high lipid content and contrast medium washout characteristics. An inverse relationship between lipid content and CT attenuation has been shown [79], and lipid-rich adenomas typically have density measurements of less than 20 HU on

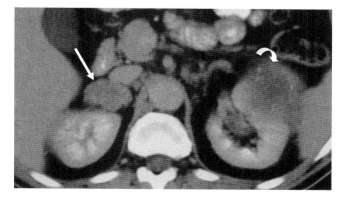

Fig. 7.19 Stage 4b renal cell carcinoma. Axial CT scan post-contrast medium administration showing a renal cell carcinoma arising from the mid-pole of the left kidney (*curved arrow*) and a contralateral metastasis within the right adrenal gland (*arrow*)

unenhanced CT [80]. When a threshold of 18 HU is taken, a diagnosis of an adrenal adenoma can be made with 85% sensitivity and 100% specificity [81]. Sensitivity increases when lower attenuation thresholds are taken and in clinical practice 10 HU or less is usually taken as the cutoff point for confident diagnosis.

However, up to 30% of adrenal adenomas are lipid poor and have attenuation values of greater than 20 HU on unenhanced CT. A confident diagnosis of both lipid-rich and lipid-poor adenomas can be made on a basis of lesion contrast medium enhancement and washout characteristics. Adenomas typically enhance early with rapid washout of contrast medium, compared with metastases which demonstrate much slower contrast washout. Quantitative evaluation can be made if lesion attenuation value measurements are taken at 0 s (unenhanced), 60 s (initial enhancement), and 15 min (delayed enhancement) following contrast medium administration. The absolute percentage contrast washout can then be calculated:

$$\text{absolute \% washout} = \frac{\text{initial enhancement} - \text{delayed enhancement}}{\text{initial enhancement} - \text{unenhanced}} \times 100$$

Alternatively, if unenhanced images are unavailable, as if often the case in clinical practice, the relative washout can be calculated:

$$\text{relative \% washout} = \frac{\text{initial enhancement} - \text{delayed enhancement}}{\text{initial enhancement}} \times 100$$

Absolute percentage washout of >60% and relative percentage washout >40% are used to make a diagnosis of adrenal adenoma with sensitivity/specificity of 88/96% and 96/100%, respectively [82].

A small percentage of adrenal adenomas, however, remains indeterminate following both unenhanced and contrast medium-enhanced CT. For this group of patients, where distinction between a benign adrenal adenoma and metastasis is vital, MRI has a role in lesion characterization. MRI sequences optimized for the detection of intracellular lipid can characterize those lipid-poor adenomas which remain indeterminate on CT. Chemical shift MRI exploits the normal difference in precessional frequency between protons in fat and water molecules within a given voxel. The protons can be made to precess, or spin, at the same frequency and are "in phase" with each other, generating an additive signal. When they are made to precess "out of phase" the signal is reduced in those voxels which contain both fat and water protons (Fig. 7.20). Loss of signal on the out-of-phase compared with the in-phase images confirms the presence of both intracellular lipid and water, only seen in adrenal adenomas, which can be diagnosed with up to 100% specificity [82].

The degree of signal intensity loss can be assessed visually or quantitatively by using region of interest (ROI) measurements of the adrenal lesion on the in-phase ($\text{SI}_{\text{adrenal IP}}$) and out-of-phase ($\text{SI}_{\text{adrenal OP}}$) images. The signal intensity index (SII) calculates percentage signal loss within the lesion:

$$\text{SII} = \frac{\text{SI}_{\text{adrenal IP}} - \text{SI}_{\text{adrenal OP}}}{\text{SI}_{\text{adrenal IP}}} \times 100$$

(a)   (b)

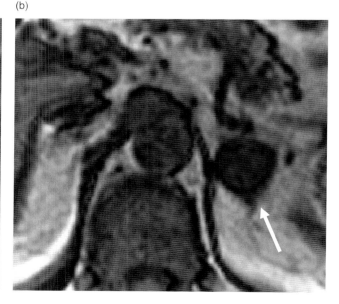

Fig. 7.20 Adrenal adenoma. Chemical shift MRI (**a**) in phase and (**b**) out of phase. There is a well-defined mass related to the left adrenal gland (*arrows*) which demonstrates homogeneous loss of signal on the out-of-phase images, in keeping with and adrenal adenoma

SII of greater than 16.5% diagnoses adrenal adenomas with up to 100% accuracy [84]. Some authors advocate comparing signal loss against an internal standard and the spleen is usually used for this purpose as it is not subject to fatty infiltration unlike the liver or skeletal muscle. The adrenal to spleen ration (ASR) is calculated by taking ROI measurements of the adrenal lesion and spleen at similar levels on the in- and out-of-phase images:

$$ASR = \frac{SI_{adrenal\ OP}/SI_{spleen\ OP}}{SI_{adrenal\ IP}/SI_{spleen\ IP}} \times 100$$

ASR of 70 or less has been shown to be 100% specific for diagnosing adenomas but only 78% specific [85]. Specificity increases to 100% when a threshold ASR of 80 or less is taken [86]. Most authors however agree that simple visual assessment of signal loss is as accurate as quantitative methods [87].

The Role of Multidetector CT (MDCT) in Nephron Sparing Surgery Planning

The aim of nephron sparing surgery is to achieve complete resection of the tumor so as to prevent local recurrence, while preserving as much renal parenchyma so as not to compromise renal function. Nephron sparing surgery involves either enucleation of the tumor with a thin 5–10 mm rim of renal parenchyma or partial nephrectomy. Image-guided radiofrequency ablation techniques are also being developed [88–90]. The selection of suitable candidates therefore requires detailed preoperative staging and knowledge of the renal anatomy, and this can be best achieved with a combination of CT and MRI. Traditionally nephron sparing surgery was considered in patients with a functional solitary kidney, severely compromised renal function, or bilateral tumors but is now also being considered in patients with small incidental tumors with normal renal function. Tumors considered suitable for this technique include small (<4 cm) usually peripheral, preferably exophytic lesions. They should be located away from the collecting system and renal hilum with no renal vein invasion or distant metastases [91]. In addition to the role of cross-sectional imaging in staging renal cell carcinoma described above, a number of authors describe the use of three-dimensional imaging generated from MDCT for preoperative surgical planning [91–94]. MDCT allows imaging of a whole volume of tissue with multiple thin overlapping slices, in a single breath hold, thus reducing misregistration and motion artifact. Two-dimensional (2D) images can be reconstructed in any plane enabling the relationship to surrounding structures to be better visualized. Volume-rendered three-dimensional (3D) images can be reformatted from the original data set and overlapping structures

can be subtracted out (Fig. 7.21). The final image, when reviewed on a dedicated workstation, can be rotated in any plane and images generated which are more favorable to the surgeon. The anatomical detail provided allows accurate depiction of the spatial relationship between tumor, collecting system, renal hilum, and vasculature [92, 93]. Three-dimensional volume-rendered or maximum intensity projection angiographic images can be generated from contrast-enhanced images to demonstrate renal vascular anatomy (Figs. 7.4 and 7.22). Similarly MRI angiographic images

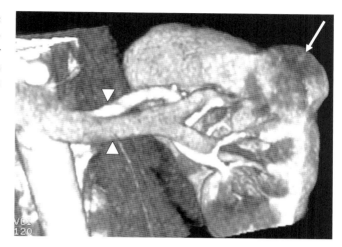

Fig. 7.21 Volume-rendered multi-row detector CT image showing a focal left renal cell carcinoma (*arrow*) and its relationship with the main renal artery and vein (*arrow heads*)

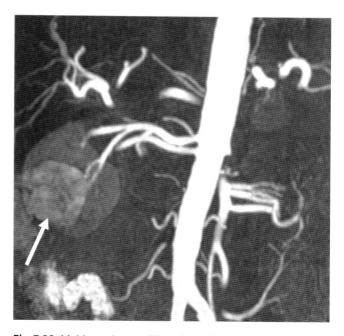

Fig. 7.22 Multi-row detector CT angiographic images showing the vascular supply of the right renal cell carcinoma (*arrow*)

(a)

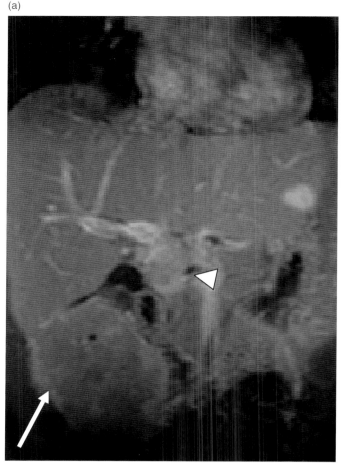

(b)

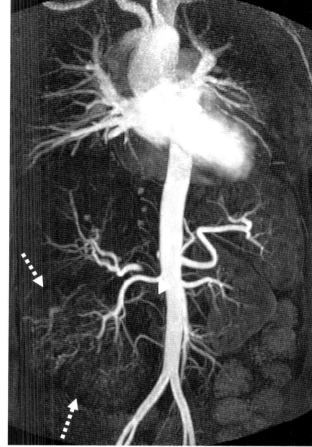

Fig. 7.23 (**a**) Coronal post-contrast T1-weighted fat-saturated MRI showing right renal cell carcinoma (*arrow*) with infrahepatic IVC inva-

sion (*arrow head*). (**b**) Coronal contrast-enhanced MR angiographic images demonstrate the arterial supply to the tumor (*hashed arrows*)

can be acquired (Fig. 7.23). The presence of accessory renal arteries and variations in renal venous anatomy are well demonstrated.

Recurrence

Surgery remains the only effective treatment option for the majority of patients with renal cell carcinoma. Tumor recurrence following radical nephrectomy occurs in approximately 20–30% [58, 95]. Isolated local recurrence in the nephrectomy bed is uncommon, seen in less than 4% [58, 96]. Risk factors for local recurrence include positive surgical margins and involved regional lymph nodes at the time of surgery. The majority of local recurrences are asymptomatic and earlier detection with cross-sectional imaging is associated with less post-surgical morbidity [96, 96]. Surgical resection of isolated recurrent disease has resulted in improved 5-year survival rates of 33–50% [63, 96, 98].

Increased survival following local recurrence resection is associated with smaller recurrent tumor size and longer time to recurrence after radical nephrectomy [97].

The most important predictor of both local and distant recurrence is the pathological stage of the primary tumor, with more frequent and earlier recurrence associated with T3 compared with T1 or T2 tumors [58, 99, 100]. Overall 5-year survival has been reported around 91% for pathologically staged T1 tumors, and is reduced to around 52% for pT3 tumors. Improved survival with lower stage disease is related to longer time to recurrence with development of metastases a mean of 43 months post-nephrectomy for pT1 tumors compared with 17.8 months for pT3 [95]. Other risk factors for recurrence include locally invasive tumor, venous tumor thrombus, high pathological grade, and sarcomatoid histological type.

The commonest site for recurrent disease is the lungs, seen in 37–61% with recurrent disease following nephrectomy for initially localized disease [58–60]. Bone metastases are the next most frequent in 22–32%, followed by liver in 9–32%. Brain metastases are reported in around 2–8% [58–60, 95]. With up to 64% of recurrent disease being asymptomatic [99], post-operative surveillance imaging is important for the early detection of resectable disease. This is primarily achieved with interval CT scanning. In planning a surveillance imaging strategy, knowledge of the natural history of recurrent renal cell carcinoma is needed. The median time to recurrence is 15–23 months following nephrectomy [58, 95, 99, 100]. Up to 85% of recurrences are diagnosed within 3 years and 93% within 5 years [58, 95]. Late recurrences occurring more than 10 years after primary surgery are well recognized. Longer overall survival is associated with a longer time interval between surgery and disease recurrence.

Recurrent tumor resembles the primary tumor radiologically, typically being hypervascular and enhancing (101). Pulmonary metastases may be hemorrhagic or lymphangitic. Hypervascular liver metastases will be best visualized on CT during the arterial phase of contrast medium enhancement (discussed above). Brain metastases are also typically hypervascular, characterized by high attenuation on unenhanced CT and avid contrast medium enhancement. Bone metastases are typically lytic and expansile. Less common but well recognized sites include the pancreas and soft tissue or skeletal muscle. Pancreatic metastases may occur late, more commonly occurring in the pancreatic tail for left-sided renal cell carcinomas.

Surveillance strategies following radical nephrectomy vary between institutions but should be based on the pathological stage of the primary tumor. T1 tumors may not need routine cross-sectional imaging but follow-up with chest radiographs and liver function tests may be advocated. Pulmonary and abdominal metastases are commonly asymptomatic, and it is recommended that patients with T2 and T3 tumors have additional CT of the chest and abdomen at 6 monthly intervals for 2–3 years, starting at 3–6 months following surgery [99, 100]. In addition to detecting recurrent local or distant disease attention must be made to the detection of metachronous tumor in the contralateral kidney. Bone scan and brain imaging should be performed in the presence of symptoms or when resection of an apparently solitary metastasis is considered.

References

1. Jemal A, Murray T, Ward E, Samuels A, Tiwari RC, Ghafoor A, et al. Cancer statistics, 2005. CA Cancer J Clin. 2005;55:10–30
2. Motzer, RJ, Bander NH, Nanus DM. Renal cell carcinoma. N Engl J Med. 1996;335:865–75.
3. Curry NS. Small renal masses (lesions smaller than 3 cm): imaging evaluation and management. Am J Roentgenol. 1995;164: 355–62.
4. Pantuck AJ, Zisman A, Belldegrun AS. The changing natural history of renal cell carcinoma. J Urol. 2001;166:1611–23.
5. Konnak JW, Grossman HB. Renal cell carcinoma as an incidental finding. J Urol. 1985;134:1094–6.
6. Smith SJ, Bosniak MA, Megibow AJ, Hulnick DH, Horii SC, Raghavendra BN. Renal cell carcinoma: earlier discovery and increased detection. Radiology. 1989;170:699–703.
7. Thompson IM, Peek M. Improvement in survival pattern of patients with renal cell carcinoma - the role of the serendipitously detected tumor. J Urol. 1988;140:487–90.
8. Jayson M, Sanders H. Increased incidence of serendipitously discovered renal cell carcinoma. Urology. 1998;51:203–5.
9. Hajdu SI, Thomas AG. Renal cell carcinoma at autopsy. J Urol. 1967;97:978–82.
10. Amis ES, Cronan JJ, Pfister RC. Needle puncture of cystic renal masses: a survey of the Society of Uroradiology. Am J Roentgenol. 1987;148:297–9.
11. Amendola MA, Bree RL, Pollack HM, Francis IR, Glazer GM, Jafri SZ, et al. Small renal cell carcinomas: resolving a diagnostic dilemma. Radiology. 1988;166:637–641.
12. Levine E, Huntrakoon M, Wetzel LH. Small renal neoplasms: clinical, pathologic and imaging features. Am J Roentgenol. 1989;153:69–73.
13. Bosniak MA. The small (<3.0 cm) renal parenchymal tumour: detection, diagnosis, and controversies. Radiology. 1991;179:307–17.
14. Silverman SG, Lee BY, Seltzer SE, Bloom DA, Corless CL, Adams DF. Small (<3 cm) renal masses: correlation of spiral CT features and pathologic findings. Am J Roentgenol. 1994;163:597–605.
15. Birnbaum BA, Bosniak MA, Megibow AJ, Lubat E, Gordon RB. Observations on the growth of renal neoplasms. Radiology. 1990;176:695–701.
16. Israel GM, Bosniak MA. How I do it: evaluating renal masses. Radiology. 2005;236:441–50.
17. Herts BR, Coll DM, Novick AC, Obuchowski N, Linnell G, Wirth SL, et al. Enhancement characteristics of papillary renal neoplasms revealed on triphasic helical CT of the kidneys. Am J Roentgenol. 2002;178:367–72.
18. Kim JK, Kim TK, Anh HJ, Kim CS, Kim KR, Cho KS. Differentiation of subtypes of renal cell carcinoma on helical CT scans. Am J Roentgenol. 2002;178:1499–506.
19. Tsuda K, Kinouchi T, Tanikawa G, Yasuhara Y, Yanagawa M, Kakimoto K, et al. Imaging characteristics of papillary renal cell carcinoma by computed tomography scan and magnetic resonance imaging. Int J Urol. 2005;12:795–800.
20. Howard RCL, Marmery H, Houghton R, Rockall AG, Rankin SC, Reznek RH. Papillary renal cell carcinoma: a review of the CT imaging characteristics. RSNA. 2004;0664UR:726.
21. Davidson AJ, Hartman DS, Choyke PL, Wagner BJ. Radiologic assessment of renal masses: implications for patient care. Radiology. 1997;202:297–305.
22. Bosniak MA. The current radiological approach to renal cysts. Radiology. 1986;158:1–10.
23. Israel GM, Bosniak MA. Follow-up CT of moderately complex cystic lesions of the kidney (Bosniak category IIF). Am J Roentgenol. 2003;181:627–33.
24. Hartman DS, Choyke PL, Hartman MS. A practical approach to the cystic renal mass. Radiographics. 2004;24:S101–15.
25. Harisinghani MG, Maher MM, Gervais DA, McGovern F, Hahn P, Jhaveri K, et al. Incidence of malignancy in complex cystic renal masses (Bosniak category III): should imaging-guided biopsy precede surgery? Am J Roentgenol. 2003;180:755–8.
26. Israel GM, Bosniak MA. MR imaging of cystic renal masses. Magn Reson Imaging Clin N Am. 2004;12:403–12.
27. Rominger MB, Kenney PJ, Morgan DE, Bernreuter WK, Listinsky JJ. Gadolinium-enhanced MR imaging of renal masses. Radiographics. 1992;12:1097–1116.

28. Clayman RV, Gonzalez R, Fraley EE. Renal cell cancer invading the inferior vena cava: clinical review and anatomical approach. J Urol. 1980;123:157–63.

29. Hatcher PA, Anderson EE, Paulson DF, Carson CC, Robertson JE. Surgical management and prognosis of renal cell carcinoma invading the vena cava. J Urol. 1991;145:20–3.

30. Johnson CD, Dunnick NR, Cohan RH, Illescas FF. Renal adenocarcinoma: CT staging of 100 tumors. Am J Roentgenol. 1987;148:59–63.

31. Hricak H, Thoeni RF, Carroll PR, Demas BE, Marotti M, Tanagho EA. Detection and staging of renal neoplasms: a reassessment of MR imaging. Radiology. 1988;166:643–649.

32. Fein AB, Lee JK, Balfe DM, Heiken JP, Ling D, Glazer HS, et al. Diagnosis and staging of renal cell carcinoma: a comparison of MR imaging and CT. Am J Roentgenol. 1987;148: 749–53.

33. Hricak H, Demas BE, Williams RD, McNamara MT, Hedgcock MW, Amparo EG, et al. Magnetic resonance imaging in the diagnosis and staging of renal and perirenal neoplasms. Radiology. 1985;154:709–15.

34. Amendola MA, King LR, Pollack HM, Gefter W, Kressel HY, Wein AJ. Staging of renal carcinoma using magnetic resonance imaging at 1.5 Tesla. Cancer. 1990;66:40–4.

35. Kabala JE, Gillatt DA, Persad RA, Penry JB, Gingell JC, Chadwick D. Magnetic resonance imaging in the staging of renal cellcarcinoma. Br J Radiol. 1991;64:683–9.

36. Kamel IR, Hochman MG, Keogan MT, Eng J, Longmaid HE 3rd, DeWolf W, et al. Accuracy of breath-hold magnetic resonance imaging in preoperative staging of organ-confined renal cell carcinoma. J Comput Assist Tomogr. 2004;28:327–32.

37. Hallscheidt PJ, Bock M, Riedasch G, Zuna I, Schoenberg SO, Autschbach F, et al. Diagnostic accuracy of staging renal cell carcinomas using multidetector-row computed tomography and magnetic resonance imaging. A prospective study with histopathological correlation. J Comput Assist Tomogr. 2004;28:333–9.

38. Ergen FB, Hussain HK, Caoili EM, Korobkin M, Carlos RC, Weadock WJ, et al. MRI for preoperative staging of renal cell carcinoma using the 1997 TNM classification: comparison with surgical and pathologic staging. Am J Roentgenol. 2004;182: 217–25.

39. Aslam Sohaib SA, Teh J, Nargund VH, Lumley JS, Hendry WF, Reznek RH. Assessment of tumour invasion of the vena caval wall in renal cell carcinoma cases by magnetic resonance imaging. J Urol. 2002;167:1271–5.

40. Reznek RH, Webb J. Renal tumours. In: Husband JE, Reznek RH, editors. Imaging in oncology. London: Taylor and Francis; 2004. pp. 273–305.

41. Pretorius ES, Siegelman ES, Ramchandani P, Cangiano T, Banner MP. Renal neoplasms amenable to partial nephrectomy: MR imaging. Radiology. 1999;212:28–34.

42. Yamashita Y, Honda S, Nishiharu T, Urata J, Takahashi M. Detection of pseudocapsule of renal cell carcinoma with MR imaging and CT. Am J Roentgenol. 1996;166:1151–5.

43. Palapattu GS, Pantuck AJ, Dorey F, Said JW, Figlin RA, Belldegrun AS. Collecting system invasion in renal cell carcinoma: impact on prognosis and future staging strategies. J Urol. 2003;170:768–72.

44. Waters WB, Richie JP. Aggressive surgical approach to renal cell carcinoma: review of 130 cases. J Urol. 1979;122:306–9.

45. Kallman DA, King BF, Hattery RR, Charboneau JW, Ehman RL, Guthman DA, et al. Renal vein and inferior vena cava tumour thrombus in renal cell carcinoma: CT, US, MRI and venacavography. J Comput Assist Tomogr. 1992;16:240–7.

46. Goncharenko V, Gerlock AJ, Kadir S, Turner B. Incidence and distribution of venous extension in 10 hypernephromas. Am J Roentgenol. 1979;133:263–5.

47. Zeman RK, Cronan JJ, Rosenfield AT, Lynch JH, Jaffe MH, Clark LR. Renal cell carcinoma: dynamic thin-section CT assessment of vascular invasion and tumour vascularity. Radiology. 1988;167:393–6.

48. Horan JJ, Robertson CN, Choyke PL, Frank JA, Miller DL, Pass HI, et al. The detection of renal carcinoma extension into the renal vein and inferior vena cava: a prospective comparison of vencavography and magnetic resonance imaging. J Urol. 1989;142:943–8.

49. Myneni L, Hricak H, Carroll PR. Magnetic resonance imaging of renal carcinoma with extension into the vena cava: staging accuracy and recent advances. Br J Urol. 1991;68:571–8.

50. Roubidoux MA, Dunnick NR, Sostman HD, Leder RA. Renal carcinoma: detection of venous extension with gradient –echo MR imaging. Radiology. 1992;182:269–72.

51. Catalano C, Fraioli F, Laghi A, Napoli A, Pediconi F, Danti M, et al. High-resolution multidetector CT in the preoperative evaluation of patients with renal cell carcinoma. Am J Roentgenol. 2003;180:1271–1277.

52. Studer UE, Scherz S, Scheidegger J, Kraft R, Sonntag R, Ackermann D, et al. Enlargement of regional lymph nodes in renal cell carcinoma is often not due to metastases. J Urol. 1990;144: 243–5.

53. Harisinghani MG, Barentsz J, Hahn PF, Deserno WM, Tabatabaei S, van de Kaa CH, et al. Non-invasive detection of clinically occult lymph-node metastases in prostate cancer. N Engl J Med. 2003;348:2491–99.

54. Rockall AG, Sohaib SA, Harisinghani MG, Babar SA, Singh N, Jeyarajah AR, et al. Diagnostic performance of nanoparticle-enhanced magnetic resonance imaging in the diagnosis of lymph node metastases in patients with endometrial and cervical cancer. J Clin Oncol. 2005;23:2813–21.

55. Johnsen JA, Hellsten S. Lymphatogenous spread of renal cell carcinoma: an autopsy study. J Urol. 1997;157:450–3.

56. Campbell SC, Flanigan RC, Clark JL. Nephrectomy in metastatic renal cell carcinoma. Curr Treat Options Oncol. 2003;4:363–72.

57. Flanigan RC. Debulking nephrectomy in metastatic renal cancer. Clin Cancer Res 2004;10:6335s–6341s.

58. Sandock DS, Seftel AD, Resnick M. A new protocol for the followup of renal cell carcinoma based on pathological stage. J Urol. 1995;154:28–31.

59. Harada Y, Nonomura N, Kondo M, Nishimura K, Takahara S, Miki T, et al. Clincial study of brain metastasis of renal cell carcinoma. Eur Urol. 1999;36:230–5

60. Sivaramakrishna B, Gupta NP, Wadhwa P, Hemal AK, Dogra PN, Seth A, et al. Pattern of metastases in renal cell carcinoma: a single institution study. Indian J Cancer. 2005;42:173–7.

61. Pfannschmidt J, Hoffmann H, Muley T, Krysa S, Trainer C, Dienemann H. Prognostic factors for survival after pulmonary resection of metastatic renal cell carcinoma. Ann Thorac Surg. 2002;74:1653–7.

62. Murthy SC, Kim K, Rice TW, Rajeswaran J, Bukowski R, DeCamp MM, et al. Can we predict long-term survival after pulmonary metastasectomy for renal cell carcinoma? Ann Thorac Surg. 2005;79:996–1003.

63. Hofmann HS, Neef H, Krohe K, Andreev P, Silber RE. Prognostic factors and survival after pulmonary resection of metastatic renal cell carcinoma. Eur Urol. 2005;48:77–81.

64. Danet IM, Semelka RC, Leonardou P, Braga L, Vaidean G, Woosley JT, et al. Spectrum of appearances of untreated metastases of the liver. Am J Roentgenol. 2003;181:809–17.

65. Reimer P, Jähnke N, Fiebich M, Schima W, Deckers F, Marx C, et al. Hepatic lesion detection and characterization: value of nonenhanced MR imaging, superparamagnetic iron oxide-enhanced MR imaging and spiral CT-ROC analysis. Radiology. 2000;217: 152–8.

66. Kim MJ, Kim JH, Lim JS, Oh YT, Chung JJ, Choi JS, et al. Detection and characterization of focal hepatic lesions: mangafodipir vs. superparamagnetic iron oxide-enhanced magnetic resonance imaging. J Magn Reson Imaging. 2004;20:612–21.

67. Ward J, Robinson PJ, Guthrie JA, Downing S, Wilson D, Lodge JP, et al. Liver metastases in candidates for hepatic resection: comparison of helical CT and Gadolinium and SPIO-enhanced MR imaging. Radiol. 2005;237:170–80.

68. Regge D, Campanella D, Anselmetti GC, Cirillo S, Gallo TM, Muratore A, et al. Diagnostic accuracy of portal-phase CT and MRI with mangafodipir trisodium in detecting liver metastases from colorectal carcinoma. Clin Radiol. 2006;61:338–47.

69. Sagalowsky AI, Kadesky KT, Ewalt DM, Kennedy TJ. Factors influencing adrenal metastasis in renal cell carcinoma. J Urol. 1994;151:1181–4.

70. Sandock DS, Seftel AD, Resnick MI. Adrenal metastases from renal cell carcinoma: role of ipsilateral adrenalectomy and definition of stage. Urology. 1997;49:28–31.

71. Han KR, Bui MH, Pantuck AJ, Freitas DG, Leibovich BC, Dorey FJ, et al. TNM T3a renal cell carcinoma: adrenal gland involvement is not the same as renal fat invasion. J Urol. 2003;169:899–904.

72. Gill IS, McClennan BL, Kerbl K, Carbone JM, Wick M, Clayman RV. Adrenal involvement from renal cell carcinoma: predictive value of computerised tomography. J Urol. 1994;152:1082–5.

73. Sawai Y, Kinouchi T, Mano M, Meguro N, Maeda O, et al. Ipsilateral adrenal involvement from renal cell carcinoma: retrospective study of the predictive value of computed tomography. Urology. 2002;59:28–31.

74. Glazer HS, Weyman PJ, Sagel SS, Levitt RG, McClennan BL. Nonfunctioning adrenal masses: incidental discovery on computed tomography. AJR Am J Roentgenol. 1982;139(1):81–5.

75. Dunnick NR, Korobkin M, Francis I. Adrenal radiology: distinguishing benign from malignant adrenal masses. Am J Roentgenol. 1996;167:861–7.

76. Francis IR, Smid A, Gross MD, Shapiro B, Naylor B, Glazer GM. Adrenal masses in oncologic patients: functional and morphologic evaluation. Radiology. 1988;166(2):353–6.

77. Krestin GP, Freidmann G, Fishbach R, Neufang KF, Allolio B. Evaluation of adrenal masses in oncologic patients: dynamic contrast-enhanced MR vs CT. J Comput Assist Tomogr. 1991;15(1):104–10.

78. Frilling A, Tecklenborg K, Weber F, Kuhl H, Muller S, Stamatis G, et al. Importance of adrenal incidentaloma in patients with a history of malignancy. Surgery 2004;136(6):1289–96.

79. Korobkin M, Giordano TJ, Brodeur FJ, Francis IR, Siegelman ES, Quint LE, et al. Adrenal adenomas: relationship between histologic lipid and CT and MR findings. Radiology. 1996;200(3):743–7.

80. Boland GW, Lee MJ, Gazelle GS, Halpern EF, McNicholas MM, Mueller PR. Characterization of adrenal masses using unenhanced CT: an analysis of the CT literature. Am J Roentgenol. 1998;171(1):201–4.

81. Korobkin M, Brodeur FJ, Yutzy GG, Francis IR, Quint LE, Dunnick NR, et al. Differentiation of adrenal adenomas from nonadenomas using CT attenuation values. Am J Roentgenol. 1996;166:531–6.

82. Korobkin M, Brodeur FJ, Francis IR, Quint LE, Dunnick NR, Londy F. CT time-attenuation washout curves of adrenal adenomas and nonadenomas. Am J Roentgenol. 1998;170(3):747–52.

83. Korobkin M, Lombardi TJ, Aisen AM, Francis IR, Quint LE, Dunnick NR, et al. Characterization of adrenal masses with chemical shift and gadolinium-enhanced MR imaging. Radiology. 1995;197(2):411–8.

84. Fujiyoshi F, Nakajo M, Fukukura Y, Tsuchimochi S. Characterisation of adrenal tumours by chemical shift fast low-angle shot MR imaging: comparison of four methods of quantitative evaluation. Am J Roentgenol. 2003;180:1649–57.

85. McNichols MM, Lee MJ, Mayo-Smith WW, Hahn PF, Boland GW, Mueller PR. An imaging algorithm for the differential diagnosis of adrenal adenomas and metastases. Am J Roentgenol. 1995;165:1453–9.

86. Bilbey JH, McLoughlin RF, Kurkjian PS, Wilkins GE, Chan NH, Schmidt N, et al. MR imaging of adrenal masses: value of chemical-shift imaging for distinguishing adenomas from other tumours. Am J Roentgenol. 1995;164:637–42.

87. Hussain HK, Korobkin M. MR imaging of the adrenal glands. Magn Reson Imaging Clin N Am. 2004;12:515–44.

88. Farrell MA, Charboneau WJ, DiMarco DS, Chow GK, Zincke H, Callstrom MR, et al. Imaging-guided radiofrequency ablation of solid renal tumors. Am J Roentgenol. 2003;180:1509–13.

89. Zagoria RJ, Hawkins AD, Clark PE, Hall MC, Matlaga BR, Dyer RB, et al. Percutaneous CT-guided radiofrequency ablation of renal neoplasms: factors influencing success. Am J Roentgenol. 2004;183:201–7.

90. Veltri A, De Fazio G, Malfitana V, Isolato G, Fontana D, Tizzani A, et al. Percutaneous US-guided RF thermal ablation for malignant renal tumors: preliminary results in 13 patients. Eur Radiol. 2004;14:2303–10.

91. Smith PA, Marshall FF, Corl FM, Fishman EK. Planning nephron-sparing renal surgery using 3D helical CT angiography. J Comput Assist Tomogr. 1999;23:649–54.

92. Coll DM, Uzzo RG, Herts BR, Davros WJ, Wirth SL, Novick AC. 3-dimensional volume rendered computerised tomography for preoperative evaluation and intraoperative treatment of patients undergoing nephron sparing surgery. J Urol. 1999;161:1097–102.

93. Coll DM, Herts BR, Davros WJ, Uzzo RG, Novick AC. Preoperative use of 3D volume rendering to demonstrate renal tumors and renal anatomy. Radiographics. 2000;20:431–8.

94. Sheth S, Scatarige JC, Horton KM, Corl FM, Fishman EK. Current concepts in the diagnosis and management of renal cell carcinoma: role of multidetector CT and three-dimensional CT. Radiographics. 2001;21:S237–54.

95. Ljungberg B, Alamdari FI, Rasmuson T, Roos G. Follow-up guidelines for nonmetastatic renal cell carcinoma based on the occurrence of metastases after radical nephrectomy. BJU Int. 1999;84:405–11.

96. Itano NB, Blute ML, Spotts B, Zincke H. Outcome of isolated renal cell carcinoma fossa recurrence after nephrectomy. J Urol. 2000;164:322–5.

97. Schrödter S, Hakenberg OW, Manseck A, Leike S, Wirth MP. Outcome of surgical treatment of isolated local recurrence after radical nephrectomy for renal cell carcinoma. J Urol. 2002;167:1630–33.

98. Kavolius JP, Mastorakos DP, Pavlovich C, Russo P, Burt ME, Brady MS. J Clin Oncol. 1998;16:2261–6.

99. Levy DA, Slaton JW, Swanson DA, Dinney CPN. Stage specific guidelines for surveillance after radical nephrectomy for local renal cell carcinoma. J Urol. 1998;159:1163–7.

100. Stephenson AJ, Chetner MP, Rourke K, Gleave ME, Signaevsky M, Palmer B, et al. Guidelines for the surveillance of localized renal cell carcinoma based on the patterns of relapse after nephrectomy. J Urol. 2004;172:58–62.

101. Scatarige JC, Sheth S, Corl FM, Fishman EK. Patterns of recurrence in renal cell carcinoma: manifestations on helical CT. Am J Roentgenol. 2001;177:653–8.

Chapter 8

Radionuclide Imaging in Renal Cell Carcinoma

A.H. Brouwers and P.L. Jager

Classification of a Renal Mass

Nowadays, a space-occupying lesion in the kidney is usually discovered with ultrasound, computed tomography (CT), or magnetic resonance imaging (MRI) of the abdomen. The benign or malignant nature of the lesion can usually accurately be assessed with these radiological procedures. Radionuclide imaging techniques do not play a major role in diagnosing kidney cancer, as currently there are no radiopharmaceuticals routinely available that selectively target malignant renal cells. In experimental settings, a few investigational radionuclide-labeled monoclonal antibodies specifically targeting (subsets of) renal cell carcinomas (RCCs) have been described. In this chapter the role of various nuclear medicine techniques for diagnosing kidney cancer will be discussed in more detail.

Positron Emission Tomography

Role of ^{18}F-Fluorodeoxyglucose

After the introduction of the whole-body ^{18}F-fluorodeoxyglucose (^{18}F-FDG) positron emission tomography (PET) technique for imaging many types of malignancies, reports have been published evaluating the possible role of ^{18}F-FDG for differentiating between a benign and a malignant renal lesion. Most of these reports are hampered by small patient numbers and/or selection of the included patients.

Wahl et al. were the first in 1991 to report encouraging early results in five patients who underwent early dynamic and late static ^{18}F-FDG-PET imaging preoperatively after they were scheduled for surgical resection because a solid renal mass was diagnosed on CT [1]. All primary malignancies ranging from 2.5 to 9 cm, four adenocarcinomas, and one transitional cell carcinoma were visualized, together with known metastases (Table 8.1). Subsequently, Bachor et al. reported a larger series of 29 patients with suspected primary kidney tumors (range 1.4–15 cm) [2]. Of the 26 cases with confirmed renal cell carcinoma (RCC) ^{18}F-FDG-PET detected 20 but missed 6 primary tumors (sensitivity 77%). More recently, others also reported lower sensitivities for the assessment of solid renal masses with ^{18}F-FDG-PET: a sensitivity of 32% (6/19) by Miyakita et al., 47% (14/30) versus 97% for CT by Aide et al., and 60% (9/15) (versus CT: 92%) by Kang et al. (Table 8.1) [3–5]. Only Ramdave et al. reported in a series of 17 patients with known or suspected primary tumors (range 2–15 cm) a high sensitivity for both ^{18}F-FDG-PET (94%) and CT (100%), resulting in an equal (high) accuracy for ^{18}F-FDG-PET and CT: 94% [6]. These results could not be confirmed later by the retrospective study conducted by Kang et al. (65% versus 94% accuracy for ^{18}F-FDG-PET and CT, respectively) and the prospectively performed study by Aide et al., who reported an accuracy of 51% for ^{18}F-FDG-PET and 83% for CT, in the largest prospective series of primary kidney lesions thus far (n=30) [4, 5].

Although the reported sensitivity rate is widely varying and occasionally fairly low, the reported specificity of ^{18}F-FDG for the detection of a malignant renal mass seems more constant and fairly high (Table 8.1). Reported specificities range from 80% by Aide et al. to 100% by Ramdave et al. and Kang et al. who all used a dedicated PET camera for their studies [4–6]. Only Montravers et al. and Ak and Can reported a slightly lower specificity of 75% in their series of 16 and 19 patients, respectively, that were imaged with a gamma camera adapted for detecting [18]F (equipped with coincidence detection and a thicker sodium iodine crystal) [7, 8]. Specificity can be reduced because inflammatory lesions also accumulate ^{18}F-FDG leading to false-positive results. Indeed, in the reported series, a few false-positive results have been identified in ^{18}F-FDG-PET imaging of suspected primary kidney tumors (Table 8.1). Bachor et al.

A.H. Brouwers (✉)
Nuclear Medicine Specialists, Department of Nuclear Medicine and Molecular Imaging, University Medical Center Groningen, Groningen, The Netherlands

J.J.M.C.H. de la Rosette et al. (eds.), *Imaging in Oncological Urology*,
DOI 10.1007/978-1-84628-759-6_8, © Springer-Verlag London Limited 2009

Table 8.1 Characterization of a renal mass with ^{18}F-FDG-PET.

Reference	No of pts	Inclusion (no of pts)	Detection of renal malignancy		^{18}F-FDG-PET	
			^{18}F-FDG	CT	False-negative	False positive
Wahl et al. [1]	5	Known/suspected primary renal malignancy	Se=100% (5/5)	–	0	0
Bachor et al. [2]	29	Suspected primary renal malignancy	Se=77% (20/26) Sp=0% (0/3)	–	6	3 (angiolypoma, pericytoma, pheochromocytoma)
Goldberg et al. [11]	21	Solid renal mass (10)	Se=90% (9/10) for malignancy	–	1	0
Goldberg et al. [11]	21	Bosniak indeterminate cysts (11)	Se=90% (10/11) for benignancy		1	0
Montravers et al. [7]*	22	Suspected primary renal malignancy (13)	Se=89% (8/9) Sp=75% (3/4) Acc=85%	Se=100% (9/9) Sp=50% (2/4) Acc=85%	2	1 (renal tuberculosis)
Ramdave et al. [6]	25	Known or suspected primary renal malignancy (17)	Se=94% (15/16) Sp=100% (1/1) Acc=94%	Se=100% (16/16) Sp=0% (0/1) Acc=94%	1	0
Miyakita et al. [3]	19	Suspected primary renal malignancy	Se=32% (6/19)	–	13	0
Aide et al. [4]	53	Suspected primary renal malignancy (35)	Se=47% (14/30) Sp=80% (4/5) Acc=51%	Se=97% (29/30) Sp=0% (0/5) Acc=83%	16	1 (oncocytoma)
Kang et al. [5]	66	Suspected primary renal malignancy (17)	Se=60% (9/15) Sp=100% (2/2) Acc=65%	Se=93% (14/15) Sp=100% (2/2) Acc=94%	6	0
Kumar et al. [67]	24	Solid renal mass in patients with (suspected) primary renal malignancy (10)	Se=89% (8/9) Sp=100% (1/1) Acc=90%	–	1	0
Ak and Can [8]*	19	Suspected primary renal malignancy	Se=86% (13/15) Sp=75% (3/4) Acc=84%	–	2	1 (xantogranulomatous pyelonephritis)

*Performed using coincidence detection gamma camera.

Se = sensitivity

Sp = specificity

reported three false-positive ^{18}F-FDG-PET cases: a renal angiomyolipoma, a renal pericytoma, and a pheochromocytoma where the adrenal could not clearly be delineated from the renal cortex [2]. Furthermore, occasional cases of false positivity have been identified for oncocytoma (a benign tumor of the kidney) [4, 9, 10], nephroblastoma [9], renal tuberculosis [7], and xantogranulomatous pyelonephritis [8]. In most studies, ^{18}F-FDG-PET scans were performed in patients scheduled for surgery because of a high suspicion of primary RCC. Therefore, the reported specificities should be interpreted with caution, not only since they are based on small patient series but also because even fewer patients had a benign lesion at pathology. Only Goldberg et al. examined 11 patients with 12 indeterminate cysts according to the Bosniak CT classification [11–13]. Accuracy for correctly classifying these lesions was 92%: only one small malignant lesion was missed, all other lesions were correctly PET negative.

Another dilemma in the current knowledge on the value of ^{18}F-FDG-PET for diagnosing kidney cancer is the variation in histology and the different classifying systems used in the reported series. The vast majority of kidney tumors consist of RCCs, the remainder consisting of renal pelvic tumors in adults and nephroblastoma or Wilm's tumor in children. Nowadays, for pathological classification of RCCs the WHO 2004 classification is recommended [14]. According to this classification, most RCCs are of the clear cell type (80%). Unfortunately, in the reported ^{18}F-FDG-PET series for discriminating between a malignant and a benignant renal mass, older classifications systems are sometimes used or the applied pathological classifications are not always well defined. Therefore, the reported pathological classification systems do not always correlate with each other, making direct comparisons more difficult. In the present series, few histopathological subtypes of renal cancer other than clear cell RCC have been imaged with ^{18}F-FDG-PET. The number of reported cases is too small to make a definite statement on whether these subtypes are ^{18}F-FDG avid or not. A "transitional cell carcinoma" (old classification) was reported to accumulate ^{18}F-FDG [1], as well as two "carcinosarcomas" [7] and two papillary RCCs [4]. However, two chromophobe RCCs, a "chromophil" and a "mixed type" RCC [4], were ^{18}F-FDG-PET negative together with a "poorly differentiated adenocarcinoma" [6]. Larger reported series with the more rare subtypes of RCC according to the WHO classification system are needed to determine ^{18}F-FDG avidness of the various histological subtypes of RCCs.

The reasons for (non)-visualization of primary RCCs with ^{18}F-FDG need to be further elucidated. A number of possible explanations have been put forward. First, visualization of ^{18}F-FDG uptake in renal lesions can be obscured by the physiological uptake of ^{18}F-FDG in the renal cortex and urinary tract [3–5, 7]. A second reason could be that characteristics of the renal lesion itself might explain the degree of ^{18}F-FDG accumulation. Miyauchi et al. examined the expression of glucose transporters (GLUT) 1, 2, 4, and 5 in tissue samples of newly diagnosed patients (n=11) with primary RCC [15]. Preliminary results indicated that renal cancers well visualized with ^{18}F-FDG-PET had higher GLUT-1 expression, higher tumor grade, and tended to be larger than poorly imaged cancers. However, in a larger series of 19 patients with proven RCC, Miyakita et al. could not confirm a correlation between GLUT-1 expression of the primary tumor and ^{18}F-FDG-PET positivity [3]. Also, tumor size and tumor grade were analyzed by Miyauchi et al. [15]. RCC tumors that were well visualized with ^{18}F-FDG tended to be larger and of higher tumor grade. Regarding tumor grade, the results of Miyauchi et al. are contradicted by preliminary results of Shreve et al. (n=41) and the prospective study of Aide et al. (n=35) [4, 9]. No correlation between ^{18}F-FDG uptake and nuclear grade (Fuhrman) was observed in these larger series of histologically proven primary RCCs. Regarding the size of the primary RCC, most authors agree that larger RCCs tend to be more ^{18}F-FDG avid in contrast to smaller RCCs [3, 4]. This can be explained by the physical limitations of the PET technique: no matter how good a metastatic lesion takes up ^{18}F-FDG, with the current clinical PET cameras, the lower limit to detect abnormal foci is a lesion size of approximately 8 mm.

However, not all large primary RCC lesions are detected with ^{18}F-FDG. Montravers et al. observed, in a study in RCC patients using the radiopharmaceuticals ^{111}In-pentreotide and thallium-201 (^{201}Tl), a tumor-seeking radiopharmaceutical depending on blood flow, that these large primary tumors were not visualized by either one, even though some metastases were seen with both radiopharmaceuticals [16]. An in vitro autoradiographic study showed the presence of pentreotide receptors in the tumor although the primary tumor was not detected with ^{111}In-pentreotide in vivo [16]. Therefore, they postulated that inaccessibility of certain large primary renal lesions for ^{18}F-FDG also might cause the ^{18}F-FDG-PET negativity of these lesions [7]. Whether there are still other factors for non-visualization of primary tumors or what the specific contributions are of the various mechanisms previously described may be subjects for further research.

Since for the assessment of a solid renal mass the sensitivity and the accuracy of the already routinely used imaging techniques such as CT scan are high and ^{18}F-FDG-PET performs inferiorly or at the utmost the same, presently there is no place to perform ^{18}F-FDG-PET routinely for assessing the nature of a solid renal mass. It remains to be proven in case of inconclusive results with conventional imaging whether an ^{18}F-FDG-PET scan is of additional value due to the high specificity claimed by ^{18}F-FDG-PET, as was suggested by Kang et al. [5].

Role of Other Positron-Emitting Radiopharmaceuticals

To overcome the limitations of ^{18}F-FDG for PET imaging of RCC (physiological excretion of ^{18}F-FDG via the urinary system and highly variable glucose metabolism of malignant renal cells), few groups have looked into other PET tracers. Shreve et al. applied ^{11}C-acetate in 18 normal controls and patients with common renal pathologies, both benign and malignant [17]. ^{11}C-acetate is a metabolic PET tracer for the assessment of oxidative metabolism and blood flow in tissues. Dynamic ^{11}C-acetate-PET [11]imaging patients with primary RCC revealed that neoplastic renal tissue differed markedly in the clearance of tracer compared to benign renal lesions and normal subjects, but only three patients were studied [17]. Directly after injection ^{11}C-acetate uptake in renal parenchyma is high, but due to a relative retention beyond 10 min after injection of the tracer in malignant renal tissue, a clear differentiation between malignant and benign/normal was possible. Subsequently, ^{11}C-acetate-PET was performed in 26 patients suspected of having primary RCC on CT [18]. Dynamic ^{11}C-acetate-PET imaging was directly followed by a standard ^{18}F-FDG-PET procedure. Results indicated that RCC (various pathological subtypes) demonstrated on average greater avidity for ^{11}C-acetate than for ^{18}F-FDG with mean standardized uptake values (SUVs) of 7.1 and 4.2, respectively. Furthermore, high ^{11}C-acetate uptake was consistently associated with granular and oncocytic histology, while the SUV for spindle cell carcinoma was low. It was concluded that this might indicate that information on the predominant histopathological cell type of a malignant renal lesion could be non-invasively provided with ^{11}C-acetate, although standardized uptake values (SUVs) for both ^{11}C-acetate and ^{18}F-FDG were highly variable. Clearly, these preliminary results need further confirmation.

Another PET tracer tested in RCC is ^{18}F-fluoro-L-proline (^{18}F-FPro) by Langen et al. [19]. ^{18}F-FPro is a metabolic tracer to image amino acid metabolism of tissues. ^{18}F-based tracers compared to ^{11}C-based tracers are logistically attractive as they do not require a cyclotron and production facilities on-site due to the longer half-life of ^{18}F compared to [11]C: 110 min versus 20 min, respectively. Unfortunately, in none of the eight patients with urological tumors scanned after i.v. injection of ^{18}F-FPro could tracer accumulation be observed [19]. Five of these patients had proven or suspected primary RCCs. Three of these lesions could be visualized with ^{18}F-FDG-PET. Thus, ^{18}F-Fpro does not seem a suitable PET tracer for imaging of RCC. Likewise, ^{18}F-fluorothymidine (^{18}F-FLT), another PET tracer for amino acid metabolism, was reported not to accumulate in a small grade 1 renal carcinoma metastasis [20].

From these studies it becomes clear that currently, there are no PET tracers other than ^{18}F-FDG routinely available to differentiate between a benign and a malignant renal lesion in vivo.

Single-Photon Emission Techniques

Role of Somatostatine Receptor Scintigraphy

There have been a few reports regarding the use of somatostatin receptor scintigraphy in RCC (Fig. 8.1). Somatostatin receptor scintigraphy has been well established for the evaluation of neuro-endocrine tumors. Reubi and Kvols demonstrated a high incidence of somatostatin receptors in surgically removed RCC specimens [21]. Twenty-eight of 39 RCC tumor specimens were somatostatin receptor positive. They speculated that this could have diagnostic and therapeutic consequences in RCC patients.

However, subsequent in vivo studies with ^{111}In-pentreotide (Octreoscan®) scintigraphy showed conflicting results. Initially, Flamen et al. performed imaging studies in a small series of patients with metastatic disease and their primary RCCs still in situ [22]. Three out of seven primary lesions could be detected whereas 20/23 known metastases were visualized. Results of Edgren et al. showed just the opposite: most primary lesions were ^{111}In-Octreoscan positive (9/11), while only 40 out of 68 (59%) known metastases were detected [23]. In the already-mentioned study performed by Montravers et al. it was suggested that somatostatin receptor scintigraphy with ^{111}In-Octreoscan had little value for detection of RCC metastases, since most metastatic lesions were missed [16]. Furthermore, most primary RCC lesions (n= 13) also did not show uptake. Only a small (<4 cm) primary RCC lesion could be detected with ^{111}In-Octreoscan. Interestingly, in one patient with a "cold" lesion in vivo, somatostatine receptor-positive labeling of the surgically removed tumor was demonstrated by in vitro autoradiography. The authors concluded that the very large tumors in their series were in vivo "inaccessible" for the radiopharmaceutical, since uptake of ^{201}Tl, a tumor-seeking radiopharmaceutical depending on blood flow, was also absent. However, the authors do not explain this "inaccessibility" further. One might think of tumor-related factors, such as large necrotic areas, increased interstitial pressure in the tumor, absent or low receptor expression density, besides other (patient) related factors.

Role of Experimental Monoclonal Antibodies

As part of the search for new treatment modalities for advanced RCC, several monoclonal antibodies (mAbs) targeting different antigens expressed on renal carcinoma cells

(a)

(b)

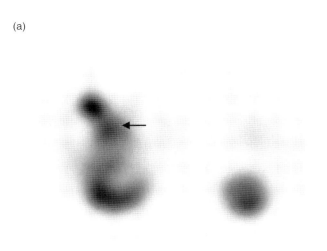

Fig. 8.1 Example of a clear cell RCC lesion imaged with[111]In-Octreoscan. Single-photon emission computed tomography (SPECT) transaxial image of abdomen showing pathological uptake in a renal mass in the right kidney (arrow), and physiological excretion via kidneys and gall bladder (a). Corresponding transaxial CT image (b)

have been developed. When labeled with a radionuclide that emits gamma rays, these radiolabeled mAbs could also be used for diagnosing renal masses or staging of RCC (Fig. 8.2). In practice, radioimmunoscintigraphy (RIS) is usually performed before radioimmunotherapy (RIT) to establish whether there is sufficient uptake of the radiolabeled mAbs in metastatic RCC lesions and/or to perform dosimetric calculations. Some of these experimental mAbs have been used in clinical studies, although these mAbs have not been specifically tested for the in vivo discrimination between a benign and a malignant renal mass.

mAb G250 and mAb MN-75 both target the carbonic anhydrase IX (CA 9)/G250 antigen which is overexpressed in the majority of clear cell RCCs [24–28]. However, different epitopes of the CA 9/G250 antigen are targeted by these two mAbs. Whereas mAb MN-75 has not been tested in humans thus far, there is experience with mAb cG250 in several clinical settings; e.g., both the murine and the murine/human chimeric forms of mAb G250 have been tested in patients with their primary RCCs still in situ (n=16 for both studies) [29, 30]. Specific localization of mAb G250 in G250-positive RCC tumors was demonstrated and primary tumors were clearly visualized. Most clear cell RCCs are G250-positive, whereas most other subtypes of RCC are usually not G250-positive [28–30]. Thus, mAb G250 is likely a very specific radiopharmaceutical for the detection of primary clear cell RCC, but, as stated earlier, no real data on sensitivity, specificity, and accuracy for the characterization of a renal mass are available.

In Minneapolis, several mAbs targeting RCC antigens have been developed of which mAb 6AH – that later

became known to recognize a cluster differentiation antigen (CD26) – looked the most promising [31–34]. Unfortunately, clinical RIS and RIT studies were hampered by unexpected fast clearance of the radiolabeled mAb [31]. Yet another mAb, mAb CE7, recognizes L1-CAM, a cell adhesion molecule present in neuroblastoma and also in a subset of RCCs [35, 36]. Like mAb MN-75, mAb CE7 has not yet been tested in humans thus far. Obviously, since these mAbs are not generally available, they do not play a role in the routine management of RCC patients.

Staging and Restaging of Patients with Suspected or Proven Renal Cell Carcinoma

Similar to the limited role in lesion characterization, the role of nuclear medicine techniques to stage and restage patients with renal cancer is also limited. The only nuclear medicine technique that for years has been applied to stage or restage patients with suspected or proven RCC is ^{99m}Tc-bone scintigraphy for the assessment of osseous metastasis. This is accepted clinical routine, although bone scintigraphy does, like most diagnostic tools, not have a perfect sensitivity and specificity score. Other techniques applied in routine practice to detect osseous metastases are CT and MRI. Since the introduction of ^{18}F-FDG-PET several reports with varying patient numbers for staging and restaging of suspected or proven RCC have been published. However, ^{18}F-FDG-PET has not earned a place in the routine work-up of these patients thus far, and most patients are staged with X-chest, CT, and,

(a)   (b)

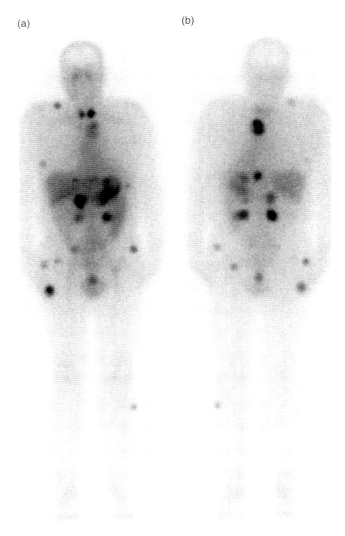

Fig. 8.2 Radioiodinated monoclonal antibody cG250 (^{131}I-cG250) uptake in a patient with numerous soft tissue RCC metastases, anterior (a) and posterior (b) planar images [56]

less frequently, with MRI and ultrasound. Lastly, a few studies regarding the performances of the experimental mAbs to detect metastases have been reported. However, most of these studies were designed as experimental therapy studies and not as primarily diagnostic studies. The value of the various nuclear medicine techniques for (re)staging of patients with RCC will be discussed in more detail in this section.

Bone-Seeking Radiopharmaceuticals

Role of Diphosphonates

Bone scintigraphy is usually performed with ^{99m}Tc-methylene diphosphonate (MDP), or less frequently with ^{99m}Tc-hydroxymethane diphosphonate (HDP) or [99m]Tc-

dicarboxypropane diphosphonate (DPD) (Fig. 8.3). The radiolabeled diphosphonates selectively localize at sites with increased bone formation, e.g., increased osteoblastic activity. The advantage of bone scintigraphy with these compounds is that it is highly sensitive to demonstrate bone pathology, whereas in general, its specificity is lower because various benign and malignant bone diseases may show elevated uptake on bone scintigraphy. A problem is that the predominantly osteolytic lesions of RCC may not be detected with bone scintigraphy because of a relative lack of increased osteoblastic activity in these areas.

In the last decade several authors have asked the question whether a bone scan should routinely be performed in the diagnostic work-up for patients with RCC to detect bone metastases. Henriksson et al. evaluated 102 consecutive patients that were treated for RCC [37]. Preoperatively, 33 patients (32%) had metastatic spread. However, only six patients (6%) had bone metastases that were found first with skeletal radiography due to local symptoms. They concluded that bone scintigraphy performed routinely in symptomless patients had no added value [37]. Staudenherz et al. assessed the diagnostic performance of bone scintigraphy in a selected series of RCC patients with a high pretest probability for bone metastases due to abnormal laboratory tests, pain, or confirmed nonosseous metastases [38]. In 14 of 36 patients skeletal metastases were confirmed with either CT, MRI, or biopsies. The bone scans were semiquantified for lesion location and intensity (cold, faint, hot). Depending on the applied visual threshold, the sensitivity of bone scintigraphy in this patient population (prevalence of bone metastases 39%) varied between 7 and 79% [38]. In a larger series of 205 patients Koga et al. also retrospectively evaluated the benefit of performing bone scans in all patients that presented with RCC [39]. Only a minority of the patients (n=56) had an abnormal bone scan of which less than 60% (n=32) indeed proved to have osseous metastases. Overall, the sensitivity and specificity of bone scintigraphy reached in their series as high as 94 and 86%, respectively (prevalence of bone metastases 17%). Furthermore, they concluded that bone scans can safely be omitted in patients with T1-2N0M0 disease and patients with T3aN0M0 disease without bone pain, since in their series in these cases the incidence of missed bone metastases was less than 5% [39]. This is partly in line with the analysis by Shvarts et al. of the large database of patients (n=1,357) that underwent nephrectomy and/or immunotherapy at the University of California-Los Angeles [40]. They, too, found that the incidence of osseous metastases increased with T stage: 5, 14, 15, and 28% for T1–4 tumors, respectively. However, if relying on locally advanced disease, bone pain, alkaline phosphatase, or extraosseous metastases to perform bone scans preoperatively, a substantial number of patients with bone metastases would have been missed; 22, 27, 45, and 27% of the cases, for T1–4 respectively [40].

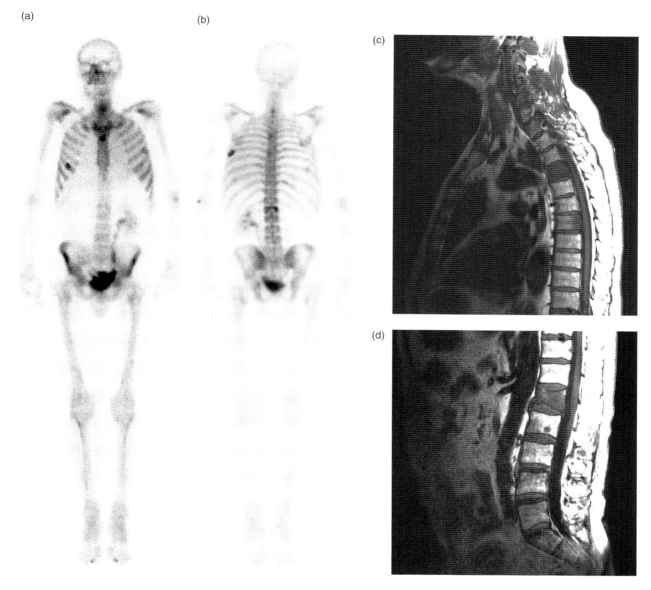

Fig. 8.3 ^{99m}Tc-MDP scintigraphy showing skeletal RCC metastases in ribs and vertebrae, anterior (a) and posterior (b) planar images. More metastatic lesions in the spine are visualized with sagittal T1-weighed MRI images (c, d): Th4, Th7, L1 (all visible with ^{99m}Tc-MDP (B)), and L2 (missed on bone scan). Patient underwent a right-sided nephrectomy

They identified a patient's performance status as the only criterion to correctly predict the absence of bone lesions. In patients with an excellent performance status of Eastern Cooperative Oncology Group (ECOG) 0, the prevalence of osseous metastases was only 1.4%. Therefore, Shvarts et al. [40] suggested to perform bone scans in patients with ECOG > 0 regardless of T stage. Preferably, this needs validation in the general population of patients with RCC, since the study was performed at a tertiary referral center [40].

Others have investigated whether there is a relationship between the level of serum alkaline phosphatase and the presence or absence of bone metastases as detected by bone scintigraphy. In several studies it was concluded that alkaline phosphatase is not a good prognosticator in these patients [38–43]. The majority of patients with an elevated alkaline phosphatase do not show osseous metastases with bone scintigraphy and most patients with bone metastases have normal alkaline phosphatase levels [42, 43].

In conclusion, most authors agree that bone scintigraphy should not be routinely performed in patients with RCC. Only in selected patients, based on presence of bone pain, elevated serum alkaline phosphatase, and nonosseous metastases, or performance status ECOG > 0 bone scintigraphy may be of additional value [40, 41].

Role of ^{18}F-Sodium Fluoride

For assessment of bone metastases another bone-seeking PET radiopharmaceutical can be used: ^{18}F-labeled sodium fluoride (^{18}F-NaF) (Fig. 8.4). Recently, there is renewed interest in this radiopharmaceutical. Although not used or studied as extensively as the ^{99m}Tc-labeled diphosphonates, like these, ^{18}F-NaF also seems to suffer from lack of specificity [44]. However, sensitivity is increased due to the better spatial resolution that can be achieved with the PET technique compared to single-photon gamma emission scintigraphy, and more favorable pharmacokinetics of ^{18}F-NaF compared to the radiolabeled diphosphonates [44]. It has been suggested that the increased sensitivity of ^{18}F-NaF-PET is mainly due to an increased sensitivity for predominantly osteolytic bone metastases, as is usually the case in metastatic RCC [44]. Thusfar, there are no reports of the use of ^{18}F-NaF-PET for the detection of osseous metastases in RCC patients.

Role of ^{18}F-Fluorodeoxyglucose

Although ^{18}F-FDG is not as specific as the ^{99m}Tc-MDP or ^{18}F-NaF for localization in bone, and strictly not "bone-seeking", ^{18}F-FDG is known to be capable of the detection of osseous metastases in various malignancies. Wu et al. were the first to directly compare ^{99m}Tc-MDP scintigraphy with ^{18}F-FDG-PET in 18 patients with biopsy-proven RCC [45]. On either scan a total of 52 bone lesions were identified. Lesions were confirmed histopathologically or with clinical and radiological follow-up of at least 1 year. Forty lesions proved to be malignant and 12 benign. ^{99m}Tc-MDP bone scan was false-negative in 9 lesions (5 patients) and false-positive in 12 lesions (7 patients). This resulted in a sensitivity and accuracy of 78 and 60%, respectively, for bone scintigraphy. It should be noted that the ^{99m}Tc-MDP bone scan was read rather sensitive and not very specific, in respect of the fact that all lesions with increased uptake were called metastatic lesions. It is often possible due to the pattern of

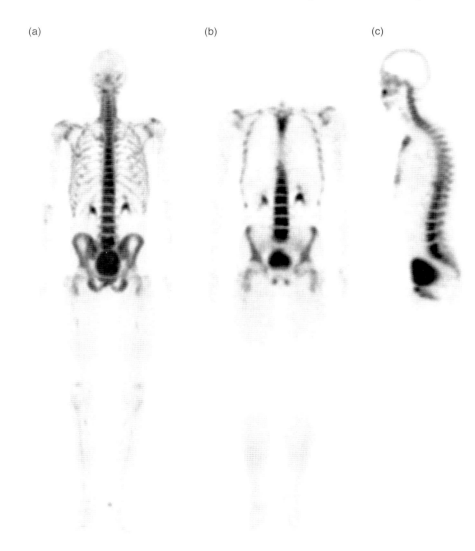

Fig. 8.4 Whole-body PET images with ^{18}F-sodium fluoride (^{18}F-NaF), a bone-seeking radiopharmaceutical showing a normal distribution pattern. Projection (a), coronal (b), and sagital images (c)

increased ^{99m}Tc-MDP uptake to differentiate more precisely between malignant and degenerative lesions. On the contrary, ^{18}F-FDG-PET correctly identified all lesions resulting in a sensitivity and accuracy of 100 and 100%, respectively [45]. These results are partly in line with the observations of Kang et al., who also noted a relatively high sensitivity (77%) with ^{18}F-FDG-PET for the detection of bone metastases compared to other sites with RCC metastases [5]. However, in the latter study, the sensitivity of combined CT and ^{99m}Tc-MDP scintigraphy was still higher (94%) [5]. Also, Brouwers et al. observed a relatively high detection rate of bone metastases with ^{18}F-FDG-PET: of 34 known skeletal RCC lesions, 29 (85%) were detected with ^{18}F-FDG [46].

Based on these few observations it may be that ^{18}F-FDG-PET is superior to ^{99m}Tc-MDP scintigraphy for the detection of osseous metastases. This needs further confirmation. Also, what the exact role of ^{18}F-FDG-PET is in comparison to other imaging techniques (CT, MRI, with or without the combination of ^{99m}Tc-MDP bone scan) or whether ^{18}F-FDG-PET can replace ^{99m}Tc-MDP bone scintigraphy in selected patients that need evaluation for bone involvement should be topics for further research.

^{18}F-Fluorodeoxyglucose – Positron Emission Tomography

One of the potential major advantages of the use of ^{18}F-FDG-PET for staging and restaging of cancer patients is that it provides a whole-body analysis in one examination, although areas with high physiological ^{18}F-FDG uptake such as the brain and the urinary tract are less evaluable for malignant disease. Especially the latter may cause uncertainty while interpreting ^{18}F-FDG-PET scans in patients with RCC. Despite this potential drawback, several studies have been published describing the role of ^{18}F-FDG-PET in (re)staging patients with suspected or proven RCC.

Local Recurrence and Locoregional Lymph Node Metastases

After nephrectomy, local recurrence may occur in up to 5% of the RCC patients. Post-treatment tissue changes can be difficult to differentiate from viable recurrence tissue via CT or MRI, so this may be more accurately assessed with ^{18}F-FDG-PET (Fig. 8.5).

A few reports have been published describing the performance of ^{18}F-FDG-PET in detecting local recurrences (Table 8.2). Case reports are published by Montravers et al. and Ramdave et al. regarding the detection of local recurrence with ^{18}F-FDG-PET [6, 7]. Montravers et al. described

two patients in whom ^{18}F-FDG-PET scan correctly identified a local recurrence and one with an incomplete removal of a RCC, while CT scan findings were either equivocal or normal [7]. Comparable good results were demonstrated by Ramdave et al.: three patients underwent ^{18}F-FDG-PET scanning for the detection of local recurrence [6]. In three patients ^{18}F-FDG uptake was increased in the renal bed, while CT was normal in one case and suggestive of radiation necrosis in the second case. In the third patient, CT scan also showed a mass in the renal bed. Based on these small patient numbers, the authors find it likely that ^{18}F-FDG-PET may be superior to CT for the detection of local recurrences.

On the other hand, in the largest patient series so far (73 follow-up PET scans in 49 patients), Kang et al. showed with ^{18}F-FDG-PET a sensitivity of 75% and specificity of 100% for retroperitoneal lymph node metastases and/or renal bed recurrence [5]. However, CT abdomen was more sensitive (93%) and as specific (98%). Therefore, the routine use of ^{18}F-FDG-PET after nephrectomy is discouraged by this group [5]. Unfortunately, separate data on the detection of local recurrence versus locoregional lymph node metastases with ^{18}F-FDG-PET are not given by this group.

In the case of locoregional lymph node metastases, CT and MRI are dependent on the artificial size criterion to discriminate between benign or malignant tissue. It has been shown that preoperative enlarged lymph nodes (CT criterion > 1 cm) not always harbor metastatic disease (42% in the study of Studer et al.) [47]. Since ^{18}F-FDG-PET is based on a difference in glucose metabolism between benign and malignant tissues, potentially this may be an advantage of the PET technique over the other techniques to stage the locoregional lymph nodes. However, it should be kept in mind that the benefit of locoregional lymph node dissection for improvement of patients' survival is not yet clear [48–50].

Data on the performance of ^{18}F-FDG-PET for detecting locoregional lymph node metastases are also scarce (Table 8.2). Probably the largest series addressing this issue is a German study of 29 patients with 26 proven RCCs and 3 benign renal lesions in which the ^{18}F-FDG uptake in the regional lymph nodes was systematically scored in addition to the primary renal lesion [2]. They reported 25 truly negatives, 3 truly positives, 1 false-positive and no false-negatives in staging of the lymph nodes. However, these were primarily low-stage tumors, and no data on the performance of CT or MRI on the detection of lymph nodes were reported.

In conclusion, based on these scarce data, the exact value of ^{18}F-FDG-PET in comparison to CT and/or MRI for the detection of local regional spread at initial staging and the recurrence of local disease at restaging has still not been determined. Therefore, currently ^{18}F-FDG-PET should not be routinely performed in RCC patients for these indications.

Perhaps, the advantage of ^{18}F-FDG-PET is its high specificity in cases in which it is unclear from other imaging modalities whether there is a local recurrence or not: Enhanced ^{18}F-FDG uptake is subsequently very suspicious for local recurrence. However, this preferably needs confirmation in studies with larger patient numbers.

Distant Metastases

More studies have investigated whether patients could be correctly staged or restaged with ^{18}F-FDG-PET for detecting distant metastases (Tables 8.3 and 8.4) (Fig. 8.5). First reports in small numbers of RCC patients showed merely the

(a)

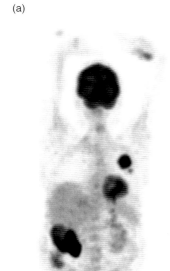

(b)

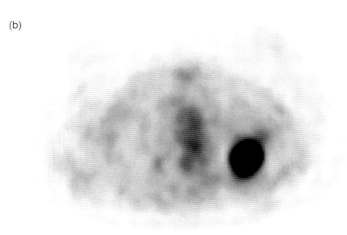

(c)

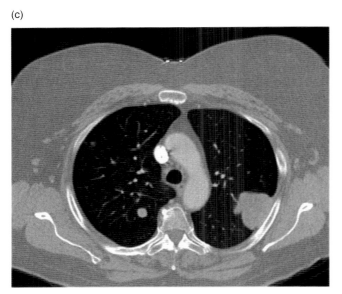

(d)

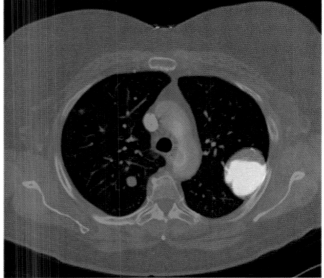

Fig. 8.5 Whole-body ^{18}F-FDG-PET image of a patient with a right-sided local recurrence and lung lesions (a, b). However, more lung lesions are visualized on the CT-chest (c). Image fusion of a transaxial slice of the FDG-PET and the CT scan (d)

Table 8.2 Detection of local recurrence and/or locoregional lymph node metastases of RCC with ^{18}F-FDG

Reference	No of pts	Indication (no of pts)	True-positive	True-negative	False-negative	False-positive
Wahl et al. [1]	5	Staging locoregional (lymph node) metastases	2 (lymph node, renal vein and inferior vena cava) (renal vein only)	3	0	0
Bachor et al. [2]	29	Staging locoregional lymph node metastases	3	25	0	1
Ak and Can [8]*	19	Staging locoregional lymph node metastases (15)	2	12	1 (lymph node)	0
Montravers et al. [7]*	22	Restaging local recurrence (3)	2	1	0	0
Montravers et al. [7]	22	Staging (locoregional) lymph node metastases (2)	2	0	0	0
Ramdave et al. [6]	25	Staging locoregional metastases (17)	1 (lymph node, CT false-negative)	15	1 (renal vein, CT false-negative)	0
Ramdave et al. [6]	25	Restaging local recurrence (3)	3 (CT inconclusive)	0	0	0
Kang et al. [5]	66	Local recurrence and/or locoregional lymph node metastases (49)	^{18}F-FDG: sens=75%, spec=100%		CT: sens=93% spec=98%	

*Performed using coincidence detection gamma camera.

Table 8.3 Patient-based detection of distant metastases of RCC with ^{18}F-FDG.

Reference	No of pts	Indication (no of pts)	True-positive	True-negative	False-negative	False-positive
Wahl et al. [1]	5	Primary staging	1	4	0	0
Montravers et al. [7]*	22	Primary staging (12)	5	7	0	0
Montravers et al. [7]*	22	Restaging (7)	4	3	0	0
Ramdave et al. [6]	25	Primary staging (17)	2 (unsuspected on CT)	15	0	0
Ramdave et al. [6]	25	Restaging (8)	5	3 (1 false-positive on CT)	0	0
Safaei et al. [51]	36	Restaging	27	5	4	0
Aide et al. [4]	53	Primary staging (35) and early restaging (18)	10 (2 false-negative on CT)	40 (4 false-positive on CT)	0	3 (2 pulmonary infections, 1 physiological ureteral uptake)
Kang et al. [5]	66	Restaging (54)	Lesion-based analysis per body-region only, see Table 8.4			
Jadvar et al. [53]	25	Restaging	15 (2 more lesions on PET compared to CT)	3	6 (lung, mediastinal, adrenal, lytic bone metastases)	1 (lumbar facet arthropathy)
Majhail et al. [52]	24	Restaging	12	3 (in all CT false-positive)	9 (lung, chest wall, mediastinal, adrenal, brain metastases)	0

*Performed using coincidence detection gamma camera.

Table 8.4 Lesion-based detection of distant metastases of RCC with ^{18}F-FDG

Reference	No of ls	Verification	Imaging	Location of metastatic RCC	TP	TN	FN	FP	sens, spec, acc, PPV, NPV
Safaei et al. [51]	25	biopsy proven	PET	–	15	6	2	2	88%, 75%, 84%
			CT	–	15	0	2	8	88%, 0%,60%
Brouwers et al. [46]	112	Follow-up	PET	bone	–	–	–	–	85%
			^{131}I-cG250						47%
			PET	thoracic (lung, pleural, mediastinal)					59%
			^{131}I-cG250						19%
			PET	abdominal (organs, local recurrence, lymph nodes)					56%
			^{131}I-cG250						19%
			PET	soft tissue (extremities, lymph nodes head and neck)					89%
			^{131}I-cG250						56%
Aide et al. [4]	–	biopsy proven/ follow-up	PET	thoracic (lung, mediastinal) and extrathoracic (skeleton, liver, abdomen other than liver)	–	–	–	–	100%, 99%, 99%
			CT						68%, 98%, 96%
Kang et al. [5]	126	biopsy proven/ follow-up	PET	contralateral kidney, second primary	–	–	–	–	50%, 99%
			CT						100%, 99%
			PET	Lung parenchyma					75%, 97%
			CT						91%, 73%
			PET	Mediastinal/hilar lymph nodes					69%, 98%
			CT						88%, 95%
			PET	Liver					62%, 100%
			CT						77%, 94%
			PET	All other soft tissue sites					65%, 97%, –, 98%, 30%
			CT						69%, 93%
			PET	Skeleton					77%, 100%, –, 100%, 93%
			CT/bone scan						94%, 87%
Jadvar et al. [53]	–	follow-up	PET	–	–	–	–	–	71%, 75%, 72%, 94%, 33%
Majhail et al. [52]	37	biopsy proven	PET	Overall	22	3	12	0	64%, 100%, 67%, 100%, 20%
				Lesion size > 1 cm					76%
				Lesion size > 1.5 cm					83%
				Lesion size > 2 cm					93%
				Lung parenchyma (n= 19)					63%, –, –, 100% (12 of 12)

feasibility of detecting distant metastases [6, 7]. In the only prospective study Aide et al. staged 53 patients before or just after (partial) nephrectomy [4]. This early staging resulted in no detection of distant metastases by ^{18}F-FDG-PET and CT in 36 patients (M0 disease). In two patients ^{18}F-FDG-PET correctly discovered disseminated disease missed by CT. In eight patients known with distant RCC lesions, all lesions were also detected with ^{18}F-FDG-PET and additionally five more lesions in three patients. In four patients ^{18}F-FDG-PET proved to be true-negative with false-positive CT scans, whereas in three patients the PET scan was falsely positive with true-negative CT scans. For the ^{18}F-FDG-PET scan this resulted in a sensitivity of 100%, specificity of 93%, and an accuracy of 94% for the detection (patient-based) of distant metastases. For the CT scan, these figures were 80, 91, and 89%, respectively (Table 8.3). The authors concluded that indeed ^{18}F-FDG-PET offers no advantage over CT for the characterization of a renal mass, but that it appears to be an efficient tool for the detection of distant metastases of RCC [4].

Safaei et al. restaged 36 patients with ^{18}F-FDG-PET and compared the PET results with other imaging studies and biopsies of 25 lesions in 20 patients [51]. Before the PET study, 4 patients had no evidence of disseminated disease, whereas the other 32 patients were suspected of having metastases. ^{18}F-FDG-PET correctly upstaged one out of four patients in the first group. In the second group 2 out of 32 patients were correctly downstaged, whereas 4 out of 32 were wrongly downstaged by PET (Table 8.3). Overall, with ^{18}F-FDG-PET the accuracy of classifying patient stage was 89% (32/36 patients) with a sensitivity of 87% and a specificity of 100%. Of the 25 suspected lesions that were biopsied, 17 proved to be malignant and 8 were benign. PET was correct in 21 of these lesions (accuracy 84%) with a sensitivity of 88% and a specificity of 75% (Table 8.4). The authors' conclusion was that PET can be useful in the characterization of anatomic lesions of unknown significance in patients with RCC [51]. However, Majhail and colleagues concluded just the opposite that ^{18}F-FDG-PET is not a sensitive imaging modality for the evaluation of metastatic RCC in a comparable study [52]. Before PET scanning was performed, in 24 patients 36 distant metastatic sites were identified with conventional imaging. Afterward, pathology for all sites was obtained by biopsy or surgical resection. Distant RCC metastases were histologically proven in 33 sites in 21 patients. PET was true-positive in 21 sites and false-negative in 12 sites. Mostly, lung lesions were missed with ^{18}F-FDG-PET. There were no false-positive PET scans. This resulted in an overall sensitivity, specificity, positive predictive value, and accuracy of 64, 100, 100, and 67%, respectively, for the detection (lesion-based) of distant metastases with ^{18}F-FDG-PET (Table 8.4). Furthermore, the authors analyzed the size of the metastases.

Not surprisingly, they noticed a significant difference in size between true-positive and false-negative PET lesions: mean size of 2.2 cm versus 1.0 cm, respectively [52]. The results of Majhail et al. were confirmed by Jadvar et al., although not biopsy-proven in most cases [52, 53]. In the latter study, 25 patients underwent ^{18}F-FDG-PET scanning for restaging and PET results were compared to CT scans. Diagnostic validation was mostly clinical and with follow-up via imaging for up to 1 year. PET was concordant with CT in most cases (n= 18) and discordant in 7. In one case PET was considered false-positive due to lumbar facet arthropathy, whereas in six patients PET was false-negative. No enhanced ^{18}F-FDG uptake was noticed in pulmonary (n= 4), mediastinal (n= 2), adrenal (n= 1), and lytic osseous metastases (n= 2). This resulted in a sensitivity of 71%, specificity of 75%, accuracy of 72%, positive predictive value of 94%, and a negative predictive value of 33% (Table 8.4). Thus, according to the authors, a positive ^{18}F-FDG-PET study is highly suspicious for malignancy, whereas a negative PET scan does not exclude metastatic disease [53].

The largest series to date has been described by Kang et al. [5]. In 66 patients in total 90 ^{18}F-FDG-PET scans were performed because of suspected or known RCC. The authors report the detection capabilities of ^{18}F-FDG-PET compared to CT on a lesion-based analysis (n=126) per region/organ system (Table 8.4). In all sites, the sensitivity of ^{18}F-FDG-PET was lower compared to CT. However, the specificity of ^{18}F-FDG-PET was superior to CT in all regions. Interestingly, they noticed that within a single patient multiple metastases showed differing levels of metabolic activity, as has also been observed by Brouwers et al. and which may have implications for prognosis, therapy, and monitoring response (see on Prognostic Value and Prediction of Response to Therapy paragraph) [5, 46]. Also, in both series detection of bone metastases is relatively high (77 and 85%, respectively), as has been mentioned previously, while the reported detection rates are lower and differ more widely for other body regions (Table 8.4). Furthermore, both Kang et al. and Aide et al. observed that ^{18}F-FDG-PET was much more sensitive to detect metastases than primary tumors (Tables 8.1 and 8.4) [4, 5]. This again supports that this technique should not be applied to characterize primary renal lesions.

Based on the currently published reports, it can be concluded that ^{18}F-FDG-PET is not yet recommended for routine application for the detection of metastatic RCC. Due to the relatively low sensitivity, a negative ^{18}F-FDG-PET study does not rule out metastatic disease. Also, it should be emphasized that lesion size appears to be an important factor regarding the sensitivity of ^{18}F-FDG-PET; only a sensitivity of >90% of lesions > 2 cm corresponds with reported sensitivities of CT (Table 8.4) [52]. For smaller lesions sensitivity drops accordingly (Table 8.4) [52]. On the other hand, several authors agree on the high specificity of ^{18}F-FDG-PET compared to CT. Therefore, currently this technique may be advocated as a problem-solving tool in cases in which other imaging modalities show inconclusive results for specific lesions: When ^{18}F-FDG uptake in these lesions is high, most likely, it is a recurrent RCC disease. Perhaps, in the future when combined PET-CT scanners have become more available, the sensitivity and specificity for the detection of metastatic RCC can be increased due to the combined presumed advantages of both imaging techniques. To date, no paper has been published on this matter in patients with RCC.

Clinical Management

Although the reported series with ^{18}F-FDG-PET in RCC patients were not primarily designed as clinical management studies, several authors have studied the effect of the ^{18}F-FDG-PET scan on clinical management [4–6, 51]. In the only prospective study by Aide et al. treatment was altered in 5 of 53 (9%) patients [4]. This is in line with the reported low percentages of changes in management because of the ^{18}F-FDG-PET scans by Kang et al. (12 of 90 scans (13%)) and Safaei et al. (3 of 36 scans (8%)) [5, 51]. Only Ramdave et al. described a direct change in treatment due to the ^{18}F-FDG-PET scan in 35% of their patients for primary staging and 50% for restaging [6]. However, especially in the latter group, the patient number was very small, 17 versus 8 patients, respectively.

Therefore, more research regarding the true clinical impact of ^{18}F-FDG-PET scans and/or the use of combined PET-CT scanners in patients with RCC is warranted.

Role of Experimental Monoclonal Antibodies

As mentioned in the first paragraph, scintigraphic studies with radiolabeled mAbs are usually performed within the framework of RIT studies. A low-activity radiolabeled mAb dose preceding a therapeutic (high) dose is often administered to determine sufficient uptake in metastatic lesions and to generate dosimetric data: how much radiation-dose is absorbed in the body, specific organs, and known metastases. Also, after high doses of radiolabeled mAbs scintigraphic images are recorded, which serve again, among others, to visualize tumor lesions. Experiences with the only clinically applied mAb G250 in RCC patients have been described in the literature, although most studies were not primarily designed for diagnostic detection of RCC metastases. These studies are highly experimental, since only few groups worldwide have this mAb at their disposal. Obviously, these do not play a role in the routine management of RCC patients.

Initially, the murine form of mAb G250 labeled with ^{131}I was used [29, 54]. In a protein-dose escalation study with low activity-dose ^{131}I-mG250 Oosterwijk et al. reported visualization of > 90% of primary and metastatic RCC lesions known from previous CT and MRI scans and the detection of additional metastases later confirmed at surgery [29]. In the subsequent phase I/II activity–dose escalation study performed by Divgi et al. all RCC lesions > 2 cm were visualized, and also smaller subcutaneous metastases were detected [54]. However, the number of missed lesions is unknown. Also, Steffens et al. reported visualization of all known RCC metastases (n=5) in a protein-dose escalation study with the human-mouse chimeric mAb ^{131}I-cG250 [30]. In the subsequent activity–dose escalation study with ^{131}I-cG250, metastases were adequately visualized in 9 of 12 patients and 4 new lesions in 3 patients were detected, confirmed radiologically [55]. Also, metastases were visualized after injection of both the low-dose and the high-dose activity of ^{131}I-cG250. This is in line with the subsequent phase I/II trial performed by Brouwers et al. in which two high-dose ^{131}I-cG250 injections were given to patients with a 3-monthly interval and both therapeutic injections were preceded by a low-dose ^{131}I-cG250 injection [56]. In general, the metastases were more clearly visualized on the images after the high-dose injection compared with the diagnostic scintigraphic images and in most cases the scans were congruent. In some patients, however, additional metastatic lesions were detected on the post high-dose images, especially in the chest. Furthermore, ^{131}I-cG250 detected new metastatic lesions, especially if located outside the field of view of routine radiological techniques. On the other hand, not all previously known metastatic lesions were visualized with ^{131}I-cG250 [56].

Since from the previous studies iodinated mAb G250 seemed rather sensitive and specific for the detection of RCC metastases, Brouwers et al. conducted a diagnostic imaging study to compare ^{18}F-FDG-PET with radioimmunoscintigraphy with ^{131}I-cG250 [46]. In 20 patients, in total 112 RCC lesions were detected with these scintigraphic techniques and with routinely performed radiological studies (CT, MRI, and ultrasound). The detection rate of RCC metastases was only 30% with ^{131}I-cG250, compared to 69% with ^{18}F-FDG and 71% for the combined routinely used imaging techniques (Table 8.4) [46]. The reason for the relatively low observed detection rate with ^{131}I-cG250 is not clear, but the patient population was highly selected. Most patients had end-stage, rapid progressive disease, which may have negatively influenced the G250 antigen expression on the metastases, partly explaining these results [28, 46]. Also, the used radionuclide in this study may not have been optimal. In subsequent studies, Brouwers et al. showed that internalizing radiolabeled mAb cG250 complexes, such as [111]In-, [177]Lu-, or

(a)   (b)

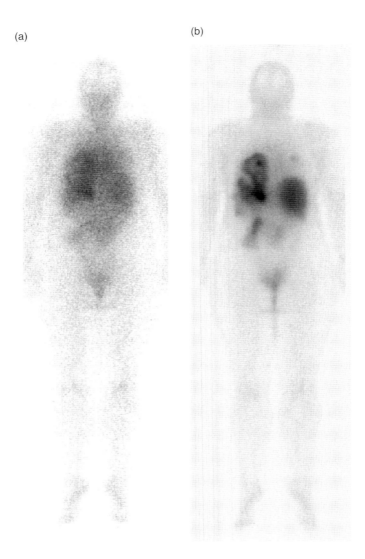

Fig. 8.6 Radioimmunoscintigraphy with mAb cG250 labeled with [131]I (^{131}I-cG250, A) or [111]In (^{111}In-SCN-DTPA-cG250, B) within the same patient, posterior views. RCC metastatic lesions in the lungs are more clearly visualized with ^{111}In-cG250 than ^{131}I-cG250 [57]. Physiological uptake in liver, spleen, and intestines

[90]Y-labeled cG250, may show higher detection rates for RCC metastases [57, 58] (Fig. 8.6). This needs further clinical confirmation.

Prognostic Value and Prediction of Response to Therapy

Not much data are available concerning whether molecular imaging techniques are helpful in informing on the prognosis of the (natural) course of metastatic RCC disease and in predicting or determining a response to anti-RCC therapy, such as can be the case in other tumor types with ^{18}F-FDG-PET (e.g., lymphoma and gastro-intestinal stroma cell

tumors (GIST)). Here the limited data that are available will be discussed.

It is known from RCC that the clinical course of the disease can be highly unpredictable with patients showing rapid progressive disease versus patients with a much more indolent course of their disease. Lang et al. studied the sensitivity of ^{18}F-FDG-PET in patients (n=46) with an indolent course of RCC and with a more aggressive form of the disease [59]. For these two groups on a patient-based analysis, the sensitivity of slow-growing RCC was 44% (7/16) versus 90% (27/30) for rapid-growing RCC. Interestingly, in a subset of these patients with predominantly high ^{18}F-FDG uptake in the RCC lesions and subsequently showing rapid progressive disease, the uptake of mAb ^{131}I-cG250 in the RCC metastases was mostly poor, as shown by Brouwers et al. [46]. mAb cG250 is directed against the CA 9/G250 antigen and is usually overexpressed in clear cell RCCs. It was speculated that rapid progressive RCCs are of higher grade and with lower G250 antigen expression [46]. Preferably, these observations need to be confirmed by others. In this light, the recent work of Bui et al. and Atkins et al. is of special interest [60, 61]. Both studied CA 9 expression on renal cell carcinoma specimens with mAb MN-75, which is also directed against the CA 9/G250 antigen. Bui et al. using immunohistochemical analysis with mAb MN-75 on tissue microarrays constructed from paraffin-embedded primary RCC tumors observed that decreased CA 9 levels are independently associated with poor survival in advanced RCC and stated that CA 9 is the most significant molecular marker for RCC cancer described to date [60]. The work of Atkins et al. expanded this observation and linked the clinical outcome and response to IL-2 therapy to the CA 9 expression levels of renal cancer tissue obtained from 66 patients: high-positively CA 9 staining of mostly primary RCC tumors correlated with a significantly better survival rate after IL-2 therapy [61].

It is tempting to hypothesize that prediction of response to therapy in the future may be assessed by scintigraphic imaging techniques visualizing non-invasively, for example, the CA 9/G250 antigen expression in individual patients and metastases [62]. The latter may also be of importance since it has been described that uptake of ^{18}F-FDG and radiolabeled mAb cG250 varies not only between patients, but also within the same patient, between metastatic lesions [46, 63]. Thus, the CA 9/G250 status, positive or negative, of the primary tumor may not always give the correct information about the CA 9/G250 status of RCC metastases and/or it may be that during the course of the disease RCC lesions change their antigen status (become CA 9/G250 negative) or their metabolism (from ^{18}F-FDG negative to ^{18}F-FDG positive). This may have implications for directing the patient toward an optimal treatment scheme. In this regard it is of interest that a new PET tracer targeting CA 9 has been recently developed and tested in vitro: ^{18}F-2,3,5,6-tetrafluoro-3'-sulfamoylbenzanilide (^{18}F-TFSB), a CA 9 inhibitor [64]. In the future, this may become another radiopharmaceutical to image non-invasively metastatic RCC lesions in patients.

Regarding prediction of response to therapy with ^{18}F-FDG-PET Hoh et al. reported preliminary data of RCC patients while being treated with IL-2-based therapy [65]. Whole-body PET images were scored as positive or negative for lesions and were compared to anatomical lesion size from various anatomical imaging techniques. In all patients (n=10) with clinically proven progressive disease ^{18}F-FDG-PET was positive whereas in only seven patients increase in lesion size was detected. ^{18}F-FDG-PET was negative in all five patients with absence of disease or complete response. In the patient with stable disease and in the five patients

with a partial response, mixed results were observed for ^{18}F-FDG-PET and anatomical imaging [65]. Kang et al. reported anecdotally on response assessed with ^{18}F-FDG-PET after a first course of immunotherapy on a lesion-based analysis from their large patient series (n=66) who underwent ^{18}F-FDG-PET scanning (n=90) [5]. All four lesions responding to immunotherapy were positive on ^{18}F-FDG-PET, whereas no PET-negative lesions responded to therapy. Based on the preliminary data of these studies, further clinical investigations are warranted concerning the prognostic value and assessment of response of ^{18}F-FDG-PET in a therapeutic setting for RCC with either immunotherapy (IL-2, IFN-α) or novel evolving treatments that are being tested recently with surprisingly good results in RCC patients (e.g., bevacizumab, a monoclonal antibody directed against vascular endothelial growth factor (VEGF) and the class of tyrosine kinase inhibitors such as sorafenib and sunitinib) [5, 65, 66].

Thus, it becomes clear that PET and other scintigraphic imaging techniques may have the advantage to inform on certain tumor characteristics such as glucose metabolism (^{18}F-FDG) or tumor receptor expression (CA 9/G250) of individual patients and even of individual metastases in patients in vivo, without the need to perform multiple biopsies, which are often clinically not feasible. This, in turn, may add to the prediction of the prognosis of individual patients noninvasively; it could help in the selection of the most appropriate anti-tumor therapy based on tumor characteristics (e.g., absence or presence of antigen expression), especially with the development of expensive but promising new anti-RCC drugs, and it could give information on the response of individual metastases to anti-tumor therapy. Clearly, further exploration in this area is warranted.

Conclusions

Regarding the role of various radionuclide imaging techniques in RCC, several conclusions can be drawn as discussed earlier.

For the classification of a renal mass, currently there are no radionuclide imaging techniques that play a role in the routine work-up of such patients. The most widely used radiopharmaceutical in oncology, ^{18}F-FDG, for PET seems to be hampered by lack of accuracy, as both sensitivity and specificity are suboptimal (range 32–100% and 75–100%, respectively). Also, no widely available single-photon-emitting radiopharmaceuticals target RCC selectively enough to have a role in this clinical setting. Unless pharmaceuticals for radionuclide imaging are being developed that specifically target RCC lesions with a high accuracy, the preferred method of identifying the nature of a renal mass is based on ultrasound, CT, and/or MRI scanning.

However, for the staging and restaging of patients with suspected or proven RCC ^{18}F-FDG-PET may play a role. In larger patient studies, the sensitivity of ^{18}F-FDG-PET for RCC lesions is less high compared to the sensitivity of CT (range 50–77% versus 69–100%, respectively). Especially small-size RCC lesions, e.g., nodules in the lung, are frequently not identified by ^{18}F-FDG-PET. However, the reported specificities of ^{18}F-FDG-PET for RCC lesions are usually as high or slightly higher than the reported figures of CT (75–100% versus 73–99%, respectively). Therefore, in cases of inconclusive results from other imaging techniques, ^{18}F-FDG-PET can be of value because of its high specificity. In this regard, also for (re)staging of RCC patients it is interesting to await the results of combined PET/CT scanners that arrive more and more in imaging departments. The high sensitivity of CT may then be combined with the high specificity of ^{18}F-FDG-PET. Furthermore, it should be noticed that data addressing the clinical impact of ^{18}F-FDG-PET in patient management or the cost-effectiveness of this technique in RCC patients are currently lacking.

Although for the detection of RCC metastases generally the sensitivity of ^{18}F-FDG-PET is lower than the sensitivity of CT, examination of the skeleton may be an exception. There are a few reports suggesting that the sensitivity of ^{18}F-FDG-PET for skeletal metastases of RCC is as high or even higher than the sensitivity of (combined) CT and bone scintigraphy with ^{99m}Tc-labeled diphosphonates (74 and 100% versus 78 and 94%, respectively). This needs to be further evaluated. Perhaps in the future, also for bone metastases of RCC, the sensitivity and specificity can be raised by combining a PET scan after an intravenous injection of ^{18}F-NaF, a PET radiopharmaceutical that attaches to bone similar to the ^{99m}Tc-labeled diphosphonates, with CT in one PET/CT modality. Also, this needs to be further evaluated. However, ^{18}F-NaF is currently not widely available.

For decades the most prominent nuclear medicine technique for the evaluation of the skeletal status of patients suspected of or with proven RCC has been bone scintigraphy with ^{99m}Tc-labeled diphosphonates. This technique should not be used routinely in all patients, since sensitivity and specificity are too low in patients without signs or symptoms that can be attributed to skeletal metastases. Sensitivity is relatively low in RCC metastases because these bone lesions are predominantly osteolytic. These lesions are better detected with MRI; however, a whole-body MRI is not generally available and not often made or advocated for this indication in daily practice.

Regarding assessment of prognosis and/or prediction of response to therapy in RCC patients, currently there is no role for ^{18}F-FDG or any other radiopharmaceutical due to insufficient data in the literature. Again, this may be addressed in future research. Of interest seems the development of a new PET radiopharmaceutical for more specific targeting of the RCC lesions by means of the CA 9/G250 antigen, which is overexpressed in the vast majority of clear cell RCCs, the most prevalent subtype of RCC.

Thus, in conclusion the role of radionuclide imaging in RCC is currently limited but may increase due to the development of new radiopharmaceuticals (for PET and/or single-photon emission techniques) and/or the development and/or increasing availability of new imaging techniques, e.g., PET/CT.

References

1. Wahl RL, Harney J, Hutchins G, et al. Imaging of renal cancer using positron emission tomography with 2-deoxy-2-(18F)-fluoro-D-glucose: pilot animal and human studies. J Urol. 1991;146:1470–4.
2. Bachor R, Kotzerke J, Gottfried HW, et al. Positron emission tomography in diagnosis of renal cell carcinoma. Urologe A. 1996;35:146–50.
3. Miyakita H, Tokunaga M, Onda H, et al. Significance of ^{18}F-fluorodeoxyglucose positron emission tomography (FDG-PET) for detection of renal cell carcinoma and immunohistochemical glucose transporter 1 (GLUT-1) expression in the cancer. Int J Urol. 2002;9:15–8.
4. Aide N, Cappele O, Bottet P, et al. Efficiency of [(18)F]FDG PET in characterising renal cancer and detecting distant metastases: a comparison with CT. Eur J Nucl Med Mol Imaging. 2003;30:1236–45.
5. Kang DE, White RL Jr, Zuger JH, et al. Clinical use of fluorodeoxyglucose F 18 positron emission tomography for detection of renal cell carcinoma. J Urol. 2004;171:1806–9.
6. Ramdave S, Thomas GW, Berlangieri SU, et al. Clinical role of F-18 fluorodeoxyglucose positron emission tomography for detection and management of renal cell carcinoma. J Urol. 2001;166:825–30.
7. Montravers F, Grahek D, Kerrou K, et al. Evaluation of FDG uptake by renal malignancies (primary tumor or metastases) using a coincidence detection gamma camera. J Nucl Med. 2000;41:78–84.
8. Ak I, Can C. F-18 FDG PET in detecting renal cell carcinoma. Acta Radiol. 2005;46:895–9.
9. Shreve P, Miyauchi T, Wahl RL. Characterization of Primary Renal Cell Carcinoma by FDG PET. Radiology. 1998;209:94P.
10. Blake MA, McKernan M, Setty B, et al. Renal Oncocytoma Displaying Intense Activity on ^{18}F-FDG PET. Am J Roentgenol. 2006;186:269–70.
11. Goldberg MA, Mayo Smith WW, Papanicolaou N, et al. FDG PET characterization of renal masses: preliminary experience. Clin Radiol. 1997;52:510–5.
12. Bosniak MA. The current radiological approach to renal cysts. Radiology. 1986;158:1–10.
13. Bosniak MA. Diagnosis and management of patients with complicated cystic lesions of the kidney. Am J Roentgenol. 1997;169:819–21.
14. WHO classification of tumours, pathology and genetics. Tumours of the urinary system and male genitale organs. Lyon: IARC Press; 2004.
15. Miyauchi T, Brown RS, Grossman HB, et al. Correlation between visualization of primary renal cancer by FDG-PET and histopathological findings. J Nucl Med. 1996;37:64P.
16. Montravers F, Rousseau C, Doublet JD, et al. In vivo inaccessibility of somatostatin receptors to ^{111}In-pentreotide in primary renal cell carcinoma. Nucl Med Commun. 1998;19:953–61.

17. Shreve P, Chiao PC, Humes HD, et al. Carbon-11-acetate PET imaging in renal disease. J Nucl Med. 1995;36:1595–601.

18. Shreve PD, Wahl RL. Carbon-11 acetate PET imaging of renal cell carcinoma. J Nucl Med. 1999;40:257P.

19. Langen KJ, Borner AR, Muller-Mattheis V, et al. Uptake of cis-4-[18F]fluoro-L-proline in urologic tumors. J Nucl Med. 2001;42:752–4.

20. Dittmann H, Dohmen BM, Paulsen F, et al. [18F]FLT PET for diagnosis and staging of thoracic tumours. Eur J Nucl Med Mol Imaging. 2003;30:1407–12.

21. Reubi JC, Kvols L. Somatostatin receptors in human renal cell carcinomas. Cancer Res. 1992;52:6074–8.

22. Flamen P, Bossuyt A, De Greve J, et al. Imaging of renal cell cancer with radiolabelled octreotide. Nucl Med Commun. 1993;14:873–7.

23. Edgren M, Westlin JE, Kalkner KM, et al. [111In-DPTA-D-Phe1]-octreotide scintigraphy in the management of patients with advanced renal cell carcinoma. Cancer Biother Radiopharm. 1999;14:59–64.

24. Oosterwijk E, Ruiter DJ, Hoedemaeker PJ, et al. Monoclonal antibody G 250 recognizes a determinant present in renal-cell carcinoma and absent from normal kidney. Int J Cancer. 1986;38:489–94.

25. Grabmaier K, Vissers JL, De Weijert MC, et al. Molecular cloning and immunogenicity of renal cell carcinoma- associated antigen G250. Int J Cancer. 2000;85:865–70.

26. Chrastina A, Pastorekova S, Pastorek J. Immunotargeting of human cervical carcinoma xenograft expressing CA IX tumor-associated antigen by (125)I-labeled M75 monoclonal antibody. Neoplasma. 2003;50:13–21.

27. Chrastina A, Zavada J, Parkkila S, et al. Biodistribution and pharmacokinetics of ^{125}I-labeled monoclonal antibody M75 specific for carbonic anhydrase IX, an intrinsic marker of hypoxia, in nude mice xenografted with human colorectal carcinoma. Int J Cancer. 2003;105:873–81.

28. Uemura H, Nakagawa Y, Yoshida K, et al. MN/CA IX/G250 as a potential target for immunotherapy of renal cell carcinomas. Br J Cancer. 1999;81:741–6.

29. Oosterwijk E, Bander NH, Divgi CR, et al. Antibody localization in human renal cell carcinoma: a phase I study of monoclonal antibody G250. J Clin Oncol. 1993;11:738–50.

30. Steffens MG, Boerman OC, Oosterwijk Wakka JC, et al. Targeting of renal cell carcinoma with iodine-131-labeled chimeric monoclonal antibody G250. J Clin Oncol. 1997;15:1529–37.

31. Vesella RL. Radioimmunoconjugates in renal cell carcinoma. In: Debruyne FM, Bukowski R, Pontes JE, editors. Immunotherapy of renal cell carcinoma. Heidelberg: Springer Verlag; 1991. pp. 38–46.

32. Chiou RK. Biodistribution and radioimmunoscintigraphy studies of renal cell carcinoma using tumor-preferential monoclonal antibodies and F(ab')2 fragments. J Urol. 1989;142:1584–8.

33. Lange PH, Vessella RL, Chiou RK, et al. Monoclonal antibodies in human renal cell carcinoma and their use in radioimmune localization and therapy of tumor xenografts. Surgery. 1985;98:143–50.

34. Hass GM, Meyer JL, Newitt RA, et al. Identification of the target of monoclonal antibody A6H as dipeptidyl peptidase IV/CD26 by LC MS\MS. Hybridoma. 2001;20:231–6.

35. Zimmermann K, Grunberg J, Honer M, et al. Targeting of renal carcinoma with (67/64)Cu-labeled anti-L1-CAM antibody chCE7: selection of copper ligands and PET imaging. Nucl Med Biol. 2003;30:417–27.

36. Meli ML, Carrel F, Waibel R, et al. Anti-neuroblastoma antibody chCE7 binds to an isoform of L1-CAM present in renal carcinoma cells. Int J Cancer. 1999;83:401–8.

37. Henriksson C, Haraldsson G, Aldenborg F, et al. Skeletal metastases in 102 patients evaluated before surgery for renal cell carcinoma. Scand J Urol Nephrol. 1992;26:363–6.

38. Staudenherz A, Steiner B, Puig S, et al. Is there a diagnostic role for bone scanning of patients with a high pretest probability for metastatic renal cell carcinoma? Cancer. 1999;85:153–5.

39. Koga S, Tsuda S, Nishikido M, et al. The diagnostic value of bone scan in patients with renal cell carcinoma. J Urol. 2001;166:2126–8.

40. Shvarts O, Lam JS, Kim HL, et al. Eastern Cooperative Oncology Group performance status predicts bone metastasis in patients presenting with renal cell carcinoma: implication for preoperative bone scans. J Urol. 2004;172:867–70.

41. Seaman E, Goluboff ET, Ross S, et al. Association of radionuclide bone scan and serum alkaline phosphatase in patients with metastatic renal cell carcinoma. Urology. 1996;48:692–5.

42. Kriteman L, Sanders WH. Normal alkaline phosphatase levels in patients with bone metastases due to renal cell carcinoma. Urology. 1998;51:397–9.

43. Bos SD, Piers DA, Mensink HJ. Routine bone scan and serum alkaline phosphatase for staging in patients with renal cell carcinoma is not cost-effective. Eur J Cancer. 1995;31A:2422–3.

44. Even-Sapir E. Imaging of malignant bone involvement by morphologic, scintigraphic, and hybrid modalities. J Nucl Med. 2005;46:1356–67.

45. Wu HC, Yen RF, Shen YY, et al. Comparing whole body ^{18}F-2-deoxyglucose positron emission tomography and technetium-99m methylene diphosphate bone scan to detect bone metastases in patients with renal cell carcinomas – a preliminary report. J Cancer Res Clin Oncol. 2002;128:503–6.

46. Brouwers AH, Dorr U, Lang O, et al. ^{131}I-cG250 monoclonal antibody immunoscintigraphy versus [18 F]FDG-PET imaging in patients with metastatic renal cell carcinoma: a comparative study. Nucl Med Commun. 2002;23:229–36.

47. Studer UE, Scherz S, Scheidegger J, Kraft R, Sonntag R, Ackermann D, et al. Enlargement of regional lymph nodes in renal cell carcinoma is often not due to metastases. J Urol. 1990;144(2 Pt 1):243–5.

48. Schafhauser W, Ebert A, Brod J, et al. Lymph node involvement in renal cell carcinoma and survival chance by systematic lymphadenectomy. Anticancer Res. 1999;19:1573–8.

49. Blom JH, Van Poppel H, Marechal JM, et al. Radical nephrectomy with and without lymph node dissection: preliminary results of the EORTC randomized phase III protocol 30881. EORTC Genitourinary Group. Eur Urol. 1999;36:570–5.

50. Pantuck AJ, Zisman A, Dorey F, et al. Renal cell carcinoma with retroperitoneal lymph nodes: role of lymph node dissection. J Urol. 2003;169:2076–83.

51. Safaei A, Figlin R, Hoh CK, et al. The usefulness of F-18 deoxyglucose whole-body positron emission tomography (PET) for re-staging of renal cell cancer. Clin Nephrol. 2002;57:56–62.

52. Majhail NS, Urbain JL, Albani JM, et al. F-18 fluorodeoxyglucose positron emission tomography in the evaluation of distant metastases from renal cell carcinoma. J Clin Oncol. 2003;21:3995–4000.

53. Jadvar H, Kherbache HM, Pinski JK, et al. Diagnostic role of [F-18]-FDG positron emission tomography in restaging renal cell carcinoma. Clin Nephrol. 2003;60:395–400.

54. Divgi CR, Bander NH, Scott AM, et al. Phase I/II radioimmunotherapy trial with iodine-131-labeled monoclonal antibody G250 in metastatic renal cell carcinoma. Clin Cancer Res. 1998;4:2729–39.

55. Steffens MG, Boerman OC, de Mulder PH, et al. Phase I radioimmunotherapy of metastatic renal cell carcinoma with ^{131}I-labeled chimeric monoclonal antibody G250. Clin Cancer Res. 1999;5 Suppl:3268s–3274s.

56. Brouwers AH, Mulders PF, de Mulder PH, et al. Lack of efficacy of two consecutive treatments of radioimmunotherapy with ^{131}I-cG250 in patients with metastasized clear cell renal cell carcinoma. J Clin Oncol. 2005;23:6540–8.

57. Brouwers AH, Buijs WCAM, Oosterwijk E, et al. Targeting of metastatic renal cell carcinoma with the chimeric monoclonal antibody G250 labeled with ^{131}I or [111]In: An intrapatient comparison. Clin Cancer Res. 2003;9 Suppl:3953s–3960s.

58. Brouwers AH, van Eerd JEM, Frielink C, et al. Optimization of radioimmunotherapy of renal cell carcinoma: labeling of monoclonal antibody cG250 with ^{131}I, ^{90}Y, ^{177}Lu, or [186]Re. J Nucl Med. 2004;45:327–37.

59. Lang O, Brouwers AH, Mergenthaler HG, et al. Value of wholebody ^{18}F-FDG-PET in metastatic renal cell carcinoma – correlation with tumor aggressiveness? J Nucl Med. 2000;41:117P.

60. Bui MH, Seligson D, Han KR, et al. Carbonic anhydrase IX is an independent predictor of survival in advanced renal clear cell carcinoma: implications for prognosis and therapy. Clin Cancer Res. 2003;9:802–11.

61. Atkins M, Regan M, McDermott D, et al. Carbonic anhydrase IX expression predicts outcome of interleukin 2 therapy for renal cancer. Clin Cancer Res. 2005;11:3714–21.

62. Brouwers AH, Boerman OC, Oyen WJ, et al. In vivo molecular prediction of carbonic anhydrase IX-G250MN expression on immunotherapy outcome in renal cancer. Clin Cancer Res. 2005;11:8886.

63. Kang DE, White RL Jr, Zuger JH, et al. Clinical use of fluorodeoxyglucose F 18 positron emission tomography for detection of renal cell carcinoma. J Urol. 2004;171:1806–9.

64. Zhang L, Cecic I, Cheng Z, et al. In Vitro evaluation of ^{18}F-2,3,5,6-tetrafluoro-3'-sulfamoylbenzanilide as a potential PET probe for carbonic anhydrase IX. Mol Imaging Biol. 2006;8:110P.

65. Hoh CK, Seltzer MA, Franklin J, et al. Positron emission tomography in urological oncology. J Urol. 1998;159: 347–56.

66. Vogelzang NJ. Treatment options in metastatic renal carcinoma: an embarrassment of riches. J Clin Oncol. 2006;24:1–3.

67. Kumar R, Chauhan A, Lakhani P, et al. 2-Deoxy-2-[F-18]fluoro-D-glucose-positron emission tomography in characterization of solid renal masses. Mol Imaging Biol. 2005; 7:431–9.

Chapter 9

Considerations: Imaging in Renal Cell Carcinoma

S. Sengupta and M.L. Blute

Introduction

Radiological imaging has assumed paramount importance in the modern management of renal cell carcinoma (RCC) such that currently the detection and diagnosis of RCC are almost totally dependent on radiological evaluation. Additionally, management decisions, particularly with respect to the selection and planning of surgical procedure, are often based largely on radiological findings. Herein we review the clinical role for imaging in the management of RCC.

Incidental Renal Masses

The increasing use of cross-sectional imaging has led to a concomitant increase in the incidental diagnosis of RCC [1–3], and the classical triad of flank pain, hematuria, and a palpable mass is now the exception rather than the rule. Incidentally diagnosed RCCs are characteristically of smaller size, lower stage, and more favorable grade compared to those presenting symptomatically, and as a result generally have a better prognosis [2, 4–6]. However, we have found that after adjusting for tumor size, stage, grade, and the presence of necrosis, symptoms at diagnosis are not of prognostic importance for RCC [7]. Thus, the management of incidentally diagnosed RCCs should be no different from that of comparable symptomatic tumors.

Diagnosis of RCC

RCCs typically appear radiographically as a solid mass, which are generally easily differentiated from cystic lesions. However, intermediate lesions (Fig. 9.1) exhibiting thick-

M.L. Blute, (✉)
Department of Urology, Mayo Clinic, 200 First St SW, Rochester, MN 55905, lute.michael@mayo.edu

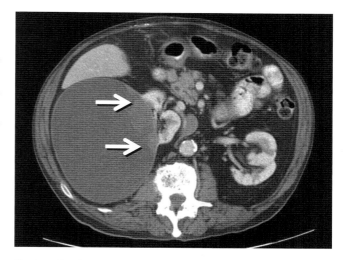

Fig. 9.1 Cystic renal cell carcinoma. 54-year-old male presented with right-sided abdominal bulge. Abdominal CT revealed large cystic lesion in right kidney with enhancing nodule in medial wall. Successfully resected by enucleation, and patient remains disease-free 10 years later

ness, nodularity, calcification or enhancement of the wall, or the presence of internal septation require careful assessment using defined criteria to estimate the risk of malignancy, such as those proposed by Bozniak [8].

RCCs represent the majority of solid renal masses detected radiologically, irrespective of the presence of symptoms [9]. Notably, the size of renal neoplasms is a critical determinant of the likelihood of malignancy, with more than 20% of lesions less than 4 cm in size being benign, compared to less than 10% of lesions larger than 4 cm [10] (Fig. 9.2). Furthermore, even for malignant tumors, small size is associated with slow growth and a low rate of metastatic progression [11]. On this basis, small renal lesions may sometimes be managed expectantly, especially among older or medically frail patients [12].

A definitive diagnosis of RCC can sometimes be made on the basis of radiological studies, while some benign tumors may also be diagnosed with certainty on the basis of pathognomonic features, such as fat content of angiomyolipomas [13, 14]. However, in many instances, the diagnosis of RCC

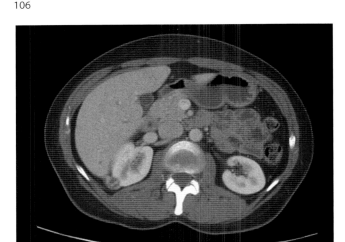

Fig. 9.2 Small incidental renal mass. 46-year-old female presenting with stress urinary incontinence also reported vague right flank pain, prompting radiological evaluation which demonstrated a solid 3 cm mass in the right kidney. The lesion was removed by partial nephrectomy at the same time as a sling procedure for her incontinence and found histologically to be an angiomyolipoma

is presumptive until pathological confirmation is obtained following nephrectomy. We have found needle biopsy to be inaccurate for the distinction of benign from malignant renal neoplasm [15, 16], and therefore do not recommend it pre-operatively.

There is a definite role for needle biopsy of renal masses in patients with a prior history of other malignancies which may give rise to renal metastases. However, in this context, the usual presentation is with multiple renal and extra-renal deposits [17]. Similarly, a suspicion of renal lymphoma, based on clinical features or imaging findings, mandates needle biopsy, since therapy is medical rather than surgical [18, 19].

Staging of RCC

Pre-operative staging of RCC is important for guiding appropriate management decisions and facilitating accurate counseling of patients and relies heavily on radiological assessment. The local staging of RCC is based on tumor size, which may be reliably estimated radiologically [20], and extra-renal extension, radiological demonstration of which is somewhat more problematic. Involvement of the ipsilateral adrenal gland by RCC can be reliably excluded on the basis of a normal radiographic appearance, thereby allowing adrenal sparing nephrectomy [21, 22].

In contrast, the detection of perinephric fat invasion on computed tomography (CT) is susceptible to both false positive and false negative results [23], but may be somewhat more accurate on magnetic resonance imaging (MRI) [24]. However, for cT1 tumors, occult invasion of perinephric fat

may be prognostically irrelevant [25]. Similarly, local extension of RCC to involve adjacent viscera such as the liver cannot always be reliably assessed radiologically because of partial volume artifact and adjacent desmoplastic adherence [23]. The definitive assessment of the involvement of adjacent structures can only be carried out intra-operatively. Occasionally, en bloc resection may be indicated (Fig. 9.3) and may result in favorable oncological results [26].

Venous extension of RCC, particularly that involving the vena cava, is usually detectable on pre-operative imaging [27, 28]. Radiological assessment is crucial in such cases, in order to assess the extent of thrombus, occlusion of the caval lumen [29], or invasion of the caval wall [30] (Fig. 9.4). Although MRI has been considered the gold standard in this setting [31, 32], CT scans with multi-planar and three-dimensional reformatting provide a comparable alternative [23, 33]. Positron emission tomography (PET) may be useful for distinguishing between bland and tumor thrombus [34].

At present, the radiological assessment of nodal spread of RCC is based purely on size criteria, with nodes greater than 1 cm considered suspicious [33] (Fig. 9.5). However, the majority of such enlarged nodes represent reactive hyperplasia [35], while up to 4% of patients with normal appearing nodes are found to harbor nodal metastases at surgery [35, 36]. Therefore, the need for lymphadenectomy is best determined on the basis of clinico-pathological rather than radiological criteria [37].

For the assessment of distant metastases, radiological evaluation of the lungs and mediastinum is mandatory. In this respect, a CT scan is more sensitive, but also less specific than a plain X-ray, and clinical outcomes appear not to be significantly impacted by a choice between the two [38].

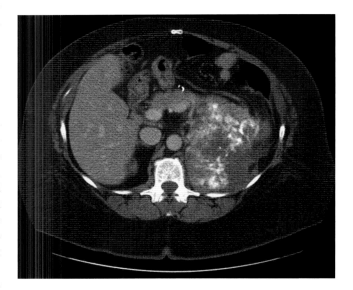

Fig. 9.3 Locally invasive RCC. 54-year-old male presented with left-sided chest and shoulder-tip pain as well as prominent constitutional symptoms, including malaise and weight loss. Abdominal CT scan revealed left renal tumor with extension into the spleen and the tail of the pancreas

(a)

(b)

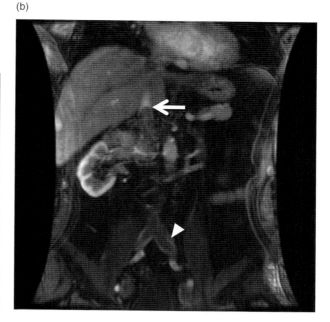

Fig. 9.4 Venous tumor thrombus. 77-year-old male presented with bilateral leg edema, consequent to deep venous thrombosis. Subsequent investigation using CT scan (**a**) revealed right-sided renal cell carcinoma with vena caval tumor thrombus (*arrow*). Coronal reconstruction on MRI (**b**) demonstrated the upper extent of tumor thrombus to be below the hepatic veins (*arrow*), with complete occlusion of vana cava infra-renally by bland thrombus (*arrow head*). Successfully managed by surgical resection of tumor and removal of thrombus

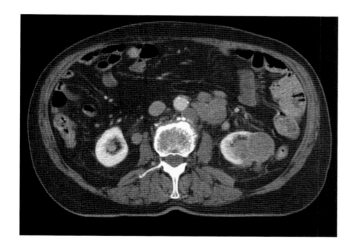

Fig. 9.5 RCC with regional lymphadenopathy. 57-year-old male with hematuria found to have left renal mass with nodal metastases. Treated by nephrectomy and nodal resection, followed by systemic therapy, but succumbed to disease after 18 months

The use of radionuclide bone scintigraphy in pre-operative staging should be selective, guided by patient performance status, symptoms, and serum alkaline phosphatase [39].

Operative Anatomy

A further crucial contribution of radiological imaging is the delineation of anatomical detail that may assist in planning the surgical approach to RCC. Occasionally, this may include the detection of congenital abnormalities such as a horseshoe kidney, ectopic kidney, or contralateral agenesis [40–42]. More critically, the demonstration of multifocal [43, 44] or bilateral [45] tumors may suggest an imperative indication for nephron sparing surgery and in rare instances lead to the diagnosis of hereditary syndromes such as von Hippel–Lindau disease or tuberous sclerosis (Fig. 9.6).

For patients in whom a nephron-sparing approach is planned, an accurate radiological assessment of the tumor, its relationship to normal structures, and the vascular anatomy is vital [46, 47] (Fig. 9.7). With three-dimensional refor-

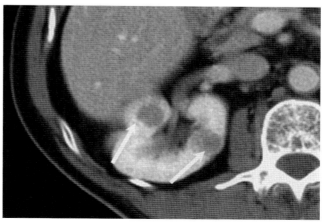

Fig. 9.6 Multifocal RCC. 65-year-old male with incidentally diagnosed multifocal RCC (*arrows*), treated by radiofrequency ablation, with no enhancement of lesions at 24-months follow-up

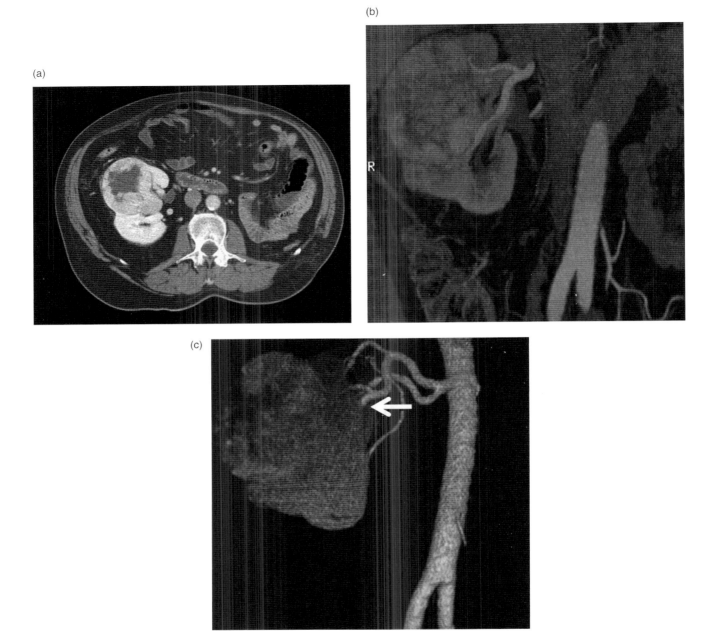

Fig. 9.7 RCC arising in a solitary functional kidney. 64-year-old male, who had previously undergone left nephrectomy in childhood for obstructed non-functioning kidney, presented with RCC arising in right kidney (**a**). Coronal (**b**) and three-dimensional (**c**) reconstructions were useful in planning operative approach at partial nephrectomy, which was successfully performed by ligating the inferior branch of the anterior division of the renal artery (*arrow*), which was the main blood supply to the tumor

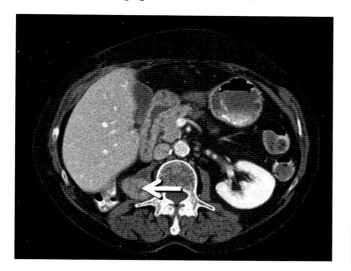

Fig. 9.8 Local recurrence of RCC. 74-year-old male status 6 months post-right radical nephrectomy for RCC found to have ipsilateral psoas recurrence (*arrow*) on surveillance CT scan. Managed by surgical excision and remains disease-free at 6 month follow-up

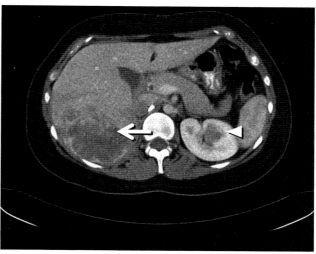

Fig. 9.9 Hepatic metastasis and metachronous contralateral RCC. 20-year-old female, status 2 years post-right radical nephrectomy for RCC, presents during pregnancy with left-sided renal tumor and hepatic secondary (*arrow*). Managed by partial nephrectomy and hemi-hepatectomy, followed by systemic immunotherapy

matting, modern CT scans can provide information regarding renal arterial anatomy that is comparable to angiography [47]. The need for detailed radiological assessment of venous tumor thrombus has already been outlined. Occasionally, variations in vascular anatomy may be found, which facilitate the surgical resection of difficult tumors [48, 49].

Surveillance for Recurrence

Patients with RCC require ongoing surveillance following nephrectomy, in order to detect local (Fig. 9.8) and systemic (Fig. 9.9) recurrences, which may be amenable to surgical resection [50] and systemic therapy, respectively [51]. There

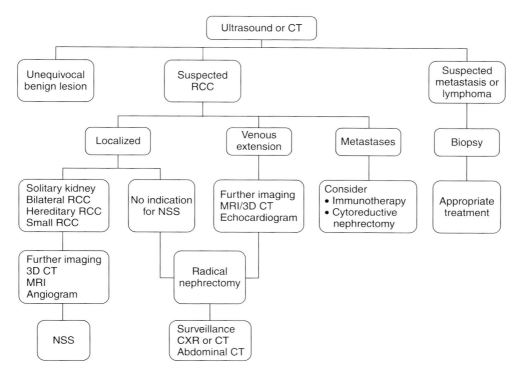

Fig. 9.10 Algorithm for the integration of imaging in the clinical management of RCC

is emerging data to suggest that the surveillance regime needs to be tailored for each patient based on pathological features [52] and surgical approach [53], both of which impact upon risk and likely site of recurrence [51]. Radiological imaging is an indispensable adjunct to clinical evaluation of such patients.

Cross-sectional imaging, usually in the form of CT scanning, provides excellent assessment of the operative bed, loco-regional lymph nodes, the liver, and other abdominal viscera. Evaluation of the lungs and mediastinum, by either plain X-ray or CT scan, is also essential. Radiological assessment of other metastatic sites, such as brain or bone, should be carried out selectively, depending on symptoms and serum markers [54]. PET may be useful for the confirmation of tumor within suspicious nodules in the operative bed or at distant sites [55, 56].

A Clinical Algorithm

One approach to the clinical integration of imaging in the management of RCCs is shown in Fig. 9.10. A key feature of this algorithm is that the imaging needs to be tailored to the individual patient. Thus, in some cases, a definitive diagnosis of a benign lesion such as a cyst or an angiomyolipoma can be made on the basis of the initial ultrasound or CT scan, which is thus sufficient. On the other hand, if a suspected RCC is to be adequately evaluated, an appropriately phased contrast CT scan is required. The staging and diagnostic information gleaned from such a study may suggest the need for more detailed examination in order to assess the arterial, venous, or other anatomy. Needle biopsy may be indicated in specific circumstances as outlined before. Finally, the post-operative patient and the occasional patient undergoing observation of a small renal mass require relevant radiological surveillance along with clinical follow-up.

References

1. Chow WH, Devesa SS, Warren JL, Fraumeni JF Jr. Rising incidence of renal cell cancer in the United States. Jama. 1999;281:1628.
2. Luciani, LG, Cestari R, Tallarigo C. Incidental renal cell carcinoma-age and stage characterization and clinical implications: study of 1092 patients (1982–1997). Urology. 2000;56:58.
3. Lightfoot N, Conlon M, Kreiger N, Bissett R, Desai M, Warde P, et al. Impact of noninvasive imaging on increased incidental detection of renal cell carcinoma. Eur Urol. 2000;37:521.
4. Duchene DA, Lotan Y, Cadeddu JA, Sagalowsky AI, Koeneman KS. Histopathology of surgically managed renal tumors: analysis of a contemporary series. Urology. 2003;62:827.
5. Ficarra V, Prayer-Galetti T, Novella G, Bratti E, Maffei N, Dal Bianco M, et al. Incidental detection beyond pathological

6. Lee CT, Katz J, Fearn PA, Russo P. Mode of presentation of renal cell carcinoma provides prognostic information. Urol Oncol. 2002;7:135.
7. Frank I, Blute ML, Cheville JC, Lohse CM, Weaver AL, Zincke H. An outcome prediction model for patients with clear cell renal cell carcinoma treated with radical nephrectomy based on tumor stage, size, grade and necrosis: the SSIGN score. J Urol. 2002;168:2395.
8. Bosniak MA. The current radiological approach to renal cysts. Radiology. 1986;158:1.
9. Ozen H, Colowick A, Freiha FS. Incidentally discovered solid renal masses: what are they? Br J Urol. 1993;72:274.
10. Frank I, Blute ML, Cheville JC, Lohse CM, Weaver AL, Zincke H. Solid renal tumors: an analysis of pathological features related to tumor size. J Urol. 2003;170:2217.
11. Bosniak MA, Birnbaum BA, Krinsky GA, Waisman J. Small renal parenchymal neoplasms: further observations on growth. Radiology. 1995;197:589.
12. Wehle MJ, Thiel DD, Petrou SP, Young PR, Frank I, Karsteadt N. Conservative management of incidental contrast-enhancing renal masses as safe alternative to invasive therapy. Urology. 2004;64:49.
13. Bosniak MA. Angiomyolipoma (hamartoma) of the kidney: a pre-operative diagnosis is possible in virtually every case. Urol Radiol. 1981;3:135.
14. Blute ML, Malek RS, Segura JW. Angiomyolipoma: clinical metamorphosis and concepts for management. J Urol. 1988;139:20.
15. Dechet CB, Sebo T, Farrow G, Blute ML, Engen DE, Zincke H. Prospective analysis of intraoperative frozen needle biopsy of solid renal masses in adults. J Urol. 1999;162:1282.
16. Dechet CB, Zincke H, Sebo TJ, King BF, LeRoy AJ, Farrow GM, et al. Prospective analysis of computerized tomography and needle biopsy with permanent sectioning to determine the nature of solid renal masses in adults. J Urol. 2003;169:71.
17. Sanchez-Ortiz RF, Madsen LT, Bermejo CE, Wen S, Shen Y, Swanson DA, et al. A renal mass in the setting of a nonrenal malignancy: when is a renal tumor biopsy appropriate? Cancer. 2004;101:2195.
18. Urban BA, Fishman EK. Renal lymphoma: CT patterns with emphasis on helical CT. Radiographics. 2000;20:197.
19. Fernandez-Acenero MJ, Galindo M, Bengoechea O, Borrega P, Reina JJ, Carapeto R. Primary malignant lymphoma of the kidney: case report and literature review. Gen Diagn Pathol. 1998;143:317.
20. Yaycioglu O, Rutman MP, Balasubramaniam M, Peters KM, Gonzalez JA. Clinical and pathologic tumor size in renal cell carcinoma: difference, correlation, and analysis of the influencing factors. Urology. 2002;60:33.
21. Gill IS, McClennan BL, Kerbl K, Carbone JM, Wick M, Clayman RV. Adrenal involvement from renal cell carcinoma: predictive value of computerized tomography. J Urol. 1994;152:1082.
22. Moudouni SM, En-Nia I, Patard JJ, Manunta A, Guille F, Lobel B. Real indications for adrenalectomy in renal cell carcinoma. Scand J Urol Nephrol. 2002;36:273.
23. Sheth S, Scatarige JC, Horton KM, Corl FM, Fishman EK. Current concepts in the diagnosis and management of renal cell carcinoma: role of multidetector ct and three-dimensional CT. Radiographics. 2001;21 Spec No:S237.
24. Roy CSr, El Ghali S, Buy X, Lindner V, Lang H, Saussine C, et al. Significance of the pseudocapsule on MRI of renal neoplasms and its potential application for local staging: a retrospective study. AJR Am J Roentgenol. 2005;184:113.
25. Roberts WW, Bhayani SB, Allaf ME, Chan TY, Kavoussi LR, Jarrett TW. Pathological stage does not alter the prognosis for renal lesions determined to be stage T1 by computerized tomography. J Urol. 2005;173:713.
26. Johnin K, Nakai O, Kataoka A, Koizumi S, Dok An C, Okada Y, et al. Surgical management of renal cell carcinoma invading into

factors as prognostic predictor of renal cell carcinoma. Eur Urol. 2003;43:663.

the liver: radical nephrectomy en bloc with right hepatic lateral sector. Urology. 2001;57:975.

27. Welch TJ, LeRoy AJ. Helical and electron beam CT scanning in the evaluation of renal vein involvement in patients with renal cell carcinoma. J Comput Assist Tomogr. 1997;21:467.

28. Hallscheidt PJ, Fink C, Haferkamp A, Bock M, Luburic A, Zuna I, et al. Preoperative staging of renal cell carcinoma with inferior vena cava thrombus using multidetector CT and MRI: prospective study with histopathological correlation. J Comput Assist Tomogr. 2005;29:64.

29. Blute ML, Leibovich BC, Lohse CM, Cheville JC, Zincke H. The Mayo Clinic experience with surgical management, complications and outcome for patients with renal cell carcinoma and venous tumour thrombus. BJU Int. 2004;94:33.

30. Aslam Sohaib SA, Teh J, Nargund VH, Lumley JS, Hendry WF, Reznek RH. Assessment of tumor invasion of the vena caval wall in renal cell carcinoma cases by magnetic resonance imaging. J Urol. 2002;167:1271.

31. Semelka RC, Shoenut JP, Magro CM, Kroeker MA, MacMahon R, Greenberg HM. Renal cancer staging: comparison of contrast-enhanced CT and gadolinium-enhanced fat-suppressed spin-echo and gradient-echo MR imaging. J Magn Reson Imaging. 1993;3:597.

32. Kallman DA, King BF, Hattery RR, Charboneau JW, Ehman RL, Guthman DA, et al. Renal vein and inferior vena cava tumor thrombus in renal cell carcinoma: CT, US, MRI and venacavography. J Comput Assist Tomogr. 1992;16:240.

33. Israel GM, Bosniak MA. Renal imaging for diagnosis and staging of renal cell carcinoma. Urol Clin North Am. 2003;30:499.

34. Rydberg JN, Sudakoff GS, Hellman RS, See WA. Positron emission tomography-computed tomography imaging characteristics of an inferior vena cava tumor thrombus with magnetic resonance imaging correlation. J Comput Assist Tomogr. 2004; 28:517.

35. Studer UE, Scherz S, Scheidegger J, Kraft R, Sonntag R, Ackermann D, et al. Enlargement of regional lymph nodes in renal cell carcinoma is often not due to metastases. J Urol. 1990; 144:243.

36. Blom JH, van Poppel H, Marechal JM, Jacqmin D, Sylvester R, Schroder FH, et al. Radical nephrectomy with and without lymph node dissection: preliminary results of the EORTC randomized phase III protocol 30881. EORTC Genitourinary Group. Eur Urol. 1999;36:570.

37. Blute ML, Leibovich BC, Cheville JC, Lohse CM, Zincke H. A protocol for performing extended lymph node dissection using primary tumor pathological features for patients treated with radical nephrectomy for clear cell renal cell carcinoma. J Urol. 2004;172:465.

38. Lim DJ, Carter MF. Computerized tomography in the preoperative staging for pulmonary metastases in patients with renal cell carcinoma. J Urol. 1993;150:1112.

39. Shvarts O, Lam JS, Kim HL, Han KR, Figlin R, Belldegrun A. Eastern Cooperative Oncology Group performance status predicts bone metastasis in patients presenting with renal cell carcinoma: implication for preoperative bone scans. J Urol. 2004; 172:867.

40. Garner E, Raahave D, Martens S, Mogensen P. The significance of digital subtraction angiography (DSA) before operative treatment

of hypernephroma in a horseshoe kidney. Scand J Urol Nephrol. 1986;20:149.

41. Schubert RA, Soldner J, Steiner T, Schubert J, Kaiser WA. Bilateral renal cell carcinoma in a horseshoe kidney: preoperative assessment with MRI and digital subtraction angiography. Eur Radiol. 1998;8:1694.

42. Terrone C, Destefanis P, Fiori C, Savio D, Fontana D. Renal cell cancer in presacral ectopic kidney: preoperative diagnostic imaging compared to surgical findings. Urol Int. 2004;72:174.

43. Blute ML, Thibault GP, Leibovich BC, Cheville JC, Lohse CM, Zincke H. Multiple ipsilateral renal tumors discovered at planned nephron sparing surgery: importance of tumor histology and risk of metachronous recurrence. J Urol. 2003;170:760.

44. Kletscher BA, Qian J, Bostwick DG, Andrews PE, Zincke H. Prospective analysis of multifocality in renal cell carcinoma: influence of histological pattern, grade, number, size, volume and deoxyribonucleic acid ploidy. J Urol. 1995;153:904.

45. Blute ML, Itano NB, Cheville JC, Weaver AL, Lohse CM, Zincke H. The effect of bilaterality, pathological features and surgical outcome in nonhereditary renal cell carcinoma. J Urol. 2003;169:1276.

46. Ghavamian R, Zincke H. Nephron-sparing surgery. Curr Urol Rep. 2001;2:34.

47. Coll DM, Uzzo RG, Herts BR, Davros WJ, Wirth SL, Novick AC. 3-dimensional volume rendered computerized tomography for preoperative evaluation and intraoperative treatment of patients undergoing nephron sparing surgery. J Urol. 1999;161:1097.

48. Sengupta S, Zincke H, Leibovich BC, Blute ML. Surgical treatment of stage pT3b renal cell carcinoma in solitary kidneys: a case series. BJU Int. 2005;96:54.

49. Pruthi RS, Angell SK, Brooks JD, Gill H. Partial nephrectomy and caval thrombectomy for renal cell carcinoma in a solitary kidney with an accessory renal vein. BJU Int. 1999;83:142.

50. Itano NB, Blute ML, Spotts B, Zincke H. Outcome of isolated renal cell carcinoma fossa recurrence after nephrectomy. J Urol. 2000;164:322.

51. Janzen NK, Kim HL, Figlin RA, Belldegrun AS. Surveillance after radical or partial nephrectomy for localized renal cell carcinoma and management of recurrent disease. Urol Clin North Am. 2003;30:843.

52. Frank I, Blute ML, Cheville JC, Lohse CM, Weaver AL, Leibovich BC, et al. A multifactorial postoperative surveillance model for patients with surgically treated clear cell renal cell carcinoma. J Urol. 2003;170:2225.

53. Hafez KS, Novick AC, Campbell SC. Patterns of tumor recurrence and guidelines for followup after nephron sparing surgery for sporadic renal cell carcinoma. J Urol. 1997;157:2067.

54. Levy DA, Slaton JW, Swanson DA, Dinney CP. Stage specific guidelines for surveillance after radical nephrectomy for local renal cell carcinoma. J Urol. 1998;159:1163.

55. Majhail NS, Urbain JL, Albani JM, Kanvinde MH, Rice TW, Novick AC, et al. F-18 fluorodeoxyglucose positron emission tomography in the evaluation of distant metastases from renal cell carcinoma. J Clin Oncol. 2003;21:3995.

56. Ramdave S, Thomas GW, Berlangieri SU, Bolton DM, Davis I, Danguy HT, et al. Clinical role of F-18 fluorodeoxyglucose positron emission tomography for detection and management of renal cell carcinoma. J Urol. 2001;166:825.

Chapter 10

Urothelial Cell Carcinoma of the Upper Urinary Tract

S. Gudjónsson and W. Månsson

Background

The urothelium of the bladder, ureters, renal pelves, and calices forms a continuous sheath that is histologically identical at the mentioned sites. Likewise, urothelial tumors of the upper urinary tract (UUTTs) are histopathologically equivalent to those found in the bladder, and they also share many risk factors.

There is, however, a huge difference in the incidence, and especially the prevalence, of these closely linked disorders. Only 5–6% of all urothelial cell cancers arise in the upper tract which, together with the traditionally aggressive treatment strategies, explains the very low prevalence of the disease. Furthermore, due to the paucity of UUTTs, the evidence-based knowledge on various aspects of such tumors is fairly limited.

Etiology

Factors that are known to predispose to both UUTTs and bladder cancer (BC) include cigarette smoking, treatment with cyclophosphamide, and occupational exposure to a variety of chemicals [1, 2]. More specific and well-documented risk factors for UUTT are analgesic abuse (phenacitin [3] being the best known culprit), endemic Balkan nephropathy [4], and a chronic nephropathy associated with ingestion of certain Chinese herbs [5]. Chronic bacterial infection together with urinary calculi and obstruction is known to predispose to squamous cell carcinoma or even urothelial adenocarcinoma, although both these entities are extremely rare [6]. Schistosomiasis can induce squamous cell carcinoma in the upper tract as well as in the bladder.

Epidemiology

Bladder tumors account for about 95% of all urothelial tumors, and UUTTs constitute the remaining 5%. Moreover, 80% of all UUTTs arise in the renal pelvis, and 20% are ureteral tumors [7] (Figs. 10.1–10.3b). The incidence of UUTTs appears to have increased slightly in recent decades [8]. The incidence of bilateral UUTTs is low (about 2%) [9], whereas ipsilateral multiplicity is common (27–36%) [7, 10–14]. Men are more prone to UUTTs than women at a ratio of 2:1, and whites have double the risk of such tumors compared to African-American males [15]. In addition, UUTTs rarely occur before the age of 40, but thereafter the incidence increases, and the mean age of occurrence is about 65 years [16].

As expected there is substantial overrepresentation of UUTTs in patients with BC and vice versa. Reports in the literature indicate that 30–75% of patients with UUTTs have a history of primary BC or develop secondary BC later in life [7, 12, 17], which is why follow-up schedules for patients

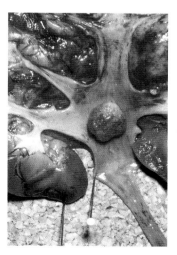

Fig. 10.1 Centrally located well/moderately differentiated tumor in the renal pelvis

S.Gudjónsson (✉)
Department of Urology, Lund University Hospital, Sweden

J.J.M.C.H. de la Rosette et al. (eds.), *Imaging in Oncological Urology*,
DOI 10.1007/978-1-84628-759-6_10, © Springer-Verlag London Limited 2009

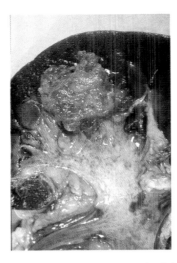

Fig. 10.2 Poorly differentiated urothelial renal pelvis tumor invading renal parenchyma

(a)

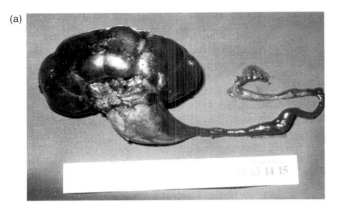

Fig. 10.3a Infact nephroureteric specimen with bladder cuff. The renal pelvis and proximal ureter are dilated

(b)

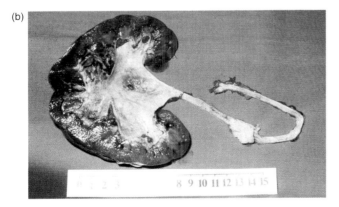

Fig. 10.3b After opening the collecting system a solitary ureteral tumor is revealed

with UUTTs include control cystoscopy. The risk of developing a UUTT is only 1–4% in patients with low-grade non-muscle invasive bladder cancer (NMIBC) [18], whereas it has been estimated to be as high as 25% in patients with high-grade NMIBC [19–22]. Consequently, a radiological investigation of the upper tract is advocated in primary diagnostic work-up of patients treated for BC and also in follow-up schedules for those with high-grade NMIBC.

The risk of developing a UUTT after radical cystectomy for invasive BC is generally low (4%) [22]. Nevertheless, patients who have multifocal disease or carcinoma in situ (CIS) of the distal ureters and undergo radical cystectomy are considered to be at increased risk of UUTT later in life, and follow-up should be tailored accordingly.

Symptoms and Diagnosis

The cardinal symptom of UUTT is macroscopic hematuria (75% of patients) [14].

In many cases (30%) flank pain caused by a clot blocking the ureter or by tumor obstruction is also seen as one of the presenting symptoms.

The methods available for radiological investigation will be covered in detail in subsequent chapters. Here it is of interest to mention that, along with cystoscopy, excretory urography (IVP) has traditionally been the first choice for investigating hematuria. Also, in doubtful cases, retrograde examination has led to better visualization of the upper tract. CT scanning of the upper tract with concomitant contrast filling (CT urography) has steadily improved in recent years and at many centers it has now replaced IVP as the preferred method of examination for patients with macroscopic hematuria.

Endoscopic examination of the upper tract is a challenging, operator-dependent procedure, which often adds very little to the radiological work-up. Constant improvements in technology have, however, contributed to enhanced endoscopic visualization of the upper tract. An important example of this is the use of flexible ureteroscopy, which allows collection of tissue samples or a brush cytology from a suspected lesion; this approach will probably become more appealing to urologists after further development of the technology.

Urine cytology is also valuable for detecting UUTTs. This method offers high specificity combined with good sensitivity for high-grade cancer cells, thus it is an effective tool for early detection of high-grade UUTTs [23] which is especially useful in patients who have a history of high-grade BC or for patients who have undergone previous conservative treatment for UUTT. Selective sampling of urine from the upper urinary tracts for cytology can be the only means of detecting

CIS in that region, and the results obtained often represent the sole basis for treatment of upper tract CIS. Urothelial cancer cells can be detected by a number of innovative methods, and one of those is fluorescent in situ hybridization (FISH), which shows promise but must be tested in larger studies to ascertain whether it is actually a suitable alternative to cytology for diagnosing UUTTs [24].

Staging

Tumor grade and stage have been shown to be the best predictors of disease-specific survival [25]. Classification is done according to the UICC TNM Classification of Malignant Tumours (6th edition, 2002) in a manner equivalent to the staging of BC. Compared to BC, upper tract tumors are more frequently associated with invasion [16] and hence the prognosis is generally worse.

Treatment

The standard treatment for UUTTs is radical nephroureterectomy with bladder cuff removal, which can be explained by the fairly high rate of ipsilateral multiplicity and a substantial recurrence rate in the remaining distal ureter (16–58%) [10], should this have been left behind. In recent years however, vast improvements in surgical technique have made minimally invasive treatments increasingly more appealing. Laparoscopic and retroperitoneoscopic nephroureterectomy have proved their value as equally effective to open procedure in terms of oncological outcomes, but with decreased morbidity and shortened hospital stay for patients as an attractive feature [26, 27].

Notwithstanding, treatment aimed at conserving renal function can be used in selected patients [28]. Renal-sparing surgery is performed by many urologists when tumors are located in the distal third of the ureter, even if the tumors are invasive [29]. Technical improvements in endourological and percutaneous methods have also made it possible to resect low-grade superficial UUTTs in selected cases, despite a relatively high rate of recurrence in the ipsilateral unit [30–32].

Local chemotherapy and immunotherapy play an important role in the prevention of recurrence of BC. In recent years, reports have demonstrated the applicability of immunotherapy with Bacillus Calmette–Guerin (BCG) for upper tract tumors and in particular CIS. BCG instillation for CIS in the upper tracts seems to be feasible and effective treatment with acceptable toxicity [33–35]. On the other hand, it has to be done properly and cautiously through a nephrostomy catheter or JJ stent, and a low pressure must be maintained in the system during the instillation period to avoid potentially serious complications.

The chemotherapeutic regimens that are indicated in systemic disease are generally the same as those used for BC patients with advanced disease, but there are no randomized prospective trials regarding the use of chemotherapy in UUTTs.

Prognosis

Tumor stage and grade are the most important determinants of the outcome in UUTT patients [7, 12, 36]. Upper tract tumors spread via lymphatic and hematogenous routes and also by direct extension into surrounding tissues, and the metastatic sites are most often the lungs, liver, bones, and regional lymph nodes [12]. Overall 5-year survival rate for patients with UUTTs seems to have improved somewhat in modern times. Current 5-year survival is reported at 75% [8]. Women have been shown to be at greater risk of dying from ureteral cancer than men [15].

Actuarial 5-year disease-free survival rates by tumor stage are 100, 92, 73, and 40% for Ta, T1, T2, and T3, respectively. Median survival for patients with T4 tumors is only 6 months [11, 12].

Surveillance Strategies

As for other tumors the follow-up after treatment of UUTTs must be individually tailored based on patient and tumor characteristics. Mode of treatment, being radical surgery of the ipsilateral upper urinary tract or a more conservative endoscopic and/or renal-sparing surgery, also comes into account. Patient factors, such as age and concomitant diseases, influence the aggressiveness of surveillance. Risk factors for recurrence include tumor stage, grade, and multifocality.

UUTTs behave biologically much in the same fashion as BCs. The recurrence rate is known to be high in the ipsilateral upper tract when conservative treatment is chosen [11, 12, 14, 37] and subsequent BCs are common as previously mentioned. In light of this fact, it is important to follow all patients with regular cystoscopy controls combined with urine cytology and, in patients who have not been treated with a radical nephroureterectomy, to do either endoscopic or radiological imaging of the ipsilateral upper tract on a regular basis. Patients who have undergone radical nephroureterectomy, where the pathological analysis shows invasion beyond the basal membrane, require follow-up imaging for local recurrence and metastasis. Patients who are candidates for chemotherapy, should recurrence occur, should be followed closely with annual CT scanning of the abdomen combined with chest radiography for at least 2–3 years. Contralateral metachronous UUTTs are uncommon, especially in patients without a history of BC [11, 38, 39], and routine imaging with IVP of the contralateral tract is therefore not indicated in those patients [39].

Conclusions

In conclusion, urothelial cell carcinoma of the upper urinary tract is a relatively uncommon type of malignancy that is closely related to bladder cancer. It often constitutes a diagnostic challenge and therefore goes undetected until late in the course of the disease, which can have serious consequences. The use of modern technology to continuously improve radiological and endoscopic assessments will undoubtedly increase the chance of early diagnosis and the quality of surveillance after treatment. It can be expected that future advances in surgical methods and medical treatment will have a major positive impact on the morbidity and prognosis of patients with UUTTs.

References

1. Brenner DW, Schellhammer PF. Upper tract urothelial malignancy after cyclophosphamide therapy: a case report and literature review. J Urol. 1987;137:1226–7.
2. Jensen OM, Knudsen JB, McLaughlin JK, Sorensen BL. The Copenhagen case-control study of renal pelvis and ureter cancer: role of smoking and occupational exposures. Int J Cancer. 1988;41:557–61.
3. McCredie M, Stewart JH, Ford JM, MacLennan RA. Phenacetin-containing analgesics and cancer of the bladder or renal pelvis in women. Br J Urol. 1983;55:220–4.
4. Petkovic SD. Epidemiology and treatment of renal pelvic and ureteral tumors. J Urol. 1975;114:858–65.
5. Cosyns JP, Jadoul M, Squifflet JP, Wese FX, van Ypersele de Strihou C. Urothelial lesions in Chinese-herb nephropathy. Am J Kidney Dis. 1999;33:1011–7.
6. Godec CJ, Murrah VA. Simultaneous occurrence of transitional cell carcinoma and urothelial adenocarcinoma associated with xanthogranulomatous pyelonephritis. Urology. 1985;26:412–5.
7. Huben RP, Mounzer AM, Murphy GP. Tumor grade and stage as prognostic variables in upper tract urothelial tumors. Cancer. 1988;62:2016–20.
8. Munoz JJ, Ellison LM. Upper tract urothelial neoplasms: incidence and survival during the last 2 decades. J Urol. 2000;164:1523–5.
9. Holmang S, Johansson SL. Synchronous bilateral ureteral and renal pelvic carcinomas: incidence, etiology, treatment and outcome. Cancer. 2004;101:741–6.
10. Racioppi M, D'Addessi A, Alcini A, Destito A, Alcini E. Clinical review of 100 consecutive surgically treated patients with upper urinary tract transitional tumours. Br J Urol. 1997;80: 707–11.
11. Krogh J, Kvist E, Rye B. Transitional cell carcinoma of the upper urinary tract: prognostic variables and post-operative recurrences. Br J Urol. 1991;67:32–6.
12. Hall MC, Womack S, Sagalowsky AI, Carmody T, Erickstad MD, Roehrborn CG. Prognostic factors, recurrence, and survival in tran-

13. sitional cell carcinoma of the upper urinary tract: a 30-year experience in 252 patients. Urology. 1998;52:594–601.
13. Babaian RJ, Johnson DE. Primary carcinoma of the ureter. J Urol 1980;123:357–9.
14. Murphy DM, Zincke H, Furlow WL. Management of high grade transitional cell cancer of the upper urinary tract. J Urol. 1981;125:25–9.
15. Greenlee RT, Murray T, Bolden S, Wingo PA. Cancer statistics. CA Cancer J Clin. 2000;50:7–33.
16. Anderstrom C, Johansson SL, Pettersson S, Wahlqvist L. Carcinoma of the ureter: a clinicopathologic study of 49 cases. J Urol. 1989;142:280–3.
17. Kakizoe T, Fujita J, Murase T, Matsumoto K, Kishi K. Transitional cell carcinoma of the bladder in patients with renal pelvic and ureteral cancer. J Urol. 1980;124:17–9.
18. Holmang S, Hedelin H, Anderstrom C, Holmberg E, Johansson SL. Long-term followup of a bladder carcinoma cohort: routine followup urography is not necessary. J Urol. 1998;160:45–8.
19. Hurle R, Losa A, Manzetti A, Lembo A. Upper urinary tract tumors developing after treatment of superficial bladder cancer: 7-year follow-up of 591 consecutive patients. Urology. 1999;53:1144–8.
20. Oldbring J, Glifberg I, Mikulowski P, Hellsten S. Carcinoma of the renal pelvis and ureter following bladder carcinoma: frequency, risk factors and clinicopathological findings. J Urol. 1989;141:1311–3.
21. Shinka T, Uekado Y, Aoshi H, Hirano A, Ohkawa T. Occurrence of uroepithelial tumors of the upper urinary tract after the initial diagnosis of bladder cancer. J Urol. 1988;140:745–8.
22. Solsona E, Iborra I, Ricos JV, Dumont R, Casanova JL, Calabuig C. Upper urinary tract involvement in patients with bladder carcinoma in situ (Tis): its impact on management. Urology. 1997;49: 347–52.
23. Chen GL, El-Gabry EA, Bagley DH. Surveillance of upper urinary tract transitional cell carcinoma: the role of ureteroscopy, retrograde pyelography, cytology and urinalysis. J Urol. 2000;164: 1901–4.
24. Bubendorf L, Grilli B. UroVysion multiprobe FISH in urinary cytology. Methods Mol Med. 2004;97:117–31.
25. McCarron JP, Mills C, Vaughn ED, Jr. Tumors of the renal pelvis and ureter: current concepts and management. Semin Urol. 1983;1:75–81.
26. Gill IS, Sung GT, Hobart MG, et al. Laparoscopic radical nephroureterectomy for upper tract transitional cell carcinoma: the Cleveland Clinic experience. J Urol. 2000;164:1513–22.
27. McNeill SA, Chrisofos M, Tolley DA. The long-term outcome after laparoscopic nephroureterectomy: a comparison with open nephroureterectomy. BJU Int. 2000;86:619–23.
28. Leitenberger A, Beyer A, Altwein JE. Organ-sparing treatment for ureteral carcinoma? Eur Urol. 1996;29:272–8.
29. Oosterlinck W, Solsona E, van der Meijden AP, et al. EAU guidelines on diagnosis and treatment of upper urinary tract transitional cell carcinoma. Eur Urol. 2004;46:147–54.
30. Keeley FX, Jr., Bibbo M, Bagley DH. Ureteroscopic treatment and surveillance of upper urinary tract transitional cell carcinoma. J Urol. 1997;157:1560–5.
31. Tawfiek ER, Bagley DH. Upper-tract transitional cell carcinoma. Urology. 1997;50:321–9.
32. Okada H, Eto H, Hara I, et al. Percutaneous treatment of transitional cell carcinoma of the upper urinary tract. Int J Urol. 1997;4:130–3.
33. Okubo K, Ichioka K, Terada N, Matsuta Y, Yoshimura K, Arai Y. Intrarenal bacillus Calmette-Guerin therapy for carcinoma in situ of the upper urinary tract: long-term follow-up and natural course in cases of failure. BJU Int. 2001;88:343–7.
34. Irie A, Iwamura M, Kadowaki K, Ohkawa A, Uchida T, Baba S. Intravesical instillation of bacille Calmette-Guerin for carcinoma

in situ of the urothelium involving the upper urinary tract using vesicoureteral reflux created by a double-pigtail catheter. Urology. 2002;59:53–7.

35. Nonomura N, Ono Y, Nozawa M, et al. Bacillus Calmette-Guerin perfusion therapy for the treatment of transitional cell carcinoma in situ of the upper urinary tract. Eur Urol. 2000;38:701–4;discussion 705.

36. Badalament RA, O'Toole RV, Kenworthy P, et al. Prognostic factors in patients with primary transitional cell carcinoma of the upper urinary tract. J Urol. 1990;144:859–63.

37. Strong DW, Pearse HD. Recurrent urothelial tumors following surgery for transitional cell carcinoma of the upper urinary tract. Cancer. 1976;38:2173–83.

38. Charbit L, Gendreau MC, Mee S, Cukier J. Tumors of the upper urinary tract: 10 years of experience. J Urol. 1991;146: 1243–6.

39. Holmang S, Johansson SL. Bilateral metachronous ureteral and renal pelvic carcinomas: incidence, clinical presentation, histopathology, treatment and outcome. J Urol. 2006;175:69–72; discussion 72–3.

Further Reading

1. Messing EM, Catalona W. Urothelial tumors of the urinary tract. In: Walsh PC, Retik AD, Vaughan ED, et al., editors. Cambell's urology, 8th ed. Philadelphia, WB Saunders; 2002. vol 4, pp. 2765–84.

2. Sagalowsky AI, Jarrett TW. Management of urothelial tumors of the renal pelvis and ureter. In: Walsh PC, Retik AD, Vaughan ED, et al., editors. Cambell's urology, 8th ed. Philadelphia, WB Saunders; 2002. vol 4, pp. 2845–75.

3. Oosterlinck W, Solsona E, van der Meijden AP, et al. EAU guidelines on diagnosis and treatment of upper urinary tract transitional cell carcinoma. Eur Urol. 2004;46:147–54.

Chapter 11

Urothelial Cell Carcinoma of the Upper Urinary Tract: Introduction

B.A. Inman, M.L. Blute, and R.P. Hartman

Introduction

Urothelium is the specialized epithelium that covers the urinary collecting system from the tips of the renal papillae to the prostatic urethra. Tumors of the urothelium can be benign but the vast majority are malignant carcinomas. Carcinomas of the urothelium are common and the upper urinary tract is the affected site in roughly 5% of cases. Similarly, 5–10% of tumors that involve the kidney actually arise from the renal collecting system. It is unusual to find an upper urinary tract tumor as a result of screening imaging. Rather, most patients present with symptoms of flank pain or hematuria and are evaluated specifically to rule out tumoral involvement of the collecting system. Nonetheless, a thorough evaluation of the collecting systems should be routinely sought in most renal imaging procedures, even if typical symptoms are not present.

This chapter discusses widely available imaging modalities used to diagnose upper urinary tract tumors: ultrasonography, intravenous pyelography, retrograde pyelography, and antegrade pyelography. For each of these imaging techniques we have attempted to present a discussion of special indications for usage, practical strengths and weaknesses, interpretation pointers and pitfalls, evidence of efficacy for diagnosing upper urinary tract tumors, and potential complications resulting from usage. References are used liberally and are meant to provide a comprehensive reading list for the reader interested in further exploring the published evidence for the imaging modalities and ideas presented herein.

Ultrasonography

The Normal Upper Urinary Tract

Kidney

Ultrasound examination of the kidney is typically performed with a 2.5–5 MHz transducer with the patient in any one of a number of positions. The kidneys are usually best viewed on deep inspiration and transverse and longitudinal images are obtained. Characteristics that should be routinely examined are the size and shape of the kidney, the echogenicity of the cortex relative to the spleen and liver, the thickness of the cortex, the degree of corticomedullary differentiation, and the structure of the intrarenal collecting system (i.e., calyces and renal pelvis).

The kidney usually has a smooth contour that resembles a bean although persistent fetal lobulation is a common normal variant. The spleen or liver may indent the upper pole of the kidney giving the impression of a dromedary hump. The adult renal cortex is thickest at the poles of the kidney where it is approximately 15 mm thick [1]. The renal medulla is principally comprised of 10–12 triangular renal pyramids that contain the collecting ducts and loops of Henle of the nephron. The pyramids are hypoechoic relative to the cortex and are separated from one another by fingers of interpyramidal renal cortex called the columns of Bertin. The rounded apex of each renal pyramid—called the papilla—projects into a minor calyx where it drains the urine flowing through its collecting ducts.

Renal Calyces and Pelvis

The 10–12 minor calyces then drain into 2–3 major calyces which coalesce to form the renal pelvis. The renal pelvis can assume a wide variety of normal shapes and may not be symmetric with the contralateral side. This pleomorphism can make diagnosing obstruction difficult at times. The renal

B.A. Inman (✉)
Assistant Professor of Urology, DUMC 2812
Duke University Medical Center, Durham, NC 27710
e-mail: brant.inman@duke.edu

J.J.M.C.H. de la Rosette et al. (eds.), *Imaging in Oncological Urology*,
DOI 10.1007/978-1-84628-759-6_11, © Springer-Verlag London Limited 2009

calyces and pelvis are located in a central concavity in the kidney that is called the renal sinus. Fatty tissue is abundant in the renal sinus of adults and accounts for its hyperechogenic appearance on ultrasound [2]. In renal ultrasonography, the normal order of increasing tissue echogenicity is renal medulla, renal cortex, liver and spleen, pancreas, and renal sinus. Demonstration of the urothelium that lines all the collecting system is not always possible but, when it is visible, it should appear as a slightly hyperechogenic layer that is smooth, thin, and regular. The renal pelvis and calyces drain into the same retroperitoneal lymph nodes as the kidney: the left side drains primarily into the para-aortic, preaortic, and postaortic nodes while the right side drains principally into the paracaval and interaortocaval nodes.

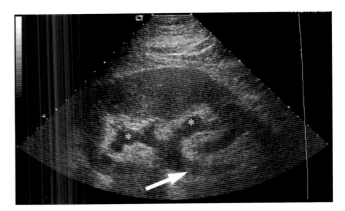

Fig. 11.1 Longitudinal ultrasound image of the left kidney demonstrates dilatation of the intrarenal collecting system (*asterisk*) with a dilated proximal ureter (*arrow*)

Ureter

Drainage of the renal pelvis into the ureter occurs at the ureteropelvic junction, a common site for both congenital and acquired obstructions. The ureter courses in the retroperitoneal space on top of the psoas muscle and is situated lateral to the vertebral pedicles until it deviates medially and crosses the common iliac artery (at the level of its bifurcation) to enter the pelvis. The retroperitoneal ureters should be at least 5 cm apart and should have a slight S shape. The pelvic portion of the ureter enters the trigone of the bladder posteriorly after passing in close proximity to the uterine artery and cervix in the female. Ureteral length varies with age, gender, and height but averages around 24 cm. Normal ureters are not routinely seen with ultrasonography but dilated ureters are. The lymphatic drainage of the ureters follows a course similar to the ureteral vasculature. The retroperitoneal portion of the left ureter drains medially into the para-aortic and presacral nodes whereas the right retroperitoneal ureter drains medially into the paracaval and interaortocaval nodes. Both pelvic ureters drain laterally into the internal iliac, external iliac, and common iliac nodes.

non-obstructive entities that produce a dilation of the collecting system that can closely mimic obstruction [6]. Technological advances in ultrasonography have helped to reverse these early problems of diagnostic accuracy and the combination of higher ultrasound frequencies, better transducers, and better software has resulted in dramatically improved image resolution. The single most important development in renal ultrasound in the last 20 years, however, has been the acquisition of the capability to perform Doppler flow analysis [7]. The expansion of early Doppler technology has led to the clinical applications of waveform Doppler sonography, power Doppler sonography, and color Doppler sonography. This, in turn, has allowed the ultrasonographer to measure the *renal resistive index* and *ureteral jets* (Fig. 11.2) [8–10], both of which can help to diagnose veritable renal obstruction.

Upper Urinary Tract Obstruction

Renal ultrasonography (RUS) may be the first imaging modality used to investigate a patient with flank pain or hematuria, both of which may be presenting signs of an upper urinary tract tumor [3, 4]. The most frequent complication of an upper urinary tract tumor that can be seen with RUS imaging is urinary tract obstruction leading to *collecting system dilation* (Fig. 11.1). Though early account of RUS described an impressive sensitivity of 98% for diagnosing obstruction, the specificity was only 74% [5]. It was quickly recognized that the cause of the high false-positive rate was a number of

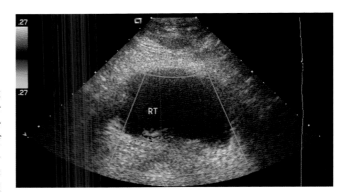

Fig. 11.2 Transverse Doppler ultrasound image of the bladder demonstrates a normal right ureteral jet. The left ureteral jet is absent suggestive of left sided obstruction

Renal Pelvic Tumors

If large enough, urothelial tumors of the renal pelvis can be visualized directly by ultrasound. Although finding a mass in the renal collecting system can sometimes be very difficult with ultrasound, an equally important task is ruling out a number of non-malignant pathologies that can cause a mass lesion in the renal pelvis (Table 11.1). A recent manuscript provides an excellent review of the diagnostic imaging features of lesions of the renal sinus [11].

Separation of the Central Echo Complex

Renal pelvic tumors can cause separation of the normally echodense central renal sinus if they are large enough [2, 12, 13]. The appearance of separation of the central echo seen in upper tract tumors is similar to what is seen in hydronephrosis but can be distinguished from the former by the presence of residual echoes and the absence of the acoustic enhancement (Fig. 11.3) [12]. The presence of a central

Table 11.1 Differential diagnosis for a collecting system filling defect

Calculi
Calyceal papilla
Cancer
Clots
Contrast air bubble
Cyclical endometriosis
Contamination/cultures
    Fungus ball (mycetoma)
    Schistosomiasis
    Tuberculosis
Chronic inflammation
    Cystic ureteropyelitis
    Malakoplakia
    Leukoplakia/cholesteatoma
Congenital
    Vascular imprint
    Kinks

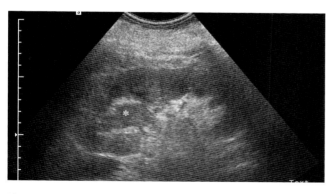

Fig. 11.3 Longitudinal ultrasound image of the right kidney demonstrates soft tissue with similar echogenicity as the renal parenchyma (*asterisk*) separating the normal renal sinus fat. The findings are due to a large TCC in the upper pole of the kidney

renal mass of moderate echogenicity that is separated from the renal parenchyma by a rim of highly echogenic renal sinus fat should be considered a malignant urothelial tumor until proven otherwise [2, 13].

Echogenicity

Urothelial tumors tend to have an echogenicity that is similar to the renal cortex but less than the normal renal sinus [12, 13]. Blood clots can have varying degrees of echogenicity and may be quite difficult to differentiate from a tumor [14, 15]. Renal calculi tend to be more echogenic than tumors and, due to their high density, calculi usually demonstrate acoustic shadowing (the cone-dome) characteristic of calcium deposition [15–18]. Calcification may also be present in tuberculous and schistosomal infection of the urinary tract [19–25]. However, it should be kept in mind that rare urothelial tumors may present with intratumoral calcification in a pattern that has been described as coarse and punctate [26]. Furthermore, certain upper urinary tract tumors—particularly squamous cell carcinomas—arise in the context of chronic irritative renal urolithiasis [27–31]. One group has even reported acoustic shadowing in a tumor [32]. Therefore, though the presence of calcification, a renal pelvic stone, or acoustic shadowing does not absolutely rule out a renal pelvic tumor, it certainly does suggest alternate diagnoses.

Mobility

One feature that can distinguish a urothelial tumor from other potential intraluminal masses is its lack of mobility. While necrotic papillae, blood clots, and certain calculi may move with a change in patient position, tumors are fixed to the urothelium and should not move [12].

Contour

Though by no means absolute, urothelial tumors of the renal pelvis tend to be poorly defined and have irregular contours while blood clots and stones tend to have sharp smooth contours [12]. Considerable overlap exists, however, and stones can be ragged and tumors smooth. Another problem is that contours are difficult to assess with ultrasonography. For these reasons contours are often of little use in diagnosing urothelial tumors by ultrasonography [33].

Blood Flow

The demonstration of blood flow within a urothelial mass is pathognomonic for a neoplastic process [33–38]. Of the few reported upper tract urothelial carcinomas that have been evaluated by Doppler ultrasonography, most have shown a Doppler shift greater than 2 kHz [34, 35].

Large Tumors

Large tumors of the central kidney that are clearly invading both the collecting system and the renal parenchyma are nearly impossible to categorize with certainty using ultrasonography [39]. These lesions can represent a renal tubular neoplasm that has invaded the collecting system or a urothelial neoplasm that has grown into the renal parenchyma. CT scanning may perform better than ultrasonography in this setting but is by no means a perfect technique [40, 41]. If treatment decisions are to be influenced by the histologic tumor type, a pretreatment biopsy should be considered.

Ureteral Tumors

Ultrasonography has not been traditionally considered a good way to assess for ureteral tumors. Whereas other imaging modalities can show a variety of imaging findings in cases of ureteral tumors, ultrasonography typically demonstrates two things: a ureteral mass or its associated hydronephrosis [37, 42, 43]. Ureteral tumors have similar features to the renal pelvic tumors described earlier in that they are of moderate echogenicity, show no acoustic shadowing, and are rarely calcified. Evidence of Doppler flow in a ureteral mass is likewise considered pathognomonic for tumor [38]. Comparative studies of the various imaging modalities for ureteral tumors are rare but at least one group has shown ultrasonography to be superior to CT in detecting these uncommon tumors [42].

Advantages of Ultrasonography

Ultrasonography is probably not the best overall method for evaluating the upper urinary tract for cancer. Nonetheless, it does have certain advantages that deserve special mention.

Noninvasive

Unlike all other methods of evaluating the upper urinary tract, ultrasonography does not require intravenous access, a percutaneous nephrostomy, or a ureteral catheter. The risk of iatrogenic injury to the body is therefore practically non-existent.

No Contrast

All other forms of urography require the administration of potentially toxic and allergenic contrast agents. Contrast-associated side effects are not a minor problem and will be discussed in more detail in the section Intravenous Pyelography.

Renal Insufficiency

Patients with impaired renal function are at high risk for contrast nephrotoxicity and should generally be spared contrast if possible. If the kidney is non-functional because of severe tumoral obstruction or some other process, contrast excretion will be markedly impaired and the quality of the imaging will suffer dramatically. Ultrasonography can be used safely and effectively in patients with renal failure.

Radiation

Ultrasonography does not use ionizing radiation to image the body and is generally considered to be free of significant side effects [44]. This important fact makes it the ideal imaging study for pregnant women. It should also be remembered that imaging-related neoplasia is a possibility for diagnostic imaging modalities that use ionizing radiation [45–48]. This may be particularly relevant for cancer patients who undergo repeated imaging tests.

Cost

Along with IVP, ultrasonography is probably the most inexpensive diagnostic test for evaluating the upper urinary tract.

Disadvantages of Ultrasonography

Calculi

Ultrasonography is not very sensitive for diagnosing renal calculi [49–52]. Since most patients with upper tract tumors are initially evaluated for flank pain or hematuria and stones are a much more common cause of these symptoms than urothelial tumors, the initial evaluation of flank pain and hematuria should employ a technique that is very sensitive for detecting stones (such as noncontrast CT) [53–55].

Staging

If a urothelial tumor is detected on initial imaging, staging the tumor then becomes a very important consideration. Conventional ultrasonography is inferior to CT and MRI for detecting retroperitoneal and pelvic lymph node enlargement [56–60], for detecting hepatic metastases [61–63], and for evaluating the lungs [64–66]. There is one particular advantage to ultrasonography for tumor staging, however: evaluation of the renal vein. Like renal cell carcinomas, urothelial carcinomas can invade the renal vein and spread to the inferior vena cava, albeit much less frequently [67]. Color Doppler imaging may be more accurate than CT in identifying tumor thrombus in the renal vein or vena cava [68–71].

Operator Dependence

Ultrasonography is operator dependent: the better the ultrasonographer, the better the accuracy [72–76]. Cross-sectional imaging modalities appear to have better interobserver reproducibility than ultrasonography.

New Advances in Ultrasonography

Endoluminal Ultrasonography

The use of intraureteral ultrasonography was first reported in the 1990s and the first report of the diagnosis of ureteral tumor occurred shortly thereafter [77, 78]. Endoluminal ultrasonography has not been widely adopted in the 15 years since it was introduced despite the refinement of smaller and more accurate probes. Its use has been principally limited to the diagnosis of crossing vessels at the ureteropelvic junction in a few select medical centers [79–83]. There have been just a few reports of its employment in diagnosing urothelial tumors of the ureter and renal pelvis [77, 84, 85]. The authors of these studies cite the principle benefit of better preoperative staging of the tumor due to more accurate identification of the ureteral mucosa and musculature. This staging advantage would only benefit the minority of patients with upper tract tumors that are considering endoscopic management. Newer modifications of the technique involve 3D reconstruction of the upper urinary tract [86, 87].

Microbubble Contrast Agents

One of the most exciting advances in ultrasonography has been the development of the technique of contrast-enhanced ultrasonography that has the potential to greatly improve diagnostic accuracy [88, 89]. The contrast agents that have been developed for ultrasound consist principally of small air bubbles measuring 3 μm in diameter that can be injected into the bloodstream or the urinary tract. At high ultrasound frequencies these microbubbles are over a thousand times more echogenic than the surrounding normal tissues [90]. Applications that are relevant to urothelial tumors include improved visualization of liver metastases [91, 92], improved imaging of tumor microvascularity [93], retrograde imaging of the ureter without radiation [94–96], molecular imaging [97], and the delivery of drugs to specific targets [88].

Intravenous Pyelography (IVP)

Brief History

After the development of medical X-rays by Roentgen in 1895, the first step toward the development of intravenous pyelogram was the development of radiocontrast. Radiocontrast was first used to visualize the urinary collecting in the form of retrograde pyelography (see discussion below) [98]. Early contrast agents—such as colloidal silver, thorium, and colloidal silver iodide—were toxic irritants that harmed the urinary tract and occasionally resulted in patient deaths. A major advance occurred in 1918 when Donald Cameron from the University of Minnesota introduced sodium iodide as a new contrast agent [99]. This agent was remarkable because it was much less toxic than other contrast agents available at the time. Mayo Clinic physicians Earl Osborne (Fig. 11.4), Charles Sutherland, Albert Scholl, and Leonard Rowntree (Fig. 11.5) used intravenous sodium iodide to produce the first intravenous pyelogram in 1918 and reported the results of their initial series in 1923 [100]. The result was a revolution in medical imaging and the next 75 years were spent trying to find contrast agents with better imaging characteristics and lower toxicity. German physician Leopold Lichtwitz was key to the development of novel contrast agents. He recruited American physician Moses Swick to a fellowship position in his laboratory in Hamburg, and the young American physician began screening multiple new agents as potential contrast agents. Swick soon moved to Berlin and began working with Alexander von Lichtenberg, the discoverer of the retrograde pyelogram, on newer and better agents. They teamed up with Arthur Binz, a Berlin chemist that had provided chemicals to Swick while he was in Hamburg,

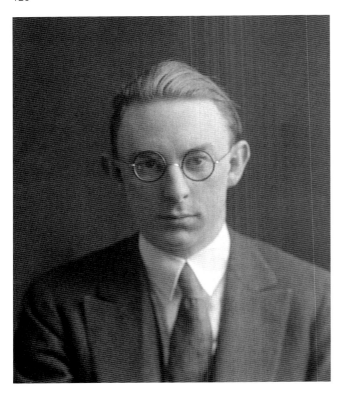

Fig. 11.4 Earl Osborne, Mayo Clinic dermatology resident, 1918–1923

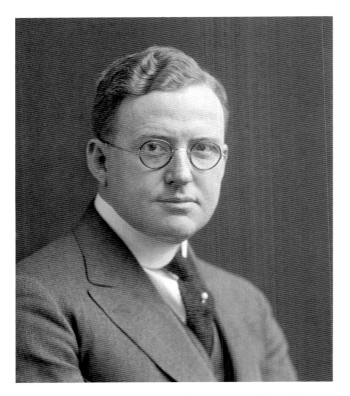

Fig. 11.5 Leonard Rowntree, Mayo Clinic internist, 1920–1932

and eventually the ionic compound Uroselectan (Iopax) was developed [101]. Uroselectan was eventually replaced by ionic monomers (e.g., diatrizoate, iothalamate) then by tri-iodinated nonionic compounds (e.g., iohexol/Omnipaque), and finally by iso-osmolar nonionic compounds (e.g., iodixans/Visipaque). With these newer agents, IVP has become a safer and better diagnostic test.

More recently, questions have surfaced as to whether IVP is dead, dying or neither [102–106]. Though IVP may no longer be the primary diagnostic modality for evaluating the urinary tract, we argue that it certainly has its place in current practice. CT and MR urography simply do not demonstrate the anatomic detail of the renal pelvis and ureter that IVP and retrograde pyelography offer [107]. These techniques are still useful and need not be abandoned.

Technique

Patient preparation is not routinely required for IVP but certain key points should be observed. Patients should be well hydrated and have adequate renal function (see section Disadvantages of IVP) and an empty bladder. The following film sequences are a suggestion for a typical case but it should be recalled that IVP should be tailored to each clinical circumstance [108]. A summary of the IVP procedure that we use at the Mayo Clinic has been previously published [109]. A scout film is first obtained and is followed by 300–600 mg/kg of contrast medium injected as a bolus into the bloodstream. An initial film coned to the kidneys can be obtained at 1 minute to demonstrate the nephrogram. A second film is obtained at 5 minutes to assess the progress of opacification of the parenchyma and collecting system. This film should include the inferior margin of the symphisis pubis and the suprarenal region. A third film is obtained at 10 minutes to view the collecting system which should be filled with contrast by this point in time. Visualization of the collecting system on this film can be improved by abdominal compression or by Trendelenberg positioning (Fig. 11.6). We routinely commence our abdominal compression shortly after contrast injection and center it at the iliac crest where the ureters can be compressed against the bony pelvis. If the collecting system is not seen perfectly, oblique films may be of use. It is recommended that at least two images of any collecting system defect be obtained. A fourth film of the ureters and full bladder can be obtained at 10–15 minutes (after release of abdominal compression) followed by a fifth post-micturition film. If there is evidence of obstruction and the collecting system has not filled adequately, delayed films should be sought.

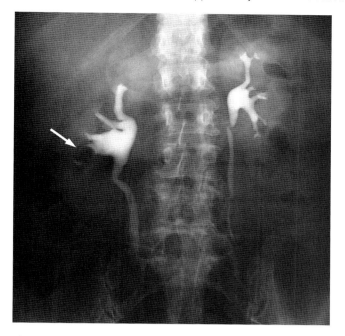

Fig. 11.6 Image from an intravenous pyelogram demonstrates a TCC in a lower pole infundibulum of the right kidney (*arrow*). External compression, as in this case, is useful for optimal distension of the intrarenal collecting system

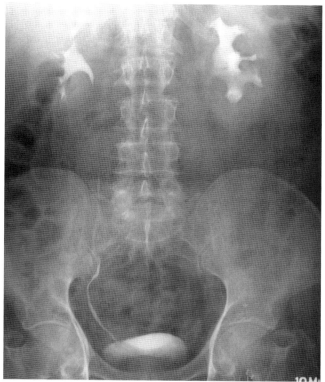

Fig. 11.7 Image from an intravenous pyelogram demonstrates left renal enlargement, dilation of the left renal collecting system and absence of filling of the left ureter

Imaging Features

Calcification

Calcification in upper tract tumors and their mimics is discussed in section Renal Pelvic Tumors. Calcification is sought on the scout film and its position confirmed following contrast injection.

Delayed Nephrogram

When the collecting system of one of two kidneys is obstructed, compensatory hemodynamic changes lead to a reduction in its glomerular filtration rate predominantly through afferent arteriolar vasoconstriction [110–114]. The reduced renal blood flow delays the passage of radiocontrast from the renal artery to the nephron and the imaging result is a delay in the nephrogram. The delay is usually best appreciated by comparing the normal unobstructed kidney to the obstructed kidney. It is noteworthy that renal units that are obstructed bilaterally or that are solitary and obstructed may not show this imaging feature because they undergo a different series of hemodynamic responses to obstruction [113].

Increased Renal Size

Obstruction of the renal collecting system usually (but not always) results in progressive dilation of the ureter and renal pelvis. The dilated kidney appears larger during the nephrographic phase of the IVP (Fig. 11.7).

Distortion of the Renal Contour

The interpapillary line is the curved line that joins the tips of the minor calyces [108]. A change in parenchymal thickness can be appreciated by comparing the distance from the interpapillary line to the edge of the renal parenchyma visualized on the nephrogram of the kidney. When the parenchyma is thickened and the underlying collecting system is abnormal, a renal mass lesion should be suspected. Renal masses can also produce a double contour that is best appreciated at tomography. Parenchymal beaking occurs when there is thickening of the parenchyma at the margins of an intraparenchymal renal lesion and indicates the presence of a slow-growing mass. Non-enhancing parenchymal thickening is typical of a renal cyst.

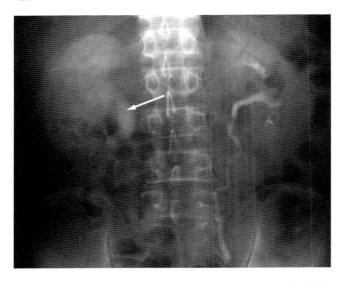

Fig. 11.8 Image from an intravenous pyelogram 45 minutes after injection demonstrates a dilated right intrarenal collecting system and upper ureter (*arrow*). There is persistence of the right nephrogram relative to the left. These secondary findings of obstruction were due to a distal right ureteral TCC (not shown)

Fig. 11.9 Image from an intravenous pyelogram demonstrates an amputated calyx in the upper pole of the right kidney (*arrow*). This was shown to be due to an obstructing TCC in the upper pole infundibulum

Pyelocaliectasis

Dilation and distortion of the calyces and renal pelvis are usually signs of obstruction though there are many other pathologies that can affect the collecting system anatomy (Fig. 11.8). Pathologies that should be considered include infection and post-infectious scarring (particularly tuberculosis, fungal infections, and schistosomiasis) [19, 24, 115], papillary necrosis [116–119], calyceal diverticulae [120, 121], and infundibular stenosis. Papillary necrosis can be diagnosed by carefully evaluating the minor calyces for a series of suggestive signs while infections are ruled out by urinalysis and urine cultures.

Phantom Calyx

A phantom calyx (a.k.a. aborted calyx) is a calyx that does not fill with contrast on imaging (Fig. 11.9) [122]. It is thought that phantom calyces generally represent serious pathology in the kidney and the differential diagnosis includes tuberculosis, urolithiasis, neoplasia (usually originating from nephron or urothelium), and congenital malformation. A tumor-filled calyx that is non-visualized has been termed an oncocalyx [108].

Filling Defects

Filling defects are likely the most common imaging feature of urothelial tumors of the renal pelvis and may be the second most common feature of ureteral tumors (after hydronephrosis) (Fig. 11.10) [18, 123–126]. The differential

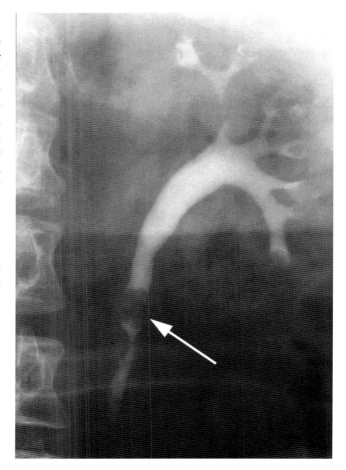

Fig. 11.10 Image from an intravenous pyelogram demonstrates a TCC in the upper left ureter (*arrow*)

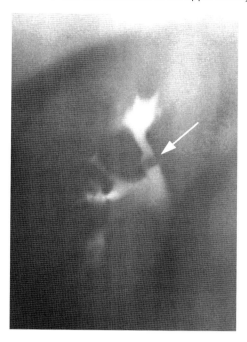

Fig. 11.11 Tomographic image from an intravenous pyelogram demonstrates a tiny TCC in an infundibulum in the upper pole of the right kidney (*arrow*)

diagnosis of collecting system filling defects is given in Table 11.1. Urothelial tumors are multifocal in 10–20% of cases and, therefore, should be high on the differential diagnosis of any process that produces multiple filling defects in the renal pelvis and ureter. Smaller filling defects may be better visualized with tomography (Fig. 11.11).

Stipple Sign

The stipple sign occurs when contrast is trapped within the interstices of a tumor and produces a stippled appearance [127, 128]. The stipple sign is highly suggestive of urothelial carcinoma but can also occur with other pathologies such as blood clots and fungus balls.

Ureteral Deviation

The course of the normal ureter is described in section The Normal Upper Urinary Tract. In most instances, the cause of ureteral deviation is ultimately determined by cross-sectional imaging. On IVP, both the direction of the ureteral deviation and the level at which it occurs are important and can suggest potential etiologies (Table 11.2).

Ureteral Dilation or Narrowing

Though the normal ureteral caliber has been defined by some uroradiologists as a ureter that is less than 8 mm in diameter,

Table 11.2 Differential diagnosis for ureteral deviation

Upper ureter
  Medial
    Renal parenchymal mass
    Renal pelvic mass
    Lateral retroperitoneal mass
    Retroperitoneal fibrosis
    Retrocaval ureter
  Lateral
    Congenital malformation of kidney
      Horseshoe kidney
      Malrotation
    Renal pelvic mass
    Retroperitoneal mass or lymph nodes
    Psoas hypertrophy or abscess
    Aortic aneurysm
    Prior retroperitoneal surgery

Lower ureter
  Medial
    Pelvic lymphadenopathy
    Pelvic mass
    Prior pelvic surgery
    Pelvic prolapse
    Bladder diverticulum
    Inguinal ureteral herniation
  Lateral
    Pelvic mass
    Iliac artery aneurysm
    Urinoma/Hematoma
    Prior pelvic surgery
    Femoral ureteral herniation

the best way to determine dilation is usually comparison to the contralateral side (Fig. 11.12) [108]. The ureter is often slightly dilated just above the area where it crosses the common iliac artery, a segment that has been called the ureteral spindle. Causes of ureteral dilation are given in Table 11.3. Narrowing of the ureter should be interpreted with caution because normal peristaltic waves may give the false impression of a narrowed segment (hence the importance of obtaining two views of any suspected pathology). Determining intrinsic from extrinsic causes of ureteral narrowing can be helpful. Intrinsic infiltration typically produces an irregular and abrupt change in ureteral caliber that resembles an apple core. Extrinsic encasement tends to produce a smooth tapering of the ureter. Causes of ureteral narrowing are given in Table 11.4.

Advantages of Ivp

Cost and Availability

Intravenous pyelography is inexpensive and can be obtained with a strict minimum of radiologic equipment. Even the most remote rural facilities can perform IVP if basic radiography is available.

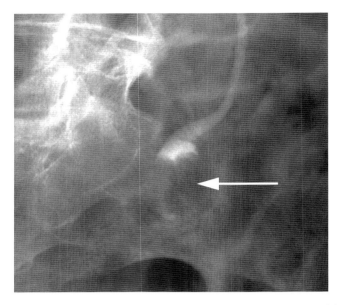

Fig. 11.12 Image from an intravenous pyelogram demonstrates a TCC filling the distal left ureter (*arrow*) with slight ureteral dilatation proximally

Table 11.3 Differential diagnosis for ureteral dilation

Obstructive
    Intraluminal ureteral mass (see Table 11.1)
    Extraluminal ureteral pathology
    Ureteral stricture
    Retroperitoneal or pelvic mass
    Retroperitoneal fibrosis
  Intravesical obstruction
    Bladder tumor
    Bladder calculus
    Bladder infection (e.g., TB, schistosomiasis)
    Neurogenic bladder (± detrusor-sphincter dysynergia)
  Infravesical obstruction
    Benign prostatic hyperplasia
    Prostatic or urethral tumor
    Urethral stricture

Non-obstructive
  Pregnancy
  Ureteral atony
    Postobstructive residual dilation
    Infection (endotoxin)
  High urine flow
    Polydipsia
    Diabetes insipidus
    Postobstructive diuresis
Congenital
  Vesicoureteral reflux
  Megaureter
  Ectopic ureter
  Ureterocele
  Prune belly syndrome
  Retrocaval ureter

Table 11.4 Differential diagnosis for ureteral narrowing

Normal
  Ureteral peristalsis
  Vascular imprinting
Neoplasia
  Urothelial tumors
  Retroperitoneal/pelvic tumor
  Lymph nodes
  Metastases
Stricture
  Iatrogenic
  Trauma
  Radiation
  Congenital
Infection
  TB
  Schistosomiasis
Inflammation
  Malakoplakia
  Endometriosis
  Inflammatory bowel disease

Image Quality

Many physicians still regard IVP as one of the best tests for visualizing ureteral anatomy.

Disadvantages of IVP

Contrast Toxicity

A full discussion of the toxicities of radiocontrast is beyond the scope of this chapter and we provide only a brief overview here. The reader is referred to Bush and Lasser for a complete discussion [129]. Nephrotoxicity is probably the most important complication of IVP—though not the only one—and its incidence depends on the type and dose of contrast used, the underlying health of the patient at study, and the medication used by the patient. Numerous clinical trials have been conducted in an attempt to find strategies to minimize this complication. European guidelines for the prevention of contrast nephrotoxicity have recently been published and propose the following important points [130]. Identifying individuals at risk of contrast nephrotoxicity prior to injecting contrast may reduce its incidence. Risk factors include diabetes, renal failure, congestive heart failure, dehydration, nephrotoxic drugs (e.g., NSAIDs, gentamicin), and age over 70. Physicians should try to minimize contrast nephrotoxicity by adopting a prevention strategy. Universal preventative measures include: ensuring adequate hydration (oral or IV), using low-osmolar contrast agents, minimizing contrast dose, maximizing time delay between contrast injections, stopping nephrotoxic drugs, avoiding diuretics, and avoiding contrast altogether if not necessary. Other interventions that have shown promise in randomized trials include intravenous bicarbonate infusions and *N*-acetylcysteine [131–134]. Another interesting investigational treatment with low toxicity is vitamin C [135].

Contrast Allergy

The incidence of anaphylactoid reactions to contrast media depends on the type of agent used and the patient's history of atopic reactions [136]. Most anaphylactoid reactions occur within minutes of contrast injection but some reactions may take up to 2 hours to develop [136]. Overall, the risk of any form of anaphylactoid reaction is 5% with ionic contrast and 1% with non-ionic contrast [136, 137]. Severe reactions are much less common, occurring in 1 in 750 patients injected with ionic contrast and in 1 in 3000 patients injected with non-ionic contrast [136, 137]. Risk factors for anaphylactoid reactions include asthma (RR=10), previous contrast reaction (RR=5), other allergies (RR=2.5), congestive heart disease, sickle cell anemia, anxiety, certain medications (β-blockers, IL-2, NSAIDs), and pheochromocytoma [136]. Patients with risk factors should receive a pre-contrast protocol of antihistamines and corticosteroids such as that supported by the European Society of Urogenital Radiology [138, 139].

Severe Obstruction

If the renal unit that is investigated is severely obstructed and no contrast is excreted into the collecting system by 10 minutes, delayed films will be required. Often these films do not adequately demonstrate the collecting system despite multiple radiation exposures, and alternative cross-sectional imaging studies become indicated. Unfortunately, the dose of contrast administered during IVP into the obstructed collecting system is quite high and may force delay of CT imaging

by 1–2 days. This delay in diagnosis may prove quite distressing for both the physician and the patient.

Retrograde Pyelography

Brief History

Retrograde pyelography was described by the German physicians Fritz Voelcker and Alexander von Lichtenberg in 1906 and was the first technique used to specifically visualize the renal collecting system [98, 140]. The initial images of the ureter were the result of vesicoureteral reflux that occurred during a cystogram but this rapidly lead to the purposeful catheterization of the ureteral orifice and the retrograde injection of contrast media. The technique of retrograde pyelography was popularized in North America by William Braasch who practiced urology at the Mayo Clinic from 1907 to 1946 (Fig. 11.13). Braasch was a major advocate of retrograde pyelography and was responsible for describing the normal pyelographic upper tract anatomy and the use of pyelography for diagnosing malignant diseases of the genitourinary tract [141–143]. Improvements in contrast agents made over the next 100 years have made retrograde pyelography much safer for the patient.

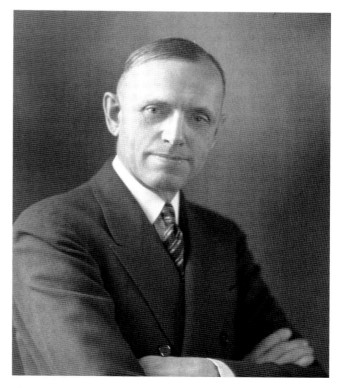

Fig. 11.13 William Braasch, Mayo Clinic urologist, 1907–1946

Technique

Standard Single-Contrast Technique

Retrograde pyelography is a minimally invasive method of imaging the renal collecting system that generally requires cystoscopic visualization of the ureteral orifice, although there have been reports of performing the technique completely under fluoroscopic guidance [144, 145]. Regardless of the method employed, sterility is important because the introduction of bacteria directly into the renal collecting system and bloodstream is a potentially catastrophic complication. A small ureteral catheter, typically 4–7 F, is then slowly advanced into the distal intramural ureter. If urine collection, brush biopsy, or saline barbotage specimens are to be sent for cytologic analysis, as should routinely be the case if a tumor is on the differential diagnosis, these samples should be obtained prior to injecting contrast media into the collecting system. This is done because contrast media, particularly ionic agents with high osmolarity, can alter the cytologic appearance of normal urothelial cells resulting in a potential false-positive urine cytology [146–149]. Newer iso-osmolar contrast agents do not appear to have this problem [146]. Air bubbles in the ureteral catheter should be purged prior to inserting the catheter into the ureter because these can create the false impression of a filling defect, and positioning the patient in the Trendelenberg position may result in better opacification of the renal calyces. A scout film should be obtained prior to contrast injection to assess for mass effects and calcification. Under fluoroscopic guidance, 5–10 mL of diluted contrast media is then slowly injected at low pressure into the ureteral catheter. The ureter and renal pelvis are then assessed systematically. Rotating the fluoroscopy head can provide alternate views of the intrarenal collecting system and prove vital to correctly diagnosing pathology.

Double-Contrast Technique

The use of gas to visualize the urinary collecting system is called gas pyelography and the combination of a gas and a liquid contrast agent is referred to as double-contrast pyelography [150–154]. Several options exist for gas pyelography including oxygen, carbon dioxide, room air, and other inert gases. Carbon dioxide is preferred because it is safest. The technique for catheterizing the ureter is the same as described above with the exception of patient positioning: the reverse Trendelenberg position is preferred [154, 155]. A volume of 15–20 mL of gas is injected into the renal pelvis immediately following the injection of 5 mL of radiocontrast media. Though the risk of gas embolism with gas pyelography is not known with certainty, it has certainly been described and should be avoided at all costs [155–157]. The risk of gas embolism and little gain in diagnostic accuracy have made gas pyelography a largely unused procedure.

Imaging Features of Ureteral and Renal Pelvic Tumors

The imaging features of ureteral and renal pelvic tumors visualized with retrograde pyelography are generally the same as described earlier with intravenous urography. Tumors appear as filling defects, irregular stenoses, non-visualized calyces, and hydronephrosis. The advantages of retrograde pyelography over other imaging modalities are discussed below. Two imaging features of ureteral tumors that are best detected with retrograde pyelography are the so-called goblet sign and Bergman's sign.

Goblet Sign

The goblet sign (a.k.a. chalice sign) refers to a cup-shaped collection of contrast media that is seen just distal to the intraluminal filling defect and suggests the presence of a tumor (Figs. 11.14 and 11.15) [158]. The slow growth of an intraluminal tumor causes proximal as well as distal expansion of the ureter [159]. Additionally, a pedunculated tumor may also be pushed distally during peristalsis only to return to its normal cephalad position between contractions [160]. Presence of the goblet sign suggests a superficial (i.e., less aggressive) tumor [158].

Bergman's Sign

Bergman's sign (a.k.a. catheter coiling sign) refers to the coiling of a ureteral catheter in the infratumoral ureter [159]. Its interpretation and cause are exactly the same as the goblet sign.

Advantages of Retrograde Pyelography

Fluoroscopic Monitoring

Fluoroscopic monitoring allows this imaging modality to better visualize the pathology in the urinary tract because the patient or fluoroscopy head can be repositioned to provide an optimal view of the problem. Often a slight change in the angle of view can result in a dramatically better picture of the pathologic process.

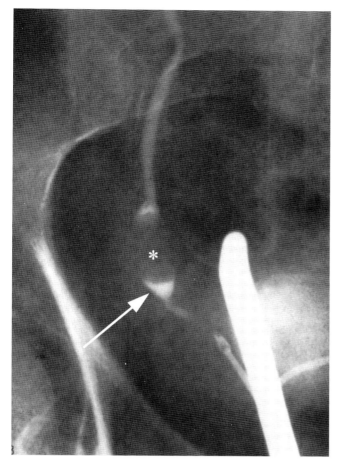

Fig. 11.14 Image from a retrograde pyelogram demonstrates a TCC filling the distal right ureter (*asterisk*) with slight ureteral dilatation distally (*arrow*). The distal ureteral dilation is known as the "chalice sign" or the "goblet sign"

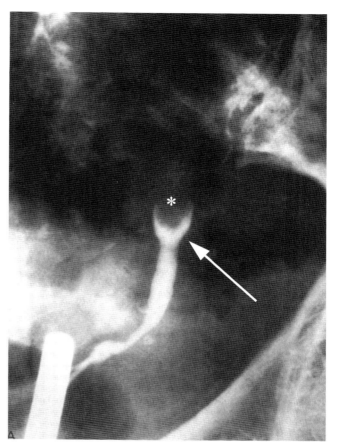

Fig. 11.15 Image from a retrograde pyelogram demonstrates a TCC filling the distal left ureter (*asterisk*) demonstrating the "goblet sign"

Intracavitary Filling

More contrast is instilled in the ureter and renal pelvis with retrograde pyelography than is possible with any intravascular imaging technique. This can sometimes be very useful in opacifying the phantom calyces seen on IVP. Many physicians feel that retrograde pyelography provides the best quality images of the renal pelvis and the most accurate measure of the extent of a ureteral tumor (i.e., length of ureteral involvement and multifocality) (Fig. 11.16).

Renal Failure

When renal function is so severely impaired that the kidney cannot excrete the contrast media or when intravascular contrast media risks worsening stable renal impairment, retrograde pyelography can be of use. As noted below, retrograde pyelography can worsen renal function, although this occurs very rarely. Most urologists and radiologists would agree that

retrograde contrast injection is unlikely to cause significant renal dysfunction.

Contrast Toxicity

The injection of contrast media into the collecting system is associated with a very low adverse event rate. Despite this, there have been reports of a variety of contrast-related complications that deserve mention. Contrast nephrotoxicity can occur after retrograde pyelography and seems to be associated with bilateral obstruction, the presence of backflow (see later), and contrast-induced mucosal edema [161–163]. The course of resolution appears similar to that observed in cases of intravenous contrast nephrotoxicity.

Contrast Allergy

There is a very low rate of anaphylactoid reactions when contrast is administered directly into the urinary collecting system via retrograde injection. Though the urothelium

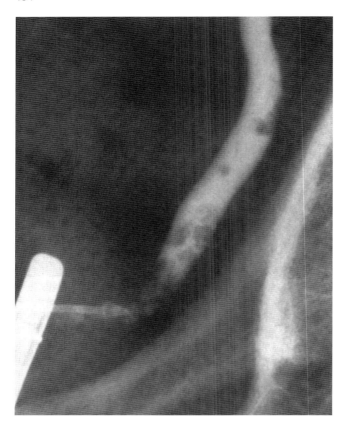

Fig. 11.16 Image from a retrograde pyelogram demonstrates multiple tiny papillary TCC in the distal left ureter

is considered a relatively impermeable barrier, contrast can be absorbed through the urothelium and enter the circulation [164–166]. Backflow mechanisms may also be involved in certain cases. A variety of allergic presentations have been described in patients undergoing cystography and retrograde pyelography, ranging from simple urticarial rashes to circulatory collapse [167–170]. Non-ionic contrast agents cause much fewer adverse reactions than ionic agents. It is unknown whether or not prophylaxis regimens are efficacious or indicated for preventing anaphylactoid reactions in patients undergoing cystography or retrograde pyelography [171]. Our bias is to err on the side of caution and administer prophylaxis to patients who have previously developed a reaction or that are at high risk of one.

Ancillary Diagnostic Procedures

Selective ureteral cytologies, saline barbotage, brush biopsy, and ureteroscopy can all be done in the same setting as retrograde pyelography. Combining all these diagnostic modalities provides a better chance of diagnosing difficult cases and is recommended in the follow-up of patients at high risk for an upper tract urothelial tumor [172].

Drainage

A ureteral stent can be placed into the ureter to relieve obstruction and symptoms caused by the tumor at the same time as retrograde pyelography.

Disadvantages of Retrograde Pyelography

Difficult Ureteral Orifice

All urologists with significant experience will recall occasions where ureteral cannulation was simply not possible. Some of the more common causes of difficult ureteral catheterization include a reimplanted ureter, the presence of a urinary diversion, a large prostate, a tumor at the ureteral orifice or previous transurethral resection thereof, a bladder diverticulum, extensive hematuria, an obstructing ureteral calculus, and looping dilated ureters. There are many tricks and tools that can assist in these situations but in certain cases the most rapid solution is to abort the procedure and obtain a percutaneous nephrostomy tract.

Iatrogenic Trauma

Though cystoscopy is a routine procedure for the urologist, inserting an instrument into the urethra should not be taken lightly. Many serious complications have occurred during cystoscopy and ureteral catheterization. Some of the more common complications include perforation of the urinary tract (urethra, bladder, ureter, or the renal pelvis) [173, 174], stricture with secondary obstruction [175–177], and infection/sepsis [178]. Although controversial, percutaneous nephrostomy is generally preferred over ureteral catheterization in the context of infected urine [179–182].

Backflow

Excessive injection pressure or trauma to the urothelium can result in the leakage of radiocontrast media into lymphovascular spaces [183–185]. This process is known as backflow and five distinct varieties have been described. *Pyelovenous backflow* occurs when contrast leaks into the venous drainage system of the kidney [186, 187]. It provides a direct route for contrast, air, and bacteria to enter the bloodstream. This is likely the point at which anaphylactoid reactions occur. Air embolism is a rare complication of retrograde pyelography that is related to pyelovenous backflow [157]. *Pyelolymphatic backflow* occurs when contrast leaks into the fine lymphatic channels that line the renal sinus and migrates toward the hilar and retroperitoneal lymph nodes [186, 188]. Renal tubular toxicity has been reported to occur through this mechanism [163]. Backflow into a tumor has been termed *pyelocancerous backflow* [189, 190]. It is rare and of unknown significance. Intrarenal backflow refers to two things: pyelotubular backflow and pyelointerstitial backflow. *Pyelotubular backflow* occurs when contrast leaks into the collecting ducts and enters the nephron in a retrograde manner whereas *pyelointerstitial backflow* occurs when contrast leaks into the renal interstitium [184, 191]. Intrarenal backflow has been associated with impending renal transplant rejection [191, 192], renal ischemia [193–195], and prolonged obstruction [184]. The last form of backflow to be discussed is *pyelosinus backflow*. This form of backflow occurs when small tears in the calyces and renal pelvis develop and allow leakage of contrast into the renal sinus and the retroperitoneal space [196, 197]. The main clinical problems associated with this type of backflow are the development of a urinoma or retroperitoneal abscess [196, 198]. Though backflow can be prevented in most instances by keeping the intrapelvic pressure below 30 mmHg, some normal individuals will have backflow despite a perfect low-pressure technique.

Staging

Retrograde pyelography cannot establish extraureteral extension or the distant spread of a detected tumor. Occasionally retrograde pyelography will identify ureteral deviation caused by retroperitoneal lymph nodes or renal parenchymal invasion by a urothelial tumor, but these are the exceptions and always require cross-sectional imaging confirmation.

Carcinogenesis

A condition of historical interest is thorium-induced urothelial carcinoma. Thorotrast and Umbrathor were contrast agents composed of thorium dioxide, first introduced in 1915 and used routinely from the 1930s to the 1950s [199]. Thorium dioxide is mildly radioactive (it emits α-particles) and has a half-life of over 400 years. Small deposits of thorium (that are detectable by CT) occasionally formed under the urothelium of patients treated with this agent and many people developed cancers of the kidney and collecting system secondarily, 20–30 years after their exposure [200–204]. Newer contrast agents have not had this problem.

Antegrade Pyelography

Brief History

Percutaneous access to the upper urinary tract had its beginning in France in 1949 and was popularized by other groups in the mid-1950s [205–209]. The technique was initially used to diagnose and treat patients with severe hydronephrosis but has since been adapted to serve a wide variety of diagnostic and therapeutic needs [210]. Ultrasound or fluoroscopy guidance is now routinely used to help place the needle in the desired calyx [211–214].

Technique

Antegrade pyelography is generally reserved for patients that cannot receive intravenous contrast and that failed an attempt at retrograde pyelography. It can also be used as a primary imaging modality for patients with an obstruction of the upper urinary tract because the obstruction can be treated and its cause diagnosed.

Antegrade Pyelography

A quick focused medical history, a urine culture, and a coagulation profile are recommended prior to commencing this procedure. The patient is placed in the prone or prone-oblique position. Some form of imaging, usually ultrasonography or fluoroscopy, is used to guide the initial needle puncture into the desired renal calyx. When imaging or manometry are the only goals, a small 22- or 24-gauge needle may be sufficient to inject the contrast material and measure intrapelvic pressures. Strict sterility must be adhered to if infectious complications are to be avoided. To minimize the risk of bleeding complications, the needle tract is ideally placed through the relatively avascular line of Brödel on the posterolateral surface of the kidney [215, 216]. It is also generally preferred to target a posterior calyx in order to minimize the risk of bleeding and colonic injury [217, 218]. Similarly, infracostal puncture of a lower pole calyces is preferred over supracostal puncture of an upper pole calyx because of the risk of puncturing the pleura and the lung [219, 220]. Direct puncture of the renal pelvis should be avoided because of the risk of trauma to the central renal vasculature and the risks of urinoma and urinary fistula formation. Local anesthetics are usually adequate for pain control and their presence in the vicinity of the renal capsule is usually appreciated by the patient. Once the needle enters the collecting system, its position can be confirmed by the respiratory motion of the needle and the appearance of the aspirated urine. Urine cultures and cytologies are almost always appropriate. Final confirmation of needle position is obtained by injecting a small dose of contrast into the collecting system and confirming its location with fluoroscopy.

Percutaneous Nephrostomy

When the renal unit in question is obstructed, it may be desirable to leave a nephrostomy tube to decompress the kidney and permit recovery of renal function. The nephrostomy tube can be used at a later date for performing antegrade pyelography or for endourologic access to the tumor. The technique for obtaining renal access is the same as that described above except that a slightly different needle is used. Once the needle is confirmed to be in the collecting system, a guidewire is inserted into the needle and positioned within the renal pelvis and ureter. The nephrostomy tract is then progressively dilated until an appropriately sized nephrostomy tube can be placed. Great care must be taken not to overdistend or puncture the renal pelvis during this procedure because serious bleeding and infection may result. The nephrostomy is then fixed to the skin in a manner that prevents inadvertent kinking, removal, or traction [221–223].

Imaging Features of Ureteral and Renal Pelvic Tumors

Urothelial tumors have essentially the same imaging characteristics with antegrade pyelography as with IVP and retrograde pyelography. As with retrograde pyelography, some physicians feel that direct injection of contrast into the collecting system provides for optimal anatomic detail (Fig. 11.17).

Advantages of Antegrade Pyelography

Success Rate

The success rate for establishing a percutaneous nephrostomy tract is over 99% and is relatively constant if the operator performs more than 10 nephrostomies per year [224–227]. The technique is therefore a very reliable way of diagnosing patients that have failed other imaging modalities.

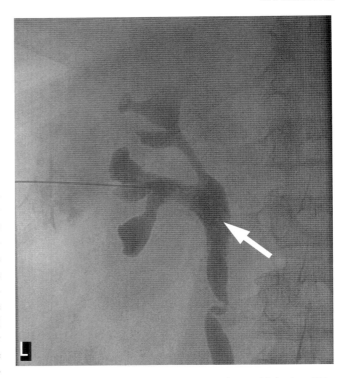

Fig. 11.17 Antegrade pyelogram demonstrating multiple tiny filling defects carpeting the right renal pelvis and upper right ureter (*arrow*) found to multifocal TCC at surgery

Drainage

The ability to leave a drainage nephrostomy catheter can be a major benefit, particularly for the patient with infected urine. There has been concern about the potential for tumor seeding along the nephrostomy tract [228–230]. This phenomenon appears to be quite rare and not all groups have observed it [231–235]. Nonetheless, for patients who eventually undergo nephroureterectomy, it may be wise to excise the nephrostomy tract. Brachytherapy has also been used to treat the nephrostomy tract in patients undergoing endourologic treatment [236].

Ancillary Diagnostic Procedures

As with retrograde pyelography, urine cultures, cytologies, and brush biopsies can all be obtained via the nephrostomy access [232]. A pressure-flow (Whittaker) study can also be performed if obstruction is questionable [237–242].

Treatment

The nephrostomy tract can be used for endourologic management of renal pelvic and upper ureteral tumors and chemotherapy and BCG can be dripped into the collecting system safely via the nephrostomy [230, 231, 233, 235, 243–245].

Disadvantages of Antegrade Pyelography

Nearly all the disadvantages of this imaging approach are due to the potential complications associated with percutaneous renal access.

Bleeding

Hematuria is nearly universal after percutaneous needle puncture of the kidney but serious hemorrhage is fortunately uncommon. The incidence of major bleeding is directly related to the size of the nephrostomy tract. For small nephrostomy tracts (<12 F) the reported transfusion and/or intervention rates generally range from 1 to 4% while large tracts (>12 F) may have rates up to 20% [224, 225, 246–250]. The estimated average blood loss from a large nephrostomy tract ranges from 16 to 28 g/L [251, 252]. Risk factors for increased blood loss other than increasing nephrostomy tract size include renal pelvic perforation [251, 252], multiple renal punctures [251, 252], anterior calyx access [217], supracostal access [217, 220], diabetes [252], dilation of the nephrostomy tract without a balloon [248], and the lack of imaging guidance [213, 252]. Most renal hemorrhages can be handled non-operatively and we suggest a stepwise approach to management. Simple maneuvers such as clamping the nephrostomy tube and balloon tamponade should be considered first [249, 253, 254]. For procedures conducted in the operative setting, simple cauterization of the bleeding vessel or the application of fibrin glue may be of value [255–258]. If these methods fail or if the bleeding is too brisk to warrant an initial conservative approach, vascular access and selective renal embolization should be attempted [247, 249, 259–264]. Renal embolization is generally well tolerated but renal infarction of varying degrees of severity can occur [265, 266]. Other complications that have been reported secondary to endovascular techniques include pseudoaneurysm or arteriovenous fistula formation at the access site [267–270], thrombosis and dissection of the aorta [271, 272], and embolization of the limbs [273].

Lastly, severe bleeding can be associated with the formation of a retroperitoneal hematoma [274, 275]. These hematomas can be a source of pain and a nidus for infection.

Arteriovenous Fistula

AV fistulae are usually clinical entities that escape clinical attention. The incidence of radiologic AV fistula occurring after nephrostomy is unknown but reaches 10–15% for renal biopsies [276–279]. Most of these cases resolve spontaneously within 6–12 months but may occasionally require embolization or surgical treatment [280, 281].

Iatrogenic Organ Injury

Any organ that lies in or near the retroperitoneum can be punctured while obtaining percutaneous access to the kidney. The most commonly injured organs are the renal pelvis [224], the colon [218, 282–285], the liver [286, 287], the spleen [286–289], and pleura/lung [219, 220, 250, 287, 290–293].

Death

The death rate from percutaneous nephrostomies is very low but is not zero. Large series report death rates in the 0.1–0.5% range [224, 250].

Conclusions

The traditional diagnostic modalities of IVP and retrograde pyelography are rapidly being replaced as first-line diagnostic modalities for flank pain and hematuria by CT and MR urography. In many circumstances, however, they may still be the optimal method of evaluating the upper urinary tract for the presence of a urothelial tumor. Table 11.5 shows the relative strengths and weaknesses of the various imaging techniques that can be used to identify upper urinary tract tumors.

Table 11.5 Strengths of various imaging modalities for upper urinary tract tumors

	IVP	Retrograde/antegrade	US	CT	MRI
Renal pelvis	+++	+++	+	++	++
Ureter	+++	+++	+	++	++
Calculi	++	++	+	+++	+
Staging	+	+	++	+++	+++
Cost	+++	+	+++	++	+
Radiation	++	++	+++	+	+++

References

1. Emamian SA, Nielsen MB, Pedersen JF, Ytte L. Kidney dimensions at sonography: correlation with age, sex, and habitus in 665 adult volunteers. AJR Am J Roentgenol. 1993;160(1):83–6.

2. Sanders RC, Conrad MR. The ultrasonic characteristics of the renal pelvicalyceal echo complex. J Clin Ultrasound. 1977;5(6):372–7.

3. Erwin BC, Carroll BA, Sommer FG. Renal colic: the role of ultrasound in initial evaluation. Radiology. 1984;152(1):147–50.

4. Szabo V, Sobel M, Legradi J, Balogh F. Diagnostic ultrasound in urology. Int Urol Nephrol. 1980;12(4):291–309.

5. Ellenbogen PH, Scheible FW, Talner LB, Leopold GR: sensitivity of gray scale ultrasound in detecting urinary tract obstruction. AJR Am J Roentgenol. 1978;130(4):731–3.

6. Amis ES Jr, Cronan JJ, Pfister RC, Yoder IC. Ultrasonic inaccuracies in diagnosing renal obstruction. Urology. 1982;19(1):101–5.

7. Harzmann R, Weckermann D. Importance of Doppler sonography in urology. Urol Int. 1990;45(4):258–63.

8. Tublin ME, Bude RO, Platt JF. Review: the resistive index in renal Doppler sonography: where do we stand? AJR Am J Roentgenol. 2003;180(4):885–92.

9. Kalmon EH, Albers DD, Dunn JH. Ureteral jet phenomenon: stream of opaque medium simulating an anomalous configuration of the ureter. Radiology. 1955;65:933–5.

10. Chiu NT, Wu CC, Yao WJ, et al. Evaluation and validation of ureteric jet index by glomerular filtration rate. Invest Radiol. 1999;34(8):499–02.

11. Rha SE, Byun JY, Jung SE, et al. The renal sinus: pathologic spectrum and multimodality imaging approach. Radiographics. 2004;24 Suppl 1:S117–31.

12. Arger PH, Mulhern CB, Pollack HM, Banner MP, Wein AJ. Ultrasonic assessment of renal transitional cell carcinoma: preliminary report. AJR Am J Roentgenol. 1979;132(3):407–11.

13. Subramanyam BR, Raghavendra BN, Madamba MR. Renal transitional cell carcinoma: sonographic and pathologic correlation. J Clin Ultrasound. 1982;10(5):203–10.

14. Wicks JD, Silver TM, Bree RL. Gray scale features of hematomas: an ultrasonic spectrum. AJR Am J Roentgenol. 1978;131(6):977–80.

15. Rosenfield AT, Taylor KJ, Dembner AG, Jacobson P. Ultrasound of renal sinus: new observations. AJR Am J Roentgenol. 1979;133(3):441–8.

16. Pollack HM, Arger PH, Goldberg BB, Mulholland SG. Ultrasonic detection of nonopaque renal calculi. Radiology. 1978;127(1):233–7.

17. Edell S, Zegel H. Ultrasonic evaluation of renal calculi. AJR Am J Roentgenol. 1978;130(2):261–3.

18. Mulholland SG, Arger PH, Goldberg BB, Pollack HM. Ultrasonic differentiation of renal pelvic filling defects. J Urol. 1979;122(1):14–6.

19. Gibson MS, Puckett ML, Shelly ME. Renal tuberculosis. Radiographics. 2004;24(1):251–6.

20. Kim SH, Yoon HK, Park JH, et al. Tuberculous stricture of the urinary tract: antegrade balloon dilation and ureteral stenting. Abdom Imaging. 1993;18(2):186–90.

21. Kollins SA, Hartman GW, Carr DT, Segura JW, Hattery RR. Roentgenographic findings in urinary tract tuberculosis. A 10 year review. Am J Roentgenol Radium Ther Nucl Med. 1974;121(3):487–99.

22. Dittrich M, Doehring E. Ultrasonographical aspects of urinary schistosomiasis: assessment of morphological lesions in the upper and lower urinary tract. Pediatr Radiol. 1986;16(3):225–30.

23. Ghoneim MA, Ashamallah A, Khalik MA. Bilharzial strictures of the ureter presenting with anuria. Br J Urol. 1971;43(4):439–43.

24. Gupta R, Kehinde EO, Sinan T, Al-Essa AA. Urinary schistosomiasis: urographic features and significance of drooping kidney appearance. Int Urol Nephrol. 2001;33(3):461–5.

25. Jorulf H, Lindstedt E. Urogenital schistosomiasis: CT evaluation. Radiology. 1985;157(3):745–9.

26. Dinsmore BJ, Pollack HM, Banner MP. Calcified transitional cell carcinoma of the renal pelvis. Radiology. 1988;167(2):401–4.

27. Li MK, Cheung WL. Squamous cell carcinoma of the renal pelvis. J Urol. 1987;138(2):269–71.

28. Blacher EJ, Johnson DE, Abdul-Karim FW, Ayala AG. Squamous cell carcinoma of renal pelvis. Urology. 1985;25(2):124–6.

29. Dumbadze I, Crawford ED, Mulvaney WP. Giant dendritic struvite calculus associated with transitional cell carcinoma of the ipsilateral renal pelvis and bladder: a case report and review of the literature. J Urol. 1979;122(5):692–3.

30. Lee TY, Ko SF, Wan YL, et al. Renal squamous cell carcinoma: CT findings and clinical significance. Abdom Imaging. 1998;23(2):203–8.

31. Katz R, Gofrit ON, Golijanin D, et al. Urothelial cancer of the renal pelvis in percutaneous nephrolithotomy patients. Urol Int. 2005;75(1):17–20.

32. Janetschek G, Putz A, Feichtinger H. Renal transitional cell carcinoma mimicking stone echoes. J Ultrasound Med. 1988;7(2):83–6.

33. Seong CK, Kim SH, Lee JS, Kim KH, Sim JS, Chang KH. Hypoechoic normal renal sinus and renal pelvis tumors: sonographic differentiation. J Ultrasound Med. 2002;21(9):993–9; quiz 1001–2.

34. Kier R, Taylor KJ, Feyock AL, Ramos IM. Renal masses: characterization with Doppler US. Radiology. 1990;176(3):703–7.

35. Kuijpers D, Jaspers R. Renal masses: differential diagnosis with pulsed doppler US. Radiology. 1989;170(1 Pt 1):59–60.

36. Horstman WG, McFarland RM, Gorman JD. Color Doppler sonographic findings in patients with transitional cell carcinoma of the bladder and renal pelvis. J Ultrasound Med. 1995;14(2):129–33.

37. Kim HJ, Lim JW, Lee DH, Ko YT, Oh JH, Kim YW. Transitional cell carcinoma involving the distal ureter: assessment with transrectal and color doppler ultrasonography. J Ultrasound Med. 2005;24(12):1625–33.

38. Killi RM, Cal C, Pourbagher A, Yurtseven O. Doppler sonographic diagnosis of primary transitional cell carcinoma of the ureter. J Clin Ultrasound. 2000;28(7):361–4.

39. Bree RL, Schultz SR, Hayes R. Large infiltrating renal transitional cell carcinomas: CT and ultrasound features. J Comput Assist Tomogr. 1990;14(3):381–5.

40. Igarashi T, Muakami S, Shichijo Y, Matsuzaki O, Isaka S, Shimazaki J. Clinical and radiological aspects of infiltrating transitional cell carcinoma of the kidney. Urol Int. 1994;52(4):181–4.

41. Fukuya T, Honda H, Nakata H, et al. Computed tomographic findings of invasive transitional cell carcinoma in the kidney. Radiat Med. 1994;12(1):6–10.

42. Hadas-Halpern I, Farkas A, Patlas M, Zaghal I, Sabag-Gottschalk S, Fisher D. Sonographic diagnosis of ureteral tumors. J Ultrasound Med. 1999;18(9):639–45.

43. Voet D, Mareels S, Oosterlinck W, Afschrift M. Sonographic diagnosis of a nonobstructive tumor in the mid-ureter. J Clin Ultrasound. 1997;25(8):459–60.

44. Barnett SB. Biophysical aspects of diagnostic ultrasound. Ultrasound Med Biol. 2000;26 Suppl 1:S68–70.

45. Dendy PP, Brugmans MJ. Low dose radiation risks. Br J Radiol. 2003;76(910):674–7.

46. Berrington de Gonzalez A, Darby S. Risk of cancer from diagnostic X-rays: estimates for the UK and 14 other countries. Lancet. 2004;363(9406):345–51.

47. Wakeford R. The cancer epidemiology of radiation. Oncogene. 2004;23(38):6404–28.

48. Brenner DJ, Doll R, Goodhead DT, et al. Cancer risks attributable to low doses of ionizing radiation: assessing what we really know. Proc Natl Acad Sci USA. 2003;100(24):13761–6.

49. Sheafor DH, Hertzberg BS, Freed KS, et al. Nonenhanced helical CT and US in the emergency evaluation of patients with renal colic: prospective comparison. Radiology. 2000;217(3):792–7.

50. Ripolles T, Agramunt M, Errando J, Martinez MJ, Coronel B, Morales M. Suspected ureteral colic: plain film and sonography vs unenhanced helical CT. a prospective study in 66 patients. Eur Radiol. 2004;14(1):129–36.

51. Fowler KA, Locken JA, Duchesne JH, Williamson MR. US for detecting renal calculi with nonenhanced CT as a reference standard. Radiology. 2002;222(1):109–13.

52. Remer EM, Herts BR, Streem SB, et al. Spiral noncontrast CT versus combined plain radiography and renal US after extracorporeal shock wave lithotripsy: cost-identification analysis. Radiology. 1997;204(1):33–7.

53. Hamm M, Wawroschek F, Weckermann D, et al. Unenhanced helical computed tomography in the evaluation of acute flank pain. Eur Urol. 2001;39(4):460–5.

54. Heidenreich A, Desgrandschamps F, Terrier F. Modern approach of diagnosis and management of acute flank pain: review of all imaging modalities. Eur Urol. 2002;41(4):351–62.

55. Grossfeld GD, Litwin MS, Wolf JS Jr, et al. Evaluation of asymptomatic microscopic hematuria in adults: the American Urological Association best practice policy—part II: patient evaluation, cytology, voided markers, imaging, cystoscopy, nephrology evaluation, and follow-up. Urology. 2001;57(4):604–10.

56. Delorme S, van Kaick G. Imaging of abdominal nodal spread in malignant disease. Eur Radiol. 1996;6(3):262–74.

57. Williams AD, Cousins C, Soutter WP, et al. Detection of pelvic lymph node metastases in gynecologic malignancy: a comparison of CT, MR imaging, and positron emission tomography. AJR Am J Roentgenol. 2001;177(2):343–8.

58. Grubnic S, Vinnicombe SJ, Norman AR, Husband JE. MR evaluation of normal retroperitoneal and pelvic lymph nodes. Clin Radiol. 2002;57(3):193–200; discussion 201–4.

59. Bellin MF, Lebleu L, Meric JB. Evaluation of retroperitoneal and pelvic lymph node metastases with MRI and MR lymphangiography. Abdom Imaging. 2003;28(2):155–63.

60. Friedland GW. Staging of genitourinary cancers. The role of diagnostic imaging. Cancer. 1987;60(3 Suppl):450–8.

61. Wernecke K, Rummeny E, Bongartz G, et al. Detection of hepatic masses in patients with carcinoma: comparative sensitivities of sonography, CT, and MR imaging. AJR Am J Roentgenol. 1991;157(4):731–9.

62. Heiken JP, Weyman PJ, Lee JK, et al. Detection of focal hepatic masses: prospective evaluation with CT, delayed CT, CT during arterial portography, and MR imaging. Radiology. 1989;171(1):47–51.

63. Hohmann J, Albrecht T, Hoffmann CW, Wolf KJ. Ultrasonographic detection of focal liver lesions: increased sensitivity and specificity with microbubble contrast agents. Eur J Radiol. 2003;46(2):147–59.

64. Davis SD. CT evaluation for pulmonary metastases in patients with extrathoracic malignancy. Radiology. 1991;180(1):1–12.

65. Chalmers N, Best JJ. The significance of pulmonary nodules detected by CT but not by chest radiography in tumour staging. Clin Radiol. 1991;44(6):410–2.

66. Herold CJ, Bankier AA, Fleischmann D. Lung metastases. Eur Radiol. 1996;6(5):596–606.

67. Miyazato M, Yonou H, Sugaya K, Koyama Y, Hatano T, Ogawa Y. Transitional cell carcinoma of the renal pelvis forming tumor thrombus in the vena cava. Int J Urol. 2001;8(10):575–7.

68. Spahn M, Portillo FJ, Michel MS, et al. Color Duplex sonography vs. computed tomography: accuracy in the preoperative evaluation of renal cell carcinoma. Eur Urol. 2001;40(3):337–42.

69. Solwa Y, Sanyika C, Hadley GP, Corr P. Colour Doppler ultrasound assessment of the inferior vena cava in patients with Wilms' tumour. Clin Radiol. 1999;54(12):811–4.

70. Bos SD, Mensink HJ. Can duplex Doppler ultrasound replace computerized tomography in staging patients with renal cell carcinoma? Scand J Urol Nephrol. 1998;32(2):87–91.

71. Habboub HK, Abu-Yousef MM, Williams RD, See WA, Schweiger GD. Accuracy of color Doppler sonography in assessing venous thrombus extension in renal cell carcinoma. AJR Am J Roentgenol. 1997;168(1):267–71.

72. Smith-Bindman R, Hosmer WD, Caponigro M, Cunningham G. The variability in the interpretation of prenatal diagnostic ultrasound. Ultrasound Obstet Gynecol. 2001;17(4):326–32.

73. Mikkonen RH, Kreula JM, Virkkunen PJ. Reproducibility of Doppler ultrasound measurements. Acta Radiol. 1996;37(4):545–50.

74. Mikkonen RH, Kreula JM, Virkkunen PJ. Reliability of Doppler ultrasound in follow-up studies. Acta Radiol. 1998;39(2):193–9.

75. Ablett MJ, Coulthard A, Lee RE, et al. How reliable are ultrasound measurements of renal length in adults? Br J Radiol. 1995;68(814):1087–9.

76. Emamian SA, Nielsen MB, Pedersen JF. Intraobserver and interobserver variations in sonographic measurements of kidney size in adult volunteers. a comparison of linear measurements and volumetric estimates. Acta Radiol. 1995;36(4):399–401.

77. Goldberg BB, Bagley D, Liu JB, Merton DA, Alexander A, Kurtz AB. Endoluminal sonography of the urinary tract: preliminary observations. AJR Am J Roentgenol. 1991;156(1):99–103.

78. Goldberg BB, Liu JB, Merton DA, Kurtz AB. Endoluminal US: experiments with nonvascular uses in animals. Radiology. 1990;175(1):39–43.

79. Zeltser IS, Liu JB, Bagley DH. The incidence of crossing vessels in patients with normal ureteropelvic junction examined with endoluminal ultrasound. J Urol. 2004;172(6 Pt 1):2304–7.

80. Bagley DH, Liu JB, Grasso M, Goldberg BB. Endoluminal sonography in evaluation of the obstructed ureteropelvic junction. J Endourol. 1994;8(4):287–92.

81. Bagley DH, Liu JB, Goldberg B. Endoluminal sonographic imaging of the ureteropelvic junction. J Endourol. 1996;10(2):105–10.

82. Siegel CL, McDougall EM, Middleton WD, et al. Preoperative assessment of ureteropelvic junction obstruction with endoluminal sonography and helical CT. AJR Am J Roentgenol. 1997;168(3):623–6.

83. Keeley FX Jr, Moussa SA, Miller J, Tolley DA. A prospective study of endoluminal ultrasound versus computerized tomography angiography for detecting crossing vessels at the ureteropelvic junction. J Urol. 1999;162(6):1938–41.

84. Holm HH, Torp-Pedersen S, Larsen T, Dorph S. Transabdominal and endoluminal ultrasonic scanning of the lower ureter. Scand J Urol Nephrol Suppl. 1994;157:19–25.

85. Liu JB, Bagley DH, Conlin MJ, Merton DA, Alexander AA, Goldberg BB. Endoluminal sonographic evaluation of ureteral and renal pelvic neoplasms. J Ultrasound Med. 1997;16(8):515–21; quiz 523–4.

86. Grotas A, Grasso M. Endoluminal sonographic imaging of upper urinary tract: three-dimensional reconstruction. J Endourol. 2001;15(5):485–8.

87. Bagley DH, Liu JB. Three-dimensional endoluminal ultrasonography of the ureter. J Endourol. 1998;12(5):411–6.

88. Blomley MJ, Cooke JC, Unger EC, Monaghan MJ, Cosgrove DO. Microbubble contrast agents: a new era in ultrasound. BMJ. 2001;322(7296):1222–5.

89. Jakobsen JA, Correas JM. Ultrasound contrast agents and their use in urogenital radiology: status and prospects. Eur Radiol. 2001;11(10):2082–91.

90. Calliada F, Campani R, Bottinelli O, Bozzini A, Sommaruga MG. Ultrasound contrast agents: basic principles. Eur J Radiol. 1998;27 Suppl 2:S157–60.

91. Cosgrove D, Blomley M. Liver tumors: evaluation with contrast-enhanced ultrasound. Abdom Imaging. 2004;29(4):446–54.

92. Nicolau C, Bru C. Focal liver lesions: evaluation with contrast-enhanced ultrasonography. Abdom Imaging. 2004;29(3):348–59.

93. Chomas JE, Pollard RE, Sadlowski AR, Griffey SM, Wisner ER, Ferrara KW. Contrast-enhanced US of microcirculation of superficially implanted tumors in rats. Radiology. 2003;229(2):439–46.

94. Kmetec A, Bren AF, Kandus A, Fettich J, Buturovic-Ponikvar J. Contrast-enhanced ultrasound voiding cystography as a screening examination for vesicoureteral reflux in the follow-up of renal transplant recipients: a new approach. Nephrol Dial Transplant. 2001;16(1):120–3.

95. Ascenti G, Zimbaro G, Mazziotti S, Chimenz R, Baldari S, Fede C. Vesicoureteral reflux: comparison between urosonography and radionuclide cystography. Pediatr Nephrol. 2003;18(8):768–71.

96. Valentini AL, De Gaetano AM, Minordi LM, et al. Contrast-enhanced voiding US for grading of reflux in adult patients prior to antireflux ureteral implantation. Radiology. 2004;233(1):35–9.

97. Liang HD, Blomley MJ. The role of ultrasound in molecular imaging. Br J Radiol. 2003;76 Spec No 2:S140–50.

98. Voelcker F, von Lichtenberg A. Pyelographie röntgenographie des neirenbeckens nach Kollargolfullung. Munch Med Wochenschr. 1906;53:105–6.

99. Cameron DF. Aqueous solutions of potassium and sodium iodides as opaque mediums in roentgenography. JAMA. 1918;70(11):754–5.

100. Osborne ED, Sutherland CG, Scholl AJ, Rowntree LG. Roentgenography of urinary tract during excretion of sodium iodide. JAMA. 1923;80(6):368–73.

101. Swick M. Intravenous urography by means of the sodium salt 5-iodo-2-pyridon-N-acetic acid. JAMA. 1930;95:1403–9.

102. Amis ES Jr. Epitaph for the urogram. Radiology. 1999;213(3):639–40.

103. Pollack HM, Banner MP. Current status of excretory urography. a premature epitaph? Urol Clin North Am. 1985;12(4):585–601.

104. Kumar R, Schreiber MH. The changing indications for excretory urography. JAMA. 1985;254(3):403–5.

105. Dalla Palma L. What is left of i.v. urography? Eur Radiol. 2001;11(6):931–9.

106. Choyke PL. The urogram: are rumors of its death premature? Radiology. 1992;184(1):33–4.

107. Hattery RR, King BF. Invited commentary. Radiographics. 2001;21(4):822–3.

108. Dyer RB, Chen MY, Zagoria RJ. Intravenous urography: technique and interpretation. Radiographics. 2001;21(4):799–21; discussion 822–4.

109. Hattery RR, Williamson B Jr, Hartman GW, LeRoy AJ, Witten DM. Intravenous urographic technique. Radiology. 1988;167(3):593–9.

110. Moody TE, Vaughn ED Jr, Gillenwater JY. Relationship between renal blood flow and ureteral pressure during 18 hours of total unilateral uretheral occlusion. Implications for changing sites of increased renal resistance. Invest Urol. 1975;13(3):246–51.

111. Vaughan ED Jr, Shenasky JH II, Gillenwater JY. Mechanism of acute hemodynamic response to ureteral occlusion. Invest Urol. 1971;9(2):109–18.

112. Vaughan ED Jr, Sorenson EJ, Gillenwater JY. Effects of acute and chronic ureteral obstruction on renal hemodynamics and function. Surg Forum. 1968;19:536–8.

113. Moody TE, Vaughan ED Jr, Gillenwater JY. Comparison of the renal hemodynamic response to unilateral and bilateral ureteral occlusion. Invest Urol. 1977;14(6):455–9.

114. Vaughan ED Jr, Sorenson EJ, Gillenwater JY. The renal hemodynamic response to chronic unilateral complete ureteral occlusion. Invest Urol. 1970;8(1):78–90.

115. Erden A, Fitoz S, Karagulle T, Tukel S, Akyar S. Radiological findings in the diagnosis of genitourinary candidiasis. Pediatr Radiol. 2000;30(12):875–7.

116. Adams FG, Murray RM. The radiological diagnosis of analgesic nephropathy. Clin Radiol. 1975;26(3):417–27.

117. Hare WS, Poynter JD. The radiology of renal papillary necrosis as seen in analgesic nephropathy. Clin Radiol. 1974;25(4):423–43.

118. Lindvall N. Radiological changes of renal papillary necrosis. Kidney Int. 1978;13(1):93–106.

119. Vijayaraghavan SB, Kandasamy SV, Mylsamy A, Prabhakar M. Sonographic features of necrosed renal papillae causing hydronephrosis. J Ultrasound Med. 2003;22(9):951–6; quiz 957–8.

120. Siegel MJ, McAlister WH. Calyceal diverticula in children: unusual features and complications. Radiology. 1979;131(1):79–82.

121. Devine CJ Jr, Guzman JA, Devine PC, Poutasse EF. Calyceal diverticulum. J Urol. 1969;101(1):8–11.

122. Brennan RE, Pollack HM. Nonvisualized ("phantom") renal calyx: causes and radiological approach to diagnosis. Urol Radiol. 1979;1(1):17–23.

123. Fein AB, McClennan BL. Solitary filling defects of the ureter. Semin Roentgenol. 1986;21(3):201–13.

124. Pollack HM, Arger PH, Banner MP, Mulhern CB Jr, Coleman BG. Computed tomography of renal pelvic filling defects. Radiology. 1981;138(3):645–51.

125. Parienty RA, Ducellier R, Pradel J, Lubrano JM, Coquille F, Richard F. Diagnostic value of CT numbers in pelvocalyceal filling defects. Radiology. 1982;145(3):743–7.

126. Lowe PP, Roylance J. Transitional cell carcinoma of the kidney. Clin Radiol. 1976;27(4):503–12.

127. McLean GK, Pollack HM, Banner MP. The "stipple sign"; - urographic harbinger of transitional cell neoplasms. Urol Radiol. 1979;1(2):77–9.

128. Gee J, Larsen CR, Silverman ML, Bihrle W III. Urothelial striations in a patient with transitional cell carcinoma in situ involving the ureter. J Urol. 1999;161(4):1279–80.

129. Bush WH, Lasser EC. Adverse reactions to intravascular iodinated contrast material. In: Pollack HM, McClennan BL, editors. Clinical urography. 2nd ed. Philadelphia: W.B. Saunders Company; 2000. pp. 43–66.

130. Thomsen HS, Morcos SK. Contrast media and the kidney: European Society of Urogenital Radiology (ESUR) guidelines. Br J Radiol. 2003;76(908):513–8.

131. Merten GJ, Burgess WP, Gray LV, et al. Prevention of contrast-induced nephropathy with sodium bicarbonate: a randomized controlled trial. JAMA. 2004;291(19):2328–34.

132. Tepel M, van der Giet M, Schwarzfeld C, Laufer U, Liermann D, Zidek W. Prevention of radiographic-contrast-agent-induced reductions in renal function by acetylcysteine. N Engl J Med. 2000;343(3):180–4.

133. Kay J, Chow WH, Chan TM, et al. Acetylcysteine for prevention of acute deterioration of renal function following elective coronary angiography and intervention: a randomized controlled trial. JAMA. 2003;289(5):553–8.

134. Pannu N, Manns B, Lee H, Tonelli M. Systematic review of the impact of N-acetylcysteine on contrast nephropathy. Kidney Int. 2004;65(4):1366–74.

135. Spargias K, Alexopoulos E, Kyrzopoulos S, et al. Ascorbic acid prevents contrast-mediated nephropathy in patients with renal

dysfunction undergoing coronary angiography or intervention. Circulation. 2004;110(18):2837–42.

136. Hagan JB. Anaphylactoid and adverse reactions to radiocontrast agents. Immunol Allergy Clin North Am. 2004;24(3):507–19, vii–viii.

137. Cochran ST. Anaphylactoid reactions to radiocontrast media. Curr Allergy Asthma Rep. 2005;5(1):28–31.

138. Thomsen HS, Morcos SK. Prevention of generalized reactions to CM. Acad Radiol. 2002;9 Suppl 2:S433–5.

139. Morcos SK, Thomsen HS, Webb JA. Prevention of generalized reactions to contrast media: a consensus report and guidelines. Eur Radiol. 2001;11(9):1720–8.

140. Skrepetis K, Siafakas I, Lykourinas M. Evolution of retrograde pyelography and excretory urography in the early 20th century. J Endourol. 2001;15(7):691–6.

141. Braasch WF, Carman RD. The pyelographic and roentgenologic diagnosis of renal tumors. Radiology. 1925;4(6):445–52.

142. Braasch WF. Pyelography (pyelo-ureterography) a study of the normal and pathologic anatomy of the renal pelvis and ureter. 1st ed. Philadelphia: Saunders; 1915.

143. Braasch WF, Hager BH. Urography. 2nd ed. Philadelphia: Saunders; 1927.

144. Babel SG, Winterkorn KG. Retrograde catheterization of the ureter without cystoscopic assistance: preliminary experience. Radiology. 1993;187(2):547–9.

145. Banner MP, Amendola MA, Pollack HM. Anastomosed ureters: fluoroscopically guided transconduit retrograde catheterization. Radiology. 1989;170(1 Pt 1):45–9.

146. Andriole GL, McClennan BL, Becich MJ, Picus DD. Effect of low osmolar, ionic and nonionic, contrast media on the cytologic features of exfoliated urothelial cells. Urol Radiol. 1989;11(3):133–5.

147. Fischer S, Nielsen ML, Clausen S, Vogelsang M, Hogsborg E. Increased abnormal urothelial cells in voided urine following excretory urography. Acta Cytol. 1982;26(2):153–8.

148. Barry JM, Murphy JB, Nassir E, Dawson P, Hodges CV. The influence of retrograde contrast medium on urinary cytodiagnosis: a preliminary report. J Urol. 1978;119(5):633–4.

149. McClennan BL, Oertel YC, Malmgren RA, Mendoza M. The effect of water soluble contrast material on urine cytology. Acta Cytologica. 1978;22(4):230–3.

150. Ricketts HJ, Rudd TG, Marcus VL, Krieger JN. Pneumopyelography: an adjunct to percutaneous nephrostomy and nephrolithotomy. AJR Am J Roentgenol. 1984;143(5):1093–5.

151. Izquierdo F, Rousaud A, Garat JM. Intraoperative pneumopyelography. Eur Urol. 1982;8(3):148–9.

152. Khan AU, Leary FJ, Greene LF. Pneumopyelography. Urology. 1976;8(1):92–3.

153. Fischel RE, Pikielny SS. Giant congenital calyceal diverticulum visualised by retrograde pneumopyelography. Br J Radiol. 1962;35:647–9.

154. Christiansen J. Retrograde pyelography with double contrast. A preliminary report. Acta Chir Scand. 1970;136(5):435–9.

155. Christiansen J. Retrograde pyelography with gas (carbon dioxide) as contrast medium. Acta Chir Scand. 1970;136(5):441–5.

156. Varkarakis J, Su LM, Hsu TH. Air embolism from pneumopyelography. J Urol. 2003;169(1):267.

157. Pyron CL, Segal AJ. Air embolism: a potential complication of retrograde pyelography. J Urol. 1983;130(1):125–6.

158. Daniels RE III. The goblet sign. Radiology. 1999;210(3):737–8.

159. Bergman H, Friedenberg RM, Sayegh V. New roentgenologic signs of carcinoma of the ureter. AJR. 1961;86(4):707–17.

160. Leder RA, Dunnick NR. Transitional cell carcinoma of the pelvicalices and ureter. AJR Am J Roentgenol. 1990; 155(4):713–22.

161. Chiu YS, Chiang HW, Huang CY, Tsai TJ. ARF after retrograde pyelography: a case report and literature review. Am J Kidney Dis. 2003;42(2):E13–6.

162. Hurley RM. Acute renal failure secondary to bilateral retrograde pyelography. Clinical Pediatrics. 1979;18(12):754–6.

163. Whalley DW, Ibels LS, Eckstein RP, Alexander JH, Smith RD. Acute tubular necrosis complicating bilateral retrograde pyelography. Aust N Z J Med. 1987;17(5):536–8.

164. Lytton B, Brooks MB, Spencer RP. Absorption of contrast material from the urinary tract during retrograde pyelography. J Urology. 1968;100(6):779–82.

165. Marshall WH Jr, Castellino RA. The urinary mucosal barrier in retrograde pyelography. The role of the ureteric mucosa. Radiology. 1970;97(1):5–7.

166. Castellino RA, Marshall WH Jr. The urinary mucosal barrier in retrograde pyelography: experimental findings and clinical implications. Radiology. 1970;95(2):403–9.

167. Weese DL, Greenberg HM, Zimmern PE. Contrast media reactions during voiding cystourethrography or retrograde pyelography. Urology. 1993;41(1):81–4.

168. Johenning PW. Reactions to contrast material during retrograde pyelography. Urology. 1980;16(4):442–4.

169. Miller KT, Moshyedi AC. Systemic reaction to contrast media during cystography. AJR Am J Roentgenol. 1995;164(6):1551.

170. Gaiser RR, Chua E. Anaphylactic/anaphylactoid reaction to contrast dye administered in the ureter. J Clin Anesth. 1993;5(6):510–2.

171. Cohan RH, Leder RA, Ellis JH. Treatment of adverse reactions to radiographic contrast media in adults. Radiol Clin North Am. 1996;34(5):1055–76.

172. Chen GL, El-Gabry EA, Bagley DH. Surveillance of upper urinary tract transitional cell carcinoma: the role of ureteroscopy, retrograde pyelography, cytology and urinalysis. J Urol. 2000;164(6):1901–4.

173. Selzman AA, Spirnak JP. Iatrogenic ureteral injuries: a 20-year experience in treating 165 injuries. J Urol. 1996;155(3):878–81.

174. Armenakas NA, Pareek G, Fracchia JA. Iatrogenic bladder perforations: longterm followup of 65 patients. J Am Coll Surg. 2004;198(1):78–82.

175. Pansadoro V, Emiliozzi P. Iatrogenic prostatic urethral strictures: classification and endoscopic treatment. Urology. 1999;53(4):784–9.

176. Stormont TJ, Suman VJ, Oesterling JE. Newly diagnosed bulbar urethral strictures: etiology and outcome of various treatments. J Urol. 1993;150(5 Pt 2):1725–8.

177. Smith AD. Management of iatrogenic ureteral strictures after urological procedures. J Urol. 1988;140(6):1372–4.

178. Howards SS, Harrison JH. Retroperitoneal phlegmon. A fatal complication of retrograde pyelography. J Urology. 1973;109(1):92–3.

179. Ku JH, Lee SW, Jeon HG, Kim HH, Oh SJ. Percutaneous nephrostomy versus indwelling ureteral stents in the management of extrinsic ureteral obstruction in advanced malignancies: are there differences? Urology. 2004;64(5):895–9.

180. Mokhmalji H, Braun PM, Martinez Portillo FJ, Siegsmund M, Alken P, Kohrmann KU. Percutaneous nephrostomy versus ureteral stents for diversion of hydronephrosis caused by stones: a prospective, randomized clinical trial. J Urol. 2001;165(4):1088–92.

181. Watson RA, Esposito M, Richter F, Irwin RJ Jr, Lang EK. Percutaneous nephrostomy as adjunct management in advanced upper urinary tract infection. Urology. 1999;54(2):234–9.

182. Pearle MS, Pierce HL, Miller GL, et al. Optimal method of urgent decompression of the collecting system for obstruction and infection due to ureteral calculi. J Urol. 1998;160(4):1260–4.

183. Thomsen HS. Pressures during retrograde pyelography. Acta Radiol Diagn. 1983;24(2):171–5.

184. Thomsen HS, Dorph S. Pyelorenal backflow during retrograde pyelography in adult patients. Scand J Urol Nephrol. 1981;15(1):65–8.

185. Thomsen HS, Larsen S. Intrarenal backflow during retrograde pyelography with graded intrapelvic pressure. a pathoanatomic study. Acta Pathol Microbiol Immunol Scand [A]. 1983;91(4):245–52.

186. Bidgood WD Jr, Cuttino JT Jr, Clark RL, Volberg FM. Pyelovenous and pyelolymphatic backflow during retrograde pyelography in renal vein thrombosis. Invest Radiol. 1981;16(1):13–9.

187. Murayama S, Shimoda Y, Kishikawa T. Pyelovenous backflow in left renal vein hypertension: case report. Radiat Med. 1989;7(2):55–7.

188. Helin I, Okmian L, Olin T. Renal blood flow and function at elevated ureteric pressure. An experimental study in the pig. Scand J Urol Nephrol. 1975;28 Suppl:53–69.

189. McAninch LN, Mostafa HM. Pyelocancerous backflow. A diagnostic radiological sign for renal cell carcinoma. J Urol. 1971;105(4):491.

190. Copeland JS, Schellhammer PF, Devine CJ Jr. Pyelocancerous backflow: a radiologic finding in renal malignancy. J Urol. 1976;115(2):214–5.

191. Thomsen HS, Dorph S. Pyelorenal backflow during retrograde pyelography after renal transplantation. Scand J Urol Nephrol. 1978;12(2):175–9.

192. Thomsen HS. Intrarenal backflow during retrograde pyelography following kidney transplantation. Acta Radiol Diagn. 1984;25(2):113–20.

193. Thomsen HS, Talner LB, Higgins CB. Intrarenal backflow during retrograde pyelography with graded intrapelvic pressure. A radiologic study. Invest Radiol. 1982;17(6):593–603.

194. Thomsen HS, Dorph S, Olsen S. Pyelorenal backflow in normal and ischemic rabbit kidneys. Invest Radiol. 1981;16(3):206–14.

195. Thomsen HS, Larsen S, Talner LB. Pyelorenal backflow during retrograde pyelography in normal and ischemic porcine kidneys. A radiologic and pathoanatomic study. Eur Urol. 1982;8(5):291–7.

196. Friedenberg RM, Moorehouse H, Gade M. Urinomas secondary to pyelosinus backflow. Urol Radiol. 1983;5(1):23–9.

197. Ihara H, Ihara Y, Sagawa S, Takaha M, Sonoda T. Pyelosinus backflow: a case with an unusual pyelographic appearance. Urol Radiol. 1980;2(4):263–4.

198. Titton RL, Gervais DA, Hahn PF, Harisinghani MG, Arellano RS, Mueller PR. Urine leaks and urinomas: diagnosis and imaging-guided intervention. Radiographics. 2003;23(5):1133–47.

199. Burns JE. Thorium, a new agent for pyelography, preliminary report. JAMA. 1915;64:2126–7.

200. Oyen RH, Gielen JL, Van Poppel HP, et al. Renal thorium deposition associated with transitional cell carcinoma: radiologic demonstration in two patients. Radiology. 1988;169(3):705–7.

201. Griffiths MH, Thomas DP, Xipell JM, Hope RN. Thorotrast-induced bilateral carcinoma of the kidney. Pathology. 1977;9(1):43–8.

202. Kauzlaric D, Barmeir E, Luscieti P, Binek J, Ramelli F, Petrovic M. Renal carcinoma after retrograde pyelography with Thorotrast. AJR Am J Roentgenol. 1987;148(5):897–8.

203. Mihatsch MJ, Rutishauser G. Thorotrast induced transitional cell carcinoma in a residual ureter after nephrectomy. Cancer. 1973;32(6):1346–9.

204. Wenz W. Tumors of the kidney following retrograde pyelography with colloidal thorium dioxide. Ann N Y Acad Sci. 1967;145(3):806–10.

205. Kapandji M. Ponction de bassinet et radiomanometrie meato-uretero-pyelocalicielle. Bull Mem Soc Med Hop Paris M. 1949;849:21–2.

206. Goodwin WE, Casey WC, Woolf W. Percutaneous trocar (needle) nephrostomy in hydronephrosis. JAMA. 1955;157(11):891–4.

207. Casey WC, Goodwin WE. Percutaneous antegrade pyelography and hydronephrosis. J Urol. 1955;74(1):164–73.

208. Weens HS, Florence TJ. The diagnosis of hydronephrosis by percutaneous renal puncture. J Urol. 1954;72(4):589–95.

209. Wickbom I. Pyelography after direct puncture of the renal pelvis. Acta Radiol. 1954;41:505.

210. Fritzsche P. Antegrade pyelography: therapeutic applications. Radiol Clin North Am. 1986;24(4):573–86.

211. Pedersen JF. Percutaneous nephrostomy guided by ultrasound. J Urol. 1974;112(2):157–9.

212. Hellsten S, Hildell J, Link D, Ulmsten U. Percutaneous nephrostomy. Aspects on applications and technique. Eur Urol. 1978;4(4):282–7.

213. Zegel HG, Pollack HM, Banner MC, et al. Percutaneous nephrostomy: comparison of sonographic and fluoroscopic guidance. AJR Am J Roentgenol. 1981;137(5):925–7.

214. Hay MS, Elyaderani MK, Belis JA. Percutaneous approach to the renal pelvis: combined use of ultrasonography and fluoroscopy. South Med J. 1981;74(1):31–3.

215. Myers RP. Brodel's line. Surg Gynecol Obstet. 1971;132(3):424–6.

216. Dyer RB, Regan JD, Kavanagh PV, Khatod EG, Chen MY, Zagoria RJ. Percutaneous nephrostomy with extensions of the technique: step by step. Radiographics. 2002;22(3):503–25.

217. Zagoria RJ, Dyer RB. Do's and don't's of percutaneous nephrostomy. Acad Radiol. 1999;6(6):370–7.

218. Boon JM, Shinners B, Meiring JH. Variations of the position of the colon as applied to percutaneous nephrostomy. Surg Radiol Anat. 2001;23(6):421–5.

219. O'Donnell A, Schoenberger C, Weiner J, Tsou E. Pulmonary complications of percutaneous nephrostomy and kidney stone extraction. South Med J. 1988;81(8):1002–5.

220. Radecka E, Brehmer M, Holmgren K, Magnusson A. Complications associated with percutaneous nephrolithotripsy: supra- versus subcostal access. A retrospective study. Acta Radiol. 2003;44(4):447–51.

221. Ostendorf N, van Ahlen H, Hertle L. Simple reinforcement for thin nephrostomy catheters. J Urol. 1998;159(2):485–6.

222. Watson G. Problems with double-J stents and nephrostomy tubes. J Endourol. 1997;11(6):413–7.

223. Paul EM, Marcovich R, Lee BR, Smith AD. Choosing the ideal nephrostomy tube. BJU Int. 2003;92(7):672–7.

224. Lewis S, Patel U. Major complications after percutaneous nephrostomy-lessons from a department audit. Clin Radiol. 2004;59(2):171–9.

225. Sim LS, Tan BS, Yip SK, et al. Single centre review of radiologically-guided percutaneous nephrostomies: a report of 273 procedures. Ann Acad Med Singapore. 2002;31(1):76–80.

226. Lee WJ, Mond DJ, Patel M, Pillari GP. Emergency percutaneous nephrostomy: technical success based on level of operator experience. J Vasc Interv Radiol. 1994;5(2):327–30.

227. Lee WJ, Patel U, Patel S, Pillari GP. Emergency percutaneous nephrostomy: results and complications. J Vasc Interv Radiol. 1994;5(1):135–9.

228. Sengupta S, Harewood L. Transitional cell carcinoma growing along an indwelling nephrostomy tube track. Br J Urol. 1998;82(4):591.

229. Huang A, Low RK, deVere White R. Nephrostomy tract tumor seeding following percutaneous manipulation of a ureteral carcinoma. J Urol. 1995;153(3 Pt 2):1041–2.

230. Gerber GS, Lyon ES. Endourological management of upper tract urothelial tumors. J Urol. 1993;150(1):2–7.

231. Thalmann GN, Markwalder R, Walter B, Studer UE. Long-term experience with bacillus Calmette-Guerin therapy of upper urinary tract transitional cell carcinoma in patients not eligible for surgery. J Urol. 2002;168(4 Pt 1):1381–5.

232. Guz B, Streem SB, Novick AC, et al. Role of percutaneous nephrostomy in patients with upper urinary tract transitional cell carcinoma. Urology. 1991;37(4):331–6.

233. Goel MC, Mahendra V, Roberts JG. Percutaneous management of renal pelvic urothelial tumors: long-term followup. J Urol. 2003;169(3):925–9; discussion 929–30.

234. Clark PE, Streem SB, Geisinger MA. 13-year experience with percutaneous management of upper tract transitional cell carcinoma. J Urol. 1999;161(3):772–5; discussion 775–6.

235. Elliott DS, Segura JW, Lightner D, Patterson DE, Blute ML. Is nephroureterectomy necessary in all cases of upper tract transitional cell carcinoma? Long-term results of conservative endourologic management of upper tract transitional cell carcinoma in individuals with a normal contralateral kidney. Urology. 2001;58(2):174–8.

236. Shepherd SF, Patel A, Bidmead AM, Kellett MJ, Woodhouse CR, Dearnaley DP. Nephrostomy track brachytherapy following percutaneous resection of transitional cell carcinoma of the renal pelvis. Clin Oncol (R Coll Radiol). 1995;7(6):385–7.

237. Whitaker RH. Pressure-controlled nephrostography. Eur Urol. 1977;3(3):145–9.

238. Witherow RO, Whitaker RH. The predictive accuracy of antegrade pressure flow studies in equivocal upper tract obstruction. Br J Urol. 1981;53(6):496–9.

239. Wahlin N, Magnusson A, Persson AE, Lackgren G, Stenberg A. Pressure flow measurement of hydronephrosis in children: a new approach to definition and quantification of obstruction. J Urol. 2001;166(5):1842–7.

240. Gonzalez R, Chiou R. The diagnosis of upper urinary tract obstruction in children: comparison of diuresis renography and pressure flow studies. J Urol. 1985;133(4):646–9.

241. Jakobsen H, Nordling J, Munck O, Iversen P, Nielsen SL, Holm HH. Sensitivity of 131I-hippuran diuresis renography and pressure flow study (Whitaker test) in upper urinary tract obstruction. Urol Int. 1988;43(2):89–92.

242. Kashi SH, Irving HC, Sadek SA. Does the Whitaker test add to antegrade pyelography in the investigation of collecting system dilatation in renal allografts? Br J Radiol. 1993;66(790):877–81.

243. Yokogi H, Wada Y, Mizutani M, Igawa M, Ishibe T. Bacillus Calmette-Guerin perfusion therapy for carcinoma in situ of the upper urinary tract. Br J Urol. 1996;77(5):676–9.

244. Patel A, Soonawalla P, Shepherd SF, Dearnaley DP, Kellett MJ, Woodhouse CR. Long-term outcome after percutaneous treatment of transitional cell carcinoma of the renal pelvis. J Urol. 1996;155(3):868–74.

245. See WA. Continuous antegrade infusion of adriamycin as adjuvant therapy for upper tract urothelial malignancies. Urology. 2000;56(2):216–22.

246. Sacha K, Szewczyk W, Bar K. Massive haemorrhage presenting as a complication after percutaneous nephrolithotomy (PCNL). Int Urol Nephrol. 1996;28(3):315–8.

247. Martin X, Murat FJ, Feitosa LC, et al. Severe bleeding after nephrolithotomy: results of hyperselective embolization. Eur Urol. 2000;37(2):136–9.

248. Davidoff R, Bellman GC. Influence of technique of percutaneous tract creation on incidence of renal hemorrhage. J Urol. 1997;157(4):1229–31.

249. Kessaris DN, Bellman GC, Pardalidis NP, Smith AG. Management of hemorrhage after percutaneous renal surgery. J Urol. 1995;153(3 Pt 1):604–8.

250. Lee WJ, Smith AD, Cubelli V, et al. Complications of percutaneous nephrolithotomy. AJR Am J Roentgenol. 1987;148(1):177–80.

251. Stoller ML, Wolf JS Jr, St Lezin MA. Estimated blood loss and transfusion rates associated with percutaneous nephrolithotomy. J Urol. 1994;152(6 Pt 1):1977–81.

252. Kukreja R, Desai M, Patel S, Bapat S. Factors affecting blood loss during percutaneous nephrolithotomy: prospective study. J Endourol. 2004;18(8):715–22.

253. Routh WD, Tatum CM, Lawdahl RB, Rosch J, Keller FS. Tube tamponade: potential pitfall in angiography of arterial hemorrhage associated with percutaneous drainage catheters. Radiology. 1990;174(3 Pt 2):945–9.

254. Kaye KW, Clayman RV. Tamponade nephrostomy catheter for percutaneous nephrostolithotomy. Urology. 1986;27(5):441–5.

255. Jou YC, Cheng MC, Sheen JH, Lin CT, Chen PC. Electrocauterization of bleeding points for percutaneous nephrolithotomy. Urology. 2004;64(3):443–6; discussion 446–7.

256. Jou YC, Cheng MC, Sheen JH, Lin CT, Chen PC. Cauterization of access tract for nephrostomy tube-free percutaneous nephrolithotomy. J Endourol. 2004;18(6):547–9.

257. Mikhail AA, Kaptein JS, Bellman GC. Use of fibrin glue in percutaneous nephrolithotomy. Urology. 2003;61(5):910–4; discussion 914.

258. Pfab R, Ascherl R, Blumel G, Hartung R. Local hemostasis of nephrostomy tract with fibrin adhesive sealing in percutaneous nephrolithotomy. Eur Urol. 1987;13(1–2):118–21.

259. Orzel JA, Coldwell DM, Eskridge JM. Superselective embolization for renal hemorrhage with a new coaxial catheter and steerable guidewire. Cardiovasc Intervent Radiol. 1988;11(6):343–5.

260. Peene P, Wilms G, Baert AL. Embolization of iatrogenic renal hemorrhage following percutaneous nephrostomy. Urol Radiol. 1990;12(2):84–7.

261. Ueda J, Furukawa T, Takahashi S, Miyake O, Itatani H, Araki Y. Arterial embolization to control renal hemorrhage in patients with percutaneous nephrostomy. Abdom Imaging. 1996;21(4):361–3.

262. Gupta M, Bellman GC, Smith AD. Massive hemorrhage from renal vein injury during percutaneous renal surgery: endourological management. J Urol. 1997;157(3):795–7.

263. Cowan NC, Traill ZC, Phillips AJ, Gleeson FV. Direct percutaneous transrenal embolization for renal artery injury following percutaneous nephrostomy. Br J Radiol. 1998;71(851):1199–201.

264. Beaujeux R, Saussine C, al-Fakir A, et al. Superselective endo-vascular treatment of renal vascular lesions. J Urol. 1995;153(1):14–7.

265. Kernohan RM, Johnston LC, Donaldson RA. Bleeding following percutaneous nephrolithotomy resulting in loss of the kidney. Br J Urol. 1990;65(6):657–8.

266. Dorffner R, Thurnher S, Prokesch R, et al. Embolization of iatrogenic vascular injuries of renal transplants: immediate and follow-up results. Cardiovasc Intervent Radiol. 1998;21(2):129–34.

267. Demirbas O, Batyraliev T, Eksi Z, Pershukov I. Femoral pseudoaneurysm due to diagnostic or interventional angiographic procedures. Angiology. 2005;56(5):553–6.

268. Ferguson JD, Whatling PJ, Martin V, Walton J, Banning AP. Ultrasound guided percutaneous thrombin injection of iatrogenic femoral artery pseudoaneurysms after coronary angiography and intervention. Heart. 2001;85(4):E5.

269. Pejic R. Iatrogenic arteriovenous fistula of the profunda femoris artery/vein: a case report. Indiana Med. 1990;83(2):118–20.

270. Marsan RE, McDonald V, Ramamurthy S. Iatrogenic femoral arteriovenous fistula. Cardiovasc Intervent Radiol. 1990;13(5):314–6.

271. Sakamoto I, Hayashi K, Matsunaga N, et al. Aortic dissection caused by angiographic procedures. Radiology. 1994;191(2):467–71.

272. Gorog DA, Watkinson A, Lipkin DP. Treatment of iatrogenic aortic dissection by percutaneous stent placement. J Invasive Cardiol. 2003;15(2):84–5.

273. Sharma PV, Babu SC, Shah PM, Nassoura ZE. Changing patterns of atheroembolism. Cardiovasc Surg. 1996;4(5):573–9.

274. Cronan JJ, Dorfman GS, Amis ES, Denny DF Jr. Retroperitoneal hemorrhage after percutaneous nephrostomy. AJR Am J Roentgenol. 1985;144(4):801–3.

275. Merine D, Fishman EK. Perirenal hematoma following catheter removal. An unusual complication of percutaneous nephrostomy. Clin Imaging. 1989;13(1):74–6.

276. Hergesell O, Felten H, Andrassy K, Kuhn K, Ritz E. Safety of ultrasound-guided percutaneous renal biopsy-retrospective analysis of 1090 consecutive cases. Nephrol Dial Transplant. 1998;13(4):975–7.

277. Merkus JW, Zeebregts CJ, Hoitsma AJ, van Asten WN, Koene RA, Skotnicki SH. High incidence of arteriovenous fistula after biopsy of kidney allografts. Br J Surg. 1993;80(3):310–2.

278. Hubsch P, Schurawitzki H, Traindl O, Karnel F. Renal allograft arteriovenous fistula due to needle biopsy with late onset of symptoms—diagnosis and treatment. Nephron. 1991;59(3):482–5.

279. Brandenburg VM, Frank RD, Riehl J. Color-coded duplex sonography study of arteriovenous fistulae and pseudoaneurysms complicating percutaneous renal allograft biopsy. Clin Nephrol. 2002;58(6):398–404.

280. Mansy H, Khalil A, Bafaqeeh M, et al. Transplant nephrectomy for a large AV fistula following renal biopsy. Nephron. 1995;71(4):481–2.

281. deSouza NM, Reidy JF, Koffman CG. Arteriovenous fistulas complicating biopsy of renal allografts: treatment of bleeding with superselective embolization. AJR Am J Roentgenol. 1991;156(3):507–10.

282. Gerspach JM, Bellman GC, Stoller ML, Fugelso P. Conservative management of colon injury following percutaneous renal surgery. Urology. 1997;49(6):831–6.

283. Hussain M, Hamid R, Arya M, Peters JL, Kellett MJ, Philip T. Management of colonic injury following percutaneous nephrolithotomy. Int J Clin Pract. 2003;57(6):549–50.

284. Vallancien G, Capdeville R, Veillon B, Charton M, Brisset JM. Colonic perforation during percutaneous nephrolithotomy. J Urol. 1985;134(6):1185–7.

285. Wolf JS Jr. Management of intraoperatively diagnosed colonic injury during percutaneous nephrostolithotomy. Tech Urol. 1998;4(3):160–4.

286. Robert M, Maubon A, Roux JO, Rouanet JP, Navratil H. Direct percutaneous approach to the upper pole of the kidney: MRI anatomy with assessment of the visceral risk. J Endourol. 1999;13(1):17–20.

287. Hopper KD, Yakes WF. The posterior intercostal approach for percutaneous renal procedures: risk of puncturing the lung, spleen, and liver as determined by CT. AJR Am J Roentgenol. 1990;154(1):115–7.

288. Kondas J, Szentgyorgyi E, Vaczi L, Kiss A. Splenic injury: a rare complication of percutaneous nephrolithotomy. Int Urol Nephrol. 1994;26(4):399–404.

289. Hopper KD, Chantelois AE. The retrorenal spleen. Implications for percutaneous left renal invasive procedures. Invest Radiol. 1989;24(8):592–5.

290. Gouze VA, Breslow MJ. Hydrothorax as a complication of percutaneous access to the renal pelvis. Anesth Analg. 1996;83(3):652–3.

291. Radecka E, Magnusson A. Complications associated with percutaneous nephrostomies. A retrospective study. Acta Radiol. 2004;45(2):184–8.

292. Gupta R, Kumar A, Kapoor R, Srivastava A, Mandhani A. Prospective evaluation of safety and efficacy of the supracostal approach for percutaneous nephrolithotomy. BJU Int. 2002;90(9):809–13.

293. Forsyth MJ, Fuchs EF. The supracostal approach for percutaneous nephrostolithotomy. J Urol. 1987;137(2):197–8.

Chapter 12

Cross-Sectional Imaging Techniques in Transitional Cell Carcinoma of the Upper Urinary Tract

K.S. Jhaveri, P. O'Keefe, M. O'Malley, and M. Haider

Patients with hematuria or those at high risk for upper urinary tract urothelial carcinoma are often imaged with multiple modalities such as intravenous urography (IVU), ultrasound (US), computed tomography (CT), and/or magnetic resonance imaging (MRI). Multiple examination work-up causes patient discomfort as well as an incremental cost burden on the medical system. An ideal cross-sectional imaging test that comprehensively assesses the urinary tract with a high degree of sensitivity and specificity for urothelial carcinoma is very much desired.

US, CT, and MRI are the mainstay in the cross-sectional imaging armamentarium for diagnosing and staging urothelial carcinoma. US has by and large a limited role in the diagnosis of upper tract urothelial carcinoma. We will restrict the following discussion to CT and MRI, which form the dominant portion of clinical imaging for this indication.

CT has been accepted for a while to be superior to IVU and US in its ability to detect and characterize renal masses [1, 2] and recently in detecting urolithiasis [3, 4]. The final frontier is the perceived limited accuracy in the assessment of the mucosal surfaces of the renal collecting systems and ureters. With recent technical leaps in CT technology specifically with the advent of multidetector row CT (MDCT), it has become possible to acquire a large number of very thin axial CT sections through the entire urinary tract in a matter of seconds. This allows for image acquisitions during different phases of contrast excretion and allows a more detailed and comprehensive evaluation of the urinary tract. The development of techniques such as CT urography (CTU) combined with multidetector CT technology has contributed to improved resolution and multiplanar capabilities of CT. Conventional MRI and applied techniques such as T2-weighted and T1-weighted gadolinium excretory urography can also be used to assess the urinary tract for transitional cell carcinoma (TCC) in patients who are unable to undergo CT due to renal failure or contrast allergies.

CT can be used to detect TCC, assess the extent of local disease spread, presence of lymphadenopathy and metastatic disease as well as synchronous lesions, given the multicentric tendency of this tumor.

CT Urography (CTU)

MDCT technology was first introduced in 1999 and over the recent years has revolutionized the role of CT in disease imaging in various organ systems including the kidneys and collecting system. It has come to become the current standard in urinary tract CT imaging. The number of detector rows available continues to increase from 4 to the currently available generation of 64 detector row scanners; these can complete a full body scan in about 10 s (within a single breath-hold) with a tube rotation of 0.4 s and resolution of up to 0.34 mm. The recent technical advances in MDCT have led to these several following advantages: 1. Faster scanning and acquisition time. 2. Improved image resolution including improved z-axis resolution with faster scanning times. 3. Coverage of a larger patient volume during a single slice. 4. The ability to generate a true isotropic data set, which can be used in 3D imaging applications.

The application of MDCT to imaging the collecting system has been termed **"CT urography,"** a term first coined by Perlman [5] in 1996. The principal of CT urography is to perform a delayed post-contrast or excretory phase scan (between 5 and 7.5 min or longer) to opacify the collecting system with excreted contrast thereby making focal ureteric wall thickening appear more conspicuous, outline intraluminal lesions, or help identify a level of obstruction in patients with hydronephrosis. With the much higher incidence of renal cell cancer any imaging strategy to assess for an underlying neoplasm in patients with unexplained hematuria should at least include a multi-phasic urinary tract CT. A non-contrast scan of the kidneys and collecting tract can be included at the beginning of the exam to look for

K.S. Jhaveri (✉)
Department of Medical Imaging, Princess Margaret Hospital,
3-957,610 University Avenue, Toronto, ON M5G 2M9, Canada,
kartik.jhaveri@uhn.on.ca

renal calculi followed by contrast injection and scanning in cortmedullary phase (25–30 s) and nephrographic phase (parenchymal phase; 100–180 s) followed by a delayed scan of the collecting system when excreted contrast will opacify the renal pelvis and ureters (Fig. 12.1). Three-dimensional processing applications such as maximum intensity projection (MIP) can produce a series of thin slab images in the coronal plane to generate images that closely resemble traditional IVU images.

Modifications of CT urography techniques concentrate largely on how to achieve maximum opacification of the collecting tracts to enhance the detection of lesions. These include the use of abdominal compression similar to conventional excretory urography to improve calyceal opacification, split contrast boluses techniques, prehydration with

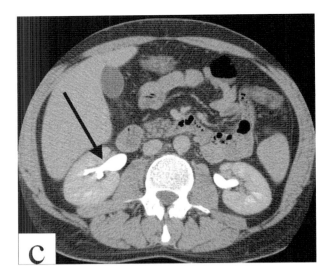

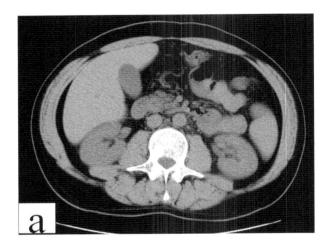

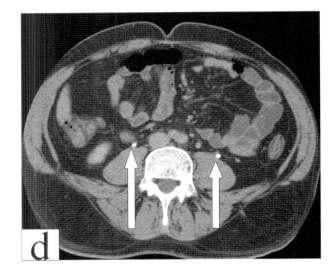

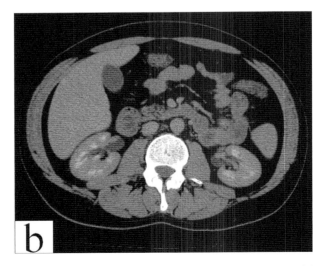

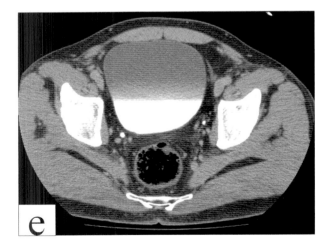

Fig. 12.1 Normal CTU : **Standard three-phase axial CT comprising of unenhanced phase** (a), **nephrographic phase** (b), **delayed excretory phase** (c,d, and e) **showing good opacification of renal calyces, pelvis** (*black arrow*), **ureters** (*white arrows*), **and urinary bladder** (e). **Coronal 3D reconstruction of excretory phase showing the pelvicaliceal systems, ureters, and bladder similar to an IVU**

Fig. 12.1 (continued)

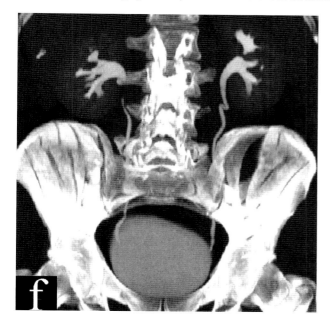

Fig. 12.1 (continued)

water, or administration of IV saline or diuretics to obtain better contrast excretion [6–9] and dynamic maneuvres such as rotating patients between renal and excretory phase scan acquisition to improve ureteric opacification. As with IVP, under-filling of segments of the distal ureter is commonly encountered. Although much research has focused on ways to maximize the opacification of the collecting system, whether this has any major influence on the rate of clinically significant lesions that are detected has yet to be proven. Excreted contrast can appear very dense within the collecting system on preset window settings; wide windowing of the images will help lessen the chance of obscuring small ureteric The most likely findings to influence clinical management are the presence of gross renal parenchymal invasion or the presence of metastatic disease. Most TCCs of the renal pelvis or calyceal urothelium are slow growing lesions. Traditionally treatment of TCC in the renal pelvis consisted of radical nephroureterctomy. Newer techniques such as endoscopic resection and laser treatment can offer more conservative treatment in selected patients such as patients with renal impairment and solitary kidneys. Accuracy in detecting early-stage lesions is of particular importance in patients in whom conservative treatment options are being considered.

CT Appearances of TCC

TCC has been described to have following types of imaging presentations [10–13]:

1. Filling defects, either single or multiple, arising from the urothelium which may have irregular stippled appearance

en face if a contrast medium is trapped on fronds (35%) (Fig. 12.2).

2. Filling defect within distended calyces, the distended calyx being secondary to partial or complete obstruction of the infundibulum by TCC (26%) (Fig. 12.3).
3. Calyceal obliteration or amputation (Fig. 12.4).
4. Hydronephrosis with renal enlargement secondary to UPJ obstruction by the tumor (6%) (Fig. 12.5).
5. Absence of excretion. Due to extensive tumor infiltration into the kidney or severe obstructive hydronephrosis (Fig. 12.6).

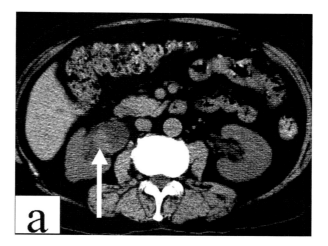

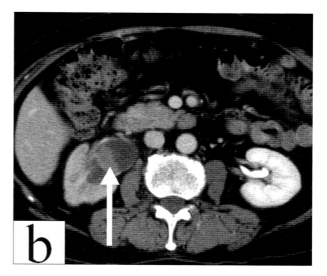

Fig. 12.2 **TCC renal pelvis:** Unenhanced (**a**) and enhanced (**b**) axial CT showing soft tissue mass arising from right renal pelvic urothelium (*arrows*) causing hydronephrosis and delayed excretion compared to left kidney. Another patient (**c**) with irregular soft tissue mass causing filling defect in left renal pelvis (*arrow*). Coronal (**d**) and oblique (**e**) reconstructions showing the irregular TCC trapping contrast medium (*arrows*)

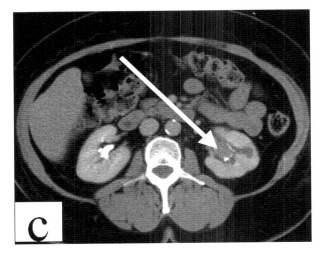

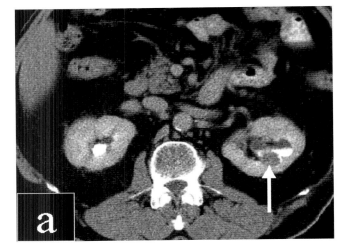

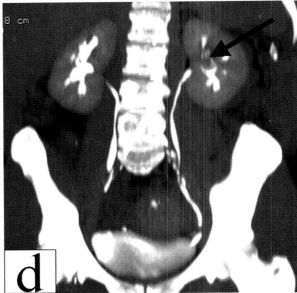

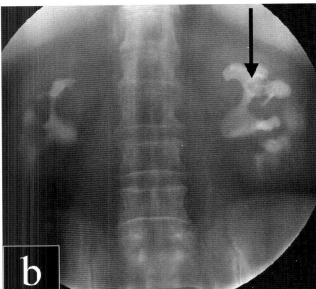

Fig. 12.3 TCC renal calyx: Soft tissue filling defect (*arrow*) in obstructed left renal calyx (**a**) and correlative imaging with IVU tomogram (**b**) showing filling defect in left upper renal calyx (*black arrow*)

CT Staging

The tumor stage at diagnosis impacts the chance of local recurrence and metastases and overall survival [14, 15]. Furthermore, treatment and prognosis are largely determined by the depth of tumor infiltration, the degree of lymph node and distant metastases, and the histological tumor type, making exact staging imperative. CT has become routine in the further characterization of upper tract lesions demonstrated with other modalities and, despite varying reports on staging accuracy, is currently the preoperative imaging modality of choice [12, 16]. Early-stage tumors (stages 0–II) confined to the muscularis are separated from the renal parenchyma by renal sinus fat or excreted contrast material and have normal

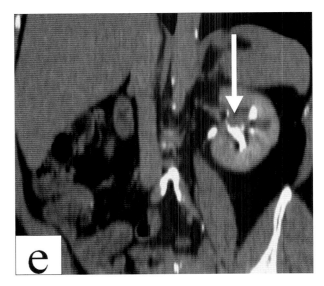

Fig. 12.2 (continued)

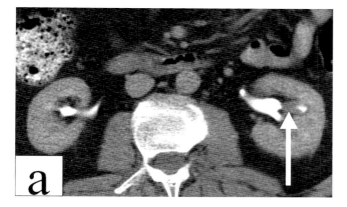

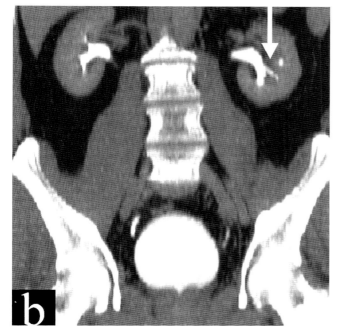

Fig. 12.4 Calyceal amputation. Axial CTU (**a**) showing soft tissue mass causing obstruction of left renal calyx with coronal CTU image (**b**) showing nonvisulization of infundibulum (*arrow*) of amputated calyx

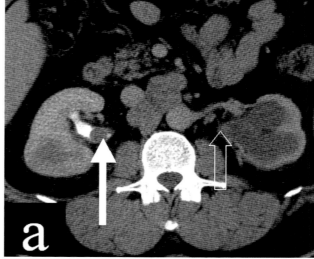

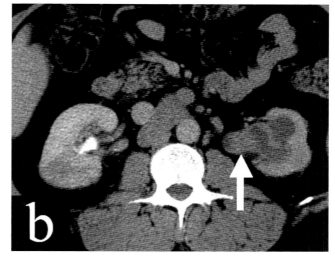

Fig. 12.5 UPJ Obstruction by TCC: Axial CT images (**a**) showing TCC at left UPJ (*open arrow*) causing left hydronephrosis (**b**). Also note TCC in contralateral right renal pelvis (longer arrow in a)

appearing peripelvic fat (Fig. 12.7). More advanced tumors infiltrating beyond the muscularis into the peripelvic fat typically show increased, inhomogeneous peripelvic attenuation (Fig. 12.8), although this finding may also be seen with superimposed infection, hmorrhage, or inflammation and should be interpreted with caution to avoid overstaging. Metastatic spread via urinary or hematogenous routes usually manifests as multifocal mucosal nodules or wall thickening, whereas direct invasion produces a short or long stricture [17]. Extrarenal spread can occur at or through the renal hilum, and common sites of metastases include the lungs, retroperitoneum, lymph nodes (Fig. 12.9), and bones [18]. Rarely, invasion of the renal vein or inferior vena cava is seen and can be well demonstrated with comprehensive CT urography protocols.

Validation of CTU

TCC is an uncommon tumor and many of the series that have reviewed the ability of CT to detect and stage TCC of the upper urinary tract are small in number and were done on older generations of axial CT or early multi-slice scanners. One group [19] reported using MDCT urography in a group of 65 patients and detecting 15 of 16 urothelial carcinomas among other abnormalities. The missed lesion was identified retrospectively. A more recent study [13] using MDCT urography (using four and eight detector scanners) showed more promising results. They were able to demonstrate 89% of upper-tract malignant foci in a group of 18 patients. Similar to previous studies they were unable to distinguish stages Ta, T1, and T2 disease, but MDCT urography was able to

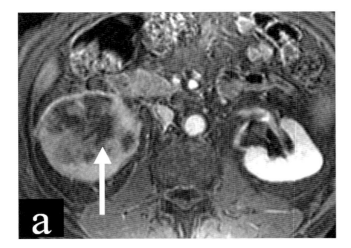

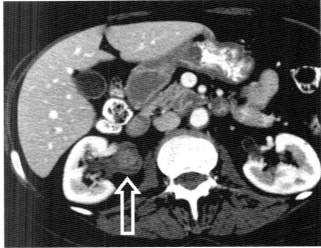

Fig. 12.7 Early-stage TCC: Tumor confined to right renal pelvis (*arrow*) with no extension to peripelvic fat

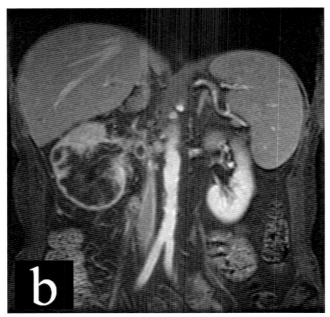

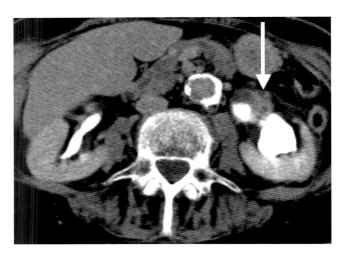

Fig. 12.8 Advanced stage TCC: Tumor infiltrated through the muscularis of the left renal pelvis into the surrounding peripelvic fat (*arrow*)

Fig. 12.6 Infiltrative TCC: Large irregular soft tissue mass infiltrating the right renal parenchyma (*arrow*) on axial (**a**) and coronal (**b**) post-contrast T1-weighted MR images

detection of renal tumor invasion [20]. The overall accuracy of CT in predicting the pathologic stage ranges from 36 to 83% in the literature [21].

CT Radiation Dose Issues

detect many low stage (Ta–T2) lesions, some small (< 5mm) lesions and areas of focal ureteric wall thickening representing foci carcinoma in situ. They also highlighted the necessity to view images on wide window settings so as not to obscure small lesions that can easily be missed on an image with dense contrast and the tendency. Several authors have reported the limitations of CT in the preoperative staging of upper-tract urothelial carcinoma with accuracy in predicting TNM stage of 59.5% (of 39 patients) [16]. Rodriguez et al. looked retrospectively at CT of upper urinary tract TCC in 82 patients and found CT to have a sensitivity of 87.5 % and a specificity of 98% in the detection of lymph node involvement and sensitivity of 64% and specificity of 97% in the

CTU can expose patients to substantial radiation doses and must be carefully considered when deciding upon performing a CTU. Estimated total effective dose in one study [8] was nearly twice for CTU compared to IVU. Caoili et al. [10] found a four-phase CTU resulted in effective radiation doses of 25–35 mSv compared to 5 10 mSv for a 10–12 film IVU. Every attempt must be made to reduce dose by either reducing tube current (mA) and or eliminating a phase if

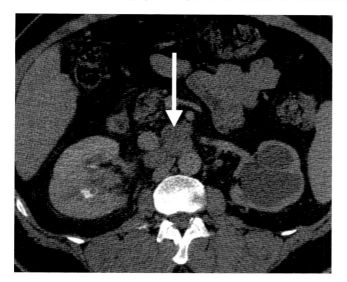

Fig. 12.9 Lymph node metastases: Axial CT showing retroperitoneal nodal metastases (*arrow*) from bilateral upper tract TCC

need be. While the carcinogenic risks of increased radiation should not be underestimated, they must be carefully weighed against the risk of missing malignant upper urinary tract pathology at an early stage when they can be optimally treated.

MR Imaging

MRI is not a first-line investigation in the assessment of hematuria or suspected upper-tract TCC. In patients with renal impairment or in patients who have a contra-indication to iodinated contrast, MRI can provide a very useful assessment of the kidney and collecting system or complimentary information in patients who have had a prior CT. MRI has the advantage of superior soft tissue contrast resolution. Similar to MDCT it can display images in multiple planes such as coronal sagittal and axial to optimally demonstrate lesions or asses a point of obstruction in hydronephrosis. On T1-weighted sequences TCC has similar or lower signal intensity to the renal parenchyma and on T2 is heterogeneous or mildly brighter compared to the renal parenchyma. Although TCC is relatively hypovascular, these lesions usually show moderate enhancement following gadolinium [22–24] and are most commonly an interureteric polypoid filling defect or a focal area of ureteric thickening (Fig. 12.10).

On MRI TCC is usually distinguishable from other causes of ureteric filling defect. Blood clots and calculi do not enhance and calculi show a signal void on T1-weighted sequences. Acute blood clots are often bright on T1-weighted sequences though this is highly variable depending on chronicity.

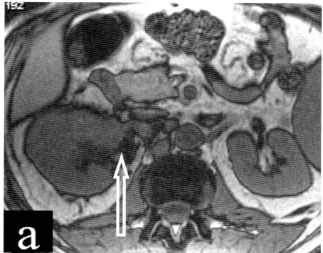

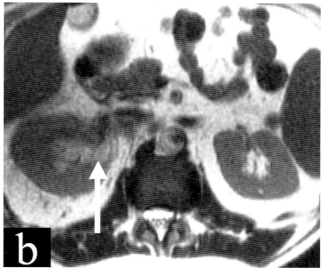

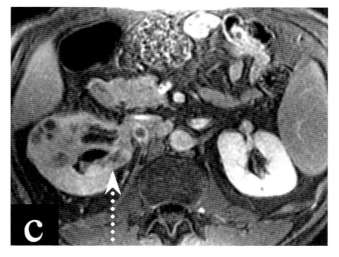

Fig. 12.10 MRI appearances of TCC: Axial T1 (**a**) showing low intensity (*arrow*) and T2-weighted MR image (**b**) showing intermediate intensity mass (*arrow*) in right renal pelvis. Axial post-gadolinium contrast T1 MRI (**c**) showing irregular enhancing mass (*dotted arrow*)

MRI has a similar sensitivity to CT in the detection of renal parenchymal lesions [25–27]; however its sensitivity in the detection of small ureteric lesion compared to other modalities such as retrograde urography and CT has not been clearly defined. Like CT, protocols designed to investigate for a neoplastic upper tract or renal cause for hematuria require the use of both conventional sequences to assess the renal parenchyma and also sequences to assess the collecting system. The combination of conventional MRI sequences with MR urography offers the advantage of a potential "all in one" assessment of the kidney and upper tract.

MR Urography (MRU)

MR urography is an evolving technique designed to assess the collecting system. Two complimentary components of MR urography have been developed in recent years using T1- and T2-weighted techniques [28–32]. In practice it makes sense to combine the advantages of both when designing protocols to assess the urinary tract.

T2-Weighted MR Urography

T2-weighted MRU relies on the inherent high signal intensity of static or slow-flowing fluids' "inherent contrast medium." It is highly sensitive and specific for the detection of hydronephrosis and localization of its level. T2 MR urography has the advantage of not relying on excreted contrast agent to opacify the collecting system and can be used in patients with a severely obstructed or non-functional kidney (Fig. 12.11). While T2 urography is sensitive to the detection of hydronephrosis it is often unable to distinguish intrinsic from extrinsic ureteric stenosis. Assessment of an undilated system can be suboptimal [33]. The administration of IV diuretics, usually frusemide, can improve visualization of the collecting tract. Over the past 10 years T2-weighted MR urography has developed into clinical practice. Turbo spin echo (TSE) sequences allow fast acquisition times. Initially described with the TSE technique of rapid acquisition with relaxation enhancement (RARE), more recent single-shot TSE techniques combined with half-Fourier acquisition such as HASTE (half-Fourier acquisition single-shot turbo spin echo) allow for the fastest acquisition times [34]. Techniques such as HASTE make it possible for single-shot sequences to be obtained in a single breath-hold to provide a coronal slab image covering several centimeters (up to 6–8 cm in 3–5 s). In patients who are unable to breath-hold this can eliminate respiratory motion artifact. Although these images do not provide good anatomical detail they have the advantage of

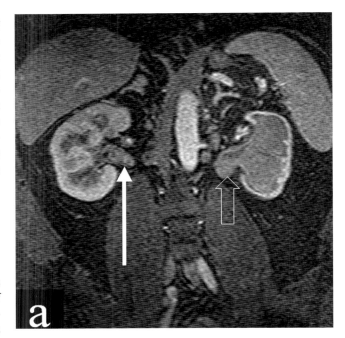

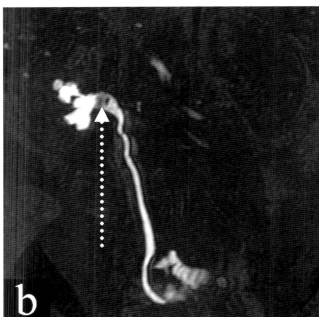

Fig. 12.11 T1 MRU: Coronal T1 post-gadolinium MR (**a**) with enhancing soft tissue in right renal pelvis (*arrow*). Delayed post-contrast T1 MRU (**b**) showing filling defect in right renal pelvis (*dotted arrow*) and non-excretion on left side due to marked obstruction

being quick to obtain and can be used as a first step to provide a rapid overview of the collecting system without the need for any post-processing. Multiple thinner overlapping slices (for example, 20–30 slices at 2–3 mm slice thickness) can be used to obtain 2D or 3D TSE sequences, with much greater anatomical detail to detect underlying pathology such as a tumor or focal ureteric stricture causing hydronephrosis.

However this technique is more time consuming and as a result requires a greater degree of patient cooperation with breath-holding. The use of respiratory triggering can help to maximize patient compliance and image quality by minimizing respiratory motion artifact [35].

T1-Weighted Excretory MR Urography

T1-weighted MRU is designed to use excreted gadolinium to outline the collecting system. Gadolinium is not nephrotoxic, making it a safer option than iodinated contrast required for CT in patients with renal impairment, provided they have sufficient renal function to excrete gadolinium. The excreted gadolinium opacifies the urinary tract allowing a point of obstruction or a filling defect to be identified (Fig. 12.12). This technique allows for both dilated and non-dilated collecting systems to be assessed but is of no use in patients with non-functional or severely obstructed collecting systems.

Unopacified urine appears black on T1-weighted sequences. A standard dose of I.V. gadolinium (0.1 mmol/kg) is usually used in excretory urography; low concentrations of excreted gadolinium create a positive contrast effect making the urine appear bright on T1-weighted images. At higher concentrations in the urine it can create an undesirable T2/T2* effect (on gradient echo sequences), resulting in a dark signal void. Frusemide 5–10 mg I.V. is an effective adjunct to help avoid this artifact (when given at or about the time of the gadolinium), by reducing the concentration of the excreted contrast in the urine.

Spoiled 3D gradient echo T1-weighted sequences such as FLASH (fast low angle shot) using low repetition and echo times can be used to obtain T1-weighted excretory images. Images are usually acquired in the coronal plane. Two-dimensional acquisitions can also be used but in general 3D sequences have better signal to noise ratio and through plane resolution.

The main disadvantage of MR imaging is the inability to reliably detect urinary tract calcifications, calculi, and air, which limits its use as a first-line test in the investigation of hematuria. Although the sensitivity of renal parenchymal MR imaging with gadolinium for assessing renal masses and abnormalities of the nephrogram is considered similar to that of CT, spatial resolution is poor compared with that of intravenous urography or CT urography, making detection of subtle urothelial malignancies less likely [28].

Summary

The emerging technique of CT urography allows detection of urinary tract tumors and calculi, assessment of perirenal tissues, and staging of lesions; it may offer the opportunity

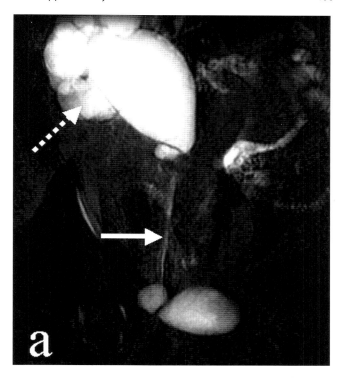

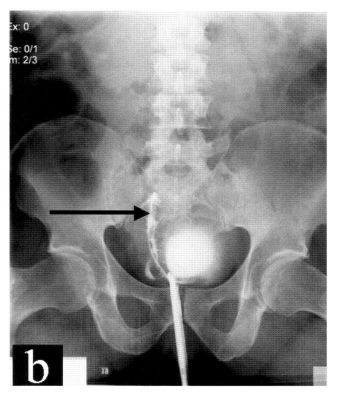

Fig. 12.12 T2 MRU: Coronal heavily T2-weighted MR (**a**) showing gross right hydronephrosis (*dotted arrow*) and irregular caliber ureter (*arrow*). Retrograde ureterogram (**b**) shows irregular narrowing of right ureter (*black arrow*)

for one-stop evaluation in the initial assessment of hematuria and in follow-up of TCC. Even as we write this review many investigators are pursuing refinements in CT technique in an attempt to maximize study accuracy while minimizing patient radiation exposure. There appears to be an emerging consensus of opinion that CTU has the potential to completely replace conventional IVU over the next few years. MR imaging, including the newer techniques of MR urography, can offer close to comparable evaluation in patients who cannot undergo a CTU and in whom multiplanar, vascular, and collecting system imaging is required.

References

1. Warshauer DM, McCarthy SM, Street L, Bookbinder MJ, Glickman MG, Richter J, et al. Detection of renal masses: sensitivities and specificities of excretory urography/linear tomography, US, and CT. Radiology. 1988;169:363–5.
2. Jamis-Dow CA, Choyke PL, Jennings SB, Linehan WM, Thakore KN, Walther MM. Small (< 3-cm) renal masses: detection with CT versus US and pathologic correlation. Radiology. 1996;198:785–8.
3. Smith RC, Verga M, McCarthy S, Rosenfield AT. Diagnosis of acute flank pain: value of unenhanced CT. Am J Roentgenol. 1996;166:97–101.
4. Levine JA, Neitlich J, Verga M, Dalrymple N, Smith RC. Ureteral calculi in patients with flank pain: correlation of plain radiography with unenhanced CT. Radiology. 1997;204: 27–31.
5. Perlman ES, Rosenfield AT, Wexler JS, Glickman MG. CT urography in the evaluation of urinary tract disease. J Comput Assist Tomogr. 1996; 20(4):620–6.
6. Chow LC, Sommer FG. Multidetector CT urography with abdominal compression and three-dimensional reconstruction. AJR Am J Roentgenol. 2001;177(4):849–55.
7. Akbar SA, Mortele KJ, Baeyens K, Kekelidze M, Silverman SG. Multidetector CT urography: techniques, clinical applications, and pitfalls. Semin Ultrasound CT MR. 2004;25(1):41–54.
8. McTavish JD, Jinzaki M, Zou KH, Nawfel RD, Silverman SG. Multi-detector row CT urography: comparison of strategies for depicting the normal urinary collecting system. Radiology. 2002;225(3):783–90.
9. Caoili EM, Inampudi P, Cohan RH, Ellis JH. Optimization of multi-detector row CT urography: effect of compression, saline administration, and prolongation of acquisition delay. Radiology. 2005;235(1):116–23.
10. Ramchandani P, Pollack H. Tumours of the urothelium. Semin Roentogenol. 1995;30(2):149–67.
11. Urban BA, Buckley J, Soyer P, Scherrer A, Fishman EK. CT appearance of transitional cell carcinoma of the renal pelvis. Am J. Roentgenol. Jul 1997;169:157–68.
12. Buckley JA, Urban BA, Soyer P, Scherrer A, Fishman EK. Transitional cell carcinoma of the renal pelvis: a retrospective look at CT staging with pathologic correlation. Radiology, 1996;201, 194–8.
13. Caoili EM, Cohan RH, Inampudi P, Ellis JH, Shah RB, Faerber GJ, Montie JE. MDCT urography of upper tract urothelial neoplasms. Am J Roentgenol. 2005;184:1873–81.
14. Hall MC, Womack S, Sagalowsky AI, Carmody T, Erickstad MD, Roehrborn CG. Prognostic factors, recurrence, and survival in transitional cell carcinoma of the upper urinary tract: a 30-year experience in 252 patients. Urology. 1998;52:594–601.

15. Chan V, Pantanowitz L, Vrachliotis TG, Rabkin DJ. CT demonstration of a rapidly growing transitional cell carcinoma of the ureter and renal pelvis. Abdom Imaging. 2002;27:222–3.
16. Scolieri MJ, Paik ML, Brown SL, Resnick MI. Limitations of computed tomography in the preoperative staging of upper tract urothetial carcinoma. Urology. 2000;56:930–4.
17. Kim JK, Cho KS. CT urography and virtual endoscopy: promising imaging modalities for urinary tract evaluation. Br J Radiol. 2003;76:199–209.
18. Urban BA, Buckley J, Soyer P, Scherrer A, Fishman EK. CT appearance of transitional cell carcinoma of the renal pelvis. II. Advanced-stage disease. AJR Am J Roentgenol. 1997;169:163–8.
19. Caoili EM, Cohan RH, Korobkin M, Platt JF, Francis IR, Faerber GJ, et al. Urinary tract abnormalities: initial experience with multi-detector row CT urography. Radiology. 2002 Feb; 222(2):353–60.
20. Millan-Rodriguez F, Palou J, de la Torre-Holguera P, Vayreda-Martija JM, Villavicencio-Mavrich H, Vicente-Rodriguez J. Conventional CT signs in staging transitional cell tumors of the upper urinary tract. Eur Urol. 1999;35:318–22.
21. Kirkali Z, Tuzel E. Transitional cell carcinoma of the ureter and renal pelvis. Crit Rev Oncol Hematol. 2003;47:155–69.
22. Walter C, Kruessell M, Gindele A, Brochhagen HG, Gossmann A, Landwehr P. Imaging of renal lesions: evaluation of fast MRI and helical CT. Br J Radiol. 2003;76:696–703.
23. Pretorius ES, Wickstrom ML, Siegelman ES. MR imaging of renal neoplasms. Magn Reson Imaging Clin N Am. 2000;8:813–36.
24. Milestone B, Friedman AC, Seidmon EJ, Radecki PD, Lev-Toaff AS, Caroline DF. Staging of ureteral transitional cell carcinoma by CT and MRI. Urology. 1990;36:346–9.
25. Cholankeril JV, Freundlich R, Ketyer S, Spirito AL, Napolitano J. Computed tomography in urothelial tumors of renal pelvis and related filling defects. J Comput Tomogr. 1986;10:263–72.
26. Walter C, Kruessell M, Gindele A, Brochhagen HG, Gossmann A, Landwehr P. Imaging of renal lesions: evaluation of fast MRI and helical CT. Br J Radiol. 2003;76:696–703.
27. Kreft BP, Müller-Miny H, Sommer T, Steudel A, Vahlensieck M, Novak D, B et al. Diagnostic value of MR imaging in comparison to CT in the detection and differential diagnosis of renal masses: ROC analysis. Eur Radiol. 1997;7:542–7.
28. Kawashima A, Glockner J, King B. CT urography and MR urography. Radiol Clin North Am. 2003;41:945–61.
29. Blandino A, Gaeta M, Minutoli F, et al. MR Urography and the ureter. AJR. 2002;179:1307–14.
30. Zielonko J, Studniarek M, Markuszewski M. MR urography of obstructive uropathy: diagnostic value of the method in selected clinical groups. Eur Radiol. 2003;13:802–9.
31. Nolte-Ernsting C, Adam G, Gunther R. MR urography: examination technique and clinical applications. Eur Radiol. 2001;11:355–72.
32. Farres M, Gattegno B, Ronco P, Flahault A, Paula-Souza R, Bigot J. Nonnephrotoxic, dynamic, contrast enhanced magnetic resonance urography: use in nephrology and urology. J Urol. 2000;164(4):1191–6.
33. Weeks SM, Brown ED, Brown JJ, Adamis MK, Eisenberg LB, Semelka RC. Transitional cell carcinoma of the upper tract: staging by MRI. Abdom Imaging. 1995;20:365–7.
34. Regan F, Bohlman ME, Khazan R, Rodriguez R, Schultze-Haakh H. MR urography using HASTE imaging in the assessment of ureteric obstruction. AJR. 1996;167:1115–20.
35. O' Malley ME, Sato JA, Yucel EK, Hussain S. MR urography: evaluation of a three-dimensional fast spin-echo technique in patients with hydronephrosis. AJR. 1997;168:387–92.

Chapter 13

Urothelial Cell Carcinoma in Upper Urinary Tract – Role of PET Imaging

J. Palou, I. Carrió, and H. Villavicencio

Clinical experience with positron emission tomography (PET) in urothelial tumors of the upper urinary tract is still very limited. The main interest of this imaging technique may be the detection and localization of lymph node and distant metastases, allowing a more precise staging and re-staging of patients with these type of tumors.

[18F]Fluorodeoxyglucose PET

PET, particularly with [18F]fluorodeoxyglucose (FDG), has undergone rapid expansion and is becoming widely used in clinical oncology. In addition, with the recent introduction of integrated PET/CT systems, the concomitantly acquired CT data have offered an anatomic reference frame for the biologic information provided by FDG-PET, and the PET/CT technique has improved the overall accuracy of data interpretation in cancer patients. In many cancers it has been useful for diagnosis, staging, assessment of recurrence, and for prognostic information. After intravenous injection, FDG is transported into cells, as is glucose, and phosphorylated to FDG-6-phosphate. It does not proceed further down the biochemical pathway and is therefore trapped in cells, in particular into those with enhanced glycolytic activity such as most cancer cells. The use of FDG-PET in urothelial tumors has been slower to develop partly due to the excretion of tracer through the urinary tract, potentially making structures and tumors difficult to see against this high physiologic background [1, 2]. PET therefore is of limited use to define the primary urological tumor. However, there is good evidence that FDG-PET may be useful in these tumors particularly for loco-regional staging and detection of recurrence. It does also have good uptake in metastatic disease, facilitating whole body assessment of eventual metastatic spread. Furthermore, for local staging one of the problems is the identification of involved lymph nodes. On CT these are generally regarded as malignant if > 1 cm and benign if < 1 cm. There are of course very small lymph nodes that contain disease and very large ones that are merely reactive. PET has the potential to assist in differentiating the composition of these nodes as it relies on metabolism of tumor cells. Enhanced FDG uptake strongly suggests malignancy despite normal lymph node dimensions.

FDG-PET has currently a central role in evaluating many malignant disorders that originate from or extend to the abdomen and pelvis. However, incidental urinary tracer accumulation and nonspecific FDG activity in the gastrointestinal tract may hamper the accuracy of abdomino-pelvic PET and PET/CT imaging. In particular, physiologic FDG activity in the urine can pose an interpretive challenge despite the improvement of simultaneous structural and biologic imaging with PET/CT [3, 4]. High levels of physiologic FDG activity in urine can mask lower levels of abnormal activity in neighboring structures such as the urinary tract and bladder. In addition, potential retention of excreted FDG in the ureters can sometimes be mistaken for active tumor foci. In an attempt to overcome these limitations, retrograde irrigation of the urinary bladder using saline irrigant and a Foley catheter has been advocated, either before or during PET data acquisition. This approach has been shown to be of some benefit in the evaluation of tumors that originate from the urinary bladder, but it may bring significant morbidity to the patient. Forced diuresis coupled with parenteral hydration, is another option that is safe and well tolerated, enhances urinary flux and allows rapid evacuation of the urinary bladder and can offer a valid alternative to improve tumor to background contrast in the assessment of urinary tract tumors [4].

Other PET Tracers with Potential in Urothelial Cancer

PET techniques are based on biologic rather than morphologic criteria, and their role in the staging and restaging of cancer has been increasingly recognized. However, the most

I. Carrió (✉)
Department of Nuclear Medicine, Hospital Sant Pau, CETIR Centre Mèdic, Barcelona

J.J.M.C.H. de la Rosette et al. (eds.), *Imaging in Oncological Urology*,
DOI 10.1007/978-1-84628-759-6_13, © Springer-Verlag London Limited 2009

widely used PET tracer, 18F-FDG, is often inappropriate for the imaging of urothelial cancer patients because its physiologic urinary excretion interferes with the imaging of tumor lesions in the urinary tract [5]. More recently, 11C-choline has been introduced as a PET tracer for the whole-body imaging of various malignancies [6]. 11C-choline generally displays high uptake in tumor tissues and is regarded as a favorable tracer for pelvic malignancies because of its negligible secretion into the urinary system.

The mechanism of 11C-choline uptake is related to the biosynthesis of phospholipids, which are essential components of all cell membranes. Carcinogenesis is characterized by enhanced cell proliferation and subsequent increased levels of phospholipids. The presence of choline transporters also seems to play a role in the process of 11C-choline uptake in tumor cells. Furthermore, one of the most studied oncogenes, ras, has been shown to activate choline kinase and phospholipase D, two enzymes responsible for the synthesis of phosphatidylcholine. In addition to their essential function as structural components of cell membranes, phospholipids are involved in the modulation of transmembrane signaling and thereby in cell proliferation and transformation [7].

If 11C-choline PET is considered for routine clinical diagnosis, then the principal disadvantage is the short half-life of 11C (20 min), limiting its use to centers with an on-site cyclotron. Therefore, 18F-labeled analogs of 11C-choline have been described and developed [8]. The mechanism of uptake of 18F-labeled choline analogs is very similar to that of 11C-choline. However, the most relevant difference is the significant secretion of radioactivity into the urinary system resulting from 18F-labeled analogs, compared with that of 11C-choline. Although urinary activity from 18F-labeled analogs could be overcome with aggressive hydration, diuresis, and irrigation catheters as mentioned above, it still represents a relevant disadvantage for imaging of urothelial cancers.

PET and PET/CT Imaging Protocols in Urothelial Cancer

18F-FDG PET

Typically, the patients are asked to fast for at least 6 h before undergoing a 18F-FDG PET examination. The radiopharmaceutical is administered by intravenous injection of approx. 5 MBq of 18F-FDG per kg of body weight and rest for 45–70 min to allow uptake of 18F-FDG by the organs and tumor. During this uptake phase, patients are asked to drink water (500–1,000 mL) and to void the bladder frequently to favor urinary excretion and at the same time to minimize radia-

tion exposure. Once this phase has been completed, a static whole-body emission PET or PET/CT scan from the pelvic floor to the head is initiated. The acquisition parameters for PET and PET/CT may vary according to the type of instrument being used in different institutions. In case a postdiuretic PET examination is performed, both the emission and the transmission times are kept the same as for the prediuretic studies. Similarly, the emission scan time for PET/CT is kept unchanged in the two acquisitions, whereas a low-dose CT may be applied for attenuation correction in the postdiuretic PET/CT study to reduce the patient's radiation burden [4, 9].

Forced Diuresis Protocol

If this technique is considered [3], immediately after the initial PET or PET/CT scan, the patients receive 0.5 mg of furosemide per kg of body weight (maximum, 40 mg) followed by infusion of 500 mL of physiologic saline through an intravenous line. During the saline infusion, which may last for 25–30 min, the patients may be encouraged to additionally drink two cups (400 mL) of water. Arterial blood pressure should be monitored during this period. For each postdiuretic PET or PET/CT study, two or three abdominopelvic cradle positions are acquired directly after the last voiding of the bladder. The length of the second acquisition may depend on the patient's clinical history or the prediuretic PET findings.

Such forced diuresis coupled with parenteral hydration may be very helpful to define confounding FDG–avid lesions in the urinary tract or its neighborhood (Fig. 13.1). Except for patients with impaired renal function, three successive voidings of the urinary bladder should suffice to decrease urinary activity to a background level, thus enhancing target to background contrast of lesions present in the urinary tract [3].

11C-Choline PET

11C-choline is usually synthesized as described by Hara et al. [6]. 11C-choline PET studies are typically performed with whole-body PET scanners same as with FDG-PET examinations. After patient positioning on the scanner table, a transmission scan is first obtained [10]. PET emission scans start 5 min after intravenous injection of approximately 370–500 MBq of 11C-choline and include several bed positions starting from the pelvis and moving to the neck. Emission imaging is usually performed in the two-dimensional mode, with 5 min for the first bed position and increasing to 12 min for the sixth bed position, and with a matrix of 128×128 pixels. Emission data are then corrected for randoms, dead

A

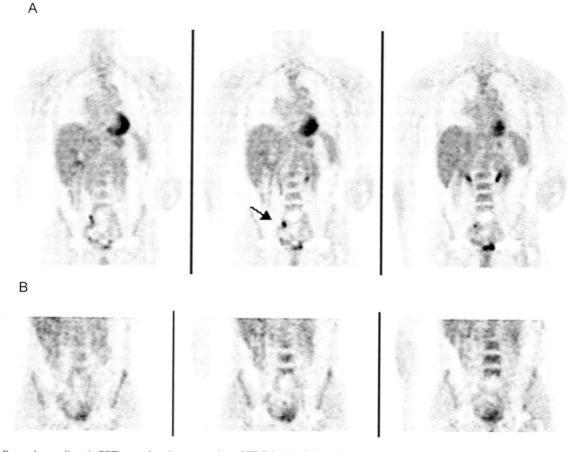

B

Fig. 13.1 Pre and post-diuretic PET scan showing stagnation of FDG in the right urether (a, see *arrow*) that clears after diuretic administration (b)

time, and attenuation, and an iterative reconstruction is performed. Images are rendered in the standard whole body and cross-sectional format.

Clinical Value of PET and PET/CT Imaging in Urothelial Cancer

FDG-PET and PET/CT imaging has high accuracy in detecting many malignant disorders of the abdomen and pelvis, however, physiologic FDG excretion along the urinary system hampers visualization of urothelial primary cancer. Continuous efforts have been devoted to overcoming this limitation inherent to FDG-PET. For instance, Kosuda et al. [11] evaluated 12 patients with suspected recurrent or residual bladder cancer. In nine of them, retrograde irrigation of the urinary bladder was applied. Although a remarkable reduction of urinary activity was observed, a background level was never reached in any patient, ending in four false-negative intravesical lesions that were masked by residual urinary activity. Likewise, in another prospective study, Koyama et al. [12] observed that at least 8 (20%) of 41 stud-

ied patients failed to eliminate all 18F-FDG activity from the urinary tract despite continuous bladder irrigation using pre-warmed physiologic saline solution. The results of these studies imply that an ideal approach to overcoming the inherent limitations must consider eliminating residual 18F-FDG activity from the entire urinary tract to avoid interference from any physiologic activity.

Kamel et al [3] observed that a furosemide dose of 0.5 mg/kg followed by parenteral infusion of 500 mL of physiologic saline over 25–30 min successfully eliminated any significant FDG activity from the bladder and both ureters. Except for one patient with chronic renal failure, a background activity level could be obtained in the lower urinary tract of 31 of 32 patients after they had voided their urinary bladder three successive times. A similar study also demonstrated that the application of diuretics significantly reduced residual FDG activity in the bladder [13]. However, in some of the patients whose kidneys were within the field of view of post-diuretic PET, renal activity did not reach a background level, potentially because of physiologic uptake of FDG by the renal tubular epithelium [14, 15]. Because of the known limited avidity of some renal cell carcinomas to FDG [16], this approach is not likely to improve the performance of PET in characterizing renal tumors. However, this technique is clearly helpful in bladder cancer [17]. The high post-diuretic 18F-FDG uptake of these lesions as seen on the PET images is helpful to clarify post-therapy radiologic findings in the bladder wall, which are often encountered in the clinical follow-up of these patients.

Approximately 15–28% of patients are found to have lymph node metastatic disease at histologic analysis [18, 19]. Recent progress in diagnostic imaging by CT and MRI with contrast enhancement has allowed the lymph node staging of bladder cancer, but the results have been generally disappointing. With cross-sectional imaging modalities, metastatic lymph node involvement is assessed by size, which can be misleading, especially after transurethral resection of bladder cancer is performed. 11C-choline has been reported to successfully visualize various tumors with a high signal-to-background ratio, including slowly growing tumors, such as prostate cancer, which are often 18F-FDG negative [20, 21]. Furthermore, with 11C-choline, a high signal-to-noise ratio can be achieved in tumors and lymph nodes located in the pelvis, in which background radioactivity is low [22].

Drieskens et al. [9] assessed in a prospective study the presence of lymph node involvement and distant metastasis in patients with invasive bladder carcinoma as a major determinant of survival. Whole-body FDG-PET and computed tomography (CT) were performed in 55 patients with non-metastatic invasive bladder cancer for preoperative staging. For the diagnosis of nodal or metastatic disease, the sensitivity, specificity, and accuracy of PET were 60, 88, and 78%, respectively. Median survival time of patients in whom PET indicated nodal or metastatic disease was 13.5 months, compared with 32.0 months in the patients with a negative PET, thus showing that addition of metabolism-based information provided by PET in the preoperative staging of invasive bladder carcinoma yields also an improved prognostic accuracy.

Liu et al. [21] evaluated the role of FDG-PET in metastatic transitional cell carcinoma. Results in these patients were compared to those in patients who had undergone prior chemotherapy. In contrast to pre-treatment findings, after chemotherapy, viable cancer cells showed a diminished metabolic rate, suggesting that PET images should be interpreted with caution in patients who have received prior chemotherapy [22].

The usefulness of 11C-choline PET for the detection of lymph node involvement has been shown for prostate cancer by de Jong et al. [23]. The reported sensitivity, specificity, and accuracy for lymph node staging of prostate cancer were 80, 96, and 93%, respectively, suggesting that this technique has a higher sensitivity than CT or MRI. False-positive results may occur because of focal bowel activity or reactive lymph nodes. False-negative findings have been described for lymph node lesions smaller than 1 cm in diameter. In addition, de Jong et al. [23] recently reported the first clinical experience on the visualization of bladder cancer with 11C-choline PET. They showed that 11C-choline uptake in bladder cancer is feasible for visualizing the extent of tumor because of the virtual absence of urinary activity. In addition, premalignant and small noninvasive tumors did not show increased 11C-choline uptake.

Pichio et al. [10] recently compared the value of 11C-choline PET and contrast-enhanced CT for the staging of advanced bladder carcinoma against histologic analysis (including lesion size measurements) as a reference. In this series, the number of correctly detected lesions was higher with 11C-choline PET than with CT. In particular, the sensitivity of 11C-choline PET was superior to that of CT for both the detection of residual bladder wall involvement and for lymph node staging. The eventual presence of false-negative results obtained for both bladder cancer sites and lymph node involvement by 11C-choline PET likely is related to its restricted spatial resolution, limiting its sensitivity for small lesions. In this study, the actual sizes of cancerous lesions within involved lymph nodes were measured. 11C-choline PET failed to demonstrate one larger (15 mm) metastatic lesion as well as two additional lesions that were below the resolution of the PET scanners used in the study (1 and 3 mm). All remaining lymph node metastatic lesions

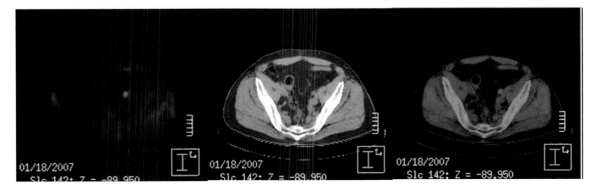

Fig. 13.2 Choline PET/CT scan (PET, CT, and fused image) showing a positive pelvic lymph node indicative of malignancy

(between 5 and 16 mm) were correctly identified. The results of this study show that the overall accuracy to detect lymph node metastatic disease is better with 11C-choline PET than with CT. This is probably due to 11C-choline PET not being affected by the inflammatory changes seen in pelvic and abdominal lymph nodes by CT when used to assess lymph

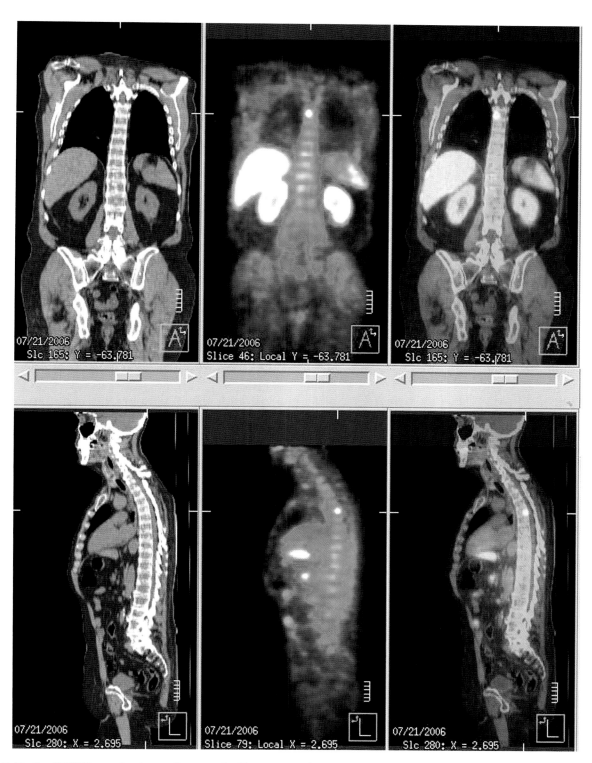

Fig. 13.3 Choline PET/CT scan showing a solitary vertebral bone metastasis

node size. At present, CT is the most commonly used non-invasive study for the staging of bladder cancer. However, despite the use of multislice CT systems and intravenous contrast medium, structural imaging of lymph node and size evaluation is only clearly limited to diagnose malignancy. It appears to be clinically relevant that 11C-choline PET yields fewer false-positive results than CT, suggesting that 11C-choline PET may be particularly useful in evaluating patients with nodal enlargement or nodes with borderline sizes. The use of integrated PET/CT will certainly provide diagnostic benefits, because focal uptake can be better delineated as resulting from lymph node involvement rather than non-specific focal bowel activity, and metastatic spread can be properly ruled out (Figs. 12.2 and 12.3). These results support the further analysis of 11C-choline for evaluating locally advanced bladder cancer and other urothelial tumors. In fact, 11C-choline imaging may allow for the selection of patients for possible neoadjuvant treatment before radical bladder resection [24, 25]. In addition, the identification of metastatic lymph nodes outside the area of standard pelvic lymph node dissection may allow their removal, which may translate to more accurate treatment and better patient outcome and survival.

Conclusions

Addition of metabolism-based information as provided by PET and PET/CT examinations using FDG or other metabolic tracers yields improved diagnostic and prognostic accuracy in patients with urothelial tumors. Although the physiologic urinary excretion of radiotracers makes structures and tumors difficult to delineate, PET imaging may be useful for local staging and recurrence, with additional value in the identification of metastatic disease.

References

1. Jimenez-Vicioso A, Torres-Isidro V, Carreras-Delgado J. The interest of PET (Positron Emission Tomography) for urothelial tumors. Arch Esp Urol. 2004;57(3):337–47.
2. Hain SF. Positron emission tomography in uro-oncology. Cancer Imaging. 2005;5(1):1–7.
3. Kamel EM, Jichlinski P, Prior J, Delaloye A, et al. Forced diuresis improves the diagnostic accuracy of 18F-FDG PET in abdominopelvic malignancies. J Nucl Med. 2006;47(11):1803–7.
4. Lopez-Gandul S, Perez-Moure G, Garcia-Garzón JR, Soler M, Simó M, et al. Intravenous furosemide injection during 18F-FDG PET acquisition. J Nucl Med Technol. 2006;34(4):228–31.
5. Shvarts O, Han KR, Seltzer M, Pantuck AJ, Belldegrun AS. Positron emission tomography in urologic oncology. Cancer Control. 2002;9:335–42.
6. Hara T. 11C-Choline and 2-deoxy-2-[18F]fluoro-D-glucose in tumor imaging with positron emission tomography. Mol Imaging Biol. 2002;4:267–73.
7. Ramirez de Molina A, Penalva V, Lucas L, Lacal JC. Regulation of choline kinase activity by Ras proteins involves Ral-GDS and PI3K. Oncogene. 2002;21:937–46.
8. Hara T, Kosaka N, Kishi H. Development of 18F-fluoroethylcholine for cancer imaging with PET: synthesis, biochemistry, and prostate cancer imaging. J Nucl Med. 2002;43:187–99.
9. Drieskens O, Oyen R, Van Poppel H, Vankan Y, Flamen P, et al. FDG-PET for preoperative staging of bladder cancer: Eur J Nucl Med Mol Imaging. 2005;32(12):1412–7.
10. Picchio M, Triber U, Beer A, Metz S, Bössner P, et al. Value of 11C-choline PET and contrast-enhanced CT for staging of bladder cancer: correlation with histopathologic findings. J Nucl Med. 2006;47(6):938–44.
11. Kosuda S, Kison PV, Greenough R, Grossman HB, Wahl RL. Preliminary assessment of fluorine-18 fluorodeoxyglucose positron emission tomography in patients with bladder cancer. Eur J Nucl Med. 1997;24:615–20.
12. Koyama K, Okamura T, Kawabe J, et al. Evaluation of 18F-FDG PET with bladder irrigation in patients with uterine and ovarian tumors. J Nucl Med. 2003;44:353–8.
13. Diehl M, Manolopoulou M, Risse J, et al. Urinary fluorine-18 fluorodeoxyglucose excretion with and without intravenous application of furosemide. Acta Med Austriaca. 2004;31:76–8.
14. Thorens B. Glucose transporters in the regulation of intestinal, renal, and liver glucose fluxes. Am J Physiol. 1996;270: G541–53.
15. Southworth R, Parry CR, Parkes HG, Medina RA, Garlick PB. Tissue-specific differences in 2-fluoro-2-deoxyglucose metabolism beyond FDG-6-P: a 19F NMR spectroscopy study in the rat. NMR Biomed. 2003;16:494–502.
16. Miyakita H, Tokunaga M, Onda H, et al. Significance of 18F-fluorodeoxyglucose positron emission tomography (FDG-PET) for detection of renal cell carcinoma and immunohistochemical glucose transporter 1 (GLUT-1) expression in the cancer. Int J Urol. 2002;9:15–8.
17. Kuczyk M, Turkeri L, Hammerer P, Ravery V, European Society for Oncological Urology. Is there a role for bladder preserving strategies in the treatment of muscle-invasive bladder cancer? Eur Urol. 2003;44:57–64.
18. Madersbacher S, Hochreiter W, Burkhard F, et al. Radical cystectomy for bladder cancer today: a homogeneous series without neoadjuvant therapy. J Clin Oncol. 2003;21:690–6.
19. Vazina A, Dugi D, Shariat SF, Evans J, Link R, Lerner SP. Stage specific lymph node metastasis mapping in radical cystectomy specimens. J Urol. 2004;171:1830–4.
20. Picchio M, Messa C, Landoni C, et al. Value of [11C]choline-positron emission tomography for re-staging prostate cancer: a comparison with [18F]fluorodeoxyglucose-positron emission tomography. J Urol. 2003;169:1337–40.
21. Liu IJ, lai YH, Espiritu JI, Segall GM, Srinivas S, et al. Evaluation of fluorodeoxyglucose positron emission tomography imaging in metastatic transitional cell carcinoma with and without prior chemotherapy. Urol Int. 2006;77(1):69–75.
22. Kaneta T, Hakamatsuka T, Yamada T, Takase K, Sato A, et al. FDG PET in solitary metastasic and secondary tumor of the kidney. Ann Nucl Med. 2006;20(1):79–82.
23. de Jong IJ, Pruim J, Elsinga PH, Jongen MM, Mensink HJ, Vaalburg W. Visualisation of bladder cancer using (11)C-choline PET: first clinical experience. Eur J Nucl Med Mol Imaging. 2002;29(10):1283–8.
24. Kotzerke J, Prang J, Neumaier B, et al. Experience with carbon-11 choline positron emission tomography in prostate carcinoma. Eur J Nucl Med. 2000;27:1415–9.
25. de Jong IJ, Pruim J, Elsinga PH, Vaalburg W, Mensink HJ. Preoperative staging of pelvic lymph nodes in prostate cancer by 11C-choline PET. J Nucl Med. 2003;44:331–5.

Chapter 14

Considerations: Imaging in Upper Urinary Tract Urothelial Carcinoma

J. Rassweiler and D. Teber

Introduction

According to the surface of both the collecting systems and the ureters in relationship to the urinary bladder, urothelial carcinoma of the upper urinary tract occurs in about 5% of all transitional cell carcinoma. Upper urinary tract tumors are rarely detected incidentally or by screening. Usually, patients present with flank pain, recurrent hematuria, and/or abnormal cytology, and are evaluated specifically to rule out tumoral involvement of the upper urinary tract (Table 14.1).

Basic Diagnostic Procedures

Principally, the diagnostic algorithm can be divided into the detection of tumor and the staging of the disease. Basic imaging modalities for tumor detection include ultrasonography, intravenous pyelography, and retrograde pyelography (Fig. 14.1).

Table 14.1 Algorithm of diagnosis of upper tract tumors

Symptoms	Flank pain, hematuria
Basic diagnosis	Urine sample (+ cytology): erythrocytes, tumor cells
	Ultrasound: hydronephrosis, pelvic tumor (hypoechoic)
	IVP: filling defect, phantom calyx
	Videocystoscopy: hematuria out of orifice
	Retrograde pyelogram (+ cytology): filling defect, phantom calyx, tumor cells
	Flexible video-ureteroscopy: visualization of tumor, biopsy
Staging diagnosis	CT-urography: tumor in collecting system, para-aortic lymph nodes, metastases
	MR-urography: hydronephrosis, para-aortic lymph nodes, metastases

J. Rassweiler (✉)
Department of Urology, SLK Kliniken Heilbronn, Am Gesundbrunnen 20, D74078 Heilbronn, Germany, jens.rassweiler@slk-kliniken.de

Ultrasonography

In contrast to parenchymal renal tumors, where ultrasound provides a high sensitivity, sonography has only secondary strengths (i.e., to exclude a calculi, detection of ureteral obstruction). Particularly in non-obstructed kidney, demonstration of the urothelium is not always possible [1]. Accordingly, only larger tumors (i.e., >15 mm) may be detected as hypoechoic or isoechoic lesions particularly in case of hydronephrosis (Fig. 14.2). In such a case, the presence of a central mass of moderate echogenicity that is separated from the renal parenchyma should be considered as a malignant urothelial tumor (Fig. 14.1). Rarely such larger tumors may present with calcifications and have to be distinguished from renal stones with the classical acoustic shadow [2].

Ultrasonography should be the first imaging modality for patients with flank pain or hematuria [3]. The most frequent complication of an upper tract urinary tumor particularly if present in the ureter is urinary tract obstruction leading to dilation of the collecting system, which can be easily identified sonographically. Unfortunately, the dilated ureter can only be demonstrated down to the level of the upper third (i.e., lower pole of the kidney) and prevesical. Because of this limited acoustic window, particularly in patients with renal colics and subsequent meteorism, ureteral tumors may usually not be clearly imaged by ultrasonography. The determination of the resistive index using color duplex sonography by determining the intrarenal blood flow may distinguish between acute obstruction and ectasia of the collecting system (i.e., RI > 0.7). However, in case of upper tract carcinoma, this information may not play an important role [4, 5].

Of course, ultrasound provides certain advantages (i.e., low costs, non-invasive procedure, no use of contrast dye, no radiation); however in case of upper tract urothelial tumors it usually offers only adjunct information. New developments such as intraureteral (endoluminal) ultrasonongraphy did not prove to be very helpful in the basic diagnosis of upper tract tumors [6–8].

Fig. 14.1 Basic diagnostic findings of a tumor in the upper urinary tract (renal pelvis): (**a**) Ultrasound: hypoechoic lesion in the central reflex zone. (**b**) Intravenous pyelography: Filling defect in renal pelvis and lower calyx. (**c**) Retrograde pyelogram: Filling defect in renal pelvis and neck of lower calyx

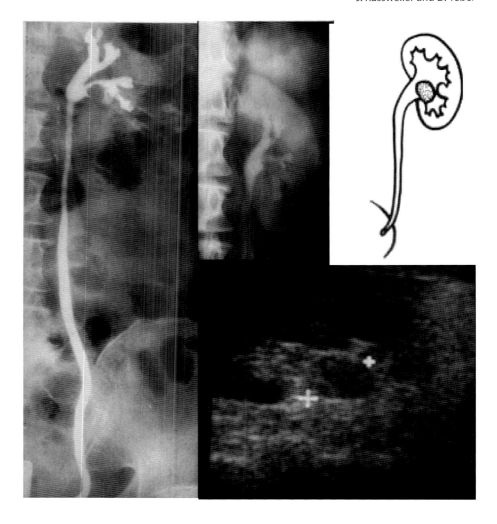

Intravenous Pyelography

Intravenous pyelography may have lost importance in the diagnostic workup of acute colic compared to sequential computed tomography; however, CT and even MRI urography simply do not demonstrate the same anatomic details of the upper urinary tract [3, 9, 10]. Therefore, intravenous pyelography is still useful and should not be abandoned (Fig. 14.1).

Due to potential contrast nephrotoxicity, certain risk factors have to be assessed prior to the examination, such as diabetes mellitus, renal insufficiency (serum creatinine!), congestive heart failure, myeloma (i.e., plasmocytoma), and dehydration. Severe allergic reactions to contrast media have to be explored. Patients with risk factors should receive pre-contrast antihistamines and corticosteroids. Moreover, non-ionic contrast media should be preferred because of a significant lower rate of anaphylactoid reactions compared to ionic contrast media (1 vs. 5%). However, in case of diagnosis of upper tract tumors usually no emergency situation is

present. Hence, all these factors can be adequately taken into consideration [11].

Proper preparation of the patient is important to receive optimal information, including bowel preparation reducing meteorism, and to avoid hyperhydration resulting in dilution of the contrast media. Under these conditions, the intravenous pyelogram allows detailed visualization of the renal collecting system and ureters. Larger tumors filling completely a calyx may result in a so-called phantom calyx. Upper tract tumors classically show as filling defects. Additionally, calcified calculi can be diagnosed. Frequent differential diagnoses of filling defects on an IVP include non-opaque calculi (i.e., uric acid), clots of patients with coagualopathy (i.e., under cumarine therapy), and papilla necrosis (i.e., diabetes mellitus).

Similar to ultrasonography, intravenous urography detects ureteral obstruction, but in addition it may help to identify exactly the localization and cause of hydronephrosis. Again a ureteral tumor is visualized as a filling defect. Frequent differential diagnoses are similar to filling defects in

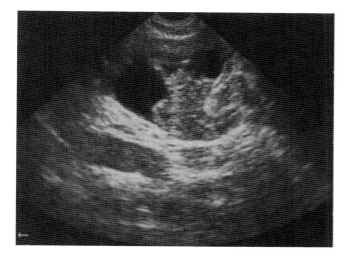

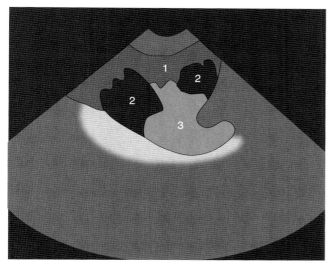

Fig. 14.2 a Sonographic picture of a papillary transitional cell carcinoma in the renal pelvis leading to hydronephrosis. b 1=renal parenchyma, 2=dilated renal pelvis, 3=tumor

the renal pelvis. Additionally, ureteral strictures of extraureteral lesions (i.e., lymphoma, lymph node metastases) may be taken into consideration.

Cystoscopy and Retrograde Pyelogram

The most important step in the diagnosis represents endoscopic imaging (i.e., cystoscopy, ureteroscopy) plus retrograde pyelogram. The procedure is essential and provides several advantages.

Cysto-urethroscopy enables diagnosis of other reasons of hematuria such as (concomitant) bladder tumors, bladder stones, benign prostatic hyperplasia, or urethral tumors. In 20–25% of upper tract urothelial tumors concomitant bladder tumors can be found. Sometimes, selective hematuria out of one of the orifices may alleviate further diagnosis. Addition-

ally to the retrograde pyelogram, selective cytology (using two different ureteral catheters) provides important information, particularly in case of high-grade tumors. Moreover, the use of fluorescent agents such as 5-amino-levulinic acid or hexyl(5-amino-4-oxopentanoat)-hydrochloride (Hexvix^R) may increase the diagnostic efficacy particularly for flat superficial lesions [12].

Similar to intravenous pyelography, imaging features of upper tract tumors include filling defects, irregular stenoses, non-visualized calyces, and hydronephrosis (Fig 14.1). One advantage of the retrograde study is the fact that the amount of filling of the collecting system can be varied to avoid overprojection of contrast dye as well as pyelosinus backflow. Additionally, there is a very low risk of anaphylactoid reactions following endoluminal injection of contrast dye [10, 13].

Flexible Ureterorenoscopy

The technical advances of instruments and video equipment lead to the development of small-caliber flexible ureteroscopes (F8-9). Such instruments allow minimally invasive exploration and endoscopic visualization of the entire urinary tract (Fig. 14.3). Nowadays, endoscopic diagnosis of the upper urinary tract to confirm the diagnosis of a tumor has become mandatory, unless in case of large tumors where the diagnosis can be based of uro-radiologic imaging techniques [14].

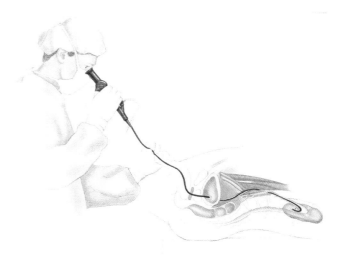

Fig. 14.3 (**a**) Flexible (video-)ureteroscopy for diagnosis of (**b**) upper tract tumors. (**c** and **d**) Visualization and documentation of the position of the endoscope by injection of contrast dye

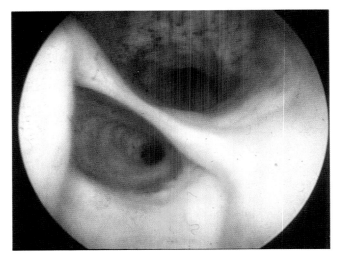

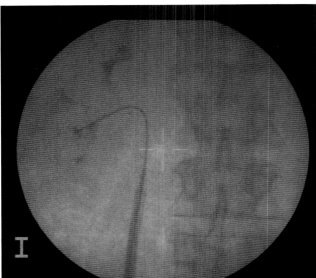

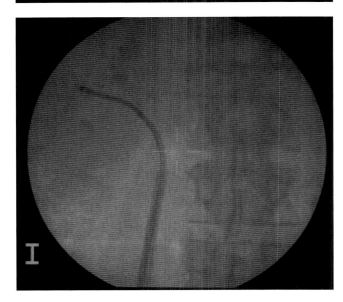

Fig. 14.3 (continued)

Antegrade Pyelography

Principally, the role of antegrade pyelography is limited. In case of a suspicious upper tract transitional cell carcinoma, percutaneous puncture of the kidney and collecting system should be avoided to minimize the risk of tumor cell spillage or seeding [15, 16]. Of course, once a percutaneous nephrostomy has been placed in an emergency situation to relieve pain, sepsis, or to preserve renal function, the access can be used for diagnostic purposes [17, 18]. Urothelial tumors have exactly the same imaging characteristics as with intravenous and retrograde pyelography.

Staging Procedures

CT-Urography

Computer tomography has been accepted to be superior in the detection of renal masses compared to IVU and ultrasonography; however, the limited accuracy in the assessment of mucosal surfaces of the upper urinary tract still represents the final frontier [19]. The introduction of multidetector row CT (MDCT) may lead to a significantly better resolution to demonstrate tumors in the collecting system; however, because of the significantly higher radiation exposure compared to the standard IVU, this imaging modality cannot be included in the primary diagnostic workup [20].

Of course, CT provides additional information besides the confirmation of the tumor diagnosis, such as involvement of lymph nodes or extension of lager tumors (i.e., infiltration depth). However, it has to be emphasized that CT-urography even using MD technology cannot be distinguished between Ta, T1, and T2 stages [21].

Future applications of CT-urography may include virtual endoscopy with visualization of the tumor [22]. This might be able to obviate flexible ureteroscopy in case of larger tumors, where biopsy is not needed (i.e., prior to laparoscopic nephroureterectomy).

Magnetic Resonance Imaging

There is consensus that MRI is not a first-line investigation in the assessment of hematuria or suspected upper tract tumors [23, 24]. Recently, MR-urography using either T1- or T2-weighted images has been introduced. While T2 MR-urography is sensitive for detection of hydronephrosis, T1-weighted MRU uses the excreted gadolinium to outline the collecting system. However, the main disadvantage of

MR imaging represents the inability to reliably detect urinary calcifications, calculi, and air, which limits its use as first-line imaging modality [24, 25]. Therefore, the main indication for MRI represents diagnosis in patients with renal impairment, because MRI-contrast media are not nephrotoxic.

Positron Emission Tomography

Whereas PET/CT using 11C-choline as tracer has become an important diagnostic modality for detection of recurrent prostatic cancer (i.e., following radical prostatectomy) distinguishing between bone, lymph node metastasis, and local recurrence [26], this imaging modality has not been proven to be helpful in primary diagnosis of upper tract tumors. This is related to its restricted spatial resolution limiting the diagnosis of small lesions. [18F]Fluorodeoxglucose (FDG) is much easier to handle compared to 11C-choline with a 20 min halftime; however physiologic excretion of FDG along the urinary system hampers the visualization of primary urinary cancer. On the other hand, early studies suggest that PET/CT may provide additional information in the identification of metastatic disease compared to CT alone [27].

Management of Upper Tract Tumors

Nowadays, therapy of upper tract transitional cell carcinoma has become multimodal, depending on the infiltration depth and localization of the tumor [28].

Standard treatment of invasive TCC still represents radical nephroureterectomy, which can be performed also laparoscopically with open removal of distal ureter including a bladder cuff [28–30]. Transurethral circumcision of the orifice or pluck-off techniques has been abandoned due to the risk of local recurrence. Long-term studies following laparoscopic nephrourectectomy have shown similar oncological efficacy, but a significantly reduced morbidity and shortened hospital stay [30].

In case of distal superficial TCC, partial ureterectomy with ureteral reimplantation may obviate ablative surgery [31]. This procedure can also be accomplished laparoscopically.

Technical improvement in endorological methods has facilitated to resect or laser-ablate low-grade superficial upper tract tumors in selected cases [32]. Such patients have to be followed carefully including regular flexible ureteroscopy and local chemoprevention with mitomycin C or immunotherapy with BCG [33].

Surprisingly the EAU and the AUA guidelines did not include recommendations on upper tract TCC. Our algorithm is a first step to come to such a work.

References

1. Mulholland SG, Arger PH, Goldberg BB, Pollack HM. Ultrasonic differentiation of renal pelvic filling defects. J Urol. 1979;122:14–6.
2. Janetschek G, Putz A, Feichtinger H. Renal transitional cell carcinoma mimicking stone echoes. J Ultrasound Med. 1988;7:83–6.
3. Heidenreich A, Desgrandschamps F, Terrier F. Modern approach of diagnosis and management of acute flank pain: review of all imaging modalities. Eur Urol. 2002;41:351–62.
4. Harzmann R, Weckermann D. Importance of Doppler sonography in urology. Urol Int. 1990;45:258–63.
5. Kim HJ, Lim JW, Lee DH, Ko YT, Oh JH, Kim YW. Transitional cell carcinoma involving the distal ureter: assessment with transrectal and color Doppler ultrasonography. J Ultrasound Med. 2005;24:1625–33.
6. Liu JB, Bagley DH, Conlin MJ, Merton DA, Alexander AA, Goldberg BB. Endoluminal sonographic evaluation of ureteral and renal pelvic neoplasm. J Ultrasound Med. 1997;16:515–21.
7. Keeley FX Jr, Moussa SA, Miller J, Tolley DA. A prospective study of endoluminal ultrasound versus computerized tomography angiography for detecting crossing vessels at the ureteropelvic junction. J Urol. 1999;162:1938–41.
8. Frede T, Hatzinger M, Rassweiler J. Ultrasound in endourology. J. Endourol. 2001;15:3–16.
9. Dalla Palma L. What is left of i.v. urography? Eur Radiol. 2001;11:931–9.
10. Skrepetis K, Siafakas I, Lykurinas M. Evolution of retrograde pyelography and excretory urography in the early 20th century. J Endourol. 2001;15:691–6.
11. Thomsen HS, Morcos SK. Contrast media and the kidney: European Society of Urogenital Radiology (ESUR) guidelines. Br J Radiol. 2003;76:513–8.
12. Kriegmair M, Zaak D, Rothenberger K-H, Rassweiler J, Jocham D, Eisenberger F, et al. Transurethral resection for bladder cancer using 5-aminolevulinic acid induced fluorescence endoscopy versus white light endoscopy. J.Urol. 2002;168:475–8.
13. Leder RA, Dunnick NR. Transitional cell carcinoma of the pelvicalices and ureter. Am J Roentgenol. 1990;155:713–22.
14. Chen GL, El-Gabry EA, Bagley DH. Surveillance of upper urinary tract transitional cell carcinoma: the role of ureteroscopy, retrograde pyelography, cytology and urinalysis. J Urol. 2000;164:1901–4.
15. Sengupta S, Harewood L. Transitional cell carcinoma growing along an indwelling nephrostomy tube track. BJU Int. 1998;82:591.
16. Patel A, Soonawalla P, Shepherd SF, Dearnaley DP, Kellet ML, Woodhouse CR. Long-term outcome after percutaneous treatment of transitional cell carcinoma of the renal pelvis. J Urol. 1996;155:868–74.
17. Rassweiler J. Letter to the editor. Re: ultrasound guided percutaneous nephrotomy for obstructive uropathy in benign and malignant disease. Int Braz J Urol. 2006;32:470.
18. Michel MS, Trojan L, Rassweiler JJ. Complications in percutaneous nephrolithotomy. Eur Urol. 2007;51:899–906.
19. Pollak HM, Arger PH, Banner MP, Mulhern CB Jr, Coleman BG. Computed tomography of renal pelvic filling defects. Radiology. 1982;145:743–7.
20. Chow LC, Sommer FG. Multidetector CT urography with abdominal compression and three-dimensional reconstruction. Am J Roentgenol. 2001;177(4):849–55.
21. Scolieri MJ, Paik ML, Brown SL, Resnick MI. Limitations of Computed Tomography in the preoperative staging of upper tract urothelial carcinoma. Urology. 2000;56:930–4.

22. Kim JK, Cho KS. CT urography and virtual endoscopy: promising imaging modalities for urinary tract evaluation. Br J Radiol. 2003;76:199–209.

23. Milestone B, Friedman AC, Seidmon EJ, Radecki PD, Lev-Toaff AS, Caroline DF. Staging of ureteral transitional cell carcinoma by CT and MRI. Urology. 1990;36:346–9.

24. Kawashima A, Glockner J, King B. CT urography and MR urography. Radiol Clin North Am. 2003;41:945–61.

25. Zielonko J, Studniarek M, Markuszewski M. MR urography of obstructive uropathy: diagnostic value of the method in selected clinical groups. Eur Radiol. 2003;13:802–9.

26. Hara T, Kosaka N, Kishi H. Development of ^{18}F-fluoroethylcholine for cancer imaging with PET: synthesis, biochemistry, and prostate cancer imaging. J Nucl Med. 2002;43:187–99.

27. Liu IJ, lai YH, Espiritu JI, Segall GM, Srinivas S, Nino-Murcia M, Terris MK. Evaluation of fluorodeoxyglucose positron emission tomography imaging in metastatic transitional cell carcinoma with and without prior chemotherapy. Urol Int. 2006;77(1):69–75.

28. Oosterlinck W, Solsona E, van der Meijden AP, Sylvester R, Böhle A, Rintala E, Lobel B. European Association of Urology (EAU) guidelines on diagnosis and treatment of upper urinary tract transitional cell carcinoma. Eur Urol. 2004;46:147–54.

29. El Fetouh HA, Rassweiler JJ, Schulze M, Salomon L, Allan J, Ramakumar S, et al. Laparoscopic radical nephroureterectomy: results of an international multicenter study. Eur Urol. 2002;42:447–52.

30. Rassweiler JJ, Schulze MM, Marrero R, Frede T, Palou Redorta J, Bassi P. Laparoscopic nephroureterectomy for upper urinary tract transitional cell carcinoma: is it better than open surgery? Eur Urol. 2004;46:690–7.

31. Rassweiler JJ, Gözen AS, Erdogru T, Sugiono M, Teber D. Ureteral reimplantation for management of ureteral strictures: a retrospective comparison of laparoscopic and open techniques. Eur Urol. 2007;51:512–23.

32. Keeley FX Jr, Bibbo M, Bagley DH. Ureteroscopic treatment and surveillance of upper urinary tract transitional cell carcinoma. J Urol. 1997;157:1560–5.

33. Irie A, Iwamura M, Kadowaki K, Ohkawa A, Uchida T, Baba S. Intravesical instillation of bacille Calmette-Guerin for carcinoma in situ of the urothelium involving the upper urinary tract using vesicoureteral reflux created by a double-pigtail catheter. Urology. 2002;59:53–7.

Chapter 15

Urothelial Carcinoma of the Lower Urinary Tract: Introduction

M. Manoharan, R. Ayyathurai, and M.S. Soloway

Introduction

Urothelial carcinoma is a heterogenous disease with an unpredictable behavior. The tumor spectrum ranges from low-grade non-invasive tumors to more lethal high-grade muscle invasive variants. More than 90% of bladder cancers are urothelial (transitional) cell carcinomas, 6–8% are squamous cell carcinomas, and 2% are adenocarcinomas. In men, urothelium extends from the tips of the renal papillae to the navicular fossa of penile urethra; in women, to halfway along the urethra. Tumors can arise at any site in this epithelium and are often multifocal. The bladder is the most common site. These tumors tend to progress and exhibit "polychronotropism" – a tendency to recur over time and in new locations in the urothelial tract. An accurate diagnosis and staging of the disease is essential to decide the optimal treatment which ultimately impacts the outcome.

Epidemiology

In the United States, over 60,000 new cases are diagnosed and over 12,000 individuals die of bladder cancer each year. Bladder cancer is the fourth most common malignancy among western men, and tenth in women. In the United States and Europe, bladder cancer accounts for 5–10% of all malignancies among males. The incidence is four times higher in men than in women and twofold higher in white than black, with a median age at diagnosis of 65 years.

The well-established risk factors are cigarette smoking and occupational exposure to aromatic amines (Table 15.1). Cigarette smoking increases risk by 2–5 fold and accounts for 30–50% of all bladder cancers. This association appears

Table 15.1 Risk factors

- Smoking
- Occupational exposure to aromatic amines
- Previous radiotherapy
- Diesel exhaust emissions

to be time and dose dependent, and the risk increases with occupational exposure to chemicals like naphthylamines.

Genetic analyses suggest that the invasive and non-invasive lesions develop along distinct pathways. This involves primary or early events like deletions of 9q followed by secondary events which lead to tumor progression. This involves activation of oncogenes and inactivation of tumor suppressor genes, such as deletions at the TP53 locus on 17p, the DCC locus in 18q, and the RB locus on 13q24. These changes have been seen only in invasive disease. Within all clinical stages, tumors with mutated TP53 have a higher risk of metastasis and death from disease. CDC91L1 is recently reported bladder cancer oncogene at location 20q11. This gene is amplified and overexpressed in a third of bladder tumors.

Pathology

Clinically urothelial tumors can be grouped into three categories: superficial or non-muscle invasive (75%), muscle invasive (20%), and de nova metastatic (5%). Non-invasive tumors are generally papillary and low grade that grow on a stalk with a feeding vessel which makes them bleed easily. The true history of untreated non-invasive disease is not fully understood. Carcinoma in situ (CIS) is a high-grade tumor confined to the urothelium which is a precursor of more lethal muscle invasive cancer (Fig. 15.1). These are flat lesions which appear as red, velvet patches.

M. Manoharan (✉)
Neobladder and bladder Cancer Center, Department of Urology, University of Miami School of Medicine, P.O. Box 016960 (M814), Miami, FL 33101, USA, mmanoharan@med.miami.edu

J.J.M.C.H. de la Rosette et al. (eds.), *Imaging in Oncological Urology*, DOI 10.1007/978-1-84628-759-6_15, © Springer-Verlag London Limited 2009

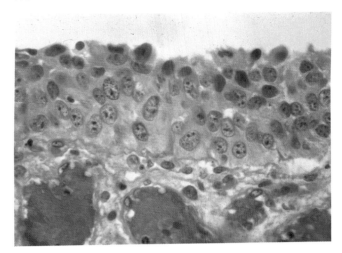

Fig. 15.1 Carcinoma in situ

Classification

Tumor grade and stage are the most important determinants of the tumor behavior. Grade reflects the degree of differentiation of tumor cells and the stage reflects the extent of the tumor. Both these factors affect prognosis, treatment choice, and outcome significantly. The depth of invasion of the bladder wall determines the clinical stage of the tumor and the widely used TNM staging system is shown in Table 15.2.

In 2004, the World Health Organization (WHO) classified urothelial tumors into non-invasive and invasive neoplasia (Table 15.3). Based on the histological features, the papillary urothelial lesions are further divided into papilloma, papillary urothelial neoplasm of low malignant potential (PUNLMP), low-grade and high-grade papillary urothelial carcinoma. The recurrence and progression rates for these lesions are given in Table 15.4. Tumor grade is a well-established prognostic factor, with strong correlation between higher grade and invasion, disease progression, metastasis, and survival.

Diagnosis

Macroscopic or microscopic hematuria is the presenting symptom in 80–90% of patients with bladder cancers. Irritative symptoms like dysuria, urgency, and frequency are the next most common symptoms and may reflect diffuse disease such as CIS. A large proportion of bladder cancer patients have no significant physical signs owing to the disease; however a small number of patients with large and invasive tumors may present with bladder wall thickening or palpable mass. All patients suspected to have bladder tumor should have urine cytology, flexible cystoscopy examination

Table 15.2 Bladder tumor staging (TNM)

Primary tumor (T)

- TX: Primary tumor cannot be assessed
- T0: No evidence of primary tumor
- Ta: Non-invasive papillary carcinoma
- Tis: Carcinoma in situ (i.e., flat tumor)
- T1: Tumor invades subepithelial connective tissue
- T2: Tumor invades muscle

    - pT2a: Tumor invades superficial muscle (inner half)
    - pT2b: Tumor invades deep muscle (outer half)

- T3: Tumor invades perivesical tissue

    - pT3a: Microscopically
    - pT3b: Macroscopically (extravesical mass)

- T4: Tumor invades any of the following: prostate, uterus, vagina, pelvic wall, or abdominal wall

    - T4a: Tumor invades the prostate, uterus, vagina
    - T4b: Tumor invades the pelvic wall, abdominal wall

Regional lymph nodes (N)

- NX: Regional lymph nodes cannot be assessed
- N0: No regional lymph node metastasis
- N1: Metastasis in a single lymph node, ≤2 cm in greatest dimension
- N2: Metastasis in a single lymph node, >2 cm but ≤5 cm in greatest dimension; or multiple lymph nodes, ≤5 cm in greatest dimension
- N3: Metastasis in a lymph node, >5 cm in greatest dimension

Distant metastasis (M)

- MX: Distant metastasis cannot be assessed
- M0: No distant metastasis
- M1: Distant metastasis

Table 15.3 WHO Classification Urothelial Neoplasia (2004)

Non-invasive urothelial neoplasia

- Urothelial carcinoma in situ (high-grade intraurothelial neoplasia)
- Urothelial papilloma
- Urothelial papilloma, inverted type
- Papillary urothelial neoplasm of low malignant potential (PUNLMP)
- Non-invasive low-grade papillary urothelial carcinoma
- Non-invasive high-grade papillary urothelial carcinoma

Invasive urothelial neoplasia

- Lamina propria invasion
- Muscularis propria (detrusor muscle) invasion

Table 15.4 Recurrence and progression of papillary lesions

	Papilloma	PUNLMP	Low grade	High grade
Recurrence	0–8%	33.3%	64.1%	56.4%
Stage progression	0%	0–4%	10.5%	27.1%
Grade progression	2%	11%	7%	–
Survival	100%	93–100%	82–96%	74–96%

of lower urinary tract, and imaging of renal tract preferably with a CT scan. Intravenous pyelogram (IVP) and ultrasonography are the choice of imaging in some centers. It is not uncommon to diagnose bladder tumors by imaging; however diagnosis is confirmed by cystoscopy. IVP is useful in identifying the tumors obstructing the ureteric orifice, concurrent upper tract lesions (0.3–2.3%).

Currently urine cytology is the standard non-invasive method for detecting bladder cancer. Diagnostic yields from UC are variable, with the sensitivity range of 35–80% and specificity range between 80 and 100%. The primary purpose of UC is to detect and monitor high-grade tumors. Urine cytology is less useful for detection of low-grade tumors due to poor expression of phenotypic features. There is a constant search going on among the researchers for a biomarker which is simple, sensitive, specific, reliable, and reproducible. Tumor markers and tests such as hemoglobin dipstick, BTA-Stat, BTA-TRAK, NMP-22, Immunocyt, survivin, Quanticyt, microsatellite analysis, telomerase, and UroVysion have been studied for their clinical usefulness. DNA-based molecular markers such as fluorescence in situ hybridization (FISH) technique are promising. FISH identifies genetic abnormalities related to cancer development before the phenotypic expression. Some molecular markers (e.g., p53, Ki-67) may be capable of predicting recurrence as well as progression of bladder cancer; however, the results of many studies are preliminary and there is no accurate marker as yet.

Endoscopic visualization of bladder tumors is the key step in diagnosis and treatment (Fig. 15.2). Cystoscopy for hematuria is an office procedure without need for anesthesia. Information such as number, size, shape, and location of tumors are easily obtained. Endoscopically, the morphology of neoplasms can be classified as papillary 70%, nodular 10%, and 20% mixed. Majority of low-grade urothelial tumors are pendunculated tumors. CIS is a flat lesion in the bladder mucosa and may appear as patchy or diffuse erythematous mucosa.

Treatment

The success in management of bladder tumor is dependent on several factors. Accurate staging, optimal timing, choice of treatment, and patient selection are vital. Once the

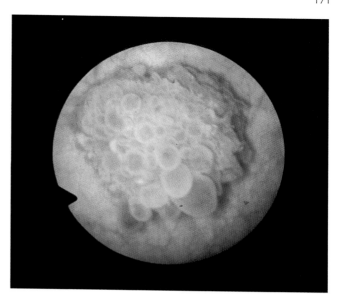

Fig. 15.2 Papillary bladder cancer – endoscopic view

presence of lesion is established, transurethral resection of bladder tumor (TUR-BT) is planned as an elective operation. Biopsy from the tumor base and suspected mucosal areas in bladder and prostate is recommended. The aim of TUR-BT is to achieve complete resection of all tumors and to obtain adequate specimen for pathology. Pathological evaluation of tumor specimen and biopsies are needed to document disease and describe grade and local stage. The high incidence of subsequent tumors after initial resection has led to the concept of intravesical instillation of chemotherapeutic agents. This could be done with a therapeutic or prophylactic intent. The decision to administer intravesical therapy depends on numerous factors including tumor stage, grade, size, the histologic subtype, number of lesions, depth of invasion, presence or absence of CIS, and patient-specific factors. One early perioperative instillation (6–24 h) with mitomycin (MMC) or epirubicin reduces recurrence rate by 40% in single as well as multiple bladder tumors and thus is recommended for all subtypes of papillary tumors. Bacillus Calmette–Guerin (BCG) is live attenuated tuberculosis organism administered in six weekly intravesical instillations, followed by maintenance, is considered standard treatment for high grade and tumors which are generally not sensitive to intravesical chemotherapy. Though it acts through T-cell-dependent immunological response, the exact mechanism of action of is unclear. Frequency, dysuria, and contact dermatitis are known side effects. Rarely, intravesical BCG may produce a systemic illness associated with granulomatous infections in multiple sites that require antituberculin therapy. The standard treatment algorithm for treatment of urothelial carcinoma of the bladder is shown in Fig. 15.3.

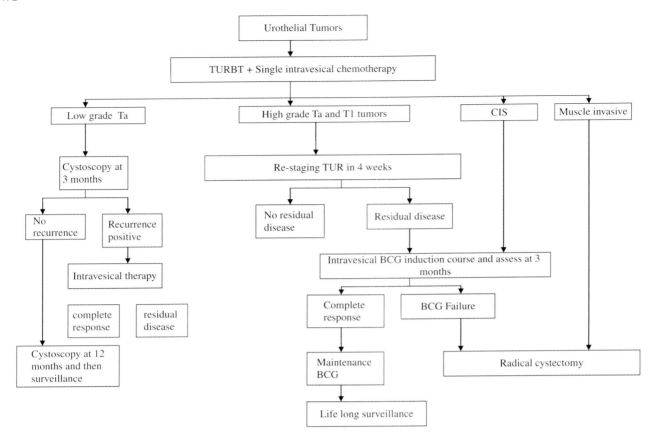

Fig. 15.3 Management of bladder tumors

Low-Grade, Non-muscle Invasive (Ta)

Complete TUR followed by single instillation of chemotherapeutic agent on the same day is the standard protocol for these tumors. Patients with solitary lesion are followed up for recurrence at 3 months and 1 year. Thereafter patient is monitored by annual cystoscopy for 5 years. For solitary recurrence, office fulguration is adequate as long as urine cytology is negative. Patients with multiple lesions are cystoscoped at 3, 6, and 12 months and yearly thereafter.

High-Grade, Non-muscle Invasive (Ta, T1)

These tumors have 20–30% chance of progression to muscle invasive disease. Standard management approach is TURBT followed by single intravesical chemotherapy and a re-staging TUR and bladder mapping/random biopsies at 2–4 week interval. If high-grade tumor is pathologically confirmed, a 6-week induction course of BCG intravesical instillations followed by 1–3-year maintenance BCG is advocated. These patients will require intense follow-up, 3 monthly for

the first 2 years, 4 monthly for the third year, 6 monthly during the fourth and fifth years, and annually thereafter. In case of failure before BCG maintenance completion or evidence of CIS or T1 disease, radical cystectomy is considered. Radical cystectomy and intravesical BCG therapy are both acceptable primary therapies for high-grade T1 disease. Regular surveillance cystoscopy and urine cytology are of paramount importance in follow-up of these patients. Interferon (IFN-alpha-2b) is the new intravesical treatment agent showing promising results. Though the efficacy is inferior to BCG, it showed synergistic effect with BCG. It is being commonly used in BCG failure patients.

Carcinoma In Situ (CIS)

CIS is a flat, high-grade carcinoma occurring in 5–10% of non-muscle invasive bladder cancers (Fig. 15.3). The marker of choice is urine cytology. Patients with CIS are at high risk (50%) of progression. A 6-week induction course of BCG followed by 1–3 year maintenance BCG is advocated with regular follow-up with cystoscopy and urine cytology. BCG provides highest rates of complete response as well as long-term disease-free survival among all intravesical treatments. BCG failure with recurrence usually warrants radical cystectomy.

Muscle Invasive (T2–T4) and Metastatic Disease

Complete metastatic evaluation is a prerequisite before definitive treatment. Radical cystectomy and bilateral lymph node dissection is the standard of care for muscle invasive bladder cancer. Radical cystectomy is major surgery that requires appropriate preoperative evaluation and planning. The procedure involves removal of the bladder and pelvic lymph nodes and creation of a conduit or reservoir for urinary flow. In males, radical cystectomy involves the removal of the bladder, prostate and seminal vesicles, and proximal urethra. In females, the procedure includes removal of the bladder, urethra, uterus, fallopian tubes, ovaries, anterior vaginal wall, and surrounding fascia. The concept of treating micro-metastases with systemic platinum-based neo-adjuvant chemotherapy prior to cystectomy or curative radiation has shown 5% survival advantage. Similarly, adjuvant chemotherapy is beneficial in patients at risk for recurrence such as T3 disease and positive lymph nodes. Common regimens include MVAC (Methotraxate, Vinblastine, Doxorubicin and Cisplatin) and a combination of Gencitabine and Cisplatin.

Radiotherapy is an effective treatment option for muscle invasive bladder tumor. The ideal candidate for curative external beam irradiation has a small, solitary muscle invasive tumor less than 5 cm in size, with no associated in situ disease or distant spread. Neo-adjuvant combination platinum-based chemotherapy followed by pelvic radiotherapy is preferred for T3–T4 disease. All patients who receive radiotherapy for muscle invasive cancer should undergo life-long cystoscopic surveillance. Salvage cystectomy should be considered following radiotherapy for residual, progressive, or recurrent muscle invasive cancer. Systemic chemotherapy is the only modality that has been shown to improve survival in responding patients with metastatic bladder cancer.

Follow-Up

Since the tumor recurrence rate is between 30 and 80%, close monitoring is mandatory to diagnose and treat early. Flexible cystoscopy and urinary cytology are essential tools in the follow-up. Urinary cytology is more valuable in following up high-grade tumors. The duration of endoscopic follow-up for patients free of recurrence is debatable. Studies reported that for a tumor-free interval of 2, 5, and 10 years, the risk of recurrence is 43, 22, and 2%, respectively. Currently various urinary markers are studied and could be the key agents in follow-up of bladder cancer in future.

Role of Radiology in Bladder Cancer

Radiologist plays a vital role in diagnosis, treatment planning, and follow-up of bladder cancer patients. Investigations such as CT scan IVP and ultrasonography are extremely helpful in the work-up of hematuria. After the initial management the staging process requires detailed input from the radiologist which helps choosing optimal treatment, especially in muscle invasive cancers. Magnetic resonance urography (MR urogram) is particularly useful in patients with renal insufficiency or contrast allergy. Though staging errors can occur with MR urography (~40%), with recent advances including endorectal coil enhancement and dynamic contrast imaging the accuracy can be improved. PET is not suitable for the evaluation of bladder tumors due to intense accumulation of fluoro-deoxy-glucose (FDG) in the urine. It can assist in the detection of positive pelvic lymph nodes or distant metastatic lesions. Bone scan is unnecessary in non-muscle invasive cancers and most muscle invasive cancers; however it is considered if symptoms or alkaline phosphatize levels are elevated. Post-cystectomy follow-up requires imaging of chest, abdomen, and pelvis to rule out local and distant recurrences.

Summary

Urothelial cancer of lower urinary tract is a common disease. A good understanding of disease behavior allows the clinicians to offer optimal treatment to the patients. The radiological imaging of the urinary tract is essential for accurate diagnosis and staging and plays a vital role in treatment decisions.

References

1. Ali-el-Dein B, Nabeeh A, Ismail EH, Ghoneim MA. Sequential bacillus Calmette-Guerin and epirubicin versus bacillus Calmette-Guerin alone for superficial bladder tumors: a randomized prospective study. J Urol. 1999;162:339–42.
2. Badalament RA, Herr HW, Wong GY, Gnecco C, Pinsky CM, Whitmore WF, et al. A prospective randomized trial of maintenance versus nonmaintenance intravesical bacillus Calmette-Guerin therapy of superficial bladder cancer. J Clin Oncol. 1987;5:441–9.

3. Boffetta P, Silverman DT. A meta-analysis of bladder cancer and diesel exhaust exposure. Epidemiology. 2001;12(1):125–30.

4. Carmack AJK, Soloway MS. The diagnosis and staging of bladder cancer: from RBCs to TURs. Urology. 2006;67(3 Suppl 1):3–8; discussion 8–10.

5. Dutta SC, Smith JA Jr, Shappell SB, Coffey CS, Chang SS, Cookson MS. Clinical under staging of high risk nonmuscle invasive urothelial carcinoma treated with radical cystectomy. J Urol. 2001;166(2):490–3.

6. Ende N, Woods LP, Shelley HS. Carcinoma originating in ducts surrounding the prostatic urethra. Amer J Clin Pathol. 1963;40:183.

7. Ferlay, Bray, Pisani, Parkin. GLOBOCAN 2000: cancer incidence, mortality and prevalence worldwide, version 1.0. IARC CancerBase No. 5. Lyon: IARC Press; 2001.

8. Fitzpatrick JM, West AB, Butler MR, Lane V, O'Flynn JD. Superficial bladder tumors (stage pTa grades 1 and 2): the importance of recurrence pattern following initial resection. J Urol. 1986;135:920–2.

9. Glas AS, Roos D, Deutekom M, Zwinderman AH, Bossuyt PMM, Kurth KH. Tumor markers in the diagnosis of primary bladder cancer. A systematic review. J Urol. 2003;169:1975–82.

10. Guo Z, Linn JF, Wu G, Anzick SL, Eisenberger CF, Halachmi S, et al. CDC91L1 (PIG-U) is a newly discovered oncogene in human bladder cancer. Nat Med. 2004;10(4):374–81.

11. Hautmann RE, de Petriconi R, Gottfried HW, Kleinschmidt K, Mattes R, Paiss T. The ileal neobladder: complications and functional results in 363 patients after 11 years of followup. J Urol. 1999;161:422–7.

12. Heney NM, Ahmed S, Flanagan MJ, Frable W, Corder MP, Hafermann MD, et al. Superficial bladder cancer: progression and recurrence. J Urol. 1983;130:1083–6.

13. Herr HW, Cookson MS, Soloway SM. Upper tract tumors in patients with primary bladder cancer followed for 15 years. J Urol. 1996;156(4):1286–7.

14. Herr HW. Does cystoscopy correlate with the histology of recurrent papillary tumors of the bladder? BJU Int. 2001;88:683–5.

15. Herr HW. The value of a second transurethral resection in evaluating patients with bladder tumors. J Urol. 1999;162(1):74–6.

16. Herr HW. The value of a second transurethral resection in evaluating patients with bladder tumors. J Urol. 1999;162(1):74–6.

17. Holmang S, Andius P, Hedelin H, Wester K. Busch C, Johansson SL. Stage progression in Ta papillary urothelial tumors: relationship to grade, immuno-histochemical expression of tumor markers, mitotic frequency and DNA ploidy. J Urol. 2001;165:1124–30.

18. Holmäng S, Hedelin H, Anderström C, Holmberg E, Johansson SL. Long-term follow-up of a bladder carcinoma cohort: routine follow up urography is not necessary. J Urol. 1998;160:45–8.

19. Jakse G, Algaba F, Malmstrom P-U, Oosterlinck WA. Secondlook TUR in T1 transitional cell carcinoma: Why? Eur Urol. 2001;45:539–46.

20. Jakse G, Hall R, Bono A, Hoeltl W, Carpentier P, Spaander JP, et al. Intravesical BCG in patients with carcinoma in situ of the urinary bladder: long-term results of EORTC GU Group hase II protocol 30861. Eur Urol. 2001;40:144–50.

21. Jewett MAS, Nieder AM. T1 Urothelial carcinoma of bladder. Bladder tumors. 2006;1:189–218.

22. Kaasinen E, Rintala E, Hellstrom P, Viitanen J, Juusela H, Rajala P, et al. Factors explaining recurrence in patients undergoing chemoimmunotherapy regimens for frequently recurring superficial bladder carcinoma. Eur Urol. 2002;42:167–74.

23. Kirk D, Hinton CE, Shaldon C. Transitional cell carcinoma of the prostate. Br J Urol. 1979;51:575–8.

24. Kirkali ZCT, Manhoharan M. Bladder cancer, epidemiology, staging, grading, and diagnosis. 2006;1:13–64.

25. Kolozsky Z. Histopathological "self control" in transurethral resection of bladder tumors. Br J Urol. 1991;67:162–4.

26. Konety BR, Getzenberg RH. Urine based markers of urological malignancy. J Urol. 2001;165:600–11.

27. Konety BR, Nguyen TS, Dhir R, Day RS, Becich MJ, Stadler WM, et al. Detection of bladder cancer using a novel nuclear matrix protein, BLCA-4. Clin Cancer Res. 2000;6:2618–25.

28. Koya MP, Simon MA, et al. Complications of intravesical therapy for urothelial cancer of the bladder. J Urol. 2006;175(6):2004–10.

29. Lamm DL, Herr HW, Jakse G, Kuroda M, Mostofi FK, Okajima E, et al. Updated concepts and treatment of carcinoma in situ. Urol Oncol. 1998;4:130–138.

30. Lamm DL. BCG immunotherapy for transitional cell carcinoma of the bladder Oncol. 1995;9:947–52.

31. Lamm DL. Carcinoma in situ. Urol Clin N Am. 1992;19:499–508.

32. Lamm DL, Blumenstein BA, Crawford ED, Crissman JD, Lowe BA, Smith JA, et al. Randomized intergroup comparison of bacillus Calmette-Guerin immunotherapy and mitomycin C chemotherapy prophylaxis in superficial transitional cell carcinoma of the bladder. A Southwest Oncology Group Study. Urol Oncol. 1995; 1:119–26.

33. Lamm DL, Blumenstein BA, Crawford ED, Montie JE, Scardino P, Grossman HB, et al. A randomized trial of intravesical doxorubicin and immunotherapy with BCG for transitional cell carcinoma of the bladder. N Engl J Med. 1991;325:1205–9.

34. Lamm DL, Blumenstein BA, Crissman JD, Montie JE, ottesman JE, Lowe BA, et al. Maintenance BCG immunotherapy for recurrent Ta, T1 and CIS transitional cell carcinoma of the bladder: a randomized SWOG study. J Urol. 2000;163:1124–9.

35. Lee R, Droller MJ. The natural history of bladder cancer. Implications for therapy. Urol Clin North Am. 2000;27:1–13, vii.

36. Lokeshwar VB. Cytology and tumor markers. Bladder Tumors. 2006;1:65–138.

37. Lokeshwar VB. Soloway MS. Current bladder tumor tests: does their projected utility fulfill clinical necessity? [Miscellaneous]. J Urol. 2001;165(4):1067–77.

38. Lokeshwar VB, Soloway MS. Re: urine based markers of urological malignancy. J Urol. 2002;167(3):1406.

39. Lokeshwar VB, Obek CAN, et al. Urinary hyaluronic acid and hyaluronidase: markers for bladder cancer detection and evaluation of grade. J Urol. 2000;163(1):348.

40. Lopez-Beltran A, Cheng L. Stage pT1 bladder carcinoma: diagnostic criteria, pitfalls and prognostic significance. Pathology. 2003;35(6):484–91.

41. Lotan Y, Roehrborn CG. Sensitivity and specificity of commonly available bladder tumor markers versus cytology: results of a comprehensive literature review and meta-analyses.Urology. 2003;61:109–18.

42. Malkowicz SB. Muscle invasive urothelial carcinoma of bladder. Bladder Tumors. 2006;1:p. 219–38.

43. Manoharan M, Soloway MS. Optimal management of the T1G3 bladder cancer. Urol Clin North Am. 2005;32(2):133–45.

44. Manoharan, Murugesan SM. Superficial transitional cell carcinoma of the bladder: management and prognosis. Urol oncol. 2005.

45. Marcus PM, Vineis P, et al. NAT2 slow acetylation and bladder cancer risk: a meta-analysis of 22 case-control studies conducted in the general population. Pharmacogenetics. 2000;10(2):115–22.

46. Miladi M, Peyromaure M, Zerbib M, Saighi D, Debré B. The value of a second transurethral resection in evaluating patients with bladder tumours. Eur Urol. 2003;43:241–5.

47. Mohr DN, Offord KP, Owen RA, Melton J III. Asymptomatic microhematuria and urologic disease. A population-based study. JAMA. 1986;256:224–9.

48. Montironi R, Lopez-Beltran A. The 2004 WHO classification of bladder tumors: a summary and commentary. Int J Surg Pathol. 2005;13(2):143–53.

49. Nieder AM. Soloway MS. Eliminate the term "superficial" bladder cancer. J Urol. 2006;175(2):417–8.

50. Nieder AM, Meinbach DS, et al. Transurethral bladder tumor resection: intraoperative and postoperative complications in a residency setting. J Urol. 2005;174(6):2307–9.

51. Nieder AM, Meinbach DS, et al. Transurethral bladder tumor resection: intraoperative and postoperative complications in a residency setting. J Urol. 2005;174(6):2307–9.

52. Oosterlinck W, Kurth K, Schröder F, Bultinck J, Hammond B, Sylvester R, et al. A prospective EORTC-GU group randomized trial comparing transurethral resection followed by a single intravesical instillation of epirubicin or water in single stage Ta, T1 papillary carcinoma of the bladder. J Urol. 1993;149: 749–52.

53. Oosterlinck W, Kurth K, Schroder F, Sylvester R. A plea for cold biopsy, fulguration and immediate bladder instillation with Epirubicin in small superficial bladder tumors. Eur Urol. 1993;23: 457–9.

54. Oosterlinck W, Lobel B, Jakse G, Malmstrom P, Stockle M, Sternberg C. The EAU working group on oncological urology. Guidelines on bladder cancer. Eur Urol. 2002;41:105–12.

55. Oosterlinck WSE. Low grade Ta, (noninvasive) urothelial carcinoma. Bladder Tumors. 2006;1:139–64.

56. Pagano F, Bassi PF, Ferranti GL, Piazza N, Abantagelo G, Pappagallo GL, et al. Is stage pT4a (D1) reliable assessing transitional cell carcinoma involvement of the prostate in patients with a concurrent bladder cancer? A necessary distinction for contiguous or noncontiguous involvement. J Urol. 1996;155: 244–7.

57. Posey JT, Soloway MS, et al. Evaluation of the prognostic potential of hyaluronic acid and hyaluronidase (HYAL1) for prostate cancer. Cancer Res. 2003;63(10):2638–44.

58. Revelo MP, Cookson MS, Chang SS, Shook MF, Smith JA Jr, Shappell SB. Incidence and location of prostate and urothelial carcinoma in prostates from cystoprostatectomies: implications for apical sparing surgery. J Urol. 2004;171:646–51.

59. Rintala E, Jauhiainen K, Rajala P, Ruutu M, Kaasinen E, lfthan O, et al. Alternating mitomycin and bacillus Calmette-Guerin instillation therapy for carcinoma in situ of the bladder. J Urol. 1995;154:2050–3.

60. Sadek S, Soloway MS, et al. (1999). The value of upper tract cytology after transurethral resection of bladder tumor in patients with bladder transitional cell cancer. J Urol. 1999;161(1):77–9.

61. Sarosdy MF, deVere White RW, et al. Results of a multicenter trial using the BTA test to monitor for and diagnose recurrent bladder cancer. J Urol. 1995;154(2):379–83.

62. Schellhammer PF, Bean MA, Whitmore WFJ. Prostatic involvement by transitional cell carcinoma: pathogenesis, patterns and prognosis. J Urol. 1997;118:399–403.

63. Scher HI, Motzer RJ. Bladder and Renal Cell Carcinomas. Harrison's Principles of Internal Medicine.

64. Shelley MD, Court JB, Kynaston H, Wilt TJ, Fish RG, Mason M. Intravesical bacillus Calmette-Guerin in Ta and T1 Bladder Cancer (Cochrane review). The Cochrane Library, Issue 4, 2003.

65. Simon MA, Lokeshwar VB, et al. Current bladder cancer tests: unnecessary or beneficial? Crit Rev Oncol Hematol. 2003;47(2): 91–107.

66. Single dose v ersus multiple instillations of epirubicin as prophylaxis for recurrence after transurethral resection of pTa and pT1 transitional cell bladder tumors: a prospective randomized controlled study. Br J Urol. 1997;79:731–5.

67. Soloway MS. Editorial comments: apparent failure of current intravesical chemotherapy prophylaxis to influence the long-term course of superficial transitional cell carcinoma of the bladder. J Urol. 1995;153(5):1450.

68. Soloway MS. Bladder tumor markers, intravesical therapy and systemic chemotherapy. J Urol. 2001;166(2):488–9.

69. Soloway MS. Editorial: bladder Cancer. How can we make a difference? [Editorial]. J Urol. 2003;170(5):1781–2.

70. Soloway MS. Expectant treatment of small, recurrent, low-grade, noninvasive tumors of the urinary bladder. Urol Oncol. 2006;24(1):58–61.

71. Soloway MS, Bruck DS, et al. Expectant management of small, recurrent, noninvasive papillary bladder tumors. J Urol. 2003;170(2, Part 1):438–41.

72. Soloway MS, Sofer M, et al. Contemporary Management Of Stage T1 Transitional Cell Carcinoma Of The Bladder. J Urol. 2002;167(4):1573–83.

73. Solsona E, Iborra I, Ricos J, Monros J, Casanova J, Dumont R. Effectiveness of a single immediate mitomycin C instillation in patients with low risk superficial bladder cancer: short and longterm follow up. J Urol. 1999;161:1120–3.

74. Steiner G, Schoenberg MP, Linn JF, Mao L, Sidransky D. Detection of bladder cancer recurrence by microsatellite analysis of urine. Nat Med. 1997;3:621–4.

75. Sylvester RJ, van der Meijden A, Lamm DL. Intravesical bacillus Calmette-Guerin reduces the risk of progression in patients with superficial bladder cancer: a meta-analysis of the published results of randomized clinical trials. J Urol. 2002;168: 1964–70.

76. Sylvester R, van der Meijden A. High grade Ta urothelial carcinoma and carcinoma in situ of the bladder. 2006;1:165–88.

77. Taguchi I, Gohji K, Hara I, Gotoh A, Yamada Y, Yamanaka K, et al. Clinical evaluation of random biopsy of urinary bladder in patients with superficial bladder cancer. Int J Urol. 1998;5(1): 30–4.

78. Vaidya A, Soloway MS, et al. De novo muscle invasive bladder cancer: is there a change in trend? [Article]. J Urol. 2001;165(1): 47–50.

79. Van der Meijden A, Oosterlinck W, Brausi M, Kurth KH, Sylvester R, de Balincourt C. Significance of bladder biopsies in Ta,T1 bladder tumors: a report from the EORTC Genito-Urinary Tract Cancer Cooperative Group. EORTC-GU Group Superficial Bladder Committee. Eur Urol. 1999;35(4):267–71.

80. Yousem DM, Gatewood OM, Goldman SM, Marshall FF. Synchronous and metachronous transitional cell carcinoma of the urinary tract: prevalence, incidence, and radiographic detection. Radiology. 1988;167:613–8.

Chapter 16

Urothelial Cell Carcinoma in Lower Urinary Tract: Conventional Imaging Techniques

C.Y. Nio

Introduction

Urothelial carcinoma of the bladder is the most common urinary tract malignancy in the United States and Europe, with a stable incidence in men over the past two decades but a slight increase in women [1]. The age-standardized incidence of bladder tumors in males is highest in the economically advanced European countries and the White population of North America (over 15/100,000). Tumor incidence rates are less in Asia (3–4/100,000) [2].

It is a disease of older patients, most being older than 65 years, but is not restricted to these groups. Of the new cases, 3.1% occur in patients under the age of 44 years and 8% occur in patients aged 45–54 years. Both the incidence and mortality increase with advancing age.

Bladder cancer is more common in men than in women, with a male-to-female ratio of 3–4:1; however, in women it is diagnosed at a more advanced stage and has a higher mortality rate. Survival of female patients at 5 years is 78%, equal to the 10-year survival for men.

Patients symptoms are all non-specific. The most common presenting symptom is gross hematuria, although microscopic hematuria may be detected at urine analysis.

The pathogenesis for urothelial tumors is direct prolonged contact of the bladder urothelium with urine containing excreted carcinogens, predominantly from cigarette smoking. Smokers have four times the risk of bladder cancer, related to both the duration and amount of smoking. Cigarette smoking accounts for one-third to one-half of all cases of bladder cancer [3]

There is also a well-documented causal link between urothelial malignancy and a variety of occupational and environmental chemicals. Other risk factors include bladder stones, chronic infection, and irritation, as well as certain drugs.

Bladder diverticula have an increased risk (25–10%) of developing cancer because of stasis. Tumors occurring in diverticula have a propensity to invade perivesical fat early because of lack of muscle in their wall.

Most urothelial tumors are located at the bladder base (80% at initial diagnosis); 60% are single and over 50% measure less than 2.5 cm at cystoscopy. They can be papillary, sessile, or nodular.

Urothelial carcinoma has a propensity to be multicentric with synchronous and metachronous bladder and upper tract tumors [1]. Multicentric bladder tumors occur in up to 30–40% of cases. Upper tract tumors occur in 2.6–4.5% of bladder tumor cases.

Pathologic stage is the most important predictor of survival. The TNM classification is in widespread use (Table 16.1) [4].

Superficial bladder cancer is confined to the mucosa and lamina propria. Once extension occurs into the detrusor muscle layer, the tumor is considered invasive (Fig. 16.1). Invasion may progress to involve local organs including prostate, vagina, uterus, and pelvic wall. Metastases most commonly involve pelvic lymph nodes and lung, liver, and bone in decreasing order of frequency.

The standard imaging work-up for gross hematuria and suspected urothelial tumor has shifted from intravenous urography to cross-sectional modalities such as ultrasound and more often computer tomography (CT) and magnetic resonance (MR) imaging. Cystoscopy and biopsy are the standard of reference for bladder evaluation, but imaging is important for accurate staging and treatment planning. Superficial tumors may not be evident with the common imaging techniques and normally are not staged radiologically. However, with invasive urothelial tumors, detection of pelvic side wall invasion or lymphadenopathy is critical, as clinical staging is inaccurate. Furthermore complete evaluation of the urothelial tract (both upper and lower) is indicated because of the propensity for multicentric disease.

Although as already mentioned above cross-sectional imaging (CT/MRI) is the imaging of choice when bladder

C.Y. Nio (✉)
Radiology Department, University of Amsterdam, Amsterdam, The Netherlands

J.J.M.C.H. de la Rosette et al. (eds.), *Imaging in Oncological Urology*,
DOI 10.1007/978-1-84628-759-6_16, © Springer-Verlag London Limited 2009

Table 16.1 TNM classification

Jewett-Strong System	TNM System	Histopathologic Findings
O	T0	No tumor
O	Tis	Carcinoma in situ
O	Ta	Papillary tumor confined to the epithelium (mucosa)
A	T1	Tumor invades subepithelial connective tissue (lamina propria)
B1	T2a	Tumor invades superficial muscle (inner half)
B2	T2b	Tumor invades deep muscle (outer half)
C	T3	Tumor invades perivesical fat
D1	T4a	Tumor invades surrounding organs
D1	T4b	Tumor invades pelvic or abdominal wall
D1	N1	Metastasis in a single pelvic lymph node ≤ 2 cm
D1	N2	Metastasis in a single pelvic lymph node >2 cm and ≤ 5 cm or in multiple nodes ≤ 5 cm
D1	N3	Metastasis in a single lymph node >5 cm
D2	N4	Lymph node metastases above the bifurcation of the common iliac arteries
D2	M1	Distant metastases

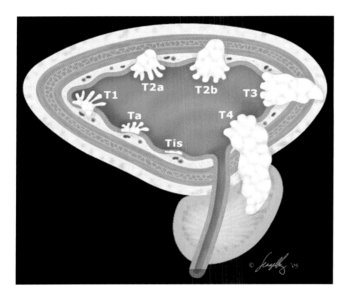

Fig. 16.1 Diagram shows stages of tumor invasion in bladder cancer (with kind permission of the RSNA and J. Wong et al., 2006) [24]

carcinoma is suspected or known, the following paragraph will discuss the findings on conventional imaging studies.

Conventional Imaging Techniques

Plain Abdominal Film

Plain abdominal radiography is of little value in the detection of bladder cancer but it may reveal focal calcification associated with urothelial cell carcinoma in 0.5% of patients. It is associated with focal dystrophic calcification, which can be linear, punctuate, or coarse in pattern [5].

Intravenous Urography (IVU)

Intravenous urography in the past was used when bladder carcinoma was suspected. Its ability to demonstrate small tumors is limited, because they are lost in the contrast medium on full bladder images. In the postvoid phase it may be difficult to recognize them as the urothelium of collapsed bladder adopts a corrugated configuration. Therefore standard and micturition cystography and the cystographic phase of IVU are notoriously insensitive (Fig. 16.2).

The reported detection rates of bladder carcinomas by IVU range from 26 to 86% [6, 7]. In addition authors vary in their confidence in detecting small carcinomas, quoting values of 0.5–1 cm as their lower limit of sensitivity (Fig. 16.3) [4, 7, 8].

When bladder cancers are visible on urography, an irregular, polypoid, or sessile filling defect is seen most often (Figs. 16.4–16.6). The bladder trigone and posterolateral bladder walls are the most frequent sites of origin of urothelial cell carcinomas. In 2% of the cases urothelial cell carcinoma originates from the wall of bladder diverticula. Mural infiltration leads to bladder wall thickening and poor distensibility (Fig. 16.7). The presence of ureterovesical junction obstruction and hydroureter usually implies muscle invasion by the neoplasm (Fig. 16.8) [9].

Synchronous and metachronous upper tract tumors are discovered with approximately 2 and 7% of primary bladder carcinomas, respectively (Figs. 16.9 and 16.10).

This was, in the past, the major argument in favor of retaining the urography [10]. For upper tract involvement

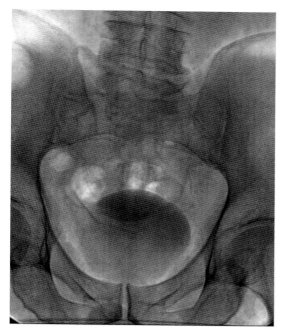

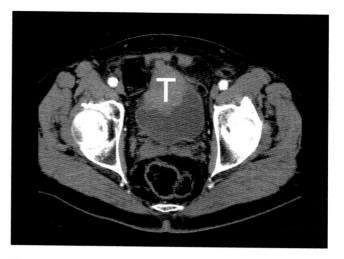

Fig. 16.2 (continued)

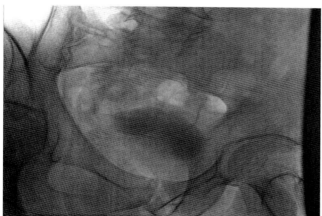

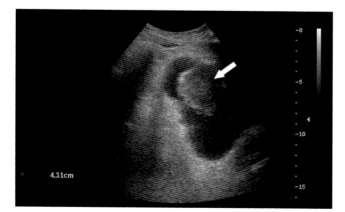

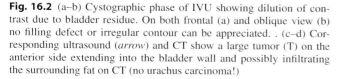

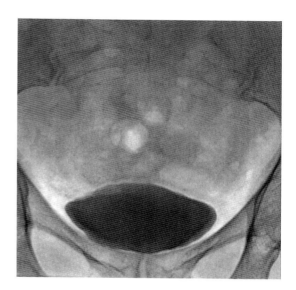

Fig. 16.2 (a–b) Cystographic phase of IVU showing dilution of contrast due to bladder residue. On both frontal (a) and oblique view (b) no filling defect or irregular contour can be appreciated. . (c–d) Corresponding ultrasound (*arrow*) and CT show a large tumor (T) on the anterior side extending into the bladder wall and possibly infiltrating the surrounding fat on CT (no urachus carcinoma!)

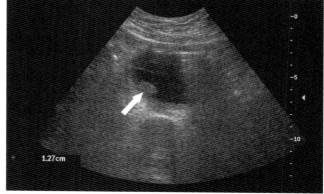

Fig. 16.3 (a) Although no optimal filling of the bladder, no lesion is visible. (b) On ultrasound of the same patient an 1-cm lesion can be detected in the bladder (*arrow*)

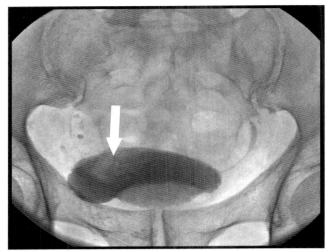

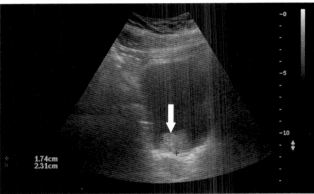

Fig. 16.4 (a) Intravenous urography (cystographic phase) with impression of an enlarged prostatic gland and multilobular irregular filling defect (*arrow*) on the right side of the bladder due to an urothelial cell carcinoma. (b) Abdominal ultrasound of the same patient reveals the corresponding soft tissue tumour originating from the posterior wall (*arrow*)

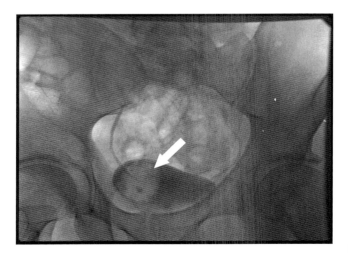

Fig. 16.5 (a) Another case with rounded filling defect (*arrow*) on the right in the bladder without obstruction of the right ureter. (b) Ultrasound of same patient supports the diagnosis of a broad-based soft tissue lesion (*arrow*)

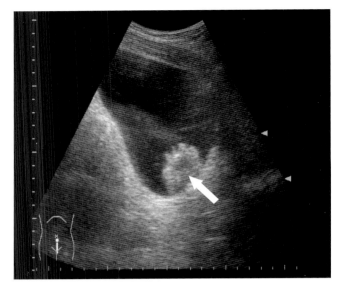

Fig. 16.5 (continued)

tomograms of the renal collecting system were used to detect irregularities or filling defects. This technique is nowadays no more available, because fluoroscopy units today lack this possibility. This decreases the sensitivity for IVU to detect upper urinary tract cancer. Miyake et al. [11] concluded in their study that routine IVU may not be required for follow-up for all patients who have had transurethral resection for

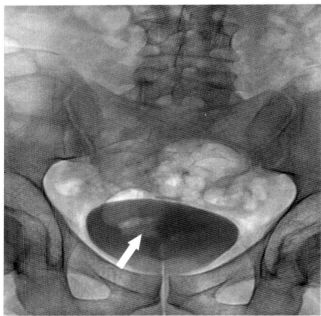

Fig. 16.6 (a–b) Overprojection of colonic air (recto-sigmoid) can mimic a filling defect. In this case below the air configuration a real lesion is present (*arrow* in a), which is better visualized on the oblique view (b). Note the irregular contour of the lesion (*arrow*) as distinct from the smooth outline of the bowel gas

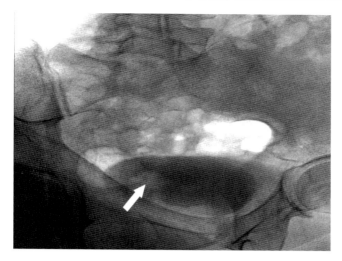

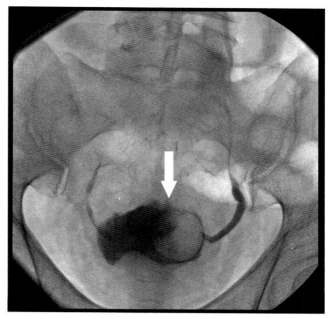

Fig. 16.6 (continued)

bladder cancer. Just in 2 (asymptomatic) of 20 positive cases IVU detected upper urinary tract cancer. In the remaining 18 symptomatic cases IVU failed to detect upper tract involvement in ten patients. Several other studies revealed that annual routine IVU following bladder carcinoma is not justified. They recommend urography at initial diagnosis of bladder carcinoma, when tumor progression occurs, and when symptoms or signs raise suspicion of upper urinary tract disease [12–15].These publications date back to1983–1998.

Transabdominal Ultrasound

Transabdominal sonography has been used to evaluate lesions of the bladder wall and lumen. Meticulous technique and adequate bladder distention are essential for optimal transabdominal sonography. The location and size of the tumor have the greatest impact on detection with sonography [16–19]. Tumors larger than 1 cm and distant from the bladder neck area are easier to image and have a relatively higher rate of detection, approaching 85% (Figs. 16.2c, 16.4b, and 16.5b). In a study by Dibb et al. 130 tumors were detected by US in 109 patients and the most frequent tumor site was the trigone (48.5%) [20].The most commonly encountered appearance of bladder tumor on US consisted of a polypoid (51.5%) and uncalcified (58.5%) mass with an irregular surface (61.5%). However, the wide variation in US features is reflected by their finding that only 11% of tumors had a combination of all these common features.

In a recent retrospective study in 100 patients abdominal sonography was compared to intravenous urography in the diagnosis of bladder carcinoma [21]. Sonography was significantly more sensitive (96%) in the detection compared

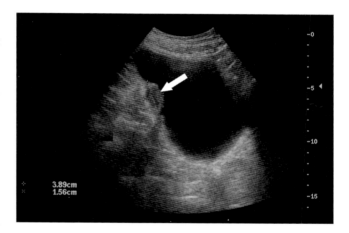

Fig. 16.7 (a) Slightly dilated distal left ureter with markedly irregular contour of the bladder dome on cystographic phase of IVU (*arrow*). The round filling defect on the left is due to a balloon catheter. (b) The ultrasound with more optimal filling of the bladder showing a less extended lesion in comparison to the cystography (*arrow*)

to urography (87%). In addition, sonography was more sensitive in clarifying the pathology in upper renal tracts, i.e., ureteric obstruction secondary to obstructing bladder carcinoma when urography failed due to none or poor excretion of contrast. Three missed lesions by sonography were smaller than 0.5 cm.

Infiltrating tumors are more likely than superficial ones to be detected. Tumors larger than 3 cm in diameter or those with associated calcification more often are overstaged. In this respect Wagner et al. staged bladder carcinoma by a new technique, three-dimensional US rendering [22]. Superficial (pTa) carcinomas were correctly staged in 66% by 3D US.

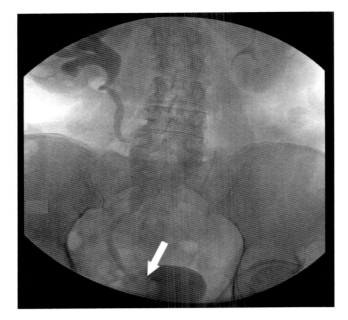

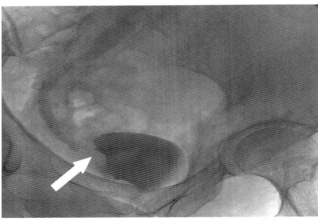

Fig. 16.8 (a) Hydronephrosis and hydro-ureter in this case of an urothelial cell carcinoma at the right vesico-ureteral junction (*arrow*). (b) The oblique view points out the acute stop in the distal ureter and the clearly visible irregularity of the bladder wall (*arrow*)

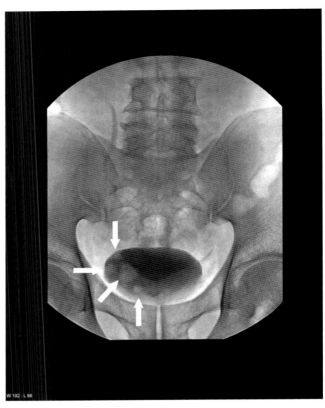

Fig. 16.9 This case illustrates the multifocality of urothelial cell carcinoma. Multiple filling defects (*arrows*) are seen on the right side of the bladder

Sonography is limited in its ability to depict extension of disease beyond the bladder wall and usually cannot detect nodal metastases. Wall edema, prominent mural folds, inflammation, muscular hypertrophy, blood clots, and postoperative changes can further reduce the specificity of ultrasound examination for the detection and staging of bladder malignancies.

Lamina propria infiltration (pT1) were correctly staged in 83% and the quota of correct staging of infiltrating carcinomas (>pT1) by 3D rendering was 100%. The overall accuracy was 79%. The conclusion is therefore that this new technique – 3D rendering – is most valuable to discriminate between superficial stages <pT1 and muscle invasive carcinoma >pT1. So this technique might improve local staging of bladder cancer.

Is color Doppler useful in staging bladder cancer? According to a study in 24 patients there was no statistical significant relationship between tumor stage and histopathological grade with presence and pattern of vascularity and spectral color Doppler findings [23].

Conclusion

Transabdominal US is the primary screening modality to evaluate patients suspected for bladder cancer. In positive cases this results in planned cystoscopy to confirm the diagnosis together with biopsy-proven pathology samples. There is no need anymore today for IVU to rule out synchronous or metachronous lesion of the upper tract. Also routine IVU in the follow-up of patients with known bladder cancer is no more justified. Cross-sectional modalities like CT with multiplanar reformatting and also MRI are nowadays used for ruling out multifocal disease and more important for staging (see other chapter).

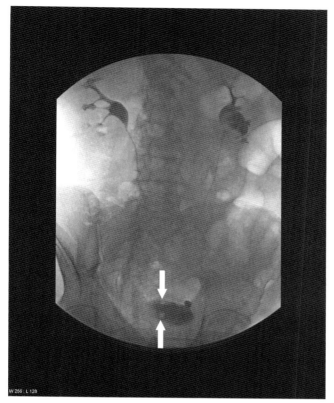

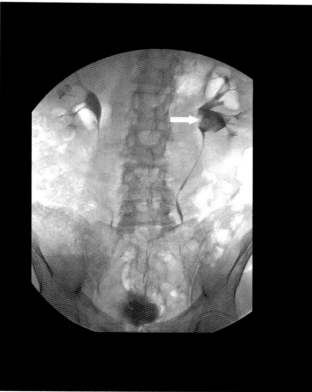

Fig. 16.10 (a–b) Apart from the round defects in the poorly filled bladder (*arrows* in a), a synchronous large lesion is found filling the dilated collecting system of the left kidney (*arrow* in b). There is no occlusion of the ureter: normal contrast drainage is visible on the left

Acknowledgment

The author wishes to express his gratitude to Professor ten Kate of the Department of Pathology who has made it possible to retrieve patients with bladder carcinoma from the pathology archive in order to review the diagnostic imaging of these patients.

References

1. Murphy WM, Grignon DJ, Perlman EJ. Tumors of the kidney, bladder, and related urinary structures. Washington, DC: American Registry of Pathology; 2004. p. 394; Ref Type: Generic.
2. McCredie M. Bladder and kidney cancers. Cancer Surv. 1994;19–20:343–68.
3. Marcus PM, Hayes RB, Vineis P, et al. Cigarette smoking, N-acetyltransferase 2 acetylation status, and bladder cancer risk: a case-series meta-analysis of a gene-environment interaction. Cancer Epidemiol Biomarkers Prev. 2000;9:461–7.
4. Eble JN, Sauter G, Epstein JI, Sesterhenn IA, editors. Pathology and genetics of tumours of the urinary system and male genital organs. World Health Organization classification of tumours. Lyon, France: IARC Press; 2004. Ref Type: Generic.
5. Zagoria RJ, Tung GA. Genitourinary radiology, The requisites. 1st ed. Mosby-Year Book Inc.; 1997. p. 219; Ref Type: Generic.
6. Mar AD, Das S. Pre-cystoscopic diagnosis of bladder tumour by modified intravenous urography. Br J Urol. 1984;56:381–4
7. Corrigan NT, Crooks J, Shand J. Are dedicated bladder films necessary as part of intravenous urography for haematuria? BJU Int. 2000;85:806–10.
8. Goessl C, Knispel HH, Miller K, Klan R. Is routine excretory urography necessary at first diagnosis of bladder cancer? J Urol. 1997;157:480–1
9. Hatch TR, Barry JM. The value of excretory urography in staging bladder cancer. J Urol. 1986;135:49.
10. Leung HY, Griffiths TR, Neal DE. Bladder cancer. Postgrad Med J. 1996;72:719–24.
11. Miyake H, Hara I, Yamanaka K, Inoue TA, Fujisawa M. Limited significance of routine excretory urography in the follow-up of patients with superficial bladder cancer after transurethral resection. BJU Int. 2006;97:720–23.
12. Hastie KJ, Hamdy FC, Collins MC, Williams JL. Upper tract tumours following cystectomy for bladder cancer. Is routine intravenous urography worthwhile? Br J Urol. 1991;67:29–31.
13. Holmang S, Hedelin H, Anderstrom C, Holmberg E, Johansson SL. Long-term followup of a bladder carcinoma cohort: routine followup urography is not necessary. J Urol. 1998;160:45–8.
14. Smith H, Weaver D, Barjenbruch O, Weinstein S, Ross G Jr. Routine excretory urography in follow-up of superficial transitional cell carcinoma of bladder. Urology. 1989;34:193–6.
15. Walzer Y, Soloway MS. Should the followup of patients with bladder cancer include routine excretory urography? J Urol. 1983;130:672–3.
16. Bessell EM, Price HM, McMillan PJ. The measurement of the regression of carcinoma of the bladder using ultrasonography and CT scanning during and after radical radiotherapy. Radiother Oncol. 1990;19:145–57.
17. Braeckman J, Denis L. The practice and pitfalls of ultrasonography in the lower urinary tract. Eur Urol. 1983;9:193–201.

18. Malone PR, Weston-Underwood J, Aron PM, Wilkinson KW, Joseph AE, Riddle PR. The use of transabdominal ultrasound in the detection of early bladder tumours. Br J Urol. 1986;58:520–2

19. Itzchak Y, Singer D, Fischelovitch Y. Ultrasonographic assessment of bladder tumors. I. Tumor detection. J Urol. 1981;126:31–3.

20. Dibb MJ, Noble DJ, Peh WC, et al. Ultrasonographic analysis of bladder tumors. Clin Imaging. 2001;25:416–20.

21. Rafique M, Javed AA. Role of intravenous urography and transabdominal ultrasonography in the diagnosis of bladder carcinoma. Int Braz J Urol. 2004;30:185–90.

22. Wagner B, Nesslauer T, Bartsch G Jr, Hautmann RE, Gottfried HW. Staging bladder carcinoma by three-dimensional ultrasound rendering. Ultrasound Med Biol. 2005;31:301–5.

23. Karahan OI, Yikilmaz A, Ekmekcioglu O, Ozturk F, Sevinc H. Color Doppler ultrasonography findings of bladder tumors: correlation with stage and histopathologic grade. Acta Radiol. 2004;45:481–6.

24. Wong-You-Cheong, Woodward PJ, Manning MA, et al. From the archives of the AFIP: neoplasms of the urinary Bladder: radiologic-pathologic correlation. RadioGraphics. 2006;26:553–80.

Chapter 17

Cross-Sectional Imaging of the Lower Urinary Tract

M.A. Blake and B.N. Setty

Introduction

Bladder cancer is a common tumor of the urinary tract, accounting for 6–8% of malignancies in men and 2–3% of malignancies in women. The majority (95%) are epithelial tumors; 95% of epithelial tumors are transitional cell carcinomas, 4% squamous cell carcinomas, 1% adenocarcinomas, with small cell carcinomas and sarcomas being relatively rare [1]. The treatment and prognosis of bladder cancer is largely determined by the tumor stage and the presence of metastases [2]. Therefore, accurate preoperative staging is imperative in determining the appropriate management of bladder carcinoma. Clinical staging is ideal for superficial tumors. Non-invasive imaging aids in the detection of local extension of the tumor, lymph node involvement, and distant metastases. Two schemes of staging are used for bladder cancer – TNM and Jewett–Strong–Marshall staging (art diagram). Superficial bladder tumors (TNM stage T1) are treated and often cured by local endoscopic resection whereas invasive carcinomas (TNM stage T2 and above) are treated by cystectomy or palliative chemotherapy or radiation therapy. Patients with extravesicular tumor spread have significantly higher recurrence rates and carry a poor prognosis [3].

Role of Cross-Sectional Imaging

Cross-sectional imaging modalities such as CT and MR are valuable in the staging of bladder cancer. However, MR imaging is superior to CT for staging carcinoma of the urinary bladder and offers several advantages over CT and sonography [4–7]. The role of any imaging technique lies in accurate delineation of the extent of tumor spread. For an imaging method to be most useful as a staging tool, it should

be able to distinguish T1 from T2 invasion particularly as over 70% of tumors present as a superficial stage (stage T1).

CT

CT is a non-invasive technique and is widely available. Advantages are short acquisition times, wide coverage in a single breath hold, and its ability for multi-organ imaging. It can detect lymph node enlargement and distant metastatic disease as well as the presence of complications such as hydronephrosis. It provides excellent inherent contrast between the bladder and extra-peritoneal fat, enabling detection of extravesical spread. Recent improvements in CT hardware have led to the development of the multi-detector row helical CT scanner, which can provide higher resolution and volume acquisition in a shorter time. With these advantages, multi-detector row helical CT is expected to improve the evaluation of patients with bladder cancer.

CT Appearance of Bladder Tumors

CT is the primary imaging modality for cancer of the urinary bladder. Stage T1 tumors typically appear pedunculated (i.e., intraluminal), but the bladder wall itself appears normal (Fig. 17.1). Hematoma and muscle trabeculations are potential mimics of these tumors. T2 lesions are characteristically sessile and appear as a smooth focal contour bulge (Fig. 17.2). CT is not capable of determining the depth of invasion of the bladder wall, i.e., differentiating stage T2a from T2b disease. Thus, CT is limited in determining the depth of bladder wall invasion. It can distinguish T3a from T3b or higher tumor. T3b tumors produce an irregular outer bladder wall or soft tissue infiltration or stranding into the perivesical fat in the region of the tumor (Fig. 17.3). It can be excluded if a clear plane of separation is preserved, although unfortunately the presence or absence of the fat plane is

M.A Blake (✉)
Division of Abdominal Imaging and Intervention, Massachusetts General Hospital, Boston, Massachusetts, USA

J.J.M.C.H. de la Rosette et al. (eds.), *Imaging in Oncological Urology*,
DOI 10.1007/978-1-84628-759-6_17, © Springer-Verlag London Limited 2009

TNM Staging of Bladder Cancer

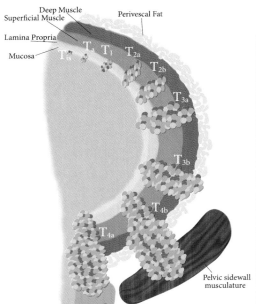

T0	No tumor
Tis	Carcinoma in situ
Ta	Papillary tumor, confined to the epithelium (mucosa)
T1	Tumor invades sub epithelial connective tissue (lamina propria)
T2a	Tumor invades superficial muscle (inner half)
T2b	Tumor invades deep muscle (outer half)
T3a	Tumor with microscopic invasion of perivesical fat
T3b	Tumor with macroscopic invasion of perivesical fat
T4a	Tumor invades surrounding organs
T4b	Tumor invades pelvic or abdominal wall

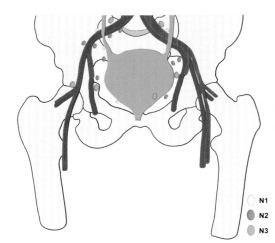

N0	No regional lymph node metastasis
N1	Metastasis to single lymph node, 2 cm or less in size
N2	Metastasis to a single lymph node, 2 to 5 cm in size, or to multiple lymph nodes, all less than 5 cm in size
N3	Metastasis to regional lymph nodes greater than 5 cm in size

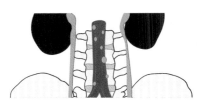

Lymph nodes above aortic bifurcation

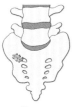

Bone

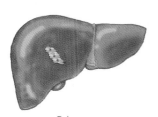

Liver

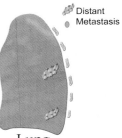

Lung

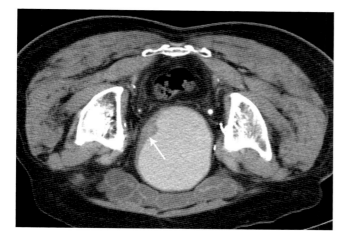

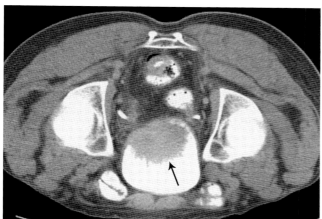

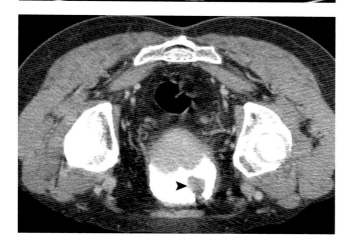

Fig. 17.1 (a) Delayed prone contrast-enhanced CT bladder images demonstrating a plaque-like thickening of the posterior left lateral bladder wall with an enhancing soft tissue mass (*white arrow*). Histopathology revealed transitional cell carcinoma in situ (stage T is). (b) A large mass with an irregular margin (*black arrow*) filling the lumen of the bladder along its posterior wall. A papillary transitional carcinoma with no invasion (stage Ta) was found on histopathology. (c) A pedunculated mass lesion (*arrowhead*) arising from the anterior wall of the bladder appearing as a filling defect within the contrast filled lumen. Transurethral resection of the mass revealed a papillary transitional cell carcinoma invading the lamina propria but not the muscularis propria (stage T1)

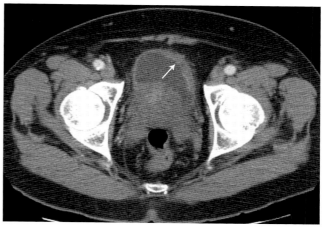

Fig. 17.2 Dynamic contrast-enhanced CT of the bladder demonstrates asymmetrical thickening of the left antero-lateral bladder wall (*arrow*) appearing as a smooth focal contour bulge (stage T2)

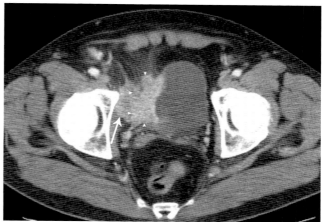

Fig. 17.3 Contrast-enhanced CT demonstrating a large, enhancing right bladder wall mass (*arrowheads*) (stage T3b) with transmural invasion and an adjacent right obturator lymph node (*arrow*) consistent with metastatic bladder cancer

not completely reliable for the determination of microscopic invasion [8, 9]. The tumor is classified as T4 disease if it invades adjacent organs or structures such as the pelvic or abdominal walls. The tumor tissue within the invaded organ enhances similarly to that of the bladder tumor with associated enlargement of the invaded organ [10] (Fig. 17.4). The disappearance of the seminal vesicle angle is a useful sign of its invasion.

Up to 5% of transitional cell carcinomas contain calcifications that can be detected on non-enhanced CT scans which appear either nodular or arched in configuration. Fifty percent of adenocarcinomas possess fine intratumoral calcifications. Bladder cancers enhance more intensely than adjacent normal bladder wall tissue on contrast-enhanced CT scans [2]. CT detects most bladder tumors, though tumors at the

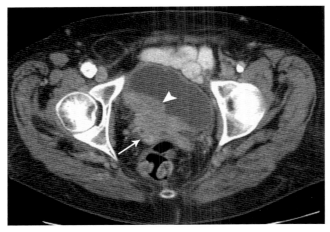

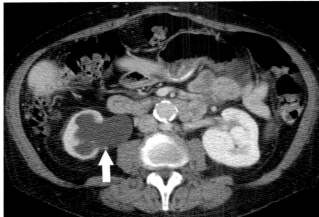

Fig. 17.4 CT images show a large bladder mass (*arrowhead*) (a) causing obstruction of the right ureteric orifice with proximal hydroureter and hydronephrosis (*thick arrow*) (b). No clear fat plane between the mass and the vagina is visualized (*thin arrow*) (stage T4a) (a). Histopathology performed following a radical cystectomy revealed an invasive transitional cell carcinoma involving the right bladder wall and ureter consistent with a mass originating from the right intravesical part of the ureter and invading the muscularis propria of the bladder, perivesical fat, and the vaginal wall and mucosa

base and dome in particular can be missed. High-quality multiplanar reconstructions improve the sensitivity of CT for these regions. Rapid scanning performed in the nephrographic phase before the excreted IV contrast reaches the bladder detects an enhancing tumor against a background of low-attenuation urine. On MDCT, the peak enhancement of bladder tumors is around 60 s following intravenous contrast administration. On delayed scanning, the lesion appears as a mural nodule against a background of high-attenuation excreted contrast material within the bladder (Fig. 17.1b). Occasionally the tumor is better seen on the non-contrast scan than on the delayed scan because of the attenuation similarity of the enhanced tumor and the excreted contrast within the bladder. The tumor can also appear plaque-like or papillary. Contrast-filled ureters may be visualized on delayed post-contrast scans. Post-micturition images may

be useful if full bladder scans suggest the involvement of bowel by adjacent tumor, as the bladder descends into the pelvis when empty resulting in an altered spatial relationship with the bowel. As the tumor grows, circumferential wall thickening may also be seen. In addition, the mass may invade the ureteral orifice, resulting in hydroureteronephrosis. With more advanced disease, bilateral hydronephrosis may be noted. Additional rectal contrast may be valuable in delineating the recto-sigmoid colon to assess advanced local disease while good opacification of the small bowel loops can be obtained with oral contrast.

CT may also be useful in assessing incomplete transurethral resection of the bladder especially when the resection is limited by complications such as bleeding. It is also an excellent method for detecting recurrent tumor following cystectomy. Potential pertinent CT findings include a mass at the cystectomy site, retroperitoneal lymphadenopathy, and liver or bone metastases [11, 12] (Fig. 17.5).

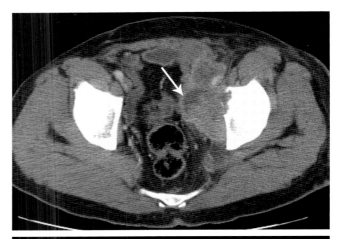

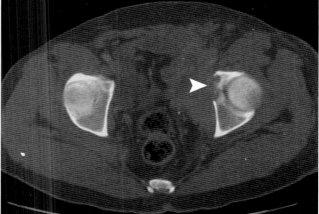

Fig. 17.5 (a) Contrast-enhanced CT demonstrates an ill-defined infiltrating mass in the left lateral pelvis following a radical cystoprostatectomy and chemotherapy (*arrow*) in a patient with known bladder cancer consistent with tumor recurrence. (b) The mass is also seen to cause progressive destruction of the medial aspect of the left acetabulum (*arrowhead*) on the bone windowed CT image

Metastases

Lymph Nodes

The major diagnostic criterion for CT evaluation of a lymph node is its size. Pelvic nodes are often considered abnormal if the minimum transverse diameter is 1 cm or more although microscopic involvement of normal-sized nodes causes false negatives and subsequent under-staging. These criteria are under ongoing review, particularly in view of advancing technology, and the upper limits of "normal" are being reduced particularly in patients with known bladder cancer. Lymph nodes tend to become rounded with metastatic involvement, and thus the maximum short-axis dimension is used for assessment on CT [13].

Pelvic nodes are more difficult to recognize than para-aortic nodes, particularly in patients with little intra-abdominal fat, although asymmetry can be helpful. Lymph nodes greater than 8 mm in the obturator and internal iliac groups are now generally considered abnormal. In addition, a number of normal pelvis structures may be unwittingly mistaken for pelvic lymph nodes including unenhanced pelvic sidewall vessels, unopacified pelvic bowel wall loops, and the normal ovary [14]. Conversely, nodal metastases from pelvic tumors may also be confused with these structures. Lymph nodes, which enhance strongly with intravenous contrast, can occur in bladder cancer [15]. In the presence of enlarged pelvic nodes, the retroperitoneum in particular should also be assessed for para-aortic adenopathy (Fig. 17.6).

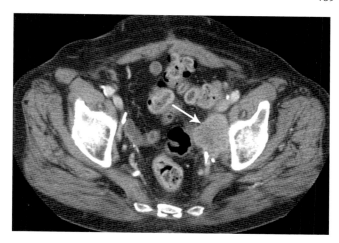

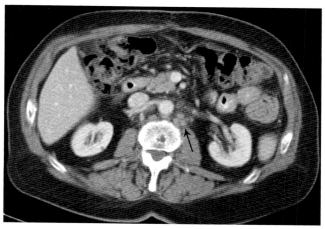

Fig. 17.6 Contrast-enhanced CT demonstrating soft issue masses in the left obturator lymph node (*white arrow*) (a) and the retroperitoneum (*black arrow*) (b) consistent with metastatic disease in a patient with stage T3 tumor

Distant Metastases

Metastases can involve the liver, bone, and lungs. CT of the abdomen should be obtained especially during follow-up because isolated metastases can occur in the recurrence of the disease (12) (Fig. 17.7).

Pitfalls of CT

Early postoperative CT especially following TURB is likely to result in pseudolesions and inaccurate staging [6, 16, 17]. This can be overcome by allowing an adequate interval between TURB and CT examination. Knowledge of the contrast enhancement pattern is necessary to differentiate cancerous tissue from non-specific wall edema, blood clots, or tissue debris that mimics the appearance of a tumor. Chronic wall thickening may also result from surgery, radiation therapy, and chemotherapy with systemic agents such

as cyclophosphamide and ifosfamide or intravesical agents such as bacillus Calmette–Guérin [18]. The bladder must be adequately distended and when a urinary catheter is present, it should be clamped before the CT examination. Over-distension of bladder may result in underestimation of bladder wall thickness with effacement of fat planes between the bladder and adjacent structures.

Another drawback of CT is its failure to demonstrate microscopic invasion of perivesical fat. The previously noted inability to detect tumor in normal-sized lymph nodes is also a major cause of under-staging. Over-staging on CT may result from misinterpretation of normal fat planes between the posterior bladder wall and the seminal vesicles in up to 27% of cases. Post-void and decubitus images may help in correct interpretation. Over-staging owing to perivesical fibrosis, particularly seen following cystoscopic biopsy, can occur and when possible CT should ideally be performed before rather than after surgical intervention [19].

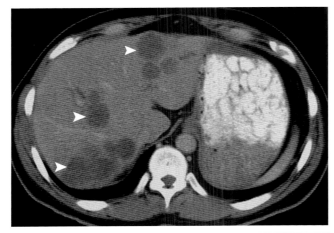

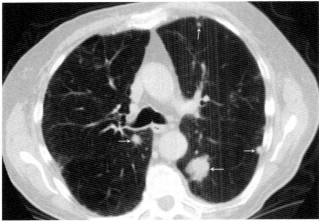

Fig. 17.7 (a) Contrast-enhanced CT of the liver demonstrating multiple hypodensities (*arrowheads*), with irregular rim enhancement throughout the liver consistent with metastases in a patient with invasive bladder cancer. (b) CT of the lung showing multiple metastatic parenchymal soft tissue nodules of varying sizes in both lung fields (*arrows*)

Accuracy of CT

The overall accuracy of CT in detecting and staging bladder cancer varies from 64–97% whereas that for perivesical invasion and for lymph node metastases ranges from 83–93 and 73–92%, respectively [6, 8, 9, 20–22]. Multi-detector row helical CT has indeed been found to improve the performance of CT with an overall higher accuracy in the evaluation of patients with bladder cancer. Cancers less than 1 cm can now be routinely detected on MDCT.

MRI

Intrinsic tissue contrast allows superior localization and characterization of bladder tumors on MRI [23]. Direct multiplanar imaging capability has also been cited as a spe-

cific MR advantage, but now MDCT also allows multiplanar reconstructions of its 3D data sets. Phased-array external surface body coils and endoluminal coils offer higher signal-to-noise ratio and a smaller field of view resulting in the acquisition of excellent image quality with high spatial resolution [24–27]. Parallel imaging techniques can also be availed to improve resolution or shorten imaging acquisition time.

MR Appearance of Bladder Cancer

Both T1- and T2-weighted images in multiple planes are required for staging bladder tumors.

On T1-weighted images, the tumor appears intermediate in signal intensity similar to muscle precluding differentiation from the adjacent bladder wall. However, T1-weighted images are useful in assessing infiltration of the perivesical fat and in the demonstration of the endoluminal component of the tumor.

On T2-weighted images, the bladder wall and perivesical fat appear low or high in signal intensity depending on the sequence used. Bladder cancers are intermediate to high in signal intensity on T2-weighted images and are greater in signal than the normal muscularis. The preservation of the low-signal bladder wall subjacent to the tumor on T2-weighted images indicates a superficial (T1) tumor [14, 28–30]. Late fibrosis appears low in signal intensity and can be distinguished from tumor on T2-weighted sequences. Invasion into the adjacent organs such as the prostate, uterus, or the vagina is also better appreciated. Depending on the echo time (TE) and repetition time (TR) used differentiating the tumor from urine and the perivesical fat may be suboptimal.

Gadolinium enhanced T1-weighted imaging demonstrates intense and immediate enhancement of the tumor compared to the uninvolved bladder wall [31, 32] (Figs. 17.8 and 17.9). The imaging should be performed within 90 s after the contrast injection to optimize tumor-bladder contrast [7, 33, 34]. Tumor can be differentiated from normal bladder wall as early as 5–15 s after contrast administration [32]. Fat saturation or subtraction techniques are used to improve tumor visualization because tumors and perivesical fat have high signal intensity on post-contrast T1-weighted images. Dynamic enhanced imaging aids in the differentiation of bladder tumor from surrounding tissues as the tumor enhances earlier to that of normal bladder wall due to the development of neovascularization [35]. Fast dynamic MR imaging acquired at least once every 2 s helps in distinguishing tumor from post-biopsy tissue. Tumors are reported to enhance earlier than post-biopsy tissue with an average of 6.5 s following contrast enhancement whereas post-biopsy

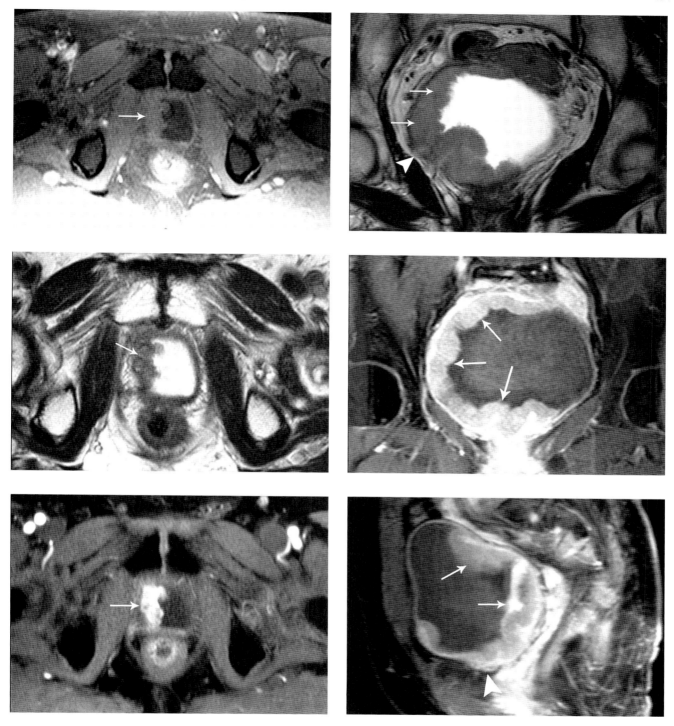

Fig. 17.8 Axial T1, T2, and gadolinium-enhanced MR images of a transmural, polypoid enhancing mass (*arrow*) arising from the right inferolateral bladder wall with no evidence of invasion into the extravesical soft tissue consistent with a stage T2 bladder cancer. The tumor has intermediate signal intensity on T1 and T2 (a, b) and demonstrates intense enhancement following administration of gadolinium (c)

Fig. 17.9 Pre-contrast T2-weighted (a) and post-contrast coronal and sagittal T1-weighted (b, c) MR images of the bladder demonstrate a large circumferential bladder mass (*arrows*). Disruption of the low signal intensity of the muscle at the right bladder base is consistent with wall invasion with focal extravesical soft tissue extension in the perivesical fat (stage T3b) (*arrow head*)

inflammation or granulation tissue enhances 13.6 s after contrast. Thus, the use of fast dynamic techniques can increase the accuracy of interpretation by up to 10% by avoiding false positives [6, 36–38].

Metastases

Lymph Nodes

T1-weighted images enable better visualization of lymph nodes from surrounding fatty tissue. However, normal and abnormal lymph nodes show similar signal intensity on unenhanced T1-weighted MR images. The detection of lymph node metastases has important clinical implications (Fig. 17.10). If lymph node metastases are present, a curative cystectomy is usually not performed. Current imaging techniques usually rely on size criteria and nodal morphology. Based on the size criteria, a number of potential pitfalls can occur due to the considerable overlap in size between benign and malignant nodes. Different sensitivities and specificities are observed based on the selection of cut-off size thresholds for lymph nodes. A 3D high-resolution MR technique has been shown to have a higher accuracy for the detection of lymph node metastases in oval nodes with a diameter larger than 10 mm and round nodes with a diameter larger than 8 mm. The presence of an asymmetric cluster of nodes is also pathological [39].

Normal-sized metastatic nodes and non-metastatic nodes unfortunately show early and similar enhancement on gadolinium-enhanced fast dynamic MR imaging. It is thus generally not possible with gadolinium to detect a metastasis in normal-sized lymph nodes due to this lack of differential enhancement between normal lymph node tissue and metastases. Novel MR imaging with ultrasmall super paramagnetic iron oxide (USPIO) particles has shown that normal nodal tissue shows uptake of this contrast material and a selective decrease in signal intensity on T2- or T2*-weighted MR images, whereas nodal areas infiltrated with metastases lack uptake and retain their high signal intensity on USPIO-enhanced MR images (Fig. 17.11). This technique promises to greatly improve MR's accuracy in the characterization of lymph nodes [40].

Distant Metastases

Liver, lung, and bone are the principal sites of distant metastases of bladder cancer. Muscle invasive tumors have a propensity for lymph node metastases at the para-aortic region and viscera. Fast dynamic MR sequences using dedicated liver protocols can detect metastases to the liver

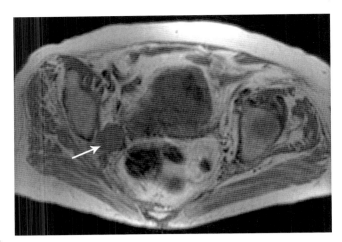

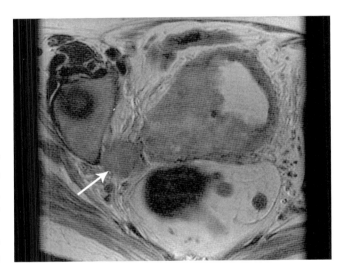

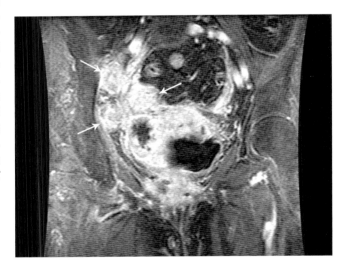

Fig. 17.10 Axial T1- and T2-weighted pre-contrast (a, b) and post-contrast coronal T1-weighted (c) MR images of the pelvis demonstrating large masses involving the right obturator and common iliac lymph nodes (arrows) which display intermediate signal on the pre-contrast T1- and T2-weighted images and marked enhancement post-contrast consistent with metastatic disease

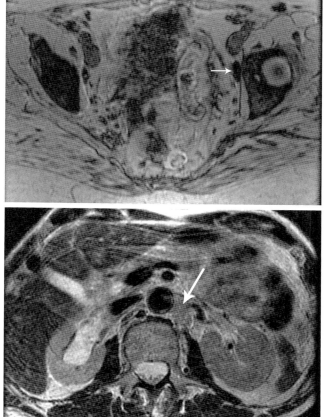

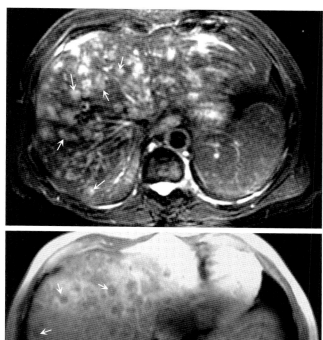

Fig. 17.11 USPIO-enhanced T2*-weighted axial MR images performed in two different patients of bladder cancers demonstrate homogenous uptake of USPIO in a benign left external iliac lymph node (*thin arrow*) causing a selective normal decrease in signal intensity (a) and an enlarged left para-aortic node (*thick arrow*) infiltrated with metastases lacking uptake of USPIO and thus abnormally retaining a high signal intensity (b) (Courtesy Dr. Mukesh Harisinghani)

Fig. 17.12 Axial T2- and contrast-enhanced T1-weighted MR images of the liver demonstrating multiple T2-weighted slightly hyperintense lesions (*arrows*) throughout the liver (a) that enhance following administration of gadolinium (b) in a known patient with bladder cancer

(Fig. 17.12). Bone marrow metastases have signal intensity equal to the primary tumor and are recognized best on T1-weighted images where there is a good contrast between them and the higher signal of the surrounding fatty bone marrow (Fig. 17.13). Peripheral enhancement can be appreciated following gadolinium administration. MR can also detect spread of the tumor through the acetabulum that requires palliative orthopedic surgery. Differentiation between radiation necrosis from tumor or infection is difficult, often requiring a biopsy for confirmation. A bone scan is indicated to assess the entire skeleton in the presence of bony metastases [32].

MR Urography

Transitional cell carcinoma is known to be multicentric in nature, so the entire urinary tract requires evaluation in patients with TCC. Multifocal disease may occur in the bladder, renal collecting system, or the ureters. With MR imaging, the entire urinary system can be visualized. Heavily T2-weighted sequences can demonstrate the urine in the pyelum and ureter especially when they are dilated due to a distal obstruction. A breath hold T1-weighted MR angiographic sequence also can be performed in delayed fashion after contrast injection to demonstrate gadolinium excretion in the ureters similar to IVU.

Accuracy of MR Staging

MR imaging is considered superior to CT scanning for local staging of carcinoma of the urinary bladder. Dedicated multiplanar imaging and superior intrinsic tissue contrast allows better visualization of the bladder dome, trigone, and adjacent structures such as the prostate and seminal vesicles. The reported accuracy of MR in overall staging of bladder cancer varies from 60 to 85% whereas that of local staging varies from 73 to 96% [5, 33, 41–43] (Table 17.1).

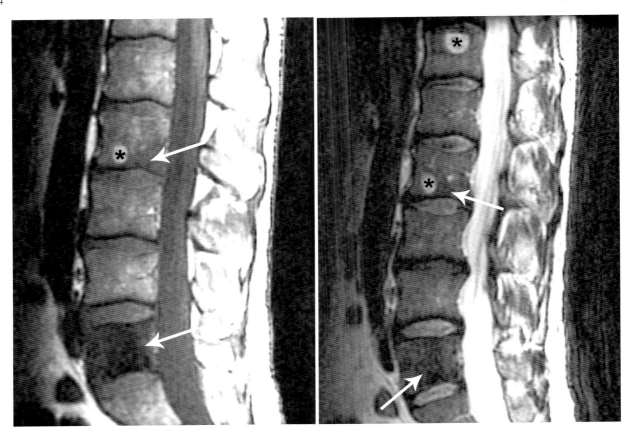

Fig. 17.13 Sagittal T1-, T2- and contrast-enhanced T1-weighted images of the lumbar spine showing multiple metastases (*arrows*) involving the L5 and lower half of the L2 vertebral bodies from a blad- der cancer. The lesions appear hypointense on T1 (a) and slightly hyper- intense on T2 (b) and enhance on gadolinium administration (c). Inci- dental vertebral hemangiomas (*asterisks*) are seen at L2 and T12 levels

Optimizing MR Images

Various ancillary measures can be taken to ensure good-quality results from an MRI study of patients with bladder cancer. Patients experiencing claustrophobia can be appropriately sedated. Attaining suitable bladder distension is crucial for accurate interpretation of images. It is difficult to appreciate small tumors in an inadequately distended bladder with a thickened bladder wall. Over-distension of the bladder also leads to patient discomfort and flat tumors can be overlooked. Ideal bladder distension can be achieved by asking the patient to void 2 h before imaging and not again until after the scan. Use of magnets with higher field strength provides superior image quality through ultrafast scanning techniques, although stronger chemical shift artifacts and lower T1 contrast can pose problems. Phased-array external surface body coils and endoluminal coils offer higher signal-to-noise ratio and a smaller field of view resulting in the acquisition of excellent image quality with high spatial resolution. They also permit parallel imaging techniques to be applied with resulting sequence advantages of shorter time or higher resolution. Endoluminal coils indeed provide higher spatial resolution and excellent images of the prostate and seminal vesicles, as well as the dorsal bladder wall for accurate recognition of tumor invasion but offer a more limited field of view. Administration of intravenous contrast as discussed above is also helpful to improve overall staging accuracy.

Recent Advances

Virtual endoscopy with CT or MR is a recent technique and preliminary studies have demonstrated its feasibility for imaging the urinary tract [49]. Cystoscopy is the standard method for the detection and direct visualization of the tumor followed by transurethral resection, which provides histology and grading. However, it is an invasive technique and associated with some patient discomfort. The other drawbacks of cystoscopy are difficulty in the detection of tumors situated in bladder diverticula and at the bladder neck and in determining extravesical tumor spread [50]. CT cystoscopy can be performed by insufflating air into the urinary tract or following intravenous contrast administration also known as

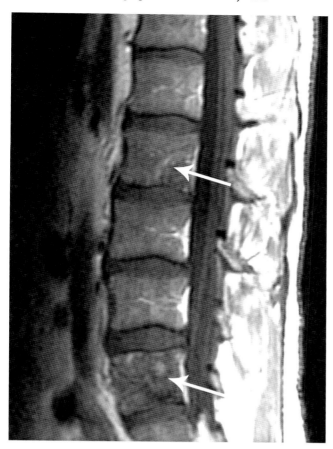

Fig. 17.13 (continued)

IVU virtual cystoscopy [51–54]. The need for repeated cystoscopies for continual surveillance of patients with a history of transitional cell carcinoma raises the concern for cumulative radiation exposures from CT cystoscopy [55]. This could be overcome by non-irradiating MR cystoscopy that has shown promising results [56].

Rare Bladder Cancers

Tumors arising from a bladder diverticulum tend to be of a higher grade and escape the bladder wall earlier because

of the lack of a muscle layer. Thus, tumors at this location have a greater potential for metastasis and a poorer prognosis. The incidence of a neoplasm in a bladder diverticulum ranges from 0.8 to 13.5% [57, 58]. Squamous cell carcinoma is the most common non-transitional cell tumor. Chronic infection caused by schistosomiasis (bilharziasis) is an important predisposing factor in endemic areas like Egypt. Non-bilharzial squamous cell carcinomas occur in association with chronic irritation from urinary calculi, long-term indwelling catheters, or chronically infected bladder diverticula. The disease is relatively more common in women, unlike transitional cell carcinoma, which is more common in men [59].

Adenocarcinoma of the urinary bladder is uncommon, accounting for 0.5–2% of all bladder malignancies [60, 61]. The base (especially the trigone) and the dome of the bladder are the common sites. Adenocarcinomas are classified into three groups: primary, urachal, and metastatic [59]. Cystitis glandularis, bladder exstrophy, and urachal remnants are also associated with adenocarcinoma of the bladder. Urachal carcinomas arise from the dome of the bladder as a mass with a superior midline extravesical component or a mass anterosuperior to the bladder dome along the course of the urachus (Fig. 17.14). Up to 90% of urachal carcinomas are mucinous adenocarcinomas [62]. It has a central low attenuation because of mucin production, with peripheral or central calcifications that are fine, arched, or nodular in pattern [50]. Signet cell adenocarcinomas characteristically produce linitis plastica of the bladder that are diffusely infiltrating by nature and tend to be of advanced stage at the time of diagnosis [63, 64].

Small cell carcinoma of the bladder is also known as undifferentiated and poorly differentiated carcinoma. Most small cell carcinomas occur as a component of mixed carcinomas. Pure small cell carcinomas are rare, representing less than 1% of all urothelial neoplasms. Age, sex, and symptoms are comparable to those of transitional cell carcinomas [64]. They can arise from anywhere in the bladder with no predilection for the base of the bladder. They are nodular or polypoidal and often ulcerated masses with mixed enhancement patterns that cannot be distinguished from other high-grade bladder cancers. Metastatic spread occurs rapidly, and the most frequent sites are the regional lymph nodes, bones, peritoneal cavity, and even the brain [65].

Carcinosarcoma of the urinary bladder is a rare neoplasm of unknown etiology. This tumor possesses epithelial and sarcomatous components on histopathology. It is more common in men, with a ratio of 3:1. These tumors usually occur at the base of the bladder and are polypoidal masses that have deeply infiltrated the wall of the bladder at the time of diagnosis. Most deaths result from complications of local growth rather than distant metastasis [64]. These tumors are usually isointense to muscle on T1-weighted images on MR and het-

Table 17.1 Overall staging accuracy of gadolinium-enhanced MRI for staging extravesical extension in bladder cancer

No. of patients	Sensitivity (%)	Specificity (%)	Accuracy (%)	Reference and year
22	82	62	73	Husband et al. – 1989 [44]
68	93	95	95	Neuerburg et al. – 1991 [45]
28	100	100	100	Barentsz et al. – 1995 [46]
71	91	87	87	Hayashi et al. – 2000 [47]
64	–	65	85	Mizuno et al. – 2003 [48]
71	82.5	81.5	82	Tekes et al. – 2005 [43]

erogeneous in signal intensity on T2-weighted images unlike transitional cell carcinoma. On contrast administration, these tumors heterogeneously enhance and lack the early arterial enhancement of transitional cell carcinoma owing to their mixed histology [66].

Ureteral Neoplasms

Epithelial neoplasms account for 75% of all primary neoplasms, with transitional cell carcinomas accounting for up to 93% of cases. Transitional cell carcinomas are divided into papillary and non-papillary subtypes based on histopathology. Of the remaining epithelial neoplasms, 5% are squamous and 2% are adenocarcinomas. Papillary tumors tend to be multicentric and in 40% of patients the tumor is found to have extended into the peri-ureteric tissues at the time of presentation. Metastases to the regional lymph nodes or hematogenous spread to distant sites such as the liver and bones may also occur. An associated transitional cell carci-

noma of the bladder is found in up to 25% of cases and in up to 70% a history of antecedent or a subsequent urothelial lesion is found elsewhere in the urinary tract. The non-papillary variety tends to be solitary by nature although most of this type has infiltrated into the submucosa by the time of diagnosis.

Transitional cell carcinomas of the ureter are staged as

Stage I: the tumor is limited to the mucosa
Stage II: invasion to the level of the ureteral muscle
Stage III: invasion of the peri-ureteral tissues
Stage IV: distant metastasis.

Ureteric tumors have a predilection for the middle and distal ureter (Fig. 17.15). Usually a diagnosis of ureteral carcinoma is obtained by an excretory urography or a retrograde pyelography. However CT is replacing excretory urography in many centers for the evaluation of patients with hematuria. Delayed post-intravenous contrast-enhanced CT can diagnose ureteric tumors as they manifest as ureteral filling defects often with proximal ureteral dilatation and thickening of the involved ureteral wall. CT also helps in determining

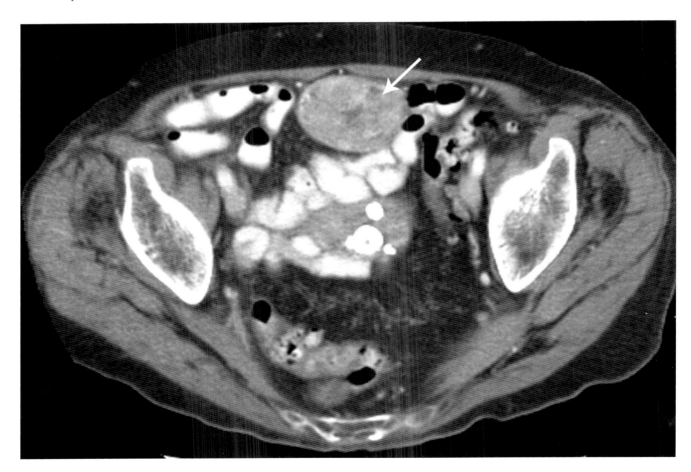

Fig. 17.14 Axial contrast enhanced (a) and coronal reformat of CT images (b) of the bladder show an moderately enhancing mass (*arrows*) anterosuperior to the bladder (*small arrows*) in the region of the urachus suggestive of an urachal tumor that was confirmed on histopathology

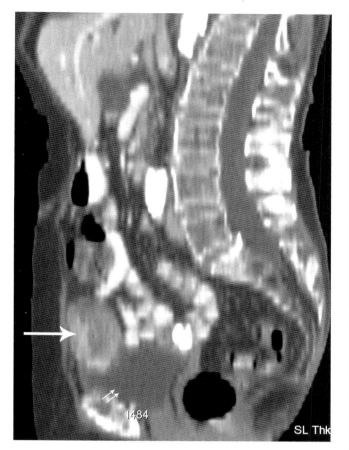

Fig. 17.14 (continued)

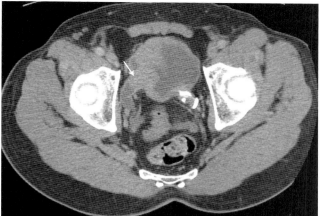

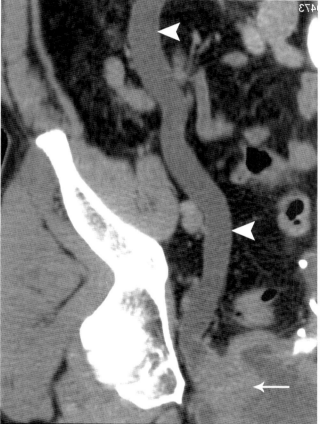

Fig. 17.15 Axial contrast-enhanced CT (a) and curved reformatted MPR images (b) showing a large soft tissue tumor (*arrow*) originating from the right intravesical part of the ureter causing obstruction of the right ureteric orifice with hydroureter (*arrow heads*) and hydronephrosis (not shown)

the extent of tumor spread. Mimics of ureteric TCC include papilloma or polyp, which commonly produce long, smooth intraluminal-filling defects. These can also occur in inflammatory conditions or ureteral metastases [67]. Squamous cell carcinomas occur in the setting of chronic urinary tract infection or calculi and present as a solitary filling defect with frequent peri-ureteral invasion. CT also helps to determine the cause of ureteral obstruction whether it is due to an intrinsic neoplasm or extrinsic disease such as idiopathic or malignant retroperitoneal fibrosis, inflammatory aortic aneurysm, or lymphomatous and metastatic retroperitoneal adenopathy [68]. MDCT urography is a novel application of MDCT to study the entire urinary tract owing to its ability to acquire thinly collimated data sets that can be used to create excellent quality 3D images of the urinary tract. It offers a promising role in the detection of urothelial wall thickening or masses, provided opacification of the entire urinary tract is obtained [69].

Conclusion

In summary, cross-sectional imaging plays an important role in defining management of patients with invasive bladder or distal ureteric cancer. It is also helpful in staging of bladder cancer despite having some limitations. CT is widely accessible and rapid advances in multi-detector technology and its far-reaching applications have allowed it to now be considered on a similar par with MR. MR is reported to have a higher accuracy for staging bladder cancer owing to its intrinsic tissue characterization. It is superior to CT in determining the depth of bladder wall invasion. CT as well as MR relies on morphological criteria and both are useful in the detection of metastases to the lymph nodes, liver, and bone. MR is however considered superior in follow-up of patients with bladder cancer post-therapy as it can distinguish biopsy changes more accurately than CT.

References

1. Barentsz JO, Witjes JA, Ruijs JH. What is new in bladder cancer imaging? Urol Clin North Am. 1997;24:583–602.
2. MacVicar AD. Bladder cancer staging. BJU Int. 2000;86 Suppl 1:111–22.
3. Stein JP, Lieskovsky G, Cote R, et al. Radical cystectomy in the treatment of invasive bladder cancer: long-term results in 1,054 patients. J Clin Oncol. 2001;19:666–75.
4. Barentsz JO, Jager GJ, Witjes JA, et al. Primary staging of urinary bladder carcinoma: the role of MRI and a comparison with CT. Eur Radiol. 1996;6:129–33.
5. Amendola MA, Glazer GM, Grossman HB, et al. Staging of bladder carcinoma: MRI-CT-surgical correlation. AJR Am J Roentgenol. 1986;146:1179–83.
6. Kim B, Semelka RC, Ascher SM, et al. Bladder tumor staging: comparison of contrast-enhanced CT, T1- and T2-weighted MR imaging, dynamic gadolinium-enhanced imaging, and late gadolinium-enhanced imaging. Radiology. 1994;193:239–45.
7. Tachibana M, Baba S, Deguchi N, et al. Efficacy of gadolinium-diethylenetriaminepentaacetic acid-enhanced magnetic resonance imaging for differentiation between superficial and muscle-invasive tumor of the bladder: a comparative study with computerized tomography and transurethral ultrasonography. J Urol. 1991;145:1169–73.
8. Koss JC, Arger PH, Coleman BG, et al. CT staging of bladder carcinoma. AJR Am J Roentgenol. 1981;137:359–62.
9. Morgan CL, Calkins RF, Cavalcanti EJ. Computed tomography in the evaluation, staging, and therapy of carcinoma of the bladder and prostate. Radiology. 1981;140(3):751–61.
10. Kundra V, Silverman PM. Imaging in oncology from the University of Texas M. D. Anderson Cancer Center. Imaging in the diagnosis, staging, and follow-up of cancer of the urinary bladder. AJR Am J Roentgenol. 2003;180(4):1045–54.
11. Oliva L, Cariati M, Reggiani L, et al. CT evaluation of the pelvic cavity after cystectomy: observation in 40 cases. J Comput Assist Tomogr. 1984;8(4):734–8.
12. Ellis JH, McCullough NB, Francis IR, et al. Transitional cell carcinoma of the bladder: patterns of recurrence after cystectomy as determined by CT. AJR Am J Roentgenol. 1991;157(5):999–1002.
13. Vinnicombe SJ, Norman AR, Nicholson V, et al. Normal pelvic lymph nodes: evaluation with CT after bipedal lymphangiography. Radiology. 1995;194:349–55.
14. Spencer JA, Swift SE. Computed tomography of the pelvis. In: Haaga JR, Lanzieri CF, Gilkeson RC, et al., editors. CT and MR imaging of the whole body. 4th ed. St Louis: Mi Mosby. Inc; 2003. pp. 1715–51.
15. Husband JE, Robinson L, Thomas G. Contrast enhancing lymph nodes in bladder cancer: a potential pitfall on CT. Clin Radiol. 1992;45(6):395–8.
16. Sager EM, Talle K, Fossa SD, et al. Contrast-enhanced computed tomography to show perivesical extension in bladder carcinoma. Acta Radiol. 1987;28:307–11
17. Salo JO, Kivisaari L, Lehtonen T. CT in determining the depth of infiltration of bladder tumors. Urol Radiol. 1985;7:88–93.
18. Ramchandani P, Pollack HM. Radiology of drug-related genitourinary disease. Semin Roentgenol. 1995;30:77–87.
19. Sager EM, Talle K, Fossa S, et al. The role of CT in demonstrating perivesical tumor growth in the preoperative staging of carcinoma of the urinary bladder. Radiology. 1983;146:443–6.
20. Kim JK, Park SY, Ahn HJ, et al. Bladder cancer: analysis of multi–detector row helical ct enhancement pattern and accuracy in tumor detection and perivesical staging. Radiology. 2004;231:725–31.
21. Lee JKT, Stanley RJ, Sagel SS, et al. Accuracy of CT in detecting intra abdominal and pelvic lymph node metastases from pelvic cancers. AJR Am J Roentgenol. 1978;131:675–9.
22. Jeffrey RB, Palubinskas AJ, Federle MP. CT evaluation of invasive lesions of the bladder. J Comput Assist Tomogr. 1981;5 (1):22–6.
23. Chen M, Lipson S, Hricak H. MR imaging evaluation of benign mesenchymal tumors of the urinary bladder. AJR Am J Roentgenol 1997;168:399–403.
24. Maeda H, Kinukawa T, Hattori R, et al. Detection of muscle layer invasion with sub millimeter pixel MR images: staging of bladder carcinoma. Magn Reson Imaging. 1995;13:9.
25. McCauley TR, McCarthy S, Lange R: Pelvic phased array coil: image quality assessment for spin-echo MR imaging. Magn Reson Imaging. 1992;10:513.
26. Outwater EK, Mitchell DG. Magnetic resonance imaging techniques in the pelvis. MRI Clin North Am. 1994;2:481.
27. Schnall MD, Connick T, Hayes CE, et al. MR imaging of the pelvis with an endorectal-external multicoil array. J Magn Reson Imaging. 1992;2:229.
28. Dershaw DD, Panicek DM. Imaging of invasive bladder cancer. Semin Oncol. 1990;17(5):544–50.
29. Fisher MR, Hricak H, Tanagho EA. Urinary bladder MR imaging. Part II. Neoplasm. Radiology. 1985;157(2):471–7.
30. Tekes A, Kamel IR, Imam K, Chan TY, et al. MR imaging features of transitional cell carcinoma of the urinary bladder. AJR Am J Roentgenol. 2003;180(3):771–7.
31. Mallampati GK. Siegelman ES. MR imaging of the bladder. MRI Clin North Am. 2004;12(3):545–55.
32. Lawler LP. MR imaging of the bladder. Radiol Clin North Am. 2003;41(1):161–77.
33. Neuerburg JM, Bohndorf K, Sohn M, et al. Urinary bladder neoplasms: evaluation with contrast-enhanced MR imaging. Radiology. 1989;172(3):739–43.
34. Venz S, Ilg J, Ebert T, et al. Determining the depth of infiltration in urinary bladder carcinoma with contrast medium enhanced dynamic magnetic resonance tomography: with reference to postoperative findings and inflammation. Urologe A. 1996;35:297.
35. Dickinson AJ, Fox SB, Persad RA, et al. Quantification of angiogenesis as an independent predictor of prognosis invasive bladder carcinomas. Br J Urol. 1994;74(6):762–6.
36. Hawnaur JM, Johnson RJ, Read G, et al. Magnetic resonance imaging with gadolinium-DTPA for assessment of bladder carcinoma and its response to treatment. Clin Radiol. 1993;47:302.
37. Dobson MJ, Carrington BM, Collins CD, et al. The assessment of irradiated bladder carcinoma using dynamic contrast-enhanced MR imaging. Clin Radiol. 2001;56:94–98.
38. Barentsz JO, Jager GJ, van Vierzen PB, et al. Staging urinary bladder cancer after transurethral biopsy: value of fast dynamic contrast-enhanced MR imaging. Radiology. 1996;201(1):185–93.

39. Jager GJ, Barentsz JO, Oosterhof G, et al. Pelvic adenopathy in prostatic and urinary bladder carcinoma: MR imaging with a three-dimensional T1-weighted magnetization-prepared rapid gradient-echo sequence. AJR Am J Roentgenol 1996;167:1503–7.

40. Deserno WM, Harisinghani MG, Taupitz M, et al. Urinary bladder cancer: preoperative nodal staging with ferumoxtran-10-enhanced MR imaging. Radiology. 2004;233(2):449–56.

41. Buy JN, Moss AA, Guinet C, et al. MR staging of bladder carcinoma: correlation with pathologic findings. Radiology 1988;169(3):695–700.

42. Tanimoto A, Yuasa Y, Imai Y, et al. Bladder tumor staging: comparison of conventional and gadolinium-enhanced dynamic MR imaging and CT. Radiology. 1992;185(3):741–7.

43. Tekes A, Kamel I, Imam K, et al. Dynamic MRI of bladder cancer: evaluation of staging accuracy. AJR Am J Roentgenol. 2005;184(1):121–7.

44. Husband JE, Olliff JF, Williams MP, et al. Bladder cancer: staging with CT and MR imaging. Radiology. 1989;173(2):435–40.

45. Neuerburg JM, Bohndorf K, Sohn M, et al. Staging of urinary bladder neoplasms with MR imaging: is Gd-DTPA helpful? J Comput Assist Tomogr. 1991;15(5):780–6.

46. Barentsz JO, Jager G, Mugler JP 3rd, et al. Staging urinary bladder cancer: value of T1-weighted three-dimensional magnetization prepared-rapid gradient-echo and two-dimensional spin-echo sequences. AJR Am J Roentgenol. 1995;164(1):109–15.

47. Hayashi N, Tochigi H, Shiraishi T, et al. A new staging criterion for bladder carcinoma using gadolinium-enhanced magnetic resonance imaging with an endorectal surface coil: a comparison with ultrasonography. BJU Int. 2000;85(1):32–6.

48. Mizuno K, Sasaki T, Saito Y, et al. Gadolinium-enhanced MR imaging, T2-weighted MR imaging, and transurethral Ultrasonography. 2001;61(9):496–501.

49. Bernhardt TM, Rapp-Bernhardt U. Virtual cystoscopy of the bladder based on CT and MRI data. Abdom Imaging. 2001;26(3):325–32. Review.

50. Lammle M, Beer A, Settles M, et al. Reliability of MR imaging-based virtual cystoscopy in the diagnosis of cancer of the urinary bladder. AJR Am J Roentgenol. 2002;178(6):1483–8.

51. Vining DJ. Virtual endoscopy: is it reality? Radiology. 1996;200(1):30–1.

52. Merkle EM, Wunderlich A, Aschoff AJ, et al. Virtual cystoscopy based on helical CT scan datasets: perspectives and limitations. Br J Radiol. 1998;71(843):262–7.

53. Kawai N, Mimura T, Nagata D, et al. Intravenous urography-virtual cystoscopy is a better preliminary examination than air virtual cystoscopy. BJU Int. 2004;94(6):832–6.

54. Tsili ACh, Tsampoulas C, Chatziparaskevas N, et al. Computed tomographic virtual cystoscopy for the detection of urinary bladder neoplasms. Eur Urol. 2004;46(5):579–85.

55. Nambirajan T, Sohaib SA, Muller-Pollard C, et al. Virtual cystoscopy from computed tomography: a pilot study. BJU Int. 2004;94(6):828–31.

56. Kawashima A, Glockner JF, King BF Jr. CT urography and MR urography. Radiol Clin North Am. 2003;41(5):945–61. Review.

57. Lowe FC, Goldman SM, Oesterling JE. Computerized tomography in the evaluation of transitional cell carcinoma in bladder diverticula. Urology. 1989;34:390–5.

58. Das S, Amar AO. Vesical diverticulum associated with bladder carcinoma: therapeutic implications J Urol. 1986;136:1013–4.

59. Messing EM, Catalona WJ. Urothelial tumors of the urinary tract. In: Walsh PC, ed. Cambell's urology. Philadelphia: Saunders, 1998:2343–2348.

60. Chan TY, Epstein JI. In situ adenocarcinoma of the bladder. Am J Surg Pathol 2001;25:892–9.

61. Tekes A, Kamel IR, Chan TY, et al. MR imaging features of non-transitional cell carcinoma of the urinary bladder with pathologic correlation. AJR Am J Roentgenol. 2003;180(3):779–84.

62. Brick SH, Friedman AC, Pollack HM, et al. Urachal carcinoma: CT findings. Radiology. 1988;169(2):377–81.

63. Blute ML, Engen DE, Travis WD, et al. Primary signet ring cell adenocarcinoma of the bladder. J Urol. 1989;141:17–21.

64. Murphy WM. Diseases of the urinary bladder, urethra, ureters, and renal pelvis. In: Murphy WM, editor. Urological pathology. Philadelphia: Saunders; 1997. pp. 98 –111.

65. Blunt DM, Sansom HE, King DM. Imaging of small cell carcinoma of the male urogenital tract. Clin Radiol. 1996;51(10):724–7.

66. Tekes A, Kamel IR, Szarf G, et al. Carcinosarcoma of the urinary bladder: Dynamic contrast-enhanced MR imaging with clinical and pathologic correlation. Am J Roentgenol. 2003;181(1):139–42.

67. Lederle FA, Wilson SE, Johnson GR, et al. Variability in measurement of abdominal aortic aneurysms. Abdominal aortic aneurysm detection and management veterans administration cooperative study group. J Vasc Surg. 1995;21(6):945–52.

68. Brown PM, Pattenden R, Gutelius JR. The selective management of small abdominal aortic aneurysms: the Kingston study. J Vasc Surg. 1992;15(1):21–5; Discussion 25–7.

69. Caoili EM, Cohan RH, Inampudi P, et al. MDCT urography of upper tract urothelial neoplasms. AJR Am J Roentgenol. 2005;184(6):1873–81.

70. Narumi Y, Kadota T, Inoue E, et al. Bladder tumors: staging with gadolinium-enhanced oblique MR imaging, Radiology. 1993;187:145.

Chapter 18

Urothelial Cell Carcinoma in Lower Urinary Tract: Radionuclide Imaging

H.R. Ham and C. van de Wiele

Introduction

Accurate tumor staging is important for determining the clinical management and prognosis of bladder cancer as radical radiotherapy or cystectomy for muscle-invasive bladder cancer has a good chance of cure for diseases confined to the bladder. Unfortunately, morphological staging with computed tomography, transrectal sonography, and MRI including gadolinium-DTPA-enhanced images may be inaccurate in up to 40% of patients. There is therefore a need for improved noninvasive staging modalities in bladder cancer.

Radionuclide methods have been widely used in the work-up of patients with malignancy. Their potential of visualizing molecular changes preceding the physical disruption of the anatomy of structures as imaged by morphological imaging constitutes a major advantage. Several radiopharmaceuticals, both single-photon emitters and positron emitters, have been evaluated for the purpose of staging bladder cancer and for detection of recurrence or for treatment monitoring.

Single-Photon Emitting Agents

Bone Scan

The role of bone scintigraphy (Fig. 18.1) in the staging of bladder cancer before attempted radical therapy was evaluated by Brismar et al. [1] and Davey et al. [2]. Brismar et al. found that from a total of 458 staging bone scans metastases were diagnosed in 4.6%, respectively, true-positive in 2.8% and false-positive in 1.7%. In addition the effect of the bone scanning results on therapy were minimal: cystectomy was performed in spite of the diagnosis of metastases in 16 of 21 patients. Surgery was avoided only in four patients because

of scintigraphy results. Out of 221 patients with invasive bladder cancer, the incidence of detectable metastases found by Davey et al. was 12% with a sensitivity of bone scintigraphy at diagnosis of only 28%.

Gallium-67 and Thallium-201

Gallium-67 is one of the first tumor-imaging agent. It is taken up by actively proliferating malignant cells. Ga-67 tumor imaging is helpful in the work-up of patients with various cancers, in lymphoma in particular. In patients with bladder cancer, however, the sensitivity and the specificity of the technique are too low to be clinically valuable [3].

Thallium-201 (Tl-201) is a potassium analog that accumulates in viable tumor cells via an active uptake mechanism. Tl-201 is a recognized tumor-imaging agent. Yang et al. [4] have evaluated the usefulness of Tl-201 single-photon emission computed tomography (SPECT) in bladder cancer. They studied 14 patients with transitional cell carcinoma (TCC) and 7 normal controls without any history of pelvic disease. In the result, Tl-201 pelvic SPECT detected bladder cancer in all 14 patients (100.0%). In contrast, all seven normal controls (100.0%) had negative results of Tl-201 pelvic SPECT. These surprisingly good results, if confirmed by others, would constitute an important step in clinical practice.

Radiolabeled Antibodies

Many authors have tried monoclonal antibodies for imaging bladder cancer. Yu et al. [5] used monoclonal antibody (BD-1) against human bladder in 19 patients. They showed that a clear immunoscintigraphy was observed in all. Intravesical administration of monoclonal antibody has also been attempted by Malamitsi et al. [6]. They showed that bladder tumors were well imaged using SPECT and Tc-99m-labeled HMFG1 monoclonal antibody. More recently, Simms et al. [7] used a conjugate of the anti-MUC1 monoclonal

H.R. Ham (✉)
Department of Nucleur Medicine, Ghent University, Ghent, Belgium

J.J.M.C.H. de la Rosette et al. (eds.), *Imaging in Oncological Urology*,
DOI 10.1007/978-1-84628-759-6_18, © Springer-Verlag London Limited 2009

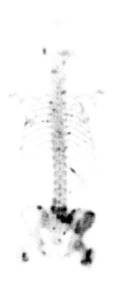

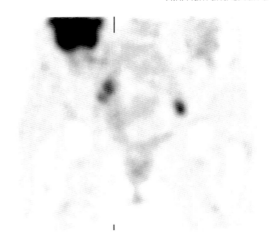

Fig. 18.2 F-18 FDG-PET showing bilateral ilical lymph nodes in a patient operated for primary bladder cancer

Fig. 18.1 Tc-99m MDP bone scintigraphy showing multiple bone metastasis in a patient with primary bladder cancer

antibody C595 and Tc-99m administered intravenously. Of the 20 patients who were found to have tumor at the time of the study, positive localization of the antibody in tumor was apparent in 16. While all these data are really encouraging, a more systematic study on a larger group of patients is required.

Positron Emitting Agents

18-Fluorodeoxyglucose(FDG)

Using F-18 FDG, PET has been shown to be a highly sensitive and specific imaging modality in the diagnosis of primary and recurrent tumors and in the control of therapies in numerous non-urologic cancers (Fig. 18.2).

The applicability of the method to bladder cancer was evaluated by Harney et al. [8]. They transplanted locally metastasizing rat bladder tumor model and evaluated the

extent of FDG uptake in bladder cancer. Significant uptake of FDG in localized bladder tumors in rats was shown, with an average tumor-to-blood ratio of 39 at 2 hours after intravenous FDG administration. Metastases also showed significant uptake of FDG, with an average metastasis-to-blood ratio of 21.7 and tumor involved-to-normal lymph node ratio of 5.3. They also performed an FDG/PET scan in a patient with biopsy-proven recurrent intravesical bladder cancer after radiation therapy. The FDG/PET scan of this patient showed significant extravesical uptake in the pelvis, confirming the abnormality noted on CT. Good images of the clinically apparent metastases in the chest also were obtained.

The potential clinical value of FDG-PET in bladder cancer was first addressed by Bachor et al. [9]. They studied 26 patients with invasive bladder cancer. The primary bladder tumor was found in 85% of cases. In a larger series from the same author [10] reporting on preoperative FDG-PET imaging in 64 patients with bladder cancer, true-positive lymph node detection was obtained in 14 patients and false-negative results observed in 7 patients. In 37 patients the PET result was true-negative and in 6 patients false-positive resulting in a sensitivity of 67%, a specificity of 86%, and an accuracy of 80%. Heicappell et al. [11] found an increase in FDG in two out of three patients with lymph nodes involvement.

The major difficulty in FDG-PET for detecting bladder tumor is the presence of the tracer accumulation in the bladder which masks the tracer uptake in the tumor.

To overcome this difficulty, Kosuda et al. [12] performed PET study with retrograde irrigation of the urinary bladder with saline during the PET study. Dynamic PET images were also obtained in addition to the static acquisition. FDG-PET scanning was true-positive in eight patients (66.7%), but false-negative in four (33.3%). They also showed that FDG-

PET scanning detected all of the 17 distant metastatic lesions and two of three proven regional lymph node metastases.

Other approaches have been made to reduce the amount of excreted FDG in the bladder including the use of diuretics but the results have largely been disappointing.

C-11 Methionine, C-11 and F18-Choline

C-11 methionine has been used as tumor-imaging agent for several years. In cancer, methionine uptake is correlated with the amount of viable tissue [13]. C-11 methionine undergoes rapid clearance from the blood pool, it is primarily metabolized in liver and pancreas with no significant renal excretion. Ahlstrom et al. [14] have attempted to detect bladder cancer using C-11 methionine PET. While the tracer uptake in the primary tumor was related to tumor grade, only 78% of all bladder cancers could be visualized.

Various studies have revealed an increased choline uptake as well as an upregulated activity of choline kinase and elevated levels of phosphorylcholine in cancer cells [15–17]. Based on these observations, Hara and coworkers [18] introduced C-11 choline for imaging of malignancies. The use of C-11 choline PET for the detection of bladder cancer has been initiated by de Jong et al. [19]. They performed PET with C-11 choline in 18 patients before cystectomy and in 5 volunteers. Normal bladder tissue showed little tracer uptake and there was only minimal urinary activity. The primary tumor was visualized in 10 patients with residual invasive disease in the cystectomy specimen. In another seven patients no residual tumor was found at the time of cystectomy. Premalignant lesions were present in three of these but were missed by PET. In the remaining patient PET was true-negative. One false-positive finding was related to inflammatory changes from an indwelling bladder catheter.

The main handicap of C-11 choline is the short half-life of C-11, an on-site cyclotron is needed for its clinical use. A fluorinated choline derivative has been recently developed that should overcome this limitation [20].

Discussion and Conclusion

The definition of the local extension of primary tumor and the detection of loco-regional lymph node or distant metastases are essential in treatment planning and outcome assessment of patients with cancer. In case of bladder cancer, correct preoperative staging is difficult because of the low sensitivity of conventional imaging techniques resulting in understaging of both local extension of the primary tumor and lymph node involvement [21].

Several nuclear medicine techniques have been evaluated for the staging of bladder cancer. Bone scintigraphy is one of the most widely employed for the detection of bone metastasis. While the technique also allows the detection of bone metastasis of a bladder cancer, its sensitivity is too low to be useful. Additionally, as its specificity is also low, a systematic use of this technique is not recommended in the work-up of patient with bladder cancer.

Ga-67 has no value for staging bladder cancer because of the presence of high abdominal activity and not enough data are available to judge an eventual utility of Tl-201 imaging and of monoclonal antibody imaging.

While results obtained using FDG-PET are better than those obtained by classical staging procedures such as CT or MRI, the sensitivity and the specificity of FDG-PET are still not good enough for its systematic use and for the time being, it has not found widespread acceptance for presurgical staging of bladder cancer. The use of combined PET–CT imaging is expected to reduce the number of false-positive findings in the lower abdomen and pelvis, which should increase the accuracy of the test [22, 23]. Similarly, not enough data are available in the literature to assess the value of other PET tracers for staging of bladder cancer.

Finally, the value of nuclear medicine techniques for detection of recurrence or to assess therapy response has not been fully addressed.

References

1. Brismar J, Gustafson T. Bone scintigraphy in staging of bladder carcinoma. Acta Radiol. 1988;29(2):251–2.
2. Davey P, Merrick MV, Duncan W, Redpath AT. Bladder cancer: the value of routine bone scintigraphy. Clin Radiol. 1985;36(1):77–9.
3. Sauerbrunn BJ, Andrews GA, Hubner KF. Ga-67 citrate imaging in tumors of the genito-urinary tract: report of cooperative study. J Nucl Med. 1978;19(5):470–5.
4. Yang CC, Shiau YC, Sun SS, Kao CH. Detection of bladder cancer using single-photon emission computed tomography of thallium-201: a preliminary report. Anticancer Res. 2003;23(3C):2977–80.
5. Yu LZ, Gu FL, Zhang CL. Radioimmunoimaging diagnosis of human bladder carcinoma. Scand J Urol Nephrol Suppl. 1994;157:13–7.
6. Malamitsi J, Zorzos J, Varvarigou AD, Archimandritis S, Dassiou C, Skarlos DV, et al. Immunolocalization of transitional cell carcinoma of the bladder with intravesically administered technetium-99m labelled HMFG1 monoclonal antibody. Eur J Nucl Med. 1995;22(1):25–31.
7. Simms MS, Perkins AC, Price MR, Scholfield DP, Bishop MC. 99mTechnetium-C595 radioimmunoscintigraphy: a potential staging tool for bladder cancer. BJU Int. 2001;88(7):686–91.
8. Harney JV, Wahl RL, Liebert M, Kuhl DE, Hutchins GD, Wedemeyer G, et al. Uptake of 2-deoxy, 2-(18F) fluoro-D-glucose in bladder cancer: animal localization and initial patient positron emission tomography. J Urol. 1991;145(2):279–83.
9. Bachor R, Kocher F, Gropengiesser F, Reske SN, Hautmann RE. Positron emission tomography. Introduction of a new procedure in

diagnosis of urologic tumors and initial clinical results. Urologe A. 1995;34(2):138–42.

10. Bachor R, Kotzerke J, Reske SN. Lymph node staging of bladder neck carcinoma with positron emission tomography. Urologe A. 1999;38:46–50.

11. Heicappell R, Muller-Mattheis V, Reinhardt M. Staging of pelvic lymph nodes in neoplasms of the bladder and prostate by positron emission tomography with 2-[(18)F]-2-deoxy-D-glucose. Eur Urol. 1999;36:582–7.

12. Kosuda S, Kison PV, Greenough R. Preliminary assessment of fluorine-18 fluorodeoxyglucose positron emission tomography in patients with bladder cancer. Eur J Nucl Med. 1997;24:615–20.

13. Kubota R, Kubota K, Yamada S, Tada M, Takahashi T, Iwata R, et al. Methionine uptake by tumor tissue: a microautoradiographic comparison with FDG. J Nucl Med. 1995;36(3):484–92.

14. Ahlstrom H, Malmstrom PU, Letocha H. Positron emission tomography in the diagnosis and staging of urinary bladder cancer. Acta Radiol. 1996;37:180–85.

15. Ratnam S, Kent C. Early increase in choline kinase activity upon induction of the H-ras oncogene in mouse fibroblast cell lines. Arch Biochem Biophys. 1995;323:313–322.

16. Ackerstaff E, Pflug BR, Nelson JB, Bhujwalla ZM. Detection of increased choline compounds with proton nuclear magnetic resonance spectroscopy subsequent to malignant transformation of human prostatic epithelial cells. Cancer Res. 2001;61(9): 3599–603.

17. Katz-Brull R, Degani H. Kinetics of choline transport and phosphorylation in human breast cancer cells; NMR application of the zero trans method. Anticancer Res. 1996;16:1375–1380.

18. Hara T, Kosaka N, Shinoura N, Kondo T. PET imaging of brain tumor with [methyl-11C]choline. J Nucl Med. 1997;38(6):842–7.

19. de Jong IJ, Pruim J, Elsinga PH, Jongen MM, Mensink HJ, Vaalburg W. Visualisation of bladder cancer using (11)C-choline PET: first clinical experience. Eur J Nucl Med Mol Imaging. 2002;29(10):1283–8.

20. Hara T. 18F-fluorocholine: a new oncologic PET tracer. J Nucl Med. 2001;42(12):1815–7.

21. Ficarra V, Dalpiaz O, Alrabi N, Novara G, Galfano A, Artibani W. Correlation between clinical and pathological staging in a series of radical cystectomies for bladder carcinoma. BJU Int. 2005;95(6):786–90.

22. Schoder H, Erdi YE, Larson SM, et al. PET/CT: a new imaging technology in nuclear medicine. Eur J Nucl Med Mol Imaging. 2003;30:1419–37.

23. Bar-Shalom R, Yefremov N, Guralnik L, et al. Clinical performance of PET/CT in evaluation of cancer: additional value for diagnostic imaging and patient management. J Nucl Med. 2003;44:1200–9.

Chapter 19

Considerations: Imaging in Urothelial Cell Carcinoma of the Lower Urinary Tract

T.M. de Reijke

The cornerstone in the treatment of patients suspected for a tumor of the lower urinary tract is optimal imaging of the inside of the urinary bladder and complete transurethral resection (TUR) of all visible lesions. Based on the findings during and following TUR, tumors can be divided in non-muscle invasive bladder cancer (NMIBC) and muscle invasive bladder cancer. In case of a NMIBC different prognostic groups can be discriminated, based on number of tumors, size, presence of carcinoma in situ (CIS), previous recurrence rate, and tumor grade. (good, intermediate, and poor prognosis groups). Using these determinants Sylvester et al. recently presented the EORTC risk tables that can be used to determine the probability for recurrence and progression [1]. In case of a NMIBC radiological imaging is not advised, since the chance of extra-vesical tumor growth or metastatic disease is very small. It is still debated whether upper tract imaging should be performed at all, because synchronous tumors are found in only 0.3–2.3% [2–4]. However, in case of follow-up of recurrent NMIBC or in patients with high-grade NMIBC imaging of the upper tract is useful. The risk of the presence of tumor(s) in the upper tract increases in these cases from 5 to 21% with a follow-up of 5–15 years [5]. Improvement on imaging of the inside of the bladder is necessary, since Brausi et al. showed that the recurrence rate at 3 months following TUR of single or multiple bladder tumors ranged from 3.4 to 20.6% and from 7.4 to 45.8%, respectively [6]. These recurrences were not all real recurrences, but there were certainly a number of "overlooked" tumors. The imaging quality has since this report been improved considerably through the introduction of flexible cystoscopy with or without digital imaging and video resection. No data are known yet whether this has resulted in a reduction in the 3-month recurrence rate.

In order to be able to perform a complete resection of all visible and non-visible tumors, several new methods have been introduced and/or are under evaluation.

Photodynamic diagnosis (PDD) is one of the methods that has now been introduced in urological clinical practice for the treatment of bladder cancer. The principle is based on the interaction between light and certain photosensitizers in tissue. The illumination of these photosensitizing agents in light of a specific wavelength results in emission of fluorescence which can be used for diagnostic purposes (Fig. 19.1). Recently, the Hexylester Hexylaminolevulinic acid (Hexvix®) has been approved for clinical use.

It has been demonstrated that by using PDD more patients were diagnosed with CIS of the bladder compared to white light cystoscopy, 97 versus 58% [7, 8]. However, also an improvement was found in the detection of Ta and T1 bladder tumors; 29 and 15% more tumors were respectively detected using PDD [9]. Finally, PDD can also be applied to perform a more complete resection by identifying all malignant areas and especially the borders of the tumor(s). Three studies have shown that during re-TUR 4–6 weeks following TUR under white light or PDD-guided TUR, less tumor areas were found using PDD compared to white light resection [10–12].

Narrow band imaging (NBI) is another technique that is now being evaluated to test whether better identification of bladder tumor(s) can be achieved. This technique has been developed by Olympus and is now ready for clinical evaluation. NBI is a high-resolution endoscopic technique that enhances the fine structure of the mucosal surface without the use of dyes. NBI is based on the phenomenon that the depth of light penetration depends on its wavelength; the longer the wavelength, the deeper the penetration. Blue light penetrates only superficially, whereas red light penetrates into the deeper layers. The first prototype NBI system (Olympus Corp., Tokyo, Japan) is based on a light source with sequential red, green, and blue (RGB) illumination. White light from a xenon lamp is passed through a rotary RGB filter that separates the white light into the colors red, green, and blue, which are used to sequentially illuminate the mucosa. The red, green, and blue reflected light is detected separately by a monochromatic charged coupled device (CCD) placed at the tip of the endoscope, and the three images are integrated into a single color image by the video processor. In addition to the

T.M. de Reijke (✉)
Department of Urology, Academic Medical Center, Amsterdam

J.J.M.C.H. de la Rosette et al. (eds.), *Imaging in Oncological Urology*,
DOI 10.1007/978-1-84628-759-6_19, © Springer-Verlag London Limited 2009

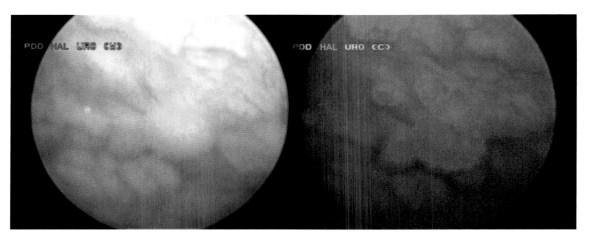

Fig. 19.1 Left: white light cystoscopy; right: PDD cystoscopy with Hexvix®

conventional RGB filters for white light endoscopy (WLE), the narrow band imaging system has special RGB filters of which the band-pass ranges have been narrowed and the relative contribution of the blue light has been increased.

The technique has been clinically tested already in gastroenterology and is now starting to be tested in bladder cancer patients [13]. The first personal experience with this NBI technique in 20 patients has shown that tumors are identified more easily, if more tumors are being detected (SKIP and) cannot be concluded from this small series. In contrast to PDD-guided TUR, NBI-guided TUR is much easier since there is no scatter image and it seems that also more complete resections can be performed. A second advantage of NBI over PDD is the lower costs compared to PDD since no agents have to be instilled into the bladder prior to TUR. Of course, this preliminary experience should be further tested in comparative studies.

Endoluminal-applied *optical coherence tomography* (OCT) offers an imaging technique, which might enhance endo-urological diagnosis by improving the estimation of tumor invasiveness and tumor grading.

OCT employs light to obtain images instead of sound waves as B-mode ultrasonography does. Light is directed into tissue where it is reflected. The back-reflected light is measured against a reference light-arm. OCT determines the optical path length, which the light has covered. Tissue layers are discriminated and determined by the time required from the light traveling from the light source through the tissue and back. The depth which can be discriminated is about 1–1.5 mm [14]. Studies using OCT to determine bladder alterations demonstrated the ability to discriminate the microstructure, such as urothelium, submucosa and muscularis of the bladder wall [15, 16] (Fig. 19.2). The resolution at 10 μm is higher than any other clinical imaging technology and provides exceptional real-time information over structural tissue alterations. The combination of a high-resolution

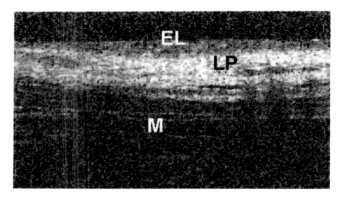

Fig. 19.2 OCT image. EL: epithelial layer, LP: lamina propria, M: muscularis

imaging technique and modern endo-urological approaches seems promising to improve diagnosis and therapy in upper urinary tract disorders. Manyak et al. have described a clinical series in 24 patients using OCT, where they found a sensitivity of 100% and an overall specificity of 89% for detecting urothelial malignancies [17]. Probably this technique should be used in combination with PDD or NBI in order to decrease false positive biopsies or resection and to guide the resection.

Another technique in development is the *Raman spectroscopy*, an optical technique that utilizes molecule-specific, inelastic scattering of light photons to interrogate biological tissues. When tissue is illuminated with laser light, photons interact with intramolecular bonds within the tissue. The photon donates energy to or receives energy from the bond, producing a change in the bond's vibrational state. When it subsequently exits the tissue, the photon has an altered energy level and, therefore, a different wavelength from the original laser light. This change in the photon's energy is known as the "Raman shift" and is measured in wave numbers. Photons interacting with different

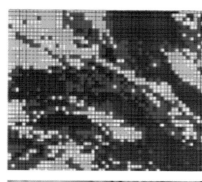

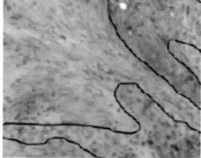

Fig. 19.3 Raman spectroscopy

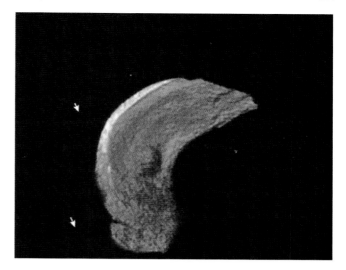

Fig. 19.4 Three-dimensional ultrasonography

biochemical bonds within the tissue undergo different Raman shifts, which, taken together, form the "Raman spectrum," a plot of intensity against Raman shift in wave numbers (Fig. 19.3). As the Raman shift is inversely proportional to the change in photons' wavelength, wave numbers are expressed in units of centimeters. The Raman spectrum is a direct function of the molecular composition of the tissue and can therefore give a truly objective picture of the pathology [18].

De Jong et al. evaluated this technique on bladder tissue samples and demonstrated that Raman spectroscopy could effectively discriminate between tumorous and non-tumorous tissue based on characterized biochemical differences [19]. This technique should also be used in combination with PDD or NBI to direct the imaging device to the region of interest.

All these techniques still use the transurethral route which can be bothersome for the patient. Nowadays, also non-invasive techniques can be used to visualize the inside of the bladder, such as virtual endoscopy. Multi-slice technology in CT and fast gradients in MRI in combination with improved data analysis could allow this technique to be introduced in clinical urological practice for specific cases where standard cystoscopy is not possible [20].

A less expensive non-invasive technique is virtual cystoscopy using 3D ultrasonography, which has been tested in animals and recently the first clinical experience was described (Fig. 19.4). In 42 patients presenting with hematuria and/or irritative symptoms, 3D ultrasonography was

more accurate compared to standard 2D ultrasonography [21, 22].

In case of demonstrated muscle invasive bladder cancer or high-risk NMIBC (T1G3 plus TIS), a metastatic work-up is essential before a potential curative approach is performed. As discussed before CT scan and MRI are the investigations of choice to detect lymphogenic or hematogenous tumor spread. If lymph node metastases could be identified more reliably, neo-adjuvant chemotherapy combination therapy could be applied.

In case a patient is not a surgical candidate, external beam radiotherapy is an alternative treatment option. In order to increase the dose to the bladder tumor and to "spare" the normal bladder mucosa and thus decrease post-radiation bladder irritative symptoms, it would be advantageous to visualize the area where the tumor is located in the blad-

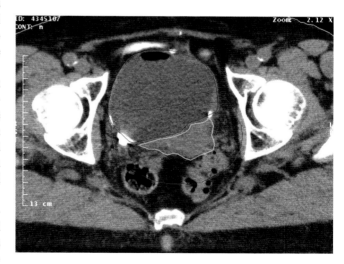

Fig. 19.5 Bladder tumor marked with endovesical lipiodol

der. This approach is now evaluated using endovesical clips or lipiodol application around the bladder tumor (Fig. 19.5). This technique was shown to be feasible and safe. A higher accuracy combined with a reduction in target volume will reduce the risk of toxicity and could allow dose escalation, hopefully leading to improvement in the outcome of bladder cancer treatment [23].

References

1. Sylvester RJ, Van der Meijden APM, Oosterlinck W, Witjes JA, Bouffioux C, Denis L, et al. Predicting recurrence and progression in individual patients with Ta T1 bladder cancer using EORTC risk tables: a combined analysis of 2596 patients from 7 EORTC trials. Eur Urol. 2006;49:466–77.
2. Goessl C, Knispel HH, Miller K, Klan R. Is routine excretory urography necessary at first diagnosis of bladder cancer? J Urol. 1997;157:480–81.
3. Harranz-Amo F, Diez-Cordero JM, Verdu-Tartajo F, Bueno-Chomon G, Leal-Hernandez F, Bielsa-Carillo A. Need for intravenous urography in patients with primary transitional cancer of the bladder? Eur Urol. 1999;36:221–4.
4. Youssem DM, Gatewood OM, Goldman SM, Marshall FF. Synchronous and metachronous transitional cell carcinoma of the urinary tract: prevalence, incidence, and radiographic detection. Radiology. 1988;167:613–8.
5. Herr HW, Cookson MS, Soloway SM. Upper tract tumors in patients with primary bladder cancer followed for 15 years. J Urol. 1996;156:1286–7.
6. Brausi M, Collette L, Kurth K, van der Meijden AP, Oosterlinck W, Witjes JA, et al. Variability in the recurrence rate at first follow-up cystoscopy after TUR in stage TaT1 transitional cell carcinoma of the bladder: a combined analysis of seven EORTC studies. Eur Urol. 2002;41:523–31.
7. Fradet Y, Grossman HB, Gomella L, Lerber S, Cookson M, Albala D, et al. A comparison of hexaminolevulinate fluorescence cystoscopy and white light cystoscopy for the detection of carcinoma in situ in patients with bladder cancer: a phase III, multicenter study. J Urol. 2007;178: 68–73.
8. Schmidbauer J, Witjes F, Schmeller N, Donat R, Susani M, Marberger M, et al. Improved detection of urothelial carcinoma in situ with hexaminolevulinate (HAL) fluorescence cystoscopy. J Urol. 2004;171:135–8.
9. Grossman HB, Gomella L, Fradet Y, Morales A, Presti J, Ritenour C, et al. A phase III, multicenter comparison of hexaminolevulinate fluorescence cystoscopy and white light cystoscopy for the detection of superficial papillary lesions in patients with bladder cancer. J Urol. 2007;178:62–7.
10. Filbeck T, Pichlmeier U, Knuechel R, Wieland WF, Roessler W. Do patients profit from 5-aminolevulinic acid-induced fluorescence diagnosis in transurethral resection of bladder carcinoma? Urology. 2002;60:1025–8.
11. Kriegmair M, Zaak D, Rothenberger KH, Rassweiler J, Jocham D, Eisenberger F, et al. Transurethral resection for bladder cancer using 5-aminolevulinic acid induced fluorescence endoscopy versus white light endoscopy. J Urol. 2002;168:475–8.
12. Riedl CR, Daniltchenko D, Koenig F, Simak R, Loening SA, Pflueger H. Fluorescence endoscopy with 5-aminolevulinic acid reduces early recurrence rate in superficial bladder cancer. J Urol. 2001;165:1121–3.
13. Hirata M, Tanaka S, Oka S, Kaneko I, Yoshida S, Yoshihara M, et al. Evaluation of microvessels in colorectal tumors by narrow band imaging magnification. Gastrointest Endosc. 2007;66:945–52.
14. Grimbergen M, Aalders MC, van Leeuwen TG. Optical imaging and diagnosis in bladder cancer. In: Imaging in oncological oncology. Springer Verlag London Limited. 2009;403–15.
15. Xie T, Xie H, Fedder GK, Pan Y. Endoscopic optical coherence tomography with a modified microelectromechanical systems mirror for detection of bladder cancers. Appl Opt. 2003;42:6422–6.
16. Jesser CA, Boppart SA, Pitris C, Stamper DL, Nielsen GP, Brezinski ME, et al. High resolution imaging of transitional cell carcinoma with optical coherence tomography: feasibility for the evaluation of bladder pathology. Br J Radiol. 1999;72:1170–6.
17. Manyak MJ, Gladkova ND, Makari JH, Schwartz AM, Zagaynova EV, Zolfaghari L, et al. Evaluation of superficial bladder transitional-cell carcinoma by optical coherence tomography. J Endourol. 2005;19:570–4.
18. Mahadevan-Jansen A, Richards-Kortum RR. Raman spectroscopy for the detection of cancers and precancers. J Biomed Optics. 1999;1:31–70.
19. De Jong BW, Schut TC, Maquelin K, van der Kwast T, Bangma CH, Kok DJ, et al.. Discrimination between nontumor bladder tissue and tumor by Raman spectroscopy. Anal Chem. 2006;78:7761–9.
20. Bernhardt TM, Rapp-Bernhardt U. Virtual cystoscopy of the bladder based on CT and MRI data. Abdom Imaging. 2001;26:325–32.
21. Moon MH, Kim SH, Lee YH, Cho JY, Jung SI, Park SH, et al. Diagnostic potential of three-dimensional ultrasound-based virtual cystoscopy: an experimental study using pig bladders. Invest Radiol. 2006; 41: 883–9.
22. Mitterberger M, Pinggera GM, Neuwirt H, Maier E, Akkad T, Strasser H, et al. Three-dimensional ultrasonography of the urinary bladder: preliminary experience of assessment in patients with haematuria. BJU Int. 2007;99:111–6.
23. Hulshof MCCM, van Andel G, Bel A, Gangel P, van de Kamer JB. Intravesical markers for delineation of target volume during external focal irradiation of bladder carcinomas. Radiother Oncol. 2007;84:49–51.

Part V
Prostate Carcinoma

Chapter 20

Prostate Carcinoma: Introduction

E.A. Klein

Epidemiology and Risk Factors

Incidence and Mortality

Prostate cancer is the fourth most common male malignancy worldwide. Its incidence varies widely between countries and ethnic populations and disease rates disease differ by more than 100-fold between populations. The lowest yearly incidence rates occur in Asia (1.9 cases per 100,000 in Tianjin, China) and the highest in North America and Scandinavia, especially in African-Americans (272 cases per 100,000) [1]. In the United States, prostate cancer has been the most common visceral malignancy in men since 1984 and now accounts for one-third of all such cancers [2]. The estimated lifetime risk of disease for U.S. males is 17.6% for Caucasians and 20.6% for African-Americans, with a lifetime risk of death of 2.8 and 4.7%, respectively. The incidence of prostate cancer peaked in 1992, approximately 5 years after introduction of PSA as a screening test, fell precipitously until 1995, and has been rising slowly since at a slope similar to that observed prior to the PSA era (Fig. 20.1). The fall in incidence between 1992 and 1995 has been attributed to the "cull effect" of identifying previously unknown cancers in the population by the use of PSA, followed by a return to baseline where fewer cases were detected in previously screened individuals [3]. As in the United States, prostate cancer incidence has increased in many countries since the early 1990s. Although much of the increase can be correlated with the introduction of PSA, some of the increase predates screening [4].

Mortality also varies widely among countries, being highest in Sweden (23 per 100,000 per year) and lowest in Asia (<5 per 100,000 per year in Singapore, Japan, and China)

E.A. Klein (✉)
Cleveland Clinic Lerner College of Medicine, Head, Section of Urologic Oncology, Glickman Urological Institute, Cleveland Clinic Foundation, Cleveland, OH, USA, kleine@ccf.org

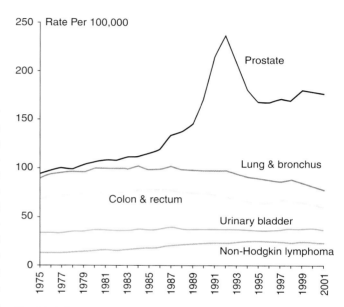

Fig. 20.1 Cancer incidence rates for men, United States, 1975–2001. Age adjusted to the 2000 US standard population.
Source: Surveillance, Epidemiology, and End Results Program, 1975–2001, Division of Cancer Control and Population Sciences, National Cancer Institute, 2004

[1]. Mortality rates across Europe are variable, with, for example, mortality twice as high in Norway as in Spain (24 per 100,000 compared with 13 per 100,000). Mortality rates increased slowly for most countries between 1985 and 1995 [1]. In the United States, prostate cancer mortality rates rose slowly between 1973 and 1990 (Fig. 20.2). This may have resulted from a gradual increase in the number of biologically lethal cancers or a decreasing use or effectiveness of therapy during this interval. Subsequent to 1991, the peak mortality year, steady declines in prostate cancer mortality were reported for the next decade. The magnitude of this decline is nearly 2.5 times larger than the increase in mortality seen as a result of attribution bias, so it seems likely that the declines in prostate cancer mortality in the United States since 1991 are real and clinically significant [3]. In 2005 the American Cancer Society estimates 30,350 prostate

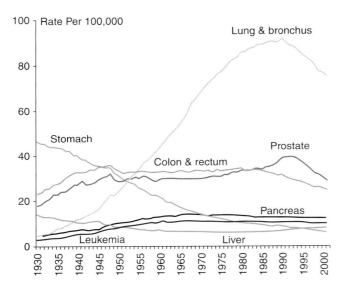

Fig. 20.2 Cancer death rates for men, United States, 1930–2001. Age adjusted to the 2000 US standard population.
Source: Surveillance, Epidemiology, and End Results Program, 1975–2001, Division of Cancer Control and Population Sciences, National Cancer Institute, 2004.

cancer-related deaths in the United States, for an approximate annual rate of 30 per 100,000 population, representing a 25% decrease from the peak in 1991 [5]. Furthermore, the mortality rate for prostate cancer in white men in the United States has declined to a level lower than that observed prior to the introduction of PSA-based screening in 1987 [6].

There are multiple complex causes for the worldwide and ethnic variations in prostate cancer incidence. Access to and quality of health care, the accuracy of cancer registries, and the penetrance of PSA screening all affect how rates of disease are reported. The observed decline in mortality in the United States since 1991 is temporally related to increased diagnostic and treatment activity in both the pre-PSA and PSA eras. Rates of both radical prostatectomy (RP) and radiation therapy rose steadily through the 1980s (pre-PSA era), whereas hormone therapy and no-treatment rates remained stable [3]. Outcomes for patients treated in the 1980s should be reflected in the mortality data of the 1990s, while outcomes for patients treated in the PSA era (the 1990s) have had less time to affect recent mortality data. Given the long natural history of low-stage cancers detected in the PSA era, their treatment would not be expected to have a substantial effect on mortality statistics for 10–15 years. Additional observation time is necessary to determine if screening, PSA-induced stage migration, and more aggressive use of therapy have contributed to declining mortality. Before reliable data were available from African countries, rates of prostate cancer in Africa were thought to be much the same as those in Asia. However, in Uganda and Nigeria prostate cancer is very common, and in Nigeria it is the

most common cancer in men [4]. Environment also plays an important role in modulating prostate cancer risk around the world. Japanese and Chinese men in the United States have a higher risk of developing and dying from prostate cancer than do their relatives in Japan and China [7]. Likewise, prostate cancer incidence and mortality have increased in Japan as the country has become more Westernized [8]. It is important to note, however, that Asian-Americans have a lower prostate cancer incidence than white or African-Americans men, indicating that genetics still plays a role in determining prostate cancer predisposition.

Racial Differences

While anthropologists accept that there are subtle biological differences between populations, commonly used categories such as African American, Caucasian, and Hispanic are social and cultural descriptors that have no defined biological basis. Observed disease-related differences between groups defined in this fashion may therefore be more reflective of common environmental exposure, diet, lifestyle, and attitudes toward health care than of differences in genetic structure or function, and attributions of biological differences between such groups should therefore be interpreted cautiously. Recognizing these caveats, it is noteworthy that African-American men have the highest reported incidence of prostate cancer in the world, with a relative incidence of 1.6 compared to white men in the United States [5]. Furthermore, age-adjusted prostate cancer-related mortality is 2.4 times higher for African Americans than whites. Recent data quantifies this difference, demonstrating a 1.8-year shorter survival for African Americans with localized disease treated by RP, 0.7 years shorter after radiation, and 1 year shorter in those choosing watchful waiting, findings that persist after adjusting for other covariates including education and income levels [9].

Many biological, environmental, and social hypotheses have been advanced to explain these differences, ranging from postulated differences in genetic predisposition; differences in mechanisms of tumor initiation, promotion and/or progression; higher fat diets, higher serum T levels, or higher body mass index; structural, financial, and cultural barriers to screening, early detection and aggressive therapy; and physician bias. Differences in screening rates between Caucasians and African Americans may play a role in explaining the differences in mortality, since a more completely screened population will have better apparent survival because of the inclusion of more individuals with nonlethal cancers. There are currently no data that clearly indicate any of these hypotheses as being the determining factor in explaining the observed differences in incidence or mortality, and it seems likely that the source of the disparity is mutlifactorial. Recent observations suggest that the incidence of organ-confined disease at diagnosis among African Americans is increasing, that the disparity in mortality is lessening in the PSA era, and that those with organ-confined disease can be cured at a high rate regardless of race [5, 10]. The incidence of prostate cancer in other ethnic groups is lower than that in whites and African Americans, with approximate age-adjusted annual rates of 50 per 100,000 for American Indians/Alaskan Natives, 105 per 100,000 for Asians or Pacific Islanders, and 140 per 100,000 for Hispanics in 2001 [11]. Comparative data for prostate cancer-related mortality is not available for these groups.

Age and Stage Migration

Prostate cancer is rarely diagnosed in men < 50 years old, accounting for only <0.1% of all patients. Peak incidence occurs between ages 70 and 74 years, with 85% diagnosed after age 65 [11]. At age 85 the cumulative risk of clinically diagnosed prostate cancer ranges from 0.5 to 20% worldwide, despite autopsy evidence of microscopic lesions in approximately 30% of men in the fourth and 50% in the sixth decade and in > 75% of men aged > 85 [4]. PSA-based screening has induced an important age migration effect, with the incidence of prostate cancer in men 50–59 years increasing by 50% between 1989 and 1992 [12], with important implications for deciding on the need for, type of, and complications after therapy.

In addition to changes in prostate cancer incidence and mortality over the last several decades, there has been a substantial shift to more favorable stage at presentation in men with newly diagnosed disease. This clinical stage migration is largely if not exclusively accounted for by PSA screening [13]. Since the introduction of PSA testing, the incidence of local-regional disease has increased, whereas the incidence of metastatic disease has decreased [14]. Diagnosis of local-regional disease increased 18.7% annually in white men between 1988 and 1992 and then decreased, on average, 9.8% annually through 1995 [12]. In contrast, the incidence of metastatic disease decreased 1.3% annually from 1988 to 1992 and then 17.9% annually through 1995. Nonpalpable cancers (AJCC clinical stage T1c) now account for 75% of newly diagnosed disease [15]. Concomitant with these changes, the percentage of men treated for clinically localized disease with RP increased substantially [12]. Clinical stage migration has also been associated with improvements in 5- and 10-year survival, which for all stages combined now are 100 and 92%, respectively [5].

The use of PSA has also resulted in a substantial downward pathological stage migration as evidenced by an increasing incidence of organ-confined disease at RP [15, 16]. The improvement in pathological stage has been seen for clinical stages T1–T3 tumors and all tumor grades, and has resulted in improved cancer-specific survival after external radiation or surgery for patients treated late in the PSA era [15–17].

Effect of Screening on Mortality

Screening for prostate cancer remains controversial because of the lack of randomized controlled trials demonstrating a reduction in mortality in screened populations. However, the observed trends in PSA-induced clinical and pathological stage migration and declining mortality where screening is common provide inferential evidence that screening is beneficial [18]. Opponents of screening contend that there is no proof that earlier detection has led to the observed declines in prostate cancer mortality, that increased treatment for screen-detected cancers do more harm than good, and that the long natural history of prostate cancer means that any beneficial effects of screening are not yet evident in mortality statistics. Screening may have led to decreased mortality rates in patients having tumors with shorter lead times (i.e., more aggressive cancers) [19]. The debate over the effect of screening on mortality is unlikely to be settled until the results of two large, randomized trials in the United States and Europe (PLCO and ERSPC) are reported later in this decade.

Risk Factors

Although the specific causes of prostate cancer initiation and progression are not yet known, considerable evidence suggests that both genetics and environment play a role in the origin and evolution of this disease. Classic and molecular epidemiology have identified a number of potential risk factors associated with the development of prostate cancer.

Familial and Genetic Influences

Ample epidemiologic evidence suggests that prostate cancer has both a familial and a genetic component. The first reports of a familial clustering were published in the mid-20th century and suggested that the risk of developing prostate cancer was higher in those with an affected first-degree relative [20]. Subsequent case–control and cohort studies have confirmed this observation, estimating the relative risk (RR) of prostate cancer in first-degree relatives of affected men at 0.64–11 [21]. Twin studies have also suggested a genetic component, with higher rates of concordance for monozygotic than dizygotic brothers [22–24]. Relative risk increases according to the number of affected family members, their degree of relatedness, and the age at which they were affected [25].

For investigative purposes prostate cancer may be conveniently divided into three phenotypes: sporadic, familial, and hereditary. Sporadic cancers occur in individuals with a negative family history. Familial prostate cancer is defined as cancer in a man with ≥ 1 affected relatives. Hereditary prostate cancer is a subset of the familial form and has been defined as nuclear families with ≥ 3 affected members, prostate cancer in 3 successive generations, or 2 affected individuals diagnosed with cancer before age 55 [26]. While most prostate cancer is likely to be polygenic in origin, the existence of a true hereditary form is suggested by three epidemiologic observations: (1) relatives of patients < 55 years old are at higher risk of getting prostate cancer than those with older affected relatives; (2) there is stronger familial clustering in families with early onset prostate cancer; and (3) the number of affected family members and their age at onset are the most important determinants of risk among relatives. Sporadic cancers account for about 85% of all prostate cancers and about 15% are familial and/or hereditary. Hereditary prostate cancer accounts for 43% of early onset disease (age 55 or younger) but only 9% of all cancers occurring by age 85 [27].

Evidence for major prostate cancer susceptibility genes that segregate into families has been obtained from several complex segregation analyses, with the majority supporting a dominant and the remainder supporting recessive or X-linked modes of inheritance [28]. At least nine candidate prostate cancer susceptibility genes have been reported, including *RNASEL/HPC1* [29], *ELAC2/HPC2* [30], *SRA/MSR1* [31], *CHEK2* [32], *BRCA2* [33], *PON1* [34], *OGG1* [35], *MIC-1* [36], and *TLR4* [37]. Individually these genes likely account for only a small fraction of the observed genetic predisposition to prostate cancer. Other segregation studies have suggested the existence of other prostate cancer susceptibility loci on chromosomes 1q42.2–43 (named *PCAP*) [38], 1p36 (named *CAPB* and linked to brain tumors) [39], and Xq27–28 [40], but the gene or genes linked to these regions have not been cloned or identified. More recent genome-wide scans in larger cohorts of hereditary prostate cancer families have identified additional chromosomal loci linked to prostate cancer, and it is likely that the number of identifiable susceptibility genes will increase [28].

Inflammation and Infection

Chronic inflammation leading to cellular hyperproliferation to replace damaged tissue contributes to the development of infection-associated cancers of the colon, esophagus, stomach, bladder, and liver [41, 42]. In 2005 the US Department of Health and Human Services added three infectious agents (hepatitis B virus, hepatitis C virus, and human papilloma virus) to the list of known cancer-causing agents [43]. The hepatic, cervical, and head and neck cancers caused by these viruses share a common pathogenesis of long latency after viral exposure and an inflammatory component to tumor promotion [43]. Accumulating epidemiologic, histologic, and genetic evidence suggests a similar process may underlie the development of prostate cancer.

Additional evidence suggests that prostate cancer may have an infectious etiology. A meta-analysis of 23 case–control studies reported a statistically significant association of prostate cancer with a history of sexually transmitted infection (relative risk [RR]= RR = 1.4; 95% CI = 1.2–1.7), including an RR of 2.30 (95% CI = 1.3–3.9) for syphilis and 1.34 (95% CI 1.2–1.6) for gonorrhea [44]. Similarly, a meta-analysis of 11 case–control studies revealed a statistically significant risk of prostate cancer (odds ratio [OR] = 1.57, 95% CI 1.0–2.4) for those reporting a history of prostatitis [45]. Supportive evidence is provided by a small number of studies demonstrating positive associations of antibodies against syphilis, human papilloma virus (HPV), and human herpes virus-8 (HHV-8) with prostate cancer [42]. Case-only or case–control studies have also reported higher plasma concentrations of acute phase reactants and proinflammatory cytokines in men with prostate cancer, including C-reactive protein, IL-6, IL-8, IL-1β, and TNF-α, especially in advanced or hormone refractory disease [42]. Two studies have demonstrated evidence of viral pathogens in human prostate tissue, including polyomavirus, human papilloma virus, and cytomegalovirus [46, 47].

Inflammatory infiltrates and a histologic lesion called proliferative inflammatory atrophy (PIA) are frequently seen in clinical prostate specimens [48]. PIA is a spectrum of lesions characterized by epithelial atrophy, low apoptotic index, and an increased proliferative index, usually associated with inflammatory infiltrates [49]. Inflammation in PIA may include mononuclear infiltrates in the periglandular stroma and macrophages and/or neutrophils in the glandular lumen or epithelium. Macrophages activated by IFN-gamma secrete proinflammatory cytokines and reactive nitrogen species (e.g., nitric oxide, NO). Inducible NO synthase, which catalyzes the generation of NO, is overexpressed in macrophages in PIA but not in normal epithelium [50]. PIA cells typically show many signs of stress, including the induction of GSTP1, GSTA1, and COX-2 expression [50]. The evidence suggests that PIA is a regenerative lesion appearing as a consequence of infection or cell trauma resulting from oxidant damage, hypoxia, infection, or autoimmunity, and that its hyperproliferative state leads to cancer. PIA is often found adjacent to high-grade prostatic intraepithelial neoplasia (HGPIN) or early cancer [49], and accumulating evidence suggests an identifiable genetic pathway between PIA, HGPIN, and cancer, with progressively frequent *TP53* mutations, gains in centromeric DNA sequences on chromosome 8, and GSTP1 CpG island hypermethylation [50–52].

The previously described genetic and histologic observations in prostate cancer strongly suggest that compromised cellular defenses against inflammatory oxidants may initiate and perpetuate prostatic carcinogenesis. Oxidative stress is mediated by reactive oxygen and nitrogen species (ROS and RNS) which bind DNA and cause mutations, and oxidant stresses from exogenous and endogenous sources are implicated in the accumulation of DNA damage that occurs with aging and subsequently leads to malignancy [41]. Cellular defense mechanisms against this process include (1) front-line antioxidant enzymes which scavenge ROS/RNS and prevent mutations; (2) enzymes to repair mutated DNA; and (3) the ability to undergo apoptosis if the DNA damage is too severe to repair. An analysis of the known prostate cancer susceptibility genes and other genetic defects in prostate cancer suggests that inherited and acquired defects in cellular defense mechanisms against infection and oxidative stress allow prostate cancer to develop.

Androgens

There is little doubt that a lifetime of variable exposure of the prostate to androgens plays an important role in prostate carcinogenesis. Long-term absence of androgen exposure to the prostate appears to protect against the development of prostate cancer, but a dose–response relationship between androgen levels and prostate cancer risk has not been established. The primary androgen of the prostate is DHT, irreversibly catalyzed from T by 5α-reductase. DHT binds to intracytoplasmic AR with much greater affinity than T, and binding of DHT to the AR enhances translocation of the steroid–receptor complex into the nucleus and activation of androgen-response elements [53]. Functional type-2 5α-reductase is a prerequisite for normal development of the prostate and external genitalia in males. Insufficient exposure of the prostate to DHT appears to protect against the development of prostate cancer. Transrectal ultrasonography of males with inherited 5α-reductase deficiency demonstrates miniscule prostatic tissue, and biopsies demonstrate prostatic stroma but no epithelium [54]. In addition to the lack of enzyme activity, a lack of T may also protect against the development of prostate cancer, as evidenced by the atrophic prostates seen in men after surgical castration [55]. Although exposure of the prostate to androgens seems to be prerequisite for later development of prostate cancer, the duration and magnitude of androgen exposure needed to set the stage for carcinogenesis is unknown.

Diet

Descriptive epidemiologic studies of migrants, geographic variations, and temporal studies suggest that dietary factors may contribute to prostate cancer development [56]. The incidence of latent prostate cancers is similar around the world, but the incidence of clinically manifest cancers differs, with Asians having among the lowest rates of clinical prostate cancer in the world. Thus, the most convincing evidence for the role of the diet and other environmental factors in modulating prostate cancer risk comes from migration studies showing an increased incidence of prostate cancer in first-generation immigrants to the United States from Japan and China [7]. These observations suggest that diet may play a role in converting latent tumors into clinically manifest ones. A strong positive correlation exists between prostate cancer incidence and the corresponding rates of several other diet-related cancers, including breast cancer and colon cancer [56]. Prostate cancer incidence and mortality rates around the world correlate highly with the average level of fat consumption, especially for polyunsaturated fats [56]. High levels of dietary fat stimulate proliferation of prostate cancer cells both in vitro and in vivo, and animal models have shown that a fat-free diet can reduce the growth of androgen-dependent tumors in the Dunning model [57].

Treatment

Localized Disease

The treatment of localized prostate cancer remains controversial because of the lack of conclusive well-controlled or randomized studies comparing outcomes of external beam radiotherapy (RT) to brachytherapy (BT) or radical prostatectomy (RP). A randomized trial published in 1982 showing an advantage of RP was never widely accepted because of randomization artifacts and worse-than previously reported RT results [58, 59]. The Southwest Oncology Group closed a randomized study comparing these two modalities in the mid-1980s due to poor accrual. More recently, an attempt to complete a randomized trial of RP vs. BT (the SPIRIT Trial) also closed because of lack of accrual. The unsettled nature of this issue is further complicated by the marked polarization of radiation oncologists and urologists in their counseling of patients with newly diagnosed localized disease, with surgeons recommending surgery and radiation therapists recommending radiation in virtually all circumstances [60].

An important issue in judging comparative outcomes is the effect of PSA-based screening on pathological stage migration. As discussed previously, the rate of organ-confined disease for a given stage, grade, and pre-treatment PSA value has increased markedly in the PSA era [61]. Year of diagnosis is an independent predictor of the likelihood for cure [62], suggesting that the observed increase in the rate of organ-confined disease has translated into improved disease-free survival for patients treated with RP. These observations also suggest that improvements in outcome for other therapies such as external RT and BT reported during this interval may be related as much to downward pathological stage migration as to improvements in specific therapeutic techniques, and that it is inappropriate to compare current outcomes with historical controls.

Another difficulty in comparing the relative efficacy of different therapies arises from differences in patient selection. The ability of pretreatment parameters including biopsy grade, clinical stage, and PSA to predict the likelihood of cure for RP and all forms of RT is well established. In the last 20 years there has been a tendency to restrict RP to those with the most favorable pre-treatment characteristics and refer the less favorable for RT, and based on these differences in patient selection, one would predict that biochemical failure rates would be worse after RT, even if the two treatments were actually equally efficacious. A comparison of different therapies for localized prostate cancer should include issues of cancer control, morbidity, quality of life, salvage of primary treatment failures, late effects, and cost. Of these, cancer control is the most important, since most patients would be willing to sacrifice some morbidity or quality of life for the best chance of cure. A detailed discussion of all of these issues is beyond the scope of this chapter, but the reader is referred to several recent primary articles and reviews that address these issues in detail [63, 64]. At present, based on single institutional experiences and published comparative series, it is fair to say that biochemical control rates at 10 years after initial therapy are similar with all three of the commonly used modalities, and that the convenience and tolerance for short-term side effects often dictate a patients' choice of therapy.

Locally Advanced Disease

Despite the beneficial effect of PSA-induced pathological stage migration to more organ-confined tumors, approximately 10% of men with newly diagnosed prostate cancer present with locally advanced disease. Such patients have a higher risk of tumor progression due to local recurrence after definitive therapy, occult nodal metastases, or systemic disease. Although there are no firmly established definitions of locally advanced disease, retrospective analysis of large radical prostatectomy (RP) and radiation cohorts have identified pretreatment characteristics that are associated with a higher likelihood of recurrence. Similarly, long-term follow-

up of RP series has defined pathological features that are associated with a higher risk of failure. Pretreatment factors which may be used to define locally advanced disease include high Gleason's grade (8 or above), high-volume palpable tumor (clinical stage T2b/c, T3, or T4), high PSA (above 15 or 20, when attributable to tumor and not a large transition zone volume), and/or involvement of more than 50% of cores by tumor or more than 50% of the length of 1 or more cores on prostate biopsy, all in the absence of clinically demonstrable lymph node or systemic metastases. Pathological features which define higher risk for recurrence include predominantly Gleason pattern ≥ 4 tumors, extracapsular extension, positive margins, seminal vesicle invasion, and/or lymph node metastasis. Various molecular markers which predict the likelihood of aggressive behavior are also under study [65]. Because relying on a single pretreatment or pathological parameter to predict the likelihood of failure for an individual patient is unreliable, the definition of locally advanced disease is usually made by combining these factors. Pretreatment parameters may be combined to define low, intermediate, and high-risk groups (D'Amico classification) [66]; the likelihood of finding adverse pathological features (Partin nomogram) [67]; or the likelihood of suffering biochemical recurrence (Kattan nomogram) [68, 69]. A nomogram for predicting the likelihood of biochemical failure based on pathological findings is also available [70].

There is currently no consensus on the best approach for treating men with locally advanced disease, and experience in the PSA era with both RP and RT has demonstrated that neither modality alone provides acceptable cure rates for these men. Long-term bRFS data from our RP series suggest that 35% of men with seminal vesicle invasion and negative margins are disease free at 15 years, an observation suggesting that the entire seminal vesicles should be removed at the time of RP; in addition, 20% of patients with positive lymph nodes are NED at 15 years, and there is emerging data that suggest an extended lymphadenectomy may prolong survival in men with positive nodes. Another advantage to an initial surgical approach is that accurate pathological staging information is obtained, identifying those patients with organ-confined disease who can be spared the morbidity of additional therapy. The disadvantages of the surgical approach is the almost certain erectile dysfunction that accompanies wide resection of the neurovascular bundles which is generally indicated in locally advanced disease and the fact that even some men with organ confined disease will fail systemically despite good local control. Advocates of a radiation-based approach point to both improved bRFS outcomes and local control with highly conformal and intensity modulated techniques which permit significant dose-escalation without increased morbidity. These techniques may permit the use of RT without or with only short course hormone therapy and thus do a better job of maintaining erectile function in the short term. A number of combined modality approaches are under actively study, including RT and BT together, and various neoadjuvant and adjuvant approaches combining systemic therapy with RP or RT.

Metastatic Disease

Androgen deprivation (ADT) in various forms remains the mainstay of therapy for metastatic disease and can achieve significant palliation and delay disease progression. Unfortunately, the emergence of androgen independence is eventually manifest in most patients and leads to progressive disease and death in the majority. Historically, androgen-independent cancer was manifested by symptoms of disease progression including bone pain, anemia, fatigue, and cachexia, and was poorly responsive to systemic therapy with a median survival of 6–12 months. As PSA became widely utilized in the late 1980s, a new class of androgen-independent patients appeared, namely those with a rising PSA following hormonal therapy without evidence of clinical metastatic disease. This subset of "biochemical" progressors has become the largest subset of this disease entity and represents a growing clinical challenge. The adverse effects of ADT are well understood, and we are beginning to understand how to address some of these side effects. Nevertheless, there is strong interest in developing ADT strategies that may be less morbid, and just as importantly, may be more durable. Intermittent ADT holds promise in this regard but no definitive conclusions can be drawn about its efficacy until completion of two large randomized studies, one in metastatic disease, the other in patients with "PSA-only" disease. New knowledge about androgen receptor signaling in castration-resistant prostate cancer is driving the development of new therapies which target this pathway distal to the initial testosterone–AR interaction which is the target of existing forms of ADT. A large inventory of novel agents targeting this and other pathways are currently in clinical trials and the remaining challenge is to develop systems to help understand biologic and clinical activity, prioritize drug development, and develop target validation strategies for these agents. In the case of immunologic therapeutics, it has become increasingly clear that prostate cancer can indeed be targeted, that immune tolerance can be broken, and that a variety of strategies hold great promise. The utility of bisphosphonates for the treatment and prevention of bone metastases is now established, but enthusiasm for their use should be tempered by the relative lack of randomized data in earlier disease states, and the small but real risk of significant complications such as osteonecrosis of the jaw. The approval of docetaxel for advanced prostate cancer based on a minor improvement in survival is a tremendous advance, raises as yet uninvestigated issues related to the timing of chemotherapy, and will result in a new disease state characterized by resistance to both hormones and chemotherapy that require development of additional therapeutic advances.

Issues in Staging

Assigning the correct stage for a newly diagnosed patient is critical to determining the best available treatment modality and the need for combined modality treatment. Unlike other cancers, where the extent of soft-tissue disease is readily evident on anatomically based scans such as CT or MRI, the available imaging modalities for prostate cancer are limited by its microscopic nature and tropism for sites not amenable to easy measurement (i.e., bone). Except for the detection of the rare individual with seminal vesicle invasion, even organ-directed modalities such as endorectal MRI have limited ability to stage the local extent of the cancer. Standard radiographic assessment of patients with metastatic prostate cancer is currently limited primarily to radionuclide bone scintigraphy, CT scan imaging of abdomen and pelvis with selected use of MRI for evaluation of bone lesions and as the de facto standard of care in evaluation of patients for spinal cord compression. Although changes in PSA kinetics are increasingly supported as an important component of response assessment, in particular in studies with cytotoxic agents, as noted above, prospective validation of this approach has not yet been accomplished. Although assessment of soft tissue disease on CT imaging using RECIST criteria is standardized, the majority of patients with advanced prostate cancer do not manifest disease amenable to this approach. Although some investigators have proposed quantifiable methods of using both radionuclide bone scintigraphy and MRI imaging for assessment of response in metastatic prostate cancer, these approaches have not been validated. New approaches to disease assessment in patients with advanced prostate cancer with special emphasis on bone metastases are also unequivocally needed. This book provides a detailed overview of the available modalities that address current shortcomings and provides a glimpse of their potential for improvement in the clinical management of patients with all stages of prostate cancer.

Future Challenges

There remain many challenges to be faced for prostate cancer. Although PSA-based screening has not been proven to reduce mortality, its high penetrance of use in the United States and the aging of the "baby boomer" population make it likely that the incidence of prostate cancer will not be declining in the near future. Furthermore, 95% of newly diagnosed men in the United States choose therapy over observation, and of those who choose observation 50% get some form of active treatment within 3 years [71]. Even striking findings from the Prostate Cancer Prevention Trial, which demonstrated that oral finasteride can reduce the risk of being diagnosed with prostate cancer by 25%, albeit with a slight increased risk of histologically appearing higher grade disease, have not appreciably changed physician or patient behavior [72]. Thus, the main questions faced today are (1) can those at risk of developing prostate cancer be identified?; (2) can prostate cancer be prevented in high-risk individuals?; (3) of those who get prostate cancer, can biologically indolent disease be distinguished from biologically aggressive tumors that require therapy?; (4) for those who choose surveillance, when is the right time to intervene?; 5) for those who choose therapy, can we improve on the ability to predict cure using biological markers added to clinical ones?; 6) can newer imaging techniques improve staging or be exploited for therapy?; and 7) for those with incurable disease, can we develop improved therapies that will prolong life or result in cure?

References

1. Quinn M, Babb P. Patterns and trends in prostate cancer incidence, survival, prevalence and mortality. Part I: international comparisons. Brit J Urol Intl. 2002;90:162–73.
2. Jemal A, Tiwari RC, Murray T, Ghafoor A, et al. American cancer society: cancer statistics. CA Cancer J Clin. 2004;54:8–29.
3. Stephenson RA. Prostate cancer overdiagnosis and overtreatment. Analysis of US mortality and SEER incidence. Trends in the PSA and Pre-PSA Eras. In: Klein EA, editors. Management of prostate cancer. 2nd ed. Totowa, NJ: Humana Press; 2005. pp. 3–13.
4. Grönberg H. Prostate cancer epidemiology. Lancet. 2003;361:859–64.
5. American Cancer Society, Cancer Facts & Figures. 2005.
6. Tarone RE, Chu KC, Brawley OW. Implications of stage-specific survival rates in assessing recent declines in prostate cancer mortality rates. Epidemiology. 11:167–70, 2000.
7. Shimizu H, Ross RK, Bernstein L, et al. Cancers of the prostate and breast among Japanese and white immigrants in Los Angeles County. Br J Cancer. 1991;63:963–6.
8. Landis SH, Murray T, Bolden S, Wingo PA. Cancer statistics, 1999. CA Cancer J Clin. 1999;49:8–31.
9. Godley PA, Schenck AP, Amamoo A, et al. Racial differences in mortality among Medicare recipients after treatment for localized prostate cancer. J Natl Cancer Inst. 2003;95:1702–10.
10. Powell IJ, Bsanerjee M, Bianco FJ, et al. The effect of race/ethnicity on prostate cancer treatment outcome is conditional: a review of Wayne State University data. J Urol. 2004;171:1508.
11. Ries LAG, Eisner MP, Kosary CL, et al. (editors). SEER Cancer Statistics Review, 1975–2001. Bethesda, MD: National Cancer Institute, 2004. http://seer.cancer.gov/csr/1975–2001/.
12. Hankey BF, Feuer EJ, Clegg LX, et al. Cancer surveillance series: interpreting trends in prostate cancer—part I: evidence of the effects of screening in recent prostate cancer incidence, mortality, and survival rates. J Natl Cancer Inst. 1999;91:1017–24.
13. Mettlin C, Murphy GP, Lee F, et al. Characteristics of prostate cancers detected in a multimodality early detection program. The Investigators of the American Cancer Society-National Prostate Cancer Detection Project. Cancer. 1993;72:1701–8.
14. Newcomer LM, Stanford JL, Blumenstein BA, Brawer MK. Temporal trends in rates of prostate cancer: Declining incidence of advanced stage disease, 1974 to 1994. J Urol. 1997;158:1427–30.
15. Derweesh IH, Kupelian PA, Zippe C, et al. Continuing trends in pathological stage migration in radical prostatectomy specimens. Urol Oncol. 2004;22:300–6.
16. Jhaveri FM, Klein EA, Kupelian PA, et al. Declining rates of extracapsular extension after radical prostatectomy: evidence for continued stage migration. J Clin Oncol. 1999;17:3167–72.
17. Kupelian P, Kuban D, Thames H, et al. Improved biochemical relapse-free survival with increased external radiation doses in patients with localized prostate cancer: the combined experience of nine institutions in patients treated in 1994 and 1995. Int J Radiat Oncol Biol Phys. 2005;61:415–509.
18. Horninger W, Berger A, Pelzer A, et al. Screening for prostate cancer: updated experience from the Tyrol study. Can J Urol. 2005;12(Suppl 1):7–13.
19. Etzioni R, Legler JM, Feuer EJ, et al. Cancer surveillance series: interpreting trends in prostate cancer—part III: Quantifying the link between population prostate-specific antigen testing and recent declines in prostate cancer mortality. J Natl Cancer Inst. 1999;91:1033–9.
20. Woolf C. An investigation of the familial aspects of carcinoma of the prostate. Cancer. 1960;13:739–44.
21. Eeles RA, Dearnaley DP, Ardern-Jones A, et al. Familial prostate cancer: the evidence and the Cancer Research Campaign/British Prostate Group (CRC/BPG) UK Familial Prostate Cancer Study. Br J Urol. 1997:79 Suppl 1:8–14.
22. Gronberg H, Damber L, Damber J-E. Studies of genetic factors in prostate cancer in a twin population. J Urol. 1994;152:1484–9.
23. Ahlbom A, Lichtenstein P, Malmstrom H, Feychting M, Hemminki K, Pedersen NL. Cancer in twins: genetic and nongenetic familial risk factors. J Natl Cancer Inst. 1994;89:287–93.
24. Page WF, Braun MM, Partin AW, Caporaso N, Walsh P. Heredity and prostate cancer: a study of World War II veteran twins. Prostate. 1997;33:240–5.
25. Bratt O. Hereditary prostate cancer: clinical aspects. J Urol. 2002;168:906–13.
26. Carter BS, Bova GS, Beaty TH, et al. Hereditary prostate cancer: epidemiologic and clinical features. J Urol. 1993;150:797–802.
27. Carter BS, Beaty TH, Steinberg GD, Childs B, Walsh PC. Mendelian inheritance of familial prostate cancer. Proc Natl Acad Sci USA. 1992;89:3367–71.
28. Gillanders EM, Xu J, Chang BL, et al. Combined genome-wide scan for prostate cancer susceptibility genes. J Natl Cancer Inst. 2004;96:1240–47.
29. Carpten J, Nupponen N, Isaacs S, et al. Germline mutations in the ribonuclease L (RNase L) gene in hereditary prostate cancer 1 (HPC1)-linked families. Nat Genet. 2002;30:181–4.
30. Tavtigian SV, Simard J, Teng DH, et al. A candidate prostate cancer susceptibility gene at chromosome 17p. Nat Genet. 2001;27:172–80.
31. Xu J, Zheng SL, Komiya A, et al. Germline mutations and sequence variants of the macrophage scavenger receptor 1 gene are associated with prostate cancer risk. Nat Genet. 2002;32:321–5.
32. Dong X, Wang L, Taniguchi K, et al. Mutations in CHEK2 associated with prostate cancer risk. Am J Hum Genet. 2003;72:270–80.
33. Edwards SM, Kote-Jarai Z, Meitz J, et al. Two percent of men with early-onset prostate cancer harbor germline mutations in the BRCA2 gene. Am J Hum Genet. 2003;72:1–12.

34. Marchesani M, Hakkarainen A, Tuomainen TP, et al. New paraoxonase 1 polymorphism I102V and the risk of prostate cancer in Finnish men. J Natl Cancer Inst. 2003;95:812–908.

35. Xu J, Zheng SL, Turner A, et al. Associations between hOGG1 sequence variants and prostate cancer susceptibility. Cancer Res. 2002;62:2253–7.

36. Lindmark F, Zheng SL, Wiklund F, et al. H6D polymorphism in macrophage-inhibitory cytokine-1 gene associated with prostate cancer. J Natl Cancer Inst. 2004;96:1248–54.

37. Zheng SL, Augustsson-Balter K, Chang B, Hedelin M, et al. Sequence variants of toll-like receptor 4 are associated with prostate cancer risk: results from the Cancer Prostate in Sweden Study. Cancer Res. 2004;64:2918–22.

38. Berthon P, Valeri A, Cohen-Akenine A, et al. Predisposing gene for early-onset prostate cancer, located on chromosome 1q42.2-43. Am J Hum Genet. 1998;62:1416–20.

39. Gibbs M, Stanford JL, McIndoe RA, et al. Evidence for a rare prostate cancer susceptibility locus at chromosome 1p36. Am J Hum Genet. 1999;64:776–80.

40. Xu J, Meyers D, Freije D, et al. Evidence for a prostate cancer susceptibility locus on the X chromosome. Nature Genet. 1998;20:175–8.

41. Coussens LM, Werb Z. Inflammation and cancer. Nature. 2002;420: 860–7.

42. Platz EA, De Marzo AM. Epidemiology of inflammation and prostate cancer. J Urol. 2004;171:S36–40.

43. U.S. Department of Health and Human Services, Public Health Service, National Toxicology Program, 11th Report on Carcinogens, 2005. http://ntp.niehs.nih.gov/ntp/roc/toc11.html (2005). Accessed 6 June 2005.

44. Dennis LK, Dawson DV. Meta-analysis of measures of sexual activity and prostate cancer. Epidemiology. 2002;13:72–9.

45. Dennis LK, Lynch CF, Torner JC. Epidemiologic association between prostatitis and prostate cancer. Urology. 2002;60:78–83.

46. Samanta M, Harkins L, Klemm K, Britt WJ, Cobbs CS. High prevalence of human cytomegalovirus in prostatic intraepithelial neoplasia and prostatic carcinoma. J Urol. 2003;170:998–1002.

47. Zambrano A, Kalantari M, Simoneau A, et al. Detection of human polyomaviruses and papillomaviruses in prostatic tissue reveals the prostate as a habitat for multiple viral infections. Prostate. 2002;53:263–76.

48. DeMarzo AM, Marchi VL, Epstein JI, Nelson WG. Proliferative inflammatory atrophy of the prostate: implications for prostatic carcinogenesis. Am J Pathol. 1999;155:1985–92.

49. Putzi MJ, De Marzo AM. Morphologic transitions between proliferative inflammatory atrophy and high-grade prostatic intraepithelial neoplasia. Urology. 2000;56:828–32.

50. Nelson WG, De Marzo AM, Isaacs WB. Prostate cancer. N Engl J Med. 2003;349:366–81.

51. Shah R, Mucci NR, Amin A, Macoska JA, Rubin MA. Postatrophic hyperplasia of the prostate gland: neoplastic precursor or innocent bystander? Am J Pathol. 2001;767–73.

52. Nakayama M, Bennett CJ, Hicks JL, et al. Hypermethylation of the human glutathione S-transferase-pi gene (GSTP1) CpG island is present in a subset of proliferative inflammatory atrophy lesions but not in normal or hyperplastic epithelium of the prostate: a detailed study using laser-capture microdissection. Am J Pathol. 2003;163:923–33.

53. Steers WD: 5-alpha-reductase activity in the prostate. Urology. 2001;58(Suppl 1):17–24.

54. Imperato-McGinley J, Gautier T, Zirinsky K, et al. Prostate visualization studies in males homozygous and heterozygous for 5 alpha-reductase deficiency. J Clin Endocrinol Metab. 1992;75:1022–6.

55. Wilson JD, Roehrborn C. Long-term consequences of castration in men: lessons from the Skoptzy and the eunuchs of the Chinese and Ottoman courts. J Clin Endocrinol Metab. 1999;84:4324–31.

56. Bostwick DG, Burke HB, Djakiew D, et al. Human prostate cancer risk factors. Cancer. 2004;101:2371–490.

57. Wang Y, Corr JG, Thaler HT, et al. Decreased growth of established human prostate LNCaP tumors in nude mice fed a low-fat diet. J Natl Cancer Inst. 1995;87:1456–9.

58. Paulson DF, Lin GH, Hinshaw W, et al. Radical surgery versus radiotherapy for adenocarcinoma of the prostate. J Urol. 1982;128:502–4.

59. Hanks GE. More on the Uro-Oncology Research Group report of radical surgery vs. radiotherapy for adenocarcinoma of the prostate. Int J Radiat Oncol Biol Phys. 1988;14:1053–4.

60. Fowler FJ, Jr., McNaughton Collins M, Albertsen PC, et al. Comparison of recommendations by urologists and radiation oncologists for treatment of clinically localized prostate cancer. JAMA. 2000;283:3217–22.

61. Jhaveri FM, Klein EA, Kupelian PA, et al. Declining rates of extracapsular extension after radical prostatectomy: evidence for continued stage migration. J Clin Oncol. 1999;17:3167–72.

62. Han M, Partin AW, Piantadosi S, Epstein JI, Walsh PC. Era specific biochemical recurrence-free survival following radical prostatectomy for clinically localized prostate cancer. J Urol. 2001;166: 416–9.

63. Kupelian PA, Elshaikh M, Reddy CA, Zippe CD, Klein EA. Comparison of the efficacy of local therapies for localized prostate cancer in the PSA era: a large single institution experience with radical prostatectomy and external beam radiotherapy. J Clin Oncol. 2002;20:3376–85.

64. Klein EA, Kupelian PA. Localized prostate cancer: radiation or surgery? Urol Clin North Am. 2003;30:315–30.

65. Trudel D, Fradet Y, Meyer F, et al. Significance of MMP-2 expression in prostate cancer: an immunohistochemical study. Cancer Res. 2003;63:8511–5.

66. D'Amico AV, Whittington R, Malkowicz SB, et al. Predicting prostate specific antigen outcome preoperatively in the prostate specific antigen era. J Urol. 2001;166:2185–8.

67. Partin AW, Kattan MW, Subong EN, et al. Combination of prostate-specific antigen, clinical stage, and Gleason score to predict pathological stage of localized prostate cancer. A multi-institutional update. JAMA. 1997;277:1445–51.

68. Kattan MW, Zelefsky MJ, Kupelian PA, et al. Pretreatment nomogram that predicts 5-year probability of metastasis following three-dimensional conformal radiation therapy for localized prostate cancer. J Clin Oncol. 2003;21:4568–71.

69. Graefen M, Karakiewicz PI, Cagiannos I, et al. International validation of a preoperative nomogram for prostate cancer recurrence after radical prostatectomy. J Clin Oncol. 2002;20:3206–12.

70. Graefen M, Karakiewicz PI, Cagiannos I, et al. Validation study of the accuracy of a postoperative nomogram for recurrence after radical prostatectomy for localized prostate cancer. J Clin Oncol. 2002;20:951–6.

71. Cooperberg MR, Broering JM, Litwin MS, Lubeck DP, Mehta SS, Henning JM, et al. CaPSURE Investigators: The contemporary management of prostate cancer in the United States: lessons from the cancer of the prostate strategic urologic research endeavor (CapSURE), a national disease registry. J Urol. 2004;171(4): 1393–401.

72. Klein EA, Tangen CM, Goodman PJ, Lippman SM, Thompson IM. Assessing benefit and risk in the prevention of prostate cancer: the prostate cancer prevention trial revisited. J Clin Oncol. 2005;[Epub ahead of print]

Chapter 21

Prostate Carcinoma: Conventional Imaging Techniques – Gray-Scale, Color, and Power Doppler Ultrasound

M. Mitterberger, L. Pallwein, and F. Frauscher

Introduction

Prostate cancer is the most common non-skin cancer in men in Europe and the United States, and is second only to lung cancer as a cause of cancer deaths in men. In the United States an estimated 230,000 men will be diagnosed with prostate cancer in 2004, and nearly 30,000 will die of the disease [1]. Nevertheless, the fact that the vast majority of tumors are now detected either localized to the prostate or regionally spread, while only a small percentage are detected at the metastatic stage, has highlighted the importance of earlier detection and diagnosis of the disease [1]. The use of prostate-specific antigen (PSA) testing has allowed physicians to detect tumors at much earlier stages of disease, and the recognition of finer points of disease pathology has enabled physicians to establish more comprehensive and detailed staging criteria [2, 3].

Current research in the areas of detection and diagnosis are primarily focusing on two main areas: identification of risk factors for disease in the general public that warrant regular screening; identification of imaging strategies for early detection of disease and disease progression, and use of these imaging strategies in predicting outcomes in different patient populations. The imaging techniques used include ultrasound (US), magnetic resonance imaging (MRI), and positron emission tomography (PET).

Prior to the widespread use of PSA screening in asymptomatic men, prostate cancer was detected via digital rectal examination (DRE), and only 25% of newly diagnosed prostate cancers were clinically organ confined [4, 5]. Since the advent of PSA testing, the percentage of newly diagnosed organ-confined and locally advanced disease has increased to upward of 80% [1]. Currently, clinical practice guidelines recommend the use of both PSA and DRE in asymptomatic men [5, 6]. Although PSA testing can detect tumors at a far earlier stage than DRE, DRE as part of a comprehensive physical exam can help physicians better assess the extent of the disease and its effect on surrounding organs. Of note, the positive predictive value of DRE increases with higher PSA levels, and the addition of DRE can more than double the predictive value in patients with a PSA level of > 4 ng/mL [7]. The use of PSA as a screening tool can be challenging. Although its name suggests that it is produced and secreted solely by the prostate gland, PSA is produced by other tissues as well – breast tissue, the periurethral glands, parotid gland, and adrenal and renal cell tumors – albeit in very low concentrations [8]. Transient or persistent elevations in serum PSA concentrations can also reflect changes in the prostate gland due to chronic or recurrent inflammation, trauma, ejaculation, urinary retention, and benign proliferation or enlargement [9–11]. Certain medications, including herbal supplements, can also cause changes in serum PSA [10–12]. A careful history and repeat PSA measurements can help distinguish between transient PSA rises due to these conditions and persistent rises due to prostate cancer, potentially minimizing unnecessary biopsy of noncancerous tissue. Of these, elevated PSA measurements due to benign conditions, particularly benign prostatic hyperplasia (BPH), most directly underscore the difficulty in making a decision about the need for biopsy in asymptomatic men. Although cancerous prostate tissue releases up to 30 times more PSA in the serum than does hyperplastic tissue [8, 13], BPH remains the most common cause of elevated serum PSA concentration [10]. However, PSA testing has shown to have a high sensitivity but lacks specificity.

The standard care in patients with an elevated PSA and or an abnormal DRE is transrectal US (TRUS)-guided systematic biopsy of the prostate. Gray-scale US has a low sensitivity and specificity for prostate cancer detection, with the chance that a hypoechoic lesion – which is the most common appearance of prostate cancer on gray-scale US – varies between 3 and 51%. Specifically, TRUS is limited

M. Mitterberger (✉)
Department of Radiology II and Urology, Medical University Innsbruck, Anichstrasse 35, Innsbruck 6020, Austria,
ferdinand.frauscher@i-med.ac.at

J.J.M.C.H. de la Rosette et al. (eds.), *Imaging in Oncological Urology*,
DOI 10.1007/978-1-84628-759-6_21, © Springer-Verlag London Limited 2009

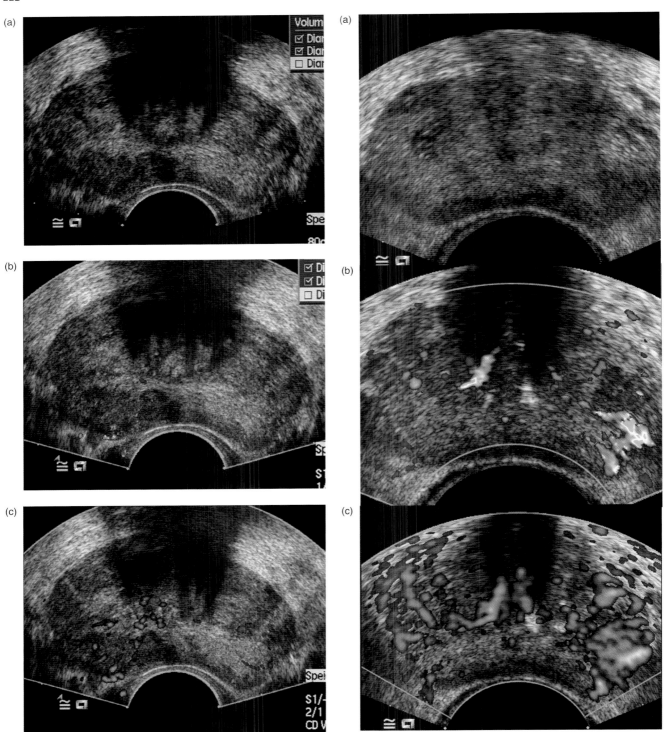

Fig. 21.1 Transrectal ultrasound (gray-scale US) in a 56-year-old patient with elevated PSA of 4.5 ng/ml. TRUS shows a hypoechoic lesion in the right mid-gland. (**a**) Targeted biopsy revealed prostate cancer (Gleason score 7). The corresponding color Doppler (**b**) and power Doppler images (**c**) show hypervascularity and flow asymmetry in this lesion

Fig. 21.2 A 65-year-old patient with an elevated PSA of 4 ng/ml. In the transcretal ultrasound (gray-scale US) a hypoechoic lesion on the left side can be seen. The targeted biopsy revealed prostate cancer (Gleason score 8). The corresponding color Doppler (**b**) and power Doppler images (**c**) show hypervascularity and flow asymmetry in this lesion

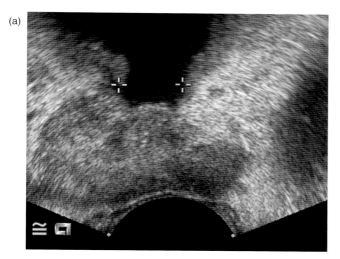

(a)

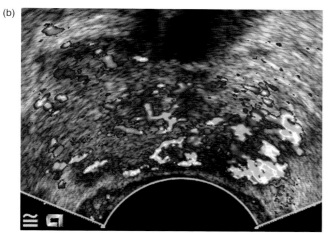

(b)

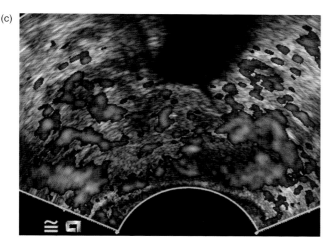

(c)

Fig. 21.3 A 72-year-old patient with an elevated PSA of 16 ng/ml and status post-TURP. In the transcretal ultrasound (gray-scale US) a hypoechoic lesion on the left side can be seen. The targeted biopsy revealed prostate cancer (Gleason score 7). The corresponding color Doppler (**b**) and power Doppler images (**c**) show hypervascularity and flow asymmetry in this lesion

by the inability to detect isoechoic tumors and by the often heterogeneous appearance of the prostate. Therefore Hodge et al. introduced the "sextant biopsy approach" in 1989, which is still a standard technique worldwide. However, numerous studies have shown that the sextant technique misses up to 35% of clinically relevant cancers. This has resulted in studies using new biopsy strategies with more laterally directed cores and overall a higher number of cores (i.e., saturation biopsies up to 45 cores). Analyzing the results, several studies have reported no significant improvement when performing a higher number of cores.

In order to improve the detection of prostate cancer, additional color and power Doppler US have been used. Color Doppler US has been applied to evaluation of vascularity within the prostate and the surrounding structures [14–21]. The motivation behind the application of color Doppler US is to detect tumor neovascularity. Cancerous tissue generally grows more rapidly than normal tissue, and demonstrates increased blood flow, as compared to normal tissue and benign lesions [22–25]. Color Doppler US may demonstrate an increased number of visualized vessels, as well as an increase in flow rate, size, and irregularity of vessels within prostate cancer [26]. Three different flow patterns may be associated with prostate cancer – diffuse flow, focal flow, and surrounding flow [14]. The most frequently identified flow pattern is diffuse flow within the lesion. Early results have suggested that up to 85% of men with prostate cancers greater than 5 mm in size have visibly increased flow in the area of tumor involvement [14]. In addition, hypervascularity may be seen in patients with more-difficult-to-identify isoechoic and hyperechoic lesions.

Clinical Application

Gray-Scale Ultrasound

TRUS of the prostate has revolutionized our ability to examine this organ [27, 28]. Among the myriad of indications for US of the prostate, the most common indication is for evaluation of suspected prostatic carcinoma. In this regard, TRUS is usually performed in conjunction with needle biopsy of the prostate. The indication for prostate ultrasound and biopsy is either an abnormality on DRE or elevation in the serum PSA level. Occasionally, men undergo TRUS owing to symptoms of bladder outlet obstruction or constitutional symptoms suggestive of metastatic prostate carcinoma. The utilization of serum assays for PSA and TRUS-guided needle biopsy has resulted, in general, in the diagnosis of prostate cancer at an earlier stage of presentation [28, 29].

Gray-scale imaging provides excellent visualization of the prostate. TRUS allows for an excellent anatomical delineation of the prostate gland in relation to the surrounding fat tissue, rectum, neurovascular bundles, and venous plexus, as well as a clear division between the inner gland (transition and central zone) and outer gland (peripheral zone) of the prostate. Advantages of TRUS-guided biopsy include the ability to direct the biopsy needle precisely into regions of interest, or to provide uniform spatial separation of biopsy cores. For these reasons, most prostate biopsies are performed under US guidance [30, 31]. TRUS may identify non-palpable malignancies. However, few studies have compared the yield of digitally directed biopsy versus those under TRUS guidance. Weaver et al. performed biopsies under both US and digital guidance in 51 men with palpable prostatic abnormality [32]. They noted carcinoma in nine patients on digitally directed biopsy. In contrast, 23 men had carcinoma detected when biopsies were performed under US guidance. Each of the men who had a positive digitally guided biopsy also had carcinoma detected on the US-guided procedure. In transrectal gray-scale US prostate cancer is classically described as a hypoechoic lesion, but may also appear as echogenic or isoechoic lesion [33]. In the early 1980s, hypoechoic nodules were seen as the main presentation of prostate cancer, and solely these nodules were targeted at biopsy. The hypoechoic appearance is believed to be due to the increased microvessel density [34]. However, up to 30% of all prostate cancers are isoechoic, and it is estimated that a hypoechoic nodule has a 17–57% chance of being identified as prostate cancer [35]. Most studies that examined the diagnostic performance of targeting hypoechoic lesions were performed at least 7 years ago. Since then, PSA-based screening has spread, and the PSA threshold for performing biopsy has decreased, resulting in earlier detection. Because of this earlier detection, the pathognomonic feature of the hypoechoic lesion as a sign of prostate cancer has decreased in value. This is supported by a recent study that reported that only 9.3% of hypoechoic nodules in the PSA era contained prostate cancer, compared with 10.4% of isoechoic prostate areas that were targeted [36]. Thus, currently targeting only hypoechoic areas is insufficient to detect prostate cancer.

However, approximately half of prostate cancer lesions are invisible by gray-scale imaging [37]. Furthermore, prostatitis and benign prostatic hyperplasia mimic the gray-scale appearance of prostate cancer. Both are common forms of prostate pathology. Prostatitis may result in a heterogeneous appearance in the prostate peripheral zone and can present with hypoechoic lesions that are indistinguishable from cancer. Although most hyperplastic prostatic nodules develop in the transition zone, BPH may also occur in the peripheral zone of the prostate [38]. A study suggests that BPH is present in the outer portion of the gland in up to 18.5% of prostate specimens [39]. Furthermore, since the peripheral zone wraps around the transition zone, hyperplastic nodules from the transition zone may protrude into the peripheral zone. Therefore given the diverse appearance of prostate cancer and the potential for benign processes to mimic the gray-scale appearance of prostate cancer, conventional prostate US has little advantage over DRE for detecting malignant areas [40]. Although conventional gray-scale US does improve the yield of needle biopsy, this technique has only limited sensitivity for the detection of cancer. Specifically, TRUS is limited by the inability to detect isoechoic tumors and by the often heterogeneous appearance of the prostate. In order to improve the detection of cancer, additional color and power Doppler imaging techniques may be used.

Color Doppler Ultrasound

Prostate cancer tends to have increased vascularity compared with healthy prostatic tissue due to the formation of new vessels or an increase in the capacity of existing vessels [41]. Also, cancer foci with higher Gleason scores have higher degrees of vascularity [42]. Because this higher degree of vascularity was reported to be correlated with a worse survival rate, the vascularity of a prostate cancer focus is an important diagnostic feature, particularly for outer gland cancers [36].

Color Doppler imaging measures blood flow velocity and direction. US Doppler techniques demonstrate the presence of blood flow by detecting a frequency/phase shift in the US radiofrequency signal reflected from moving blood. Since prostate cancer is associated with increased perfusion, the sensitivity of US for detection of prostate cancer may be increased with color Doppler imaging of blood flow within the prostate [43]. The color Doppler signal correlates positively with both stage and grade of a prostate tumor, as well as with the risk of recurrence after treatment [44]. Color Doppler US has been applied to evaluate the vascularity within the prostate and the surrounding structures [14–21]. The motivation behind the application of color Doppler US is to detect tumor neovascularity. Cancerous tissue generally grows more rapidly than normal tissue, and demonstrates increased blood flow, as compared to normal tissue and benign lesions [22–25]. Color Doppler US may demonstrate an increased number of visualized vessels, as well as an increase in flow rate, size, and irregularity of vessels within prostate cancer [26]. Three different flow patterns may be associated with prostate cancer – diffuse flow, focal flow, and surrounding flow [14]. The most frequently identified flow pattern is diffuse flow within the lesion.

Early results have suggested that up to 85% of men with prostate cancers greater than 5 mm in size have visibly increased flow in the area of tumor involvement [14].

In addition, hypervascularity may be seen in patients with more-difficult-to-identify isoechoic and hyperechoic lesions. Unfortunately, subsequent studies suggested that the combined application of gray-scale and color Doppler US will still miss a large number of cancers and is insufficient to preclude prostate biopsy.

Halpern et al. assessed the value of gray-scale, color, and power Doppler US for detection of prostatic cancer [37]. They investigated 251 patients prior to biopsy. Each biopsy site was prospectively scored for gray-scale abnormality and Doppler flow. Cancer was detected in 211 biopsy sites from 85 patients. Overall agreement between sonographic findings and biopsy results as measured with the kappa statistic was minimally superior to chance (kappa $= 0.12$ for gray-scale, kappa $= 0.11$ for color Doppler, kappa S 0.09 for power Doppler). Among patients with at least one positive biopsy for cancer, foci of increased power Doppler flow were 4.7 times more likely to contain cancer than adjacent tissues without flow. They concluded that power Doppler may be useful for targeted biopsies when the number of biopsy passes must be limited, but that there is no substantial advantage of power Doppler over color Doppler. Other investigators suggest that Doppler flow patterns may correlate with microvascular density. However, Doppler imaging may not provide sufficient sensitivity to preclude biopsy [17].

Cheng et al. evaluated color Doppler imaging (CDI) in the diagnosis of prostate cancer [45]. They retrospectively analyzed 619 consecutive patients who underwent prostate US, CDI, and biopsy because of abnormal DRE results or PSA levels. All had directed (into a specific lesion) biopsies or directed biopsies along with systematic four-quadrant or sextant biopsies, or systematic biopsy alone. Color Doppler imaging was compared with gray-scale findings and histologic results. There were 222 (35.9%) biopsy-proven cancers ($n = 197$) or prostatic intraepithelial neoplasia ($n = 25$). Of these, 106 (47.7%) had color-flow abnormalities. Of these 106 patients, 26 (24.5%), or 11.7% of all cancer patients, had relatively normal gray-scale US findings but had focal CDI abnormalities as the method of identification. Overall, 76.9% of these were moderate-to-high Gleason grades and were considered clinically significant lesions. Color Doppler imaging can identify a large number (11.7%) of clinically significant prostate cancers that are poorly seen by gray-scale US. Positive lesions on CDI are of clinical importance because 76.9% are histologically, moderately, or poorly differentiated. Therefore they recommended that CDI be used in all diagnostic and biopsy-guided US examinations of the prostate.

In another approach Ives et al. determined the effect of short-term therapy with dutasteride on the suppression of Doppler US signal in benign prostate tissue and thus on improvement in the depiction of prostate cancer with Doppler US-guided core-needle biopsy [46]. In the preliminary trial, 11 subjects scheduled for prostate biopsy were evaluated by gray-scale, color, and power Doppler at baseline and weekly for up to 3 weeks, while taking the 5-alpha-reductase inhibitor dutasteride (0.5 mg/day). Doppler flow suppression occurred in all 11 subjects after 1 week ($P < 0.01$). Further suppression was noted after 2 weeks in eight subjects ($P = 0.04$). Suppression of flow was greatest in the peripheral zone and least obvious in the periurethral zone. Cancer was detected in 20% (8/40) of targeted cores and 7.6% (5/66) of sextant cores. Cancer was detected in four subjects by targeted biopsy and in three of four by systematic biopsy. In the four men with cancer, targeted cores were 5.9 times more likely to be positive ($P = 0.027$). Selective suppression of flow in benign tissue was observed in two of the four subjects with cancer. The conclusion of the study was that short-term dutasteride therapy reduces Doppler US flow in the prostate and may improve depiction of hypervascular cancer.

Further Rouviere et al. evaluated transrectal color Doppler (CD) in guiding prostate biopsy to depict early cancer recurrence after high-intensity-focused ultrasound (HIFU) therapy [47]. Prostate CD-guided sextant biopsies were obtained in 82 patients who had undergone prostate HIFU ablation for cancer, 24 of whom had hormone therapy before the treatment. CD findings were compared with biopsy results. CD was a significant predictor of biopsy findings, according to univariate and multivariate site-by-site analysis. However, only 36 of 94 sites with residual cancer had positive CD findings, and thus, negative CD findings should not preclude random biopsy. Although, biopsies taken in CD-positive sites were 4.4 times more likely to contain cancer in patients who did not receive hormone therapy, CD could not reliably depict cancer recurrence in patients with history of hormone therapy.

Power Doppler Ultrasound

Power Doppler, a newer Doppler technique for demonstrating the presence of blood flow, reflects the amplitude of the Doppler signal. Although power Doppler does not demonstrate directionality of flow, this technique is more sensitive to small amounts of low-velocity flow. Power Doppler US, as an amplitude-based technique for the detection of flow, is more sensitive to slow flow and is less angle-dependent than color Doppler US. Power Doppler imaging is also able to visualize smaller vessels and vessels with lower flow velocity than is the case with color Doppler [24]. This newer technique has been less commonly applied to the assessment of prostate tumor vascularity, and there are few papers addressing its use [48]. However, early studies have suggested that power Doppler US may be useful in detection of prostate cancer.

Leventis et al. defined the vascular anatomy of the normal prostate by means of power Doppler US investigation [49]. The vascular anatomy of 40 subjects was studied. Power Doppler images were correlated with corresponding gray-scale images. Doppler spectral waveform measurements were obtained for the vessels identified. Separate branches of the capsular vessels were visualized clearly, distributed radially in the peripheral and central zones and converging toward the center of the gland. Urethral vessels were visualized in the transition zone coursing from bladder neck to verumontanum. The neurovascular bundles were identified posterolaterally along the length of the gland. They concluded that the vascular anatomy of the normal prostate as displayed by power Doppler demonstrates a reproducible and symmetric flow pattern. Power Doppler is highly sensitive in depicting blood flow, the number, course, and continuity of vessels more readily than other imaging modalities, such as color Doppler. These data should allow comparison of the vascular anatomy of the normal prostate with that of the prostate with diseases such as prostate cancer and BPH.

In 2004 Remzi et al. determined the utility of power Doppler US and its guided prostate biopsies in men with prostate-specific antigen (PSA) levels between 2.5 and 10 ng/ml and evaluated its impact on prostate cancer detection in men undergoing first and repeat biopsies [50]. A total of 136 consecutive referred men with serum total PSA levels between 2.5 and 10 ng/ml (mean age 64 ± 9 years, range 45–82) and a normal DRE were included; 101 underwent a first biopsy whereas 35 had repeat biopsy. Gray-scale TRUS, and power Doppler US (B&K Medical, Denmark) were performed in lithotomy position before and during the biopsy procedure. Vascularity accumulation and perfusion characteristics were recorded and graded as normal or abnormal in the peripheral zone of the prostate. In this study overall prostate cancer detection rate was 34.7 and 25.7% and abnormal accumulation on power Doppler US was identified in 42.3 and 48.6% on first and repeat biopsy, respectively. The prostate cancer detection rate, on first and repeat biopsy in patients with and without power Doppler US accumulation were 67.4 versus 10.3% ($p < 0.001$) and 47.05 versus 5.6% ($p = 0.0049$), respectively. Power Doppler US directed biopsies were positive in 5.7 and 11.1% on first and repeat biopsy whereas prostate cancer detection using the routine prostate biopsy regime was 94.3 and 88.9% on first and repeat biopsy. The sensitivity, specificity, positive predictive value, and negative predictive value of power Doppler US signal alone for prostate cancer detection on first biopsy was 82.8, 78.8, 87.9 and 89.7%, respectively, and 88.8, 68.0, 47.0 and 94.4% on repeat biopsy, respectively. They concluded that negative power Doppler US signal is able to exclude most of the patients without prostate cancer in the PSA range of 2.5–10 ng/ml. As an additional tool at TRUS biopsy power

Doppler US has a high negative predictive value and may help to reduce the number of unnecessary biopsies.

In 2002 Halpern et al. evaluated cancer detection with directed biopsy of the prostate on the basis of high-frequency Doppler US findings and determined the effect of patient position on the observed flow pattern [51]. Thirty-two patients were evaluated in the left lateral decubitus position with gray-scale, color Doppler, and power Doppler transrectal US. Both color and power Doppler US demonstrated increased flow on the left side of the prostate, with greater flow toward the base of the gland ($P < 0.002$). Consequently, 62 of 90 directed biopsy cores were obtained in the left base and mid-gland. The positive biopsy rate for directed biopsy was not significantly different from that of sextant biopsy ($P = 0.4$). Seven patients had cancer that was identified with sextant biopsy, but only four cancers were identified with directed biopsy. Each of the three healthy volunteers demonstrated increased Doppler flow on the dependent side when the subject was in the lateral decubitus position. Therefore, on the basis of observations made in healthy volunteers, the authors conclude that flow asymmetry in patients who underwent biopsy may have been related to patient position.

In a small series of 18 patients the value of power Doppler US imaging during TRUS in detecting local recurrence after radical retropubic prostatectomy (RRP) was evaluated [52]. Local recurrence of prostate cancer was suspected on the basis of elevated serum PSA levels (above 0.4 ng/ml) after RRP with no evidence of metastatic disease. The ability to detect locally recurrent prostate cancer using gray-scale TRUS alone was compared with TRUS combined with power Doppler US; 15 of the 18 patients (83%) had positive biopsies for local recurrent tumour at histological examination. TRUS alone detected gray-scale abnormalities in 15 of 18 patients (83%), of whom 14 (77%) had positive TRUS-guided biopsies. Power Doppler US during TRUS showed hypervascularity in 14 of 18 patients (77%). Biopsies of these hypervascular regions were positive in all patients (100%). The sensitivity and specificity of TRUS alone in detecting recurrent tumour were 93 and 67%, respectively, with a positive predictive value of 93% and a negative predictive value of 67%. TRUS combined with power Doppler US had a sensitivity and specificity of 93 and 100%, respectively, with a PPV and a NPV of 100 and 75%, respectively. Therefore power Doppler US, compared to TRUS alone, showed to be superior in the detection of local recurrence of prostate cancer.

In 2006 Heijmink et al. compared the diagnostic performance of systematic versus US-guided biopsies of prostate cancer [36]. They found that in a review of the current literature that imaging-guided biopsy showed better diagnostic performance than systematic biopsy with higher sensitivity. The combinations of sensitivity and specificity were highest for color Doppler and contrast-enhanced targeted biopsy. Studies targeting hypoechoic lesions had relatively high sensitivity, but specificity was low. Presently, however, with widespread PSA screening, fewer prostate cancers are hypoechoic, and the value of targeting hypoechoic lesions has diminished. Performing color or contrast-enhanced Doppler biopsy or adding these techniques to systematic biopsies improves diagnostic performance, particularly by increasing sensitivity.

Nonetheless, the up-to-date results of gray-scale, color, and power Doppler US-guided and/or targeted biopsy are not sufficient to eliminate the need for systematic biopsy.

Conclusion and Perspectives

Application of a TRUS-guided biopsy technique that targets a visual lesion increases the sensitivity of prostate cancer biopsy compared with systematic biopsy. Color Doppler- and power Doppler-targeted biopsy have shown better diagnostic performance. Targeting hypoechoic lesions achieves high sensitivity but has low specificity. As hypoechoic lesions are becoming less pathognomonic in the PSA-screening era, transrectal gray-scale US should not be used as sole biopsy guidance.

In the near future innovations like contrast-enhanced US- or elastography-guided prostate biopsy may further improve the diagnostic performance of US in prostate cancer diagnosis.

References

1. Jemal A, Tiwari RC, Murray T, Ghafoor A, Samuels A, Ward E, et al. Cancer statistics. CA Cancer J Clin. 2004;54:8–29.
2. D'Amico AV, Moul JW, Carroll PR, Sun L, Lubeck D, Chen MH. Surrogate end point for prostate cancer-specific mortality after radical prostatectomy or radiation therapy. J Natl Cancer Inst. 2003;95:1376–83.
3. D'Amico AV, Chen MH, Roehl KA, Catalona WJ. Preoperative PSA velocity and the risk of death from prostate cancer after radical prostatectomy. N Engl J Med. 2004;351:125–35.
4. Catalona WJ, Smith DS, Ratliff TL, Basler JW. Detection of organ-confined prostate cancer is increased through prostate-specific antigen-based screening. JAMA. 1993;270:948–54.
5. Smith RA, Cokkinides V, Eyre HJ. American Cancer Society guidelines for the early detection of cancer, 2003. CA Cancer J Clin. 2003;53:27–43.
6. Smith RA, von Eschenbach AC, Wender R, Levin B, Byers T, Rothenberger D, et al. American Cancer Society guidelines for the early detection of cancer: update of early detection guidelines for prostate, colorectal, and endometrial cancers. Also: update 2001—testing for early lung cancer detection. CA Cancer J Clin. 2001;51:38–75; quiz 77–80.
7. Ornish DM, Lee KL, Fair WR, Pettengill EB, Carroll PR. Dietary trial in prostate cancer: Early experience and implications for clinical trial design. Urology. 2001;57:200–1.
8. Partin AW, Hanks GE, Klein EA, Moul JW, Nelson WG, Scher HI. Prostate-specific antigen as a marker of disease activity in prostate cancer. Oncology (Williston Park). 2002;16:1218–24; discussion 1224, 1227–8 passim.
9. Gretzer MB, Partin AW. PSA markers in prostate cancer detection. Urol Clin North Am. 2003;30:677–86.
10. Caplan A, Kratz A. Prostate-specific antigen and the early diagnosis of prostate cancer. Am J Clin Pathol. 2002;117 Suppl:S104–S108.
11. De Marzo AM, DeWeese TL, Platz EA, Meeker AK, Nakayama M, Epstein JI, et al. Pathological and molecular mechanisms of prostate carcinogenesis: implications for diagnosis, detection, prevention, and treatment. J Cell Biochem. 2004;91:459–77.
12. Oh WK, George DJ, Kantoff PW. Rapid rise of serum prostate specific antigen levels after discontinuation of the herbal therapy PC-SPES in patients with advanced prostate carcinoma: report of four cases. Cancer. 2002;94:686–9.
13. Stamey TA, Kabalin JN, McNeal JE, Johnstone IM, Freiha F, Redwine EA, et al. Prostate specific antigen in the diagnosis and treatment of adenocarcinoma of the prostate. II. Radical prostatectomy treated patients. J Urol. 1989;141:1076–83.
14. Rifkin MD, Sudakoff GS, Alexander AA. Prostate: techniques, results, and potential applications of color Doppler US scanning. Radiology. 1993;186:509–13.
15. Kelly IM, Lees WR, Rickards D. Prostate cancer and the role of color Doppler US. Radiology. 1993;189:153–6.
16. Newman JS, Bree RL, Rubin JM. Prostate cancer: diagnosis with color Doppler sonography with histologic correlation of each biopsy site. Radiology. 1995;195:86–90.
17. Louvar E, Littrup PJ, Goldstein A, Yu L, Sakr W, Grignon D. Correlation of color Doppler flow in the prostate with tissue microvascularity. Cancer. 1998;83:135–40.
18. Ismail M, Gomella LG, Alexander AA. Color Doppler sonography of the prostate. Tech Urol. 1997;3:140–6.
19. Ismail M, Petersen RO, Alexander AA, Newschaffer C, Gomella LG. Color Doppler imaging in predicting the biologic behavior of prostate cancer: correlation with disease-free survival. Urology. 1997;50:906–12.
20. Alexander AA. To color Doppler image the prostate or not: that is the question. Radiology. 1995;195:11–3.
21. Rifkin MD, Alexander AA, Helinek TG, Merton DA. Color Doppler as an adjunct to prostate ultrasound. Scand J Urol Nephrol Suppl. 1991;137:85–9.
22. Sillman F, Boyce J, Fruchter R. The significance of atypical vessels and neovascularization in cervical neoplasia. Am J Obstet Gynecol. 1981;139:154–9.
23. Srivastava A, Laidler P, Davies RP, Horgan K, Hughes LE. The prognostic significance of tumor vascularity in intermediate-thickness (0.76–4.0 mm thick) skin melanoma. A quantitative histologic study. Am J Pathol. 1988;133:419–23.
24. Weidner N, Semple JP, Welch WR, Folkman J. Tumor angiogenesis and metastasis—correlation in invasive breast carcinoma. N Engl J Med. 1991;324:1–8.
25. Brawer MK, Deering RE, Brown M, Preston SD, Bigler SA. Predictors of pathologic stage in prostatic carcinoma. The role of neovascularity. Cancer. 1994;73:678–87.
26. Fleischer AC, Rodgers WH, Rao BK, Kepple DM, Worrell JA, Williams L, et al. Assessment of ovarian tumor vascularity with transvaginal color Doppler sonography. J Ultrasound Med. 1991;10:563–568.
27. Rifkin MD. Ultrasound of the prostate—applications and indications. Schweiz Med Wochenschr. 1991;121:282–91.
28. Rifkin MD. Prostate cancer: the diagnostic dilemma and the place of imaging in detection and staging. World J Urol. 1998;16:76–80.

29. Bartsch G, Egender G, Hubscher H, Rohr H. Sonometrics of the prostate. J Urol. 1982;127:1119–21.

30. Rifkin MD, Alexander AA, Pisarchick J, Matteucci T. Palpable masses in the prostate: superior accuracy of US-guided biopsy compared with accuracy of digitally guided biopsy. Radiology. 1991;179:41–2.

31. Spencer JA, Alexander AA, Gomella L, Matteucci T, Goldberg BB. Ultrasound-guided four quadrant biopsy of the prostate: efficacy in the diagnosis of isoechoic cancer. Clin Radiol. 1994;49:711–4.

32. Weaver RP, Noble MJ, Weigel JW. Correlation of ultrasound guided and digitally directed transrectal biopsies of palpable prostatic abnormalities. J Urol. 1991;145:516–8.

33. Rifkin MD, Dahnert W, Kurtz AB. State of the art: endorectal sonography of the prostate gland. AJR Am J Roentgenol. 1990;154:691–700.

34. Engelbrecht MR, Huisman HJ, Laheij RJ, Jager GJ, van Leenders GJ, Hulsbergen-Van De Kaa CA, et al. Discrimination of prostate cancer from normal peripheral zone and central gland tissue by using dynamic contrast-enhanced MR imaging. Radiology. 2003;229:248–54.

35. Borre M, Offersen BV, Nerstrom B, Overgaard J. Microvessel density predicts survival in prostate cancer patients subjected to watchful waiting. Br J Cancer. 1998;78:940–4.

36. Heijmink SW, van Moerkerk H, Kiemeney LA, Witjes JA, Frauscher F, Barentsz JO. A comparison of the diagnostic performance of systematic versus ultrasound-guided biopsies of prostate cancer. Eur Radiol. 2006;16:927–38.

37. Halpern EJ, Strup SE. Using gray-scale and color and power Doppler sonography to detect prostatic cancer. AJR Am J Roentgenol. 2000;174:623–27.

38. Oyen RH, Van de Voorde WM, Van Poppel HP, Brys PP, Ameye FE, Franssens YM, et al. Benign hyperplastic nodules that originate in the peripheral zone of the prostate gland. Radiology. 1993;189:707–11.

39. Van de Voorde WM, Oyen RH, Van Poppel HP, Wouters K, Baert LV, Lauweryns JM. Peripherally localized benign hyperplastic nodules of the prostate. Mod Pathol. 1995;8: 46–50.

40. Halpern EJ. Contrast-enhanced ultrasound imaging of prostate cancer. Rev Urol. 2006;8 Suppl 1:S29–S37.

41. Neumaier CE, Martinoli C, Derchi LE, Silvestri E, Rosenberg I. Normal prostate gland: examination with color Doppler US. Radiology. 1995;196:453–7.

42. Wilson NM, Masoud AM, Barsoum HB, Refaat MM, Moustafa MI, Kamal TA. Correlation of power Doppler with microvessel density in assessing prostate needle biopsy. Clin Radiol. 2004;59:946–50.

43. Naya Y, Ochiai A, Troncoso P, Babaian RJ. A comparison of extended biopsy and sextant biopsy schemes for predicting the pathological stage of prostate cancer. J Urol. 2004;171:2203–8.

44. Naughton CK, Miller DC, Mager DE, Ornstein DK, Catalona WJ. A prospective randomized trial comparing 6 versus 12 prostate biopsy cores: impact on cancer detection. J Urol. 2000;164:388–92.

45. Cheng S, Rifkin MD. Color Doppler imaging of the prostate: important adjunct to endorectal ultrasound of the prostate in the diagnosis of prostate cancer. Ultrasound Q. 2001;17:185–9.

46. Ives EP, Gomella LG, Halpern EJ. Effect of dutasteride therapy on Doppler US evaluation of prostate: preliminary results. Radiology. 2005;237:197–201.

47. Rouvière O, Mège-Lechevallier F, Chapelon JY, Gelet A, Bouvier R, Boutitie F, et al. Evaluation of color Doppler in guiding prostate biopsy after HIFU ablation. Eur Urol. 2006;50:490–7.

48. Cho JY, Kim SH, Lee SE. Diffuse prostatic lesions: role of color Doppler and power Doppler ultrasonography. J Ultrasound Med. 1998;17:283–7.

49. Leventis AK, Shariat SF, Utsunomiya T, Slawin KM. Characteristics of normal prostate vascular anatomy as displayed by power Doppler. Prostate. 2001;46:281–8.

50. Remzi M, Dobrovits M, Reissigl A, Ravery V, Waldert M, Wiunig C, et al. Can Power Doppler enhanced transrectal ultrasound guided biopsy improve prostate cancer detection on first and repeat prostate biopsy? Eur Urol. 2004;46:451–6.

51. Halpern EJ, Frauscher F, Forsberg F, Strup SE, Nazarian LN, O'Kane P, et al. High-frequency Doppler US of the prostate: effect of patient position. Radiology. 2002;222:634–9.

52. Tamsel S, Killi R, Apaydin E, Hekimgil M, Demirpolat G. The potential value of power Doppler ultrasound imaging compared with grey-scale ultrasound findings in the diagnosis of local recurrence after radical prostatectomy. Clin Radiol. 2006;61:325–30; discussion 323–4.

Chapter 22

Prostate Carcinoma – Cross-Sectional Imaging Techniques

E. Sala and H. Hricak

Introduction

Prostate cancer is the most common malignancy in American men and the second leading cause of cancer death in American males. An estimated 186,320 men will be diagnosed with prostate cancer in the United States in 2008 [1]. Increased use of serum prostate-specific antigen (PSA) testing has produced a dramatic stage shift in prostate cancer. In 2004, 86% of prostate cancer cases were localized to the prostate gland as compared to 58% in 1994 [2]. This stage migration has resulted in more patients being candidates for curative therapy [3, 4] and indeed, recent studies have suggested that most patients with clinically localized prostate cancer will undergo some type of local therapy in an attempt to cure the disease [5–7]. Controversy with regard to the appropriate choice of treatment, however, persists.

Ideally, the determination of treatment options should benefit from an imaging modality that allows visualization of the primary tumor and its extent. Although much progress has been made in cross-sectional and functional imaging, no imaging modality exists that can be relied on to show the primary tumor and its extent in all cases. The accepted evaluation of patients with newly diagnosed prostate cancer includes nomograms based on the clinical stage, PSA, Gleason grade, and digital rectal examination (DRE) [8, 9]. These nomograms provide risk stratification estimates that enable physicians to assess the need for further evaluation, including cross-sectional imaging with computed tomography (CT) and/or magnetic resonance (MR). CT is useful in imaging of metastatic prostate cancer and in radiotherapy treatment planning. MRI/MR spectroscopic imaging (MRSI) offers non-invasive evaluation of anatomic and metabolic features of prostate cancer, enabling accurate detection, localization, characterization, and staging of the disease and thus poten-tially playing an important role in individual treatment selection and planning.

In this chapter we describe the roles of CT and MRI/MRSI in prostate cancer management, addressing the advantages and limitations of each technique. Our objective is to give a comprehensive view of the value of cross-sectional imaging in the diagnostic work-up, treatment planning, and follow-up of patients with prostate cancer.

CT Imaging of Prostate Cancer

Indications

CT has limited value in initial tumor staging, unless advanced disease is suspected. However, CT is useful in prostate cancer treatment follow-up, its main role being the assessment of metastatic disease in the lymph nodes, visceral organs, and bones. CT is very valuable in radiotherapy treatment planning in patients with locally advanced prostate cancer. The majority of patients with newly diagnosed prostate cancer are at low risk for metastases, hence the diagnostic yield of CT is relatively low in these patients [10–12]. At the time of initial diagnosis, CT is not recommended for patients with a PSA < 20 ng/ml, a Gleason score < 7, or a clinical stage < T3 as the likelihood of lymph node metastasis and systemic disease is very low [12]. At present, according to the American Urology Association guidelines, there is no indication for CT in a patient with a PSA level ≤ 20 ng/ml [13].

Technique

Axial CT images should extend from below the symphysis pubis up to the aortic bifurcation if only imaging of the pelvis is requested. However, if visceral or lymph node metastases are suspected, imaging of the entire pelvis and

H. Hricak
Department of Radiology Memorial, Sloan-Kettering Cancer Center, 1275 York Avenue, New York, New York - 10021, hricakh@mskcc.org

J.J.M.C.H. de la Rosette et al. (eds.), *Imaging in Oncological Urology*, DOI 10.1007/978-1-84628-759-6_22, © Springer-Verlag London Limited 2009

abdomen should be performed. It is important to be aware that retroperitoneal lymphadenopathy is rare in the absence of pelvic lymphadenopathy in patients with prostate cancer. In addition, CT of the chest may be required if there is suspicion of lung involvement either as discrete metastasis or lymphangitis carcinomatosa.

CT examination of the abdomen and pelvis requires patient preparation. The routine use of intravenous contrast medium is recommended to facilitate differentiation between lymph nodes and blood vessels. Complete opacification of the gastrointestinal tract is desirable, as unopacified small bowel loops in the pelvis can be misinterpreted as abnormal lymph nodes or tumor masses. At least 1 hour before the examination, 500–1000 ml of dilute oral contrast medium should be given. The use of rectal contrast medium is not required. A full urinary bladder is preferred, as it displaces small bowel loops out of the pelvis, making it easier to identify other pelvic structures. If hydronephrosis is present, delayed images showing contrast medium excretion into the renal collecting system and urinary bladder may be useful.

Imaging Findings

Local Tumor Staging

Due to the lack of soft tissue contrast CT has a limited role in local tumor staging [10, 11]. Although there is no recent literature on the multi-detector CT appearances of organ-confined prostate cancer, in our personal experience with multi-slice CT, prostate cancer appears as an area of low attenuation compared to the surrounding normal prostate tissue. CT can be useful as a baseline examination prior to radiation or medical therapy in clinically high-risk patients with grossly advanced local disease as demonstrated by established extracapsular disease, gross seminal vesicle invasion, or invasion of surrounding structures including bladder, rectum, levator ani muscles, or pelvic floor (Fig. 22.1). Such patients will also be at risk for lymph node and bone metastases, which may be assessed concurrently.

Detection of Recurrent Disease

The role of CT in prostate cancer treatment follow-up focuses on evaluation of metastatic disease in the lymph nodes, visceral organs, and bones. The regional nodes for prostate cancer that are designated as N1 in the TNM classification are pelvic nodes, including obturator, iliac (internal and external), and sacral (lateral, presacral, promontory) nodes (Fig. 22.2a). Metastatic lymph nodes (M1) are common iliac, paraaortic, mesenteric, and mediastinal nodes (Fig. 22.2b and c). Prior to any form of therapy, nodal disease usu-

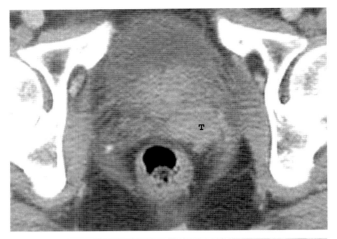

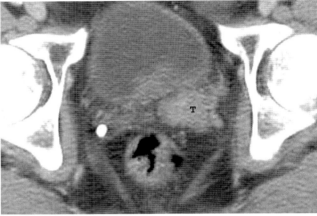

Fig. 22.1 Biopsy-proven Gleason grade 9 adenocarcinoma in a 59-year-old man with a PSA level of 15.4 ng/mL. Axial CT images (a, b) reveal a large tumor (*T*) that invades the entire prostate gland, the urinary bladder, and the left seminal vesicle

ally progresses in a step-wise fashion (Fig. 22.2), such that retroperitoneal, mesenteric, or mediastinal nodal disease is very unusual in the absence of pelvic lymphadenopathy and more likely to be due to coexistent malignancy (e.g., lymphoma) [14, 15]. However, in almost 75% of patients with disease recurrence in the lymph nodes following radical prostatectomy, the usual pattern of vertical node spread is not maintained [16]. The majority of these patients would have had previous lymph node dissection at the time of radical prostatectomy and thus only retroperitoneal lymphadenopathy would be detected at CT.

Currently, the diagnosis of nodal metastasis on CT is made only based on nodal size. However, the correlation between nodal enlargement and metastatic involvement is poor [17]. Using a short axis diameter of 1.0 cm as a cut-off has resulted in sensitivities between 25 and 85% and specificities between 66 and 100% [12, 18–20]. Oyen et al. reported a significant improvement in both sensitivity and specificity (which reached 78 and 100%, respectively) with lowering of the size threshold to 0.7 cm and fine needle aspi-

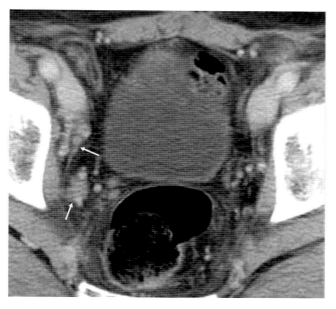

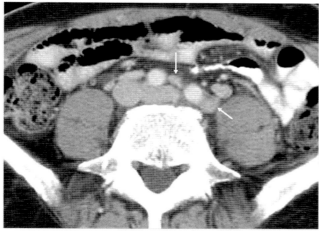

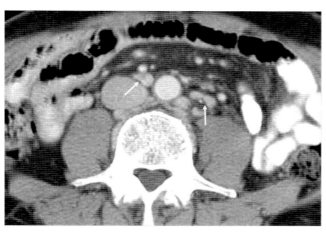

ration (FNA) of the suspicious nodes [20]. However, neither the lower size threshold nor the use of FNA has been widely accepted. Neither CT nor MRI can be used to rule out lymph node metastases, especially in lymph nodes of normal size. However, MR lymphography has demonstrated promising result in the diagnosis of metastasis within normal-sized lymph nodes (see Section on MRI).

CT is also very valuable in the evaluation of visceral and bone metastasis. Bone metastases from prostate cancer are usually sclerotic due to osteoblastic reaction (Fig. 22.3), but a mixed lytic–sclerotic pattern can occasionally be observed. However, bone scintigraphy and MRI are superior to CT in diagnosis and follow-up of bone metastases [21, 22]. One should be aware that sclerotic bone metastasis after chemo/radiation treatment can appear larger due to the effects of healing, thus leading to incorrect estimation of disease progression.

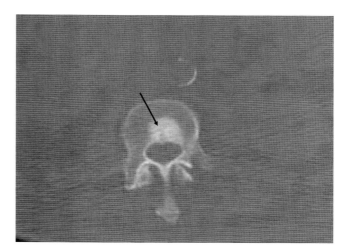

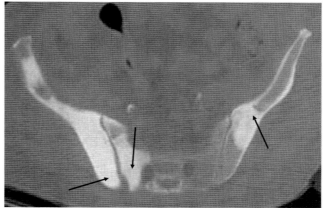

Fig. 22.2 Biopsy-proven Gleason grade 7 adenocarcinoma in a 55-year-old man with a PSA level of 5.4 ng/mL. Axial CT images of the pelvis (a) and abdomen (b, c) demonstrate enlarged right external iliac and right obturator lymph nodes (arrows in a), enlarged common iliac lymph nodes (arrows in b), and enlarged left paraaortic and aorto-caval lymph nodes (arrows in c)

Fig. 22.3 Biopsy-proven Gleason grade 9 adenocarcinoma in a 60-year-old man with a PSA level of 16.3 ng/mL. Axial CT images of the abdomen (a) and pelvis (b) reveal extensive sclerotic bone metastasis involving the vertebral body (arrow in a) as well as both iliac bones and the right sacrum (arrows in b)

MRI and MRSI of Prostate Cancer

Indications

Neither MRI nor MRSI is used as a first-line approach to diagnose prostate cancer. However, the combination of MRI/MRSI may be useful to target biopsy in patients with repeated negative biopsies but PSA levels indicative of cancer. This situation occurs most commonly in regions that are not palpable at DRE or not routinely targeted during biopsy (i.e., lesions located anteriorly in the peripheral or transition zone) [23, 24].

MRI/MRSI does, however, have great potential and high diagnostic efficacy for pretreatment staging of prostate cancer [25]. It provides useful information on the tumor as well as exquisite anatomic delineation of the pelvis. In addition, metastatic disease to lymph nodes can be accurately evaluated using MRI. MRI is also very useful in radiotherapy treatment planning and treatment follow-up, including the detection of local recurrence in prostatectomy patients with a rising PSA [25, 26].

MR Imaging and MR Spectroscopic Imaging Techniques

MRI Technique

A 1.5 T or higher strength magnet is required to perform a combined MR imaging and spectroscopy examination. Preliminary results using 3 T endorectal coil MRI/MRSI have been promising, as they have shown that an increase in spatial, temporal, and spectral resolutions can be achieved that may result in improved accuracy in localizing (detecting) and staging prostate cancer [27]. Optimal MR imaging of the prostate gland demands the use of an endorectal coil in conjunction with a pelvic-phased array coil [28]. The use of the endorectal coil improves image resolution, leading to more precise staging [28]. Patients should be carefully interviewed before endorectal coil placement, but tolerance for it is high. Contraindications include a recent history of rectal surgery, radiation therapy to the pelvis within the last 6 weeks, inflammatory bowel disease, large bowel obstruction, use of anticoagulant medication or history of bleeding disorders, and the known presence of lesions such as fistula or large hemorrhoids. MRI/MRSI should be delayed for at least 8 weeks after prostate biopsy in order to avoid under and/or overestimation of tumor extent [29].

The specific imaging parameters are dependent on the type of magnet used and the field strength. In general, the following imaging sequences are recommended:

1. TI-weighted axial imaging of the pelvis (from below the symphysis pubis up to the aortic bifurcation) is used to evaluate the presence of lymphadenopathy and post-biopsy hemorrhage in the prostate gland and seminal vesicles. Bone metastases to pelvis and lumbar spine are also well demonstrated using this sequence.
2. High-resolution T2-weighted imaging using a slice thickness of 3 mm and a small (14 cm) field of view in the axial, sagittal, and coronal planes is suggested for tumor detection, localization, and staging.

The use of dynamic contrast-enhanced MRI (DCE-MRI) is optional [30–34]. The rationale behind the use of DCE-MRI is that the increased micro-vessel density and permeability within the tumor will result in uptake being greater in the tumor than in the normal tissue. Both qualitative and quantitative methods are used to differentiate malignant lesions from benign or normal tissue. Detailed description of these methods is beyond the scope of this chapter and the reader is referred to the appropriate literature for more information on this topic [35–42].

MRSI Technique

MR spectroscopy provides non-invasive assessment of tissue metabolism. In MR spectroscopy, the nuclei of particular nuclides such as ^{1}H, ^{13}C, ^{31}P, and ^{19}F are excited with a radiofrequency (RF) pulse in the presence of a magnetic field. Different nuclei have different frequencies, which depend on (and provide information about) the chemical structure of the various molecules. By tuning in different frequencies, one can measure different concentrations of metabolites. This is known as chemical shift. MRSI exploits this chemical shift to produce a map of signal intensity versus frequency and spatial location. ^{1}H-MRSI offers higher sensitivity than the other varieties of MR spectroscopy, resulting in a better spatial resolution and signal-to-noise ratio and a decreased acquisition time. ^{1}H-MRSI yields multi-voxel data and has been used extensively, particularly in the brain and prostate. Using a 1.5 T clinical MRI scanner, it is possible to obtain a three-dimensional metabolic map of the entire gland with a resolution of 0.24 ml with excellent water and lipid suppression.

A number of ^{1}H-MRSI techniques have been described. At present, the commercially available spectroscopic imaging techniques include chemical shift imaging [43] with point-resolved spectroscopy, voxel excitation, and band-selective inversion with gradient dephasing for water and lipid suppression [44]. With point-resolved spectroscopy, a cubic or rectangular voxel is generated by acquiring three orthogonal section-selective pulses: a 90° pulse followed by two 180° pulses. Thus, the MRI image of the prostate is divided into small volumes of interest (voxels) in a grid pattern, which allows for assessment of different areas of the prostate gland. The major metabolic peaks relevant to prostate MRSI are choline, creatine, and citrate.

MRI and MRSI are usually performed as a single combined examination that takes approximately 1 hour. An endorectal coil is essential for the performance of spectroscopy [45]. In addition, a special software package is required for the performance of MRSI, which is currently available as an upgrade option.

Appearance of the Normal Prostate Gland on MRI

Knowledge of the normal MR anatomy of the prostate gland is crucial for image interpretation. On T1-weighted images, the prostate demonstrates homogeneous intermediate signal intensity. The soft tissue contrast resolution is insufficient for the visualization of either the normal zonal anatomy or areas of tumor. Conversely, the zonal anatomy of the prostate gland is well demonstrated on high-resolution T2-weighted images (Fig. 22.4) [46, 47]. The anterior fibromuscular stroma is of low signal intensity on both T1- and T2-weighted images. On T2-weighted images, the normal peripheral zone shows high signal intensity similar to or higher than the signal intensity of adjacent periprostatic fat. A thin rim of low signal intensity, which represents the anatomic or true capsule, surrounds the peripheral zone. The capsule is often incomplete especially at the apex, as has been confirmed by pathological specimen findings. The neurovascular bundles can be identified as low-signal-intensity foci posterolateral to the capsule bilaterally.

The central and transition zones have similar appearances on T2-weighted images, both having lower signal intensity than the peripheral zone. The transition and central zones are composed of more compact smooth muscle and sparser glandular tissue. Benign prostatic hyperplasia develops in the transition zone, gradually compresses the central zone, and may ultimately compress the peripheral zone, which sometimes becomes very difficult to appreciate around the hyperplastic transition zone. The central zone also atrophies with age. On contrast-enhanced MRI, the peripheral zone enhances more than the transition and central zones.

The proximal urethra is rarely identifiable unless a Foley catheter is present or a transurethral resection has been performed. The verumontanum can be identified as a higher-signal-intensity small focus on T2-weighted images. The distal prostatic urethra below the verumontanum can be seen as a low-signal-intensity ring similar to a doughnut because it is enclosed by an additional layer of muscle. The vas deferens and seminal vesicles, which have grape-like configurations,

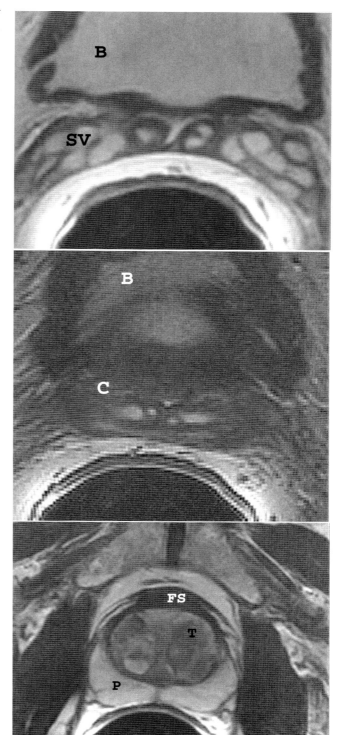

Fig. 22.4 Normal prostate zonal anatomy in a 65-year-old man depicted with T2-weighted axial MR images obtained at the levels of the seminal vesicles (a), the base of prostate (b), the mid-gland (c) and the apex/membranous urethra (d), as well as coronal (e) and parasagittal (f) MR images. The vertical line in image e indicates the membranous urethra length. B = urinary bladder, C = central zone, FS = anterior fibromuscular stroma, P = peripheral zone, SV = seminal vesicles, T = transition zone, U = urethra

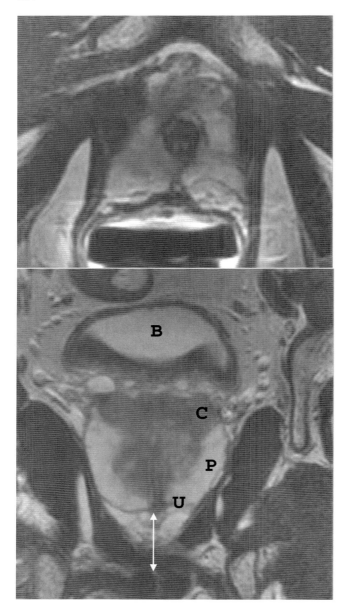

Fig. 22.4 (continued)

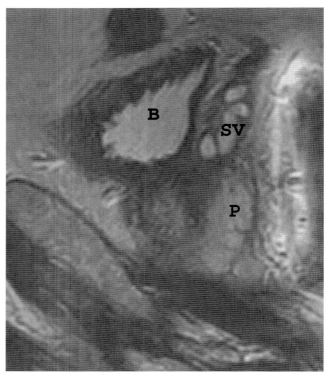

Fig. 22.4 (continued)

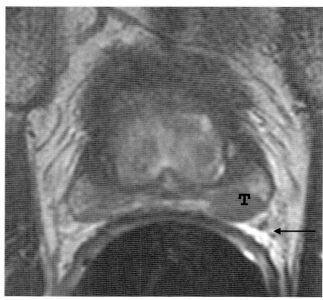

demonstrate high signal intensity on T2-weighted images (Fig. 22.4).

Appearance of Prostate Cancer on MRI

On T2-weighted images prostate cancer appears as an area of low signal intensity in contrast to the high signal intensity of the normal peripheral zone (Fig. 22.5). However, while detection is often easier on axial images, cross-correlation with T2-weighted coronal and sagittal sequences is recommended for a reliable diagnosis. One should be aware that

Fig. 22.5 Biopsy-proven Gleason grade 7 adenocarcinoma in a 67-year-old man with a PSA level of 2.3 ng/mL. T2-weighted axial (a) and coronal (b) images show a dominant tumor (*T*) within the left peripheral zone in the mid-gland. Note the smooth capsular contour adjacent to the tumor (a) and the well-defined left neurovascular bundle (arrow in a), both indicative of an organ-confined tumor. On the spectra from ^{1}H MR spectroscopy (c), voxels marked with * show an increase in choline (*Ch/Cr*) and a marked decrease in citrate (*Cit*); these voxels correspond to the low-signal-intensity region on the axial MR image (a). Findings at surgery and step-section histopathologic examination (d) show a Gleason grade 8, organ-confined tumor

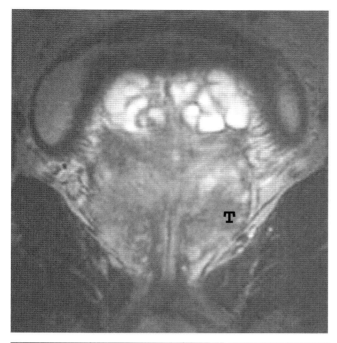

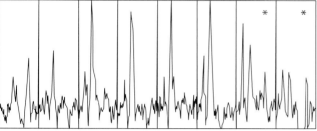

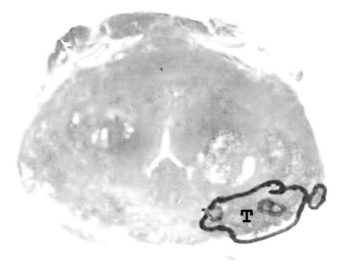

Fig. 22.5 (continued)

low signal intensity in the peripheral zone can also be seen in several benign conditions such as hemorrhage, prostatitis, hyperplastic nodules or previous radiation and hormonal therapy. Usually, areas of post-biopsy hemorrhage have a

feathery rather than a mass-like appearance. They demonstrate high signal intensity on T1-weighted images, hence correlation of T1- and T2-weighted images is crucial for accurate diagnosis.

Seventy percent of prostate carcinomas occur in the peripheral zone, while 20% originate in the transition zone and 10% develop in the central zone. Tumors in the central zone present a diagnostic challenge, as the normal central zone is of homogeneous low signal intensity on T2-weighted images and the tumor is best detected by examining anatomical appearance (i.e., shape or contour) rather than depending on signal intensity features [47]. It is very important to carefully scrutinize the transition zone (TZ) of the prostate, as in approximately 20% of patients the largest (dominant) tumor is located there [48]. Recognition of TZ tumors is important in order to avoid positive anterior margins at radical prostatectomy [48] and/or to plan disease-targeting therapies [49, 50]. Moreover, dominant TZ tumors are present in 25% of patients with impalpable T1c prostate cancers [4]. Because the transition zone is not routinely sampled during biopsy, tumors located there can result in the increasingly common clinical problem of an elevated PSA accompanied by initial negative biopsies [51–53].

Sommer et al. suggested that TZ tumors can be detected as regions of homogenous low signal intensity on T2-weighted images [54]. Our data confirm this suggestion and provide additional imaging features for the diagnosis of TZ cancers [55]. Findings indicative of TZ cancer include (1) a homogenous low-signal-intensity region in the transition zone; (2) poorly defined lesion margins; (3) lack of a low-signal-intensity rim (seen commonly in association with benign hyperplastic nodules); (4) interruption of the pseudocapsule (TZ/PZ boundary of low signal intensity); and (5) urethral or anterior fibromuscular stromal invasion (Fig. 22.6) [55]. Although these features are not pathognomonic for a TZ tumor, they are more frequently present in tumors than in benign prostatic hyperplasia. The detection rate seems to be higher for tumors with high Gleason grade, which also could be explained by the enhanced ability of aggressive tumors to disrupt the surrounding transition zone [55]. Tumors in the anterior part of the peripheral zone should also be carefully sought during MRI interpretation in patients with rising PSA and multiple negative biopsies, since this area, like the TZ, is often not routinely sampled during biopsy.

DCE-MRI was developed in an attempt to surpass the sensitivity and specificity of prostate cancer detection, localization, and staging offered by conventional high-resolution T2-weighted MR imaging (Fig. 22.7). Recent studies suggest that the peak enhancement of cancer relative to the surrounding normal prostate tissue is the most accurate parameter for cancer detection [31, 56, 57]. Ogura et al. found that detection of foci of early enhancement

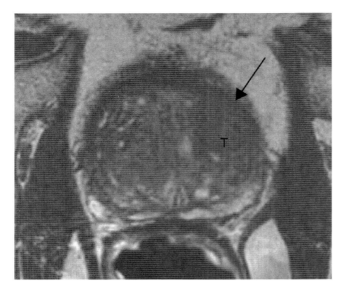

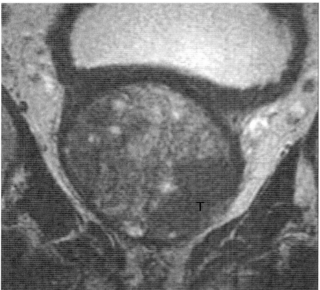

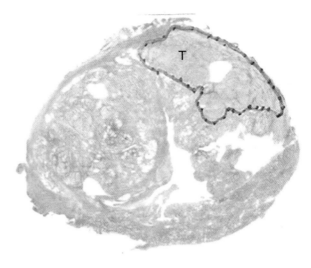

Fig. 22.6 (continued)

mation from dynamic MRI and metabolic information from MRSI has excellent potential for improving localization and characterization of prostate cancer in the clinical setting [57].

In summary, the early results using DCE-MRI in the evaluation of prostate cancer are promising, and the technique has already been incorporated in the MRI/MRSI protocol in selected centers [57]. However, more studies are necessary to optimize the technology and protocols before DCE-MRI can be used in the clinical setting routinely.

Fig. 22.6 Biopsy-proven Gleason grade 6 adenocarcinoma in a 66-year-old man with a PSA level of 9.9 ng/mL. T2-weighted axial (a) and coronal (b) images show a dominant tumor (T) within the left transition zone anteriorly extending from mid-gland to apex. Note the interruption of the low-signal-intensity fibromuscular stroma suggestive of tumor invasion (arrows in a and b). Findings at surgery and step-section histopathologic examination (c) confirm a Gleason grade 6 tumor that invades the anterior fibromuscular stroma

(30–60 seconds post-injection) had an 80% accuracy rate for PZ tumors, but for lesions in the TZ, the detection rate was 63% [58]. The results of a recent meta-analysis [59] indicated that DCE-MRI could help improve the accuracy of prostate cancer localization and staging, but the sample size was small (only eight studies were included in the analysis) and further data are needed. A recent study conducted by the same group concluded that the combination of high-resolution spatio-vascular infor-

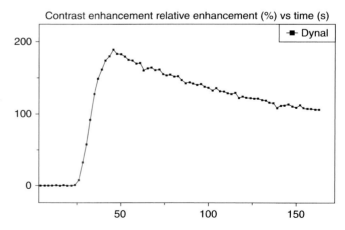

Fig. 22.7 DCE-MRI study in a patient with biopsy-proven prostate cancer in the left peripheral zone. DCE-MRI relative signal intensity contrast uptake curve (a) for the tumour region of interest is typical for malignancy due to rapid uptake and washout. Corresponding pixel color maps of gadolinium transfer rate (b) and gadolinium washout rate (c) are also shown superimposed on T2W anatomical images

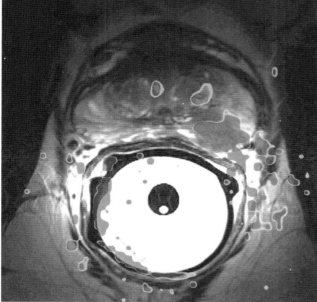

Fig. 22.7 (continued)

MRI diffusion-weighted techniques have also been used in imaging of prostate cancer. At present, the data from the literature are not uniform and the preliminary results indicate that there is an overlap of the apparent diffusion coefficient (ADC) in PZ tumors and in normal prostatic tissue [60, 61].

MR Spectroscopy of the Prostate Gland

The combination of MRI and ^{1}H-MRSI may become an important tool in the detection and staging of prostate cancer [62–65]. ^{1}H-MRSI of the prostate gland expands the diagnostic assessment of prostate cancer through the detection of cellular metabolites and may potentially lead to noninvasive differentiation of cancer from healthy tissue [66].

Normal prostate tissue contains high levels of citrate and low levels of choline and creatine. Citrate is synthesized, stored, and secreted by glandular tissue in the prostate [67–70]. The choline peak consists mainly of choline, phosphocholine, and glycerophosphocholine, which are constituents of cell membrane synthesis and degradation pathways and have been shown to be elevated in many malignancies [71–74]. The creatine peak is comprised of creatine and phosphocreatine [63]. It should be noted that citrate levels of normal prostatic tissue are higher in the peripheral zone than in the central zone and transition zone. However, glandular hyperplastic nodules of benign prostatic hypertrophy can demonstrate citrate levels as high as those observed in the peripheral zone. With improved technology, the polyamines peak which lies between choline and creatine can be resolved.

Pathology-proven prostate cancer shows a pattern of elevated choline and reduced or no citrate (Figs. 22.5 and 22.8) compared to healthy peripheral zone tissue [63, 73, 75–77]. The differences in the concentrations of metabolites are believed to be due to enhancement of phospholipid membrane turnover associated with tumor cell proliferation and increased cellularity and growth. It should be noted, however, that while the citrate level falls in prostate cancer, it is also reduced by prostatitis and post-biopsy hemorrhage [78].

The individual choline + creatine/citrate ratio is used for spectral analysis in the clinical setting because the spectral peaks of creatine and choline often overlap and may be inseparable [79]. The choline + creatine/citrate ratio for normal prostate tissue has been established as 0.22 ± 0.13. At present, there is no consensus about spectral interpretation. The most frequently used method is the classification system described by Kurhanewicz et al. [29, 63, 79]. In this system a voxel is classified as normal, suspicious, or very suspicious for cancer. Sometimes the voxel may contain non-diagnostic levels of metabolites or artifacts that may obscure the metabolite frequency range. They should not contain any metabolites with a signal-to-noise ratio greater than 5. Furthermore, in voxels in which only one metabolite is detectable, the other metabolites are assigned a value equivalent to the standard deviation (SD) of the noise. The voxels are designated as suspicious for cancer if the choline + creatine/citrate ratio is at least 2 SDs higher than the average ratio for the normal zone. Voxels are considered very suspicious if the above ratio is more than 3 SDs higher than the average ratio [63, 79]. At present, the relative size of the voxels is large in proportion to the prostate, and radiological virtual biopsies for diagnosis are not appropriate. Recently,

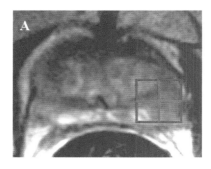

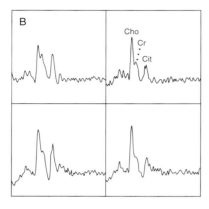

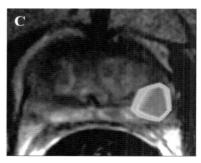

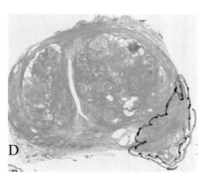

Fig. 22.8 Sixty-seven-year-old patient with PSA 5.79 ng/mL, clinical stage T1C, and biopsy Gleason grade 4+5. (a) Axial T2-weighted MR image with region of suspicion outlined by the MR spectroscopy grid, (b) MR spectroscopy grid demonstrating voxels suspicious for cancer in peripheral zone with elevated choline and reduced citrate, (c) axial T2-weighted MR image with color map overlay of the metabolic ratio (Cho + Cr / Cit), and (d) the histopathology step-section exhibiting cancer (outlined; surgical Gleason grade 4+5) in the left posterior peripheral zone

there has been increased interest in polyamine metabolism in prostate cancer, and low levels of polyamines have been reported in patients with prostate cancer [80].

Prostate Cancer Diagnosis and Characterization

Diagnosis and characterization of prostate cancer is usually achieved through histological examination following biopsy or transurethral resection of the prostate. MRI is reserved only for those patients in whom there is a clinical suspicion of cancer, often when there is an elevated PSA with two or more negative biopsies. In addition, the combination of MRI/MRSI can be useful in providing information for biopsy targeting or for quantifying the need for further biopsies [23, 51, 81]. Knowledge of pertinent clinical information such as sextant biopsy results, DRE findings, and PSA level prior to MRI/MRSI examination is important and results in increased test sensitivity.

Digital rectal examination, transrectal ultrasound (TRUS) images, and biopsy results (if the biopsies are separately labeled) can usually provide accurate information on tumor localization. However, there are limitations to this approach [82, 83]. This is confirmed by a recent study comparing DRE, TRUS-guided biopsy, and endorectal MRI in the detection and localization of prostate cancer. The investigators found that MRI performed significantly better than the DRE in detecting cancer in the apex, mid-gland, and base, and significantly better than TRUS-guided biopsy in the mid-gland and base [84]. The addition of MRSI to MRI significantly improves the specificity of tumor localization [76].

One of the most challenging characteristics of prostate cancer is its variability in biological aggressiveness. To determine the appropriate treatment options (which may include deferral of treatment), it is very important to predict the so-called indolent tumors. Kattan et al. developed nomograms for the prediction of pathologically indolent cancer [85], which they defined as organ-confined cancer with a volume of less than 0.5 cc and no elements of Gleason grade 4 or 5. The variables used in the nomograms include PSA, clinical stage, Gleason grade, proportion of cancer in a biopsy, and prostate volume on ultrasound. In a recent study, the accuracy of MRI in the detection of pathologically indolent prostate cancer was 74.4% and that of combined MRI/MRSI was 84.6% [86]. While the information from MRI/MRSI and the nomogram is not sufficient to place a patient into a surveillance program, it will assist with patient counseling and decision-making [85].

Preliminary reports on MRSI assessment of tumor aggressiveness are promising. In a recent study [77], MRI/MRSI data from a subset of 123 patients were compared to step-section histopathology. The study demonstrated that tumor detection on MRSI is dependent on Gleason score. MRSI overall sensitivity was 56% for tumor detection, increasing from 44% in Gleason pattern 3+3 lesions to 89% in lesions with Gleason pattern ≥ 4+4. There was a significant correlation between (choline+creatine)/citrate and Gleason score. Tumor volume assessed by MRSI also correlated positively with Gleason score [77]. Therefore, there is a rationale for adding MRI/MRSI to the pre-treatment evaluation of patients with prostate cancer. To date, combined use of MRI and MRSI has been limited to only a few centers, but its role is expected to increase with the dissemination of the technology.

There are controversial data on the value of DCE-MRI in assessing tumor aggressiveness. Barentz et al. suggested that very rapid enhancement occurs in very poorly differentiated tumors [34]. Although more recent studies have found a poor-to-moderate correlation between dynamic parameters/T2 relaxation rate and Gleason score [56, 87], the technique is promising and further data are needed.

Prostate Cancer Staging

Currently, the revised TNM classification is widely used in clinical practice to precisely stratify patients with newly diagnosed prostate cancer (Table 22.1) [88]. MR imaging plays an important role in the assessment of clinical T staging, being more accurate than CT, US, and DRE. The ability of MRI/MRSI to determine the location of the tumor, presence or absence of extracapsular extension (ECE), seminal vesicle involvement, and lymph node or bone metastases is very useful in the pre-treatment setting, allowing for more accurate prognostic and pathological estimations and "evidence-based" treatment decisions.

The value of MRI staging was demonstrated in a 5-year follow-up study of 1,025 cases staged radiologically before prostatectomy [89]. Tumors with established ECE on MRI had a significantly worse prognosis. A decision analysis model suggested that pre-operative MRI was cost-effective in patients with moderate and high risks of ECE [90]. MRI accuracy on prostate cancer staging ranges between 50 and 92% [59, 91–93]. In a recent study, multivariate analysis of endorectal MRI and other pre-operative variables (PSA, clinical stage, Gleason score, % cancer in biopsy cores, perineural invasion) showed that MRI findings are significant presurgical predictors of ECE in patients with prostate cancer and add incremental value to clinical variables [93]. MRI findings suggestive of ECE are (1) tumor envelopment of the neurovascular bundles; (2) asymmetry of the neurovascular bundles; (3) irregular, spiculated margins; (4) angulated con-

Table 22.1 TNM definitions for prostate cancer (AJCC Prostate Cancer Staging) [88]

Primary tumor (T)
TX: Primary tumor cannot be assessed
T0: No evidence of primary tumor
T1: Clinically the tumor is neither palpable nor visible by imaging
    T1a: Tumor incidental histologic finding in 5% or less of tissue resected
    T1b: Tumor incidental histologic finding in more than 5% of tissue resected
    T1c: Tumor identified by needle biopsy (e.g., because of elevated PSA)
T2: Tumor confined within prostate
    T2a: Tumor involves one half of 1 lobe or less
    T2b: Tumor involves more than one half of 1 lobe but not both lobes
    T2c: Tumor involves both lobes
T3: Tumor extends through the prostate capsule
    T3a: Extracapsular extension (unilateral or bilateral)
    T3b: Tumor invades seminal vesicle(s)
T4: Tumor is fixed or invades adjacent structures other than seminal vesicles: bladder neck, external sphincter, rectum, levator muscles, and/or pelvic wall

Regional lymph nodes (N)
    NX: Regional lymph nodes were not assessed
    N0: No regional lymph node metastasis
    N1: Metastasis in regional lymph node(s)

Distant metastasis (M)
MX: Distant metastasis cannot be assessed (not evaluated by any modality)
M0: No distant metastasis
M1: Distant metastasis
    M1a: Nonregional lymph node(s)
    M1b: Bone(s)
    M1c: Other site(s) with or without bone disease

tour of the prostate gland; (5) capsular retraction; and (6) obliteration of the retroprostatic angle (Fig. 22.9) [25, 94]. Despite its high specificity in the identification of organ-confined disease and extracapsular extension, owing to lower sensitivity and large interobserver variability, the routine use of MR imaging in the local staging of prostate cancer remains controversial.

Reader experience in interpretation of prostate MRI is important and remains a barrier to greater acceptance of the test for preoperative imaging in many centers. The addition of MRSI to MRI has been shown to increase staging accuracy for less experienced readers and reduce interobserver variability [76]. A recent cohort study reviewed preprostatectomy MR images of 344 consecutive patients with biopsy-proven prostate cancer [95]. They demonstrated that MRI findings are significant predictors of ECE and added significant incremental value to clinical variables when the images were interpreted by genitourinary radiologists experienced in MRI of the prostate rather than by general body MRI radiologists.

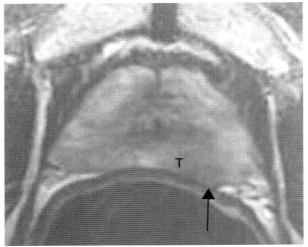

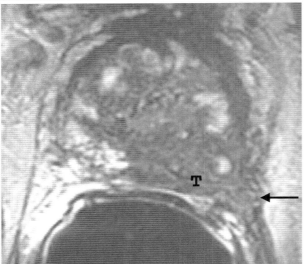

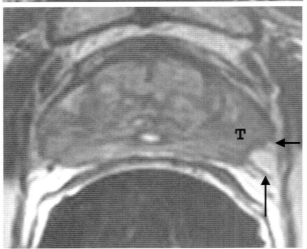

Fig. 22.9 Three different prostate cancer cases with extracapsular extension of the tumor (*T*). T2-weighted axial MR images show asymmetry of the capsule and obliteration of the rectoprostatic angle (arrow in a), breach of the capsule with direct tumor extension and envelopment of the left neurovascular bundle (arrow in b), and spiculated margin of the capsule and retraction of the left neurovascular bundle (arrows in c)

Lymph node metastasis and seminal vesicle invasion (SVI) are important predictors of tumor progression because they are associated with high rates of treatment failure [96, 97]. Bernstein et al. reviewed 124 patients with cT1c disease who were imaged by MRI prior to surgery [98]. They found that MRI and pre-operative PSA levels were predictors of SVI. In a recent cohort study of 612 consecutive patients, Wang et al. compared preoperative MRI findings to pathological specimens from radical prostatectomy and found that MRI had a positive predictive value of 78% and a negative predictive value of 94% for seminal vesicle invasion [99]. The criteria for diagnosing SVI on MR imaging are (1) focal area of low signal intensity within the seminal vesicles; (2) seminal vesicle obstruction with associated low-signal-intensity mass; (3) direct tumor extension from the base to the undersurface of the seminal vesicles; and (4) expanded, low-signal-intensity ejaculatory duct with associated low-signal-intensity seminal vesicle (Fig. 22.10) [25, 55]. Cross-referencing of images obtained in transaxial, coronal, and sagittal planes is crucial for accurate diagnosis of ECE and SVI. MR imaging is also helpful in evaluating the extension of the disease to adjacent organs such as urinary bladder and rectum. These are best appreciated on the sagittal images.

DCE-MRI may be useful for selected patients with equivocal evidence of capsular penetration [33]. A recent study demonstrated accuracy rates of 84, 97, and 97% for the detection of capsular penetration, seminal vesicle invasion, and neurovascular bundle involvement, respectively [58].

Detection of Lymph Node Metastasis – Role of MRI

The PSA levels recommended by the AUA for identifying high-risk patients with lymph node and bone metastases are 15 and 20 ng/mL, respectively. However, there is wide variation in the cut-off values for PSA reported in the literature [100, 101]. The conventional criterion for detection of metastatic lymph nodes on imaging (either CT or MRI) is a short axis of 7 mm. MRI and CT have similar efficacy in detecting lymph node metastases, with both modalities having low sensitivity. A recent study of 411 patients with clinically localized prostate cancer demonstrated that MRI was a statistically significant independent predictor of LNM, with positive and negative predictive values of 50 and 96%, respectively. On multivariate analysis, prediction of lymph node status using the model that included all MRI variables (ECE, SVI, LNM) along with the Partin nomogram results had a significantly greater AUC than the univariate model that included only MRI LNM findings (p<0.01) [102].

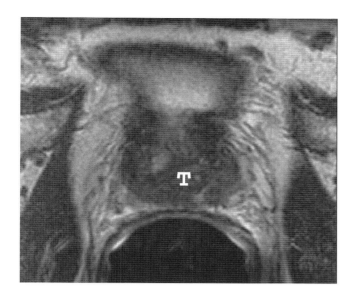

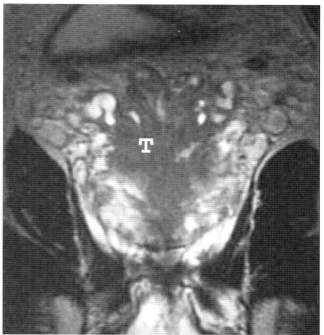

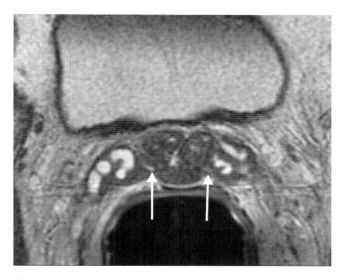

Fig. 22.10 Biopsy-proven Gleason grade 9 adenocarcinoma in a 68-year-old man with a PSA level of 3.9 ng/mL. T2-weighted axial images obtained at the levels of the base of the prostate (a) and the seminal vesicles (b) show a low-signal-intensity tumor (*T*) involving the base bilaterally, with invasion of both seminal vesicles (arrows in b). T2-weighted coronal image (c) demonstrates expansion of both ejaculatory ducts and low-signal-intensity tumor within both seminal vesicles (*T*). T2-weighted sagittal MR image (d) shows direct tumor extension from the base into the seminal vesicles (*T*)

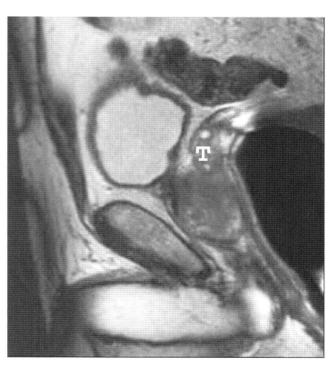

Fig. 22.10 (continued)

High-resolution MRI with lymphotropic paramagnetic ultra-small particles has demonstrated excellent results in detecting prostate cancer metastasis in normal-sized lymph nodes. Ultra-small paramagnetic iron oxide particles (USPIO) are injected intravenously 24 hours before MR imaging. They are slowly extravasated into the interstitial space and are transported to lymph nodes via the lymphatics, where they are internalized by macrophages. Due to the

T2 susceptibility effect, the normal part of the node loses signal intensity because it contains macrophages, while the metastasis remains of high signal intensity due to lack of macrophages (Fig. 22.11). Initial work reported a sensitivity of 100% and a specificity of 80% [103]. A recent study

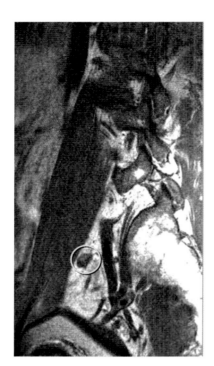

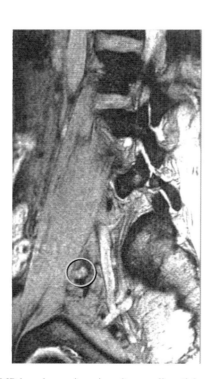

of 80 patients with prostate cancer who underwent lymph node resection or biopsy after MR lymphography demonstrated a sensitivity of 91% compared with a sensitivity of 35% for conventional MRI [104]. The use of this method in intermediate- to high-risk patients has been shown to be cost-effective [105].

Detection of Bone Metastasis – Role of MRI

Radionuclide bone scintigraphy is the initial imaging modality recommended for detection of bone metastasis in patients with prostate cancer. However, MRI is superior to bone scintigraphy in detecting bone metastasis in the axial skeleton [106] and is a useful problem-solving tool in patients with equivocal bone scintigrams [107]. A study of 200 patients with histologically proven prostate or breast cancer found that only 4 patients (2%) had peripheral bone metastases, which would have been missed by MRI [22]. Moreover, three of these metastases were painful and thus would have prompted further imaging anyway. Bone metastasis typically has low signal intensity on T1-weighted MR images and high signal intensity on T2-weighted images (Fig. 22.12).

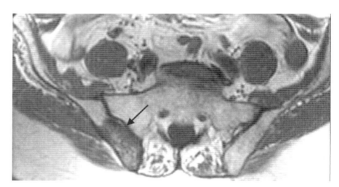

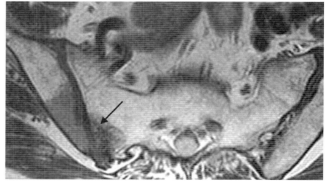

Fig. 22.11 MR lymphography using ultra-small particles of iron oxide (USPIO) in a patient with biopsy-proven prostate cancer. T1W image (a) demonstrates a small left obturator lymph node. T2*W image (b) obtained 24 hours after administration of USPIO (Sinerem) shows a high-signal-intensity node indicating lack of contrast uptake which is typical for a metastatic lymph node

Fig. 22.12 Biopsy-proven Gleason grade 8 adenocarcinoma in a 62-year-old man with a PSA level of 8.6 ng/mL. T1- (a) and T2-weighted axial images obtained at the level of the sacro-iliac joint (b) demonstrate an area of low signal intensity causing expansion of the right iliac bone and abutting the right sacro-iliac joint (arrows). Appearances are consistent with bone metastasis

However, more sclerotic lesions can have low signal intensity on both sequences.

While at present bone scintigraphy remains the test of choice for the detection of bone metastases, new MR techniques such as the whole-body MRI survey may replace bone scintigraphy in the future [108–111]. In a study by Lauenstein et al. [109], 26 patients with known or suspected bone metastases from different primary malignancies, who had undergone radionuclide scintigraphy, were examined by MRI. Patients were placed on a rolling table platform with integrated phased-array surface coils that was capable of pulling the patient through the isocenter of the magnet. T1-weighted gradient-recalled echo, half-Fourier-acquired single-shot turbo spin echo, and short tau inversion recovery images were obtained in the coronal plane. In addition, the spine was imaged in the sagittal plane. The MRI screening for bone metastases correlated well with bone scintigraphy. Using the same technique, the same group recently evaluated a total of 51 patients with known malignant tumors, among whom 24 had suspected or known bone metastasis. Whole-body MR imaging performed on a per-patient basis revealed sensitivity and specificity values of 100%. The regions missed by MRI were located mainly in the ribs and skull. MRI could identify additional bone metastases in spine, pelvis, and femur. The mean examination time for whole-body MR imaging was 14.5 minutes [110]. One limitation of MRI, however, is that other causes of altered marrow signal (trauma, infection, etc.) can mimic metastatic disease to the bone.

MR Imaging of Recurrent Prostate Cancer

Following primary treatment for prostate cancer, detection of residual or recurrent disease is crucial in order to make prompt treatment decisions for salvage prostatectomy following radiation failure or salvage radiotherapy after radical retropubic prostatectomy (RRP) failure and/or systemic therapy. In patients who are potentially cured, the PSA level should decrease to an undetectable level within a month and should remain undetectable thereafter. Serial measurements of PSA level and DRE are the standard tools used to monitor tumor recurrence. The earliest and most common indication of recurrence is a rise of serum PSA level. Biochemical relapse is defined as an increase in blood serum PSA levels in three consecutive measurements. When the PSA is elevated, the main consideration is the differentiation between local and distant recurrence. A number of clinical nomograms have been developed to predict whether a recurrence is local or metastatic [8]. They are based on clinical parameters such as tumor stage and grade at the time of diagnosis and the PSA doubling time [8]. The incidence of biochemical relapse

following RRP or radiotherapy ranges from 15 to 53% [9]. A diagnostic work-up is generated when prostate cancer recurrence is suspected due to rising PSA or a palpable nodule at DRE.

MRI can be used to evaluate both local and systemic recurrence, with endorectal MRI being capable of detecting local recurrence even in patients with rising PSA but no palpable tumor on DRE. Silverman and Krebs [112] reported excellent sensitivity (100%) and specificity (100%) of MRI in the evaluation of local recurrence following RRP. This was recently confirmed in a study by Sella et al. (sensitivity and specificity of 95 and 100%, respectively) [113]. The MR technique for detection of recurrent disease is similar to that used for the pretreatment staging of prostate cancer. Following RRP, tumor recurrence is better appreciated on T2-weighted axial images, on which it has higher signal intensity than the adjacent muscle (Fig. 22.13) [112, 113]. Cross-referencing of all three planes of imaging is important for accurate lesion localization and the use of the sagittal plane is crucial in the detection of bladder neck invasion (Fig. 22.10). Local recurrence can be detected on MRI at the peri-anastomotic and retrovesical regions. However, 30% of local recurrences can occur elsewhere in the pelvis, at the lateral or anterior surgical margins or at sites of retained seminal vesicles [113]. While seminal vesicle tissue does not contribute to serum PSA, retained seminal vesicle following RRP can be the source of confusion on rectal examination or imaging. MRI can elegantly demonstrate the retained seminal vesicles and differentiate them from fibrosis and tumor recurrence [114]. MRI has the potential to guide a transrectal biopsy to the recurrent sites and may lead to a better diagnostic yield than TRUS.

Following pelvic radiation, however, assessment of intraprostatic tumor location and parameters determining local stage, specifically ECE and SVI, may be significantly hindered by tissue changes related to radiotherapy. It has been reported that diffuse decrease of T2-weighted signal intensity within the gland and loss or indistinctness of zonal anatomy make it more difficult to distinguish cancer lesions from benign prostatic tissue [115]. On T2-weighted images, recurrent tumors appear as low-signal-intensity foci compared to the surrounding peripheral zone but have higher signal intensity than adjacent levator ani muscles.

Curative treatment options following failure of radiation therapy for localized prostate cancer are limited. Additional regimens of radiation are risky due to potential injury to the rectum, urethra, or bladder. Hormonal therapy provides limited local tumor control that is not curative. While salvage radical prostatectomy can result in prolonged disease-free survival, its routine use has not been widely accepted because of concerns for short- and long-term morbidity and because of a tendency for clinical understaging prior to surgery. In a recent study, MRI prior to salvage prostatectomy showed

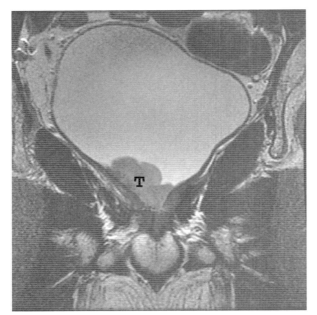

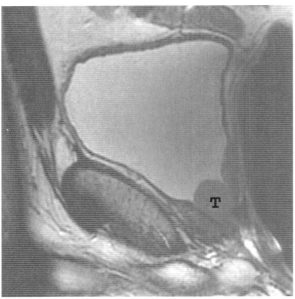

Fig. 22.13 T2-weighted axial (a) and sagittal (b) images of a 65-year-old man with increasing PSA levels after radical prostatectomy for a Gleason grade 8 adenocarcinoma of the prostate. An intermediate-signal-intensity soft tissue mass (*T*) is seen invading the bladder neck, and the appearance is consistent with recurrent tumor

substantial interobserver variability, even among readers with similar experience in MRI interpretation [116]. Nevertheless, the accuracy of MRI in tumor evaluation prior to salvage prostatectomy in this study was similar to the accuracy of MRI for pretreatment staging. Endorectal MRI prior to salvage prostatectomy achieved sensitivity/specificity values of 76%/73% for tumor detection, 86%/84% for ECE, and 58%/96% for SVI [116]. These results suggest that information obtained from MRI should be incorporated into the

criteria used to select patients appropriate for salvage radical prostatectomy

Following radiotherapy, MRSI demonstrates an absence of detectable metabolites in most voxels. However, the presence of voxels in which the only detectable metabolite is choline should raise a suspicion of recurrent or residual tumor. In a recent study of patients with biochemical failure after external beam radiotherapy, MRSI had a sensitivity of 87% and a specificity of 72% for detection of recurrent tumor [117]. Furthermore, in the same study, MRSI had a 100% negative predictive value for the exclusion of local recurrent tumor when there was no metabolic activity on spectroscopy. A further study compared sextant biopsy, DRE, MRI, and MRSI in nine patients with rising PSA after external beam radiation therapy who underwent salvage radical prostatectomy with step-section pathology. MRI and MRSI had estimated sensitivities of 68 and 77%, respectively, while the sensitivities of biopsy and DRE were 48 and 16%, respectively. MRSI was found to have lower specificity (78%) than the other three diagnostic tests, each of which had a specificity above 90% [118]. In patients who have had cryotherapy, MRSI has been shown to be superior to MRI or TRUS in determining local recurrence [50, 119].

An additional benefit of MRI over other imaging methods is the ability to concomitantly evaluate pelvic lymph nodes and osseous structures, resulting in the detection of all sites of pelvic relapse in a single examination (see Section on Prostate Cancer Staging).

Conclusions

We believe that a combination of MRI and MRSI provides detailed anatomic and metabolic information on the prostate gland and surrounding pelvic structures, leading to significant improvement in cancer detection and staging. It also results in more accurate evaluation of tumor volume and aggressiveness, allowing for better, more patient-specific therapy. At present most of the published work has come from major institutions with expertise. However, considering the benefits that MRI and MRSI have been shown to offer patients, the skills and technology required to perform these tests should be widely disseminated to make their routine use possible. Teamwork between members of radiology, pathology, urology, and radiation oncology departments is essential.

References

1. Jemal A, Murray T, Ward E, et al. Cancer statistics. CA Cancer J Clin. 2008;58:71–96.
2. American Cancer Society. Cancer facts and figures. Report No.: 5008.04. Atlanta, Ga: American Cancer Society; 2004.

3. Amling CL, Blute ML, Lerner SE, et al. Influence of prostate-specific antigen testing on the spectrum of patients with prostate cancer undergoing radical prostatectomy at a large referral practice. Mayo Clin Proc. 1998;73:401–6.

4. Stamey TA, Sozen TS, Yemoto CM, et al. Classification of localized untreated prostate cancer based on 791 men treated only with radical prostatectomy: common ground for therapeutic trials and TNM subgroups. J Urol. 1998;159:2009–12.

5. Stephenson RA, Stanford JL. Population-based prostate cancer trends in the United States: patterns of change in the era of prostate-specific antigen. World J Urol. 1997;15:331–5.

6. Kaminski JM, Hanlon AL, Horwitz EM, et al. Relationship between prostate volume, prostate-specific antigen nadir, and biochemical control. Int J Radiat Oncol Biol Phys. 2002;52:888–92.

7. Zelefsky MJ, Fuks Z, Hunt M, et al. High dose radiation delivered by intensity modulated conformal radiotherapy improves the outcome of localized prostate cancer. J Urol. 2001;166:876–81.

8. Kattan MW, Eastham JA, Stapleton AM, et al. A preoperative nomogram for disease recurrence following radical prostatectomy for prostate cancer. J Natl Cancer Inst. 1998;90:766–71.

9. Pound CR, Partin AW, Eisenberger MA, et al. Natural history of progression after PSA elevation following radical prostatectomy. Jama. 1999;281:1591–7.

10. Platt JF, Bree RL, Schwab RE. The accuracy of CT in the staging of carcinoma of the prostate. AJR Am J Roentgenol. 1987;149:315–8.

11. Engeler CE, Wasserman NF, Zhang G. Preoperative assessment of prostatic carcinoma by computerized tomography. Weaknesses and new perspectives. Urology. 1992;40:346–50.

12. Wolf JS, Jr., Cher M, Dall'era M, et al. The use and accuracy of cross-sectional imaging and fine needle aspiration cytology for detection of pelvic lymph node metastases before radical prostatectomy. J Urol. 1995;153(3 Pt 2):993–9.

13. Thompson I, Thrasher J, Aus G, et al. Guideline for the management of clinically localized prostate cancer. J Urol. 2007;177:2106–31.

14. Flocks R, Culp D, Porto R. Lymphatic spread from prostate cancer. J Urol. 1959;81:194–6.

15. Coakley FV, Lin RY, Schwartz LH, et al. Mesenteric adenopathy in patients with prostate cancer: frequency and etiology. AJR Am J Roentgenol. 2002;178:125–7.

16. Spencer JA, Golding SJ. Patterns of lymphatic metastases at recurrence of prostate cancer: CT findings. Clin Radiol. 1994;49:404–7.

17. Tiguert R, Gheiler EL, Tefilli MV, et al. Lymph node size does not correlate with the presence of prostate cancer metastasis. Urology.1999;53:367–71.

18. Walsh JW, Amendola MA, Konerding KF, et al. Computed tomographic detection of pelvic and inguinal lymph-node metastases from primary and recurrent pelvic malignant disease. Radiology. 1980;137(1 Pt 1):157–66.

19. Rorvik J, Halvorsen OJ, Albrektsen G, et al. Lymphangiography combined with biopsy and computer tomography to detect lymph node metastases in localized prostate cancer. Scand J Urol Nephrol. 1998;32:116–9.

20. Oyen RH, Van Poppel HP, Ameye FE, et al. Lymph node staging of localized prostatic carcinoma with CT and CT-guided fine-needle aspiration biopsy: prospective study of 285 patients. Radiology. 1994;190:315–22.

21. Taoka T, Mayr NA, Lee HJ, et al. Factors influencing visualization of vertebral metastases on MR imaging versus bone scintigraphy. AJR Am J Roentgenol. 2001;176:1525–30.

22. Traill ZC, Talbot D, Golding S, et al. Magnetic resonance imaging versus radionuclide scintigraphy in screening for bone metastases. Clin Radiol. 1999;54:448–51.

23. Beyersdorff D, Taupitz M, Winkelmann B, et al. Patients with a history of elevated prostate-specific antigen levels and negative transrectal US-guided quadrant or sextant biopsy results: value of MR imaging. Radiology. 2002;224:701–6.

24. Zakian KL, Eberhardt S, Hricak H, et al. Transition zone prostate cancer: metabolic characteristics at 1H MR spectroscopic imaging – initial results. Radiology. 2003;229:241–7.

25. Claus FG, Hricak H, Hattery RR. Pretreatment Evaluation of Prostate Cancer: Role of MR Imaging and 1H MR Spectroscopy. Radiographics. 2004;24 Suppl 1:S167–80.

26. Hricak H, Schoder H, Pucar D, et al. Advances in imaging in the postoperative patient with a rising prostate-specific antigen level. Semin Oncol. 2003;30:616–34.

27. Futterer JJ, Scheenen TW, Huisman HJ, et al. Initial experience of 3 tesla endorectal coil magnetic resonance imaging and 1H-spectroscopic imaging of the prostate. Invest Radiol. 2004;39:671–80.

28. Hricak H, White S, Vigneron D, et al. Carcinoma of the prostate gland: MR imaging with pelvic phased-array coils versus integrated endorectal–pelvic phased-array coils. Radiology. 1994;193:703–9.

29. Coakley FV, Qayyum A, Kurhanewicz J. Magnetic resonance imaging and spectroscopic imaging of prostate cancer. J Urol. 2003;170(6 Pt 2):S69–75;discussion S-6.

30. Rouviere O, Raudrant A, Ecochard R, et al. Characterization of time-enhancement curves of benign and malignant prostate tissue at dynamic MR imaging. Eur Radiol. 2003;13:931–42.

31. Preziosi P, Orlacchio A, Di Giambattista G, et al. Enhancement patterns of prostate cancer in dynamic MRI. Eur Radiol. 2003;13:925–30.

32. Oyen RH. Dynamic contrast-enhanced MRI of the prostate: is this the way to proceed for characterization of prostatic carcinoma? Eur Radiol. 2003;13:921–4.

33. Jager GJ, Ruijter ET, van de Kaa CA, et al. Dynamic TurboFLASH subtraction technique for contrast-enhanced MR imaging of the prostate: correlation with histopathologic results. Radiology. 1997;203:645–52.

34. Barentsz JO, Engelbrecht M, Jager GJ, et al. Fast dynamic gadolinium-enhanced MR imaging of urinary bladder and prostate cancer. J Magn Reson Imaging. 1999;10(3):295–304.

35. Padhani AR. Dynamic contrast-enhanced MRI in clinical oncology: current status and future directions. J Magn Reson Imaging. 2002;16:407–22.

36. Padhani AR, Dzik-Jurasz A. Perfusion MR imaging of extracranial tumor angiogenesis. Top Magn Reson Imaging. 2004;15:41–57.

37. Padhani AR, Hayes C, Landau S, Leach MO. Reproducibility of quantitative dynamic MRI of normal human tissues. NMR Biomed. 2002;15(2):143–53.

38. Port RE, Knopp MV, Hoffmann U, et al. Multicompartment analysis of gadolinium chelate kinetics: blood-tissue exchange in mammary tumors as monitored by dynamic MR imaging. J Magn Reson Imaging. 1999;10:233–41.

39. Taylor JS, Tofts PS, Port R, et al. MR imaging of tumor microcirculation: promise for the new millennium. J Magn Reson Imaging. 1999;10:903–7.

40. Tofts PS, Brix G, Buckley DL, et al. Estimating kinetic parameters from dynamic contrast-enhanced T(1)-weighted MRI of a diffusable tracer: standardized quantities and symbols. J Magn Reson Imaging. 1999;10:223–32.

41. Hayes C, Padhani AR, Leach MO. Assessing changes in tumour vascular function using dynamic contrast-enhanced magnetic resonance imaging. NMR Biomed. 2002;15:154–63.

42. Evelhoch JL. Key factors in the acquisition of contrast kinetic data for oncology. J Magn Reson Imaging. 1999;10:254–9.

43. Brown TR, Kincaid BM, Ugurbil K. NMR chemical shift imaging in three dimensions. Proc Natl Acad Sci USA. 1982;79: 3523–6.

44. Star-Lack J, Nelson SJ, Kurhanewicz J, et al. Improved water and lipid suppression for 3D PRESS CSI using RF band selective inversion with gradient dephasing (BASING). Magn Reson Med. 1997;38:311–21.

45. Kurhanewicz J, Swanson MG, Nelson SJ, et al. Combined magnetic resonance imaging and spectroscopic imaging approach to molecular imaging of prostate cancer. J Magn Reson Imaging. 2002;16:451–63.

46. Coakley FV, Hricak H. Radiologic anatomy of the prostate gland: a clinical approach. Radiol Clin North Am. 2000;38:15–30.

47. Hricak H, Dooms GC, McNeal JE, et al. MR imaging of the prostate gland: normal anatomy. AJR Am J Roentgenol. 1987;148:51–8.

48. Noguchi M, Stamey TA, Neal JE, et al. An analysis of 148 consecutive transition zone cancers: clinical and histological characteristics. J Urol. 2000;163:1751–5.

49. Gelet A, Chapelon JY, Bouvier R, et al. Transrectal high intensity focused ultrasound for the treatment of localized prostate cancer: factors influencing the outcome. Eur Urol. 2001;40:124–9.

50. Parivar F, Hricak H, Shinohara K, et al. Detection of locally recurrent prostate cancer after cryosurgery: evaluation by transrectal ultrasound, magnetic resonance imaging, and three-dimensional proton magnetic resonance spectroscopy. Urology. 1996;48: 594–9.

51. Perrotti M, Han KR, Epstein RE, et al. Prospective evaluation of endorectal magnetic resonance imaging to detect tumor foci in men with prior negative prostastic biopsy: a pilot study. J Urol. 1999;162:1314–7.

52. Lui PD, Terris MK, McNeal JE, et al. Indications for ultrasound guided transition zone biopsies in the detection of prostate cancer. J Urol. 1995;153(3 Pt 2):1000–3.

53. Fleshner NE, Fair WR. Indications for transition zone biopsy in the detection of prostatic carcinoma. J Urol. 1997;157:556–8.

54. Sommer FG, Nghiem HV, Herfkens R, et al. Determining the volume of prostatic carcinoma: value of MR imaging with an external-array coil. AJR Am J Roentgenol. 1993;161:81–6.

55. Akin O, Sala E, Moskowitz CS, et al. Transition zone prostate cancers: detection, localization, local staging and feature analysis with endorectal MR imaging. Radiology. 2006;239:784–92.

56. Engelbrecht MR, Huisman HJ, Laheij RJ, et al. Discrimination of prostate cancer from normal peripheral zone and central gland tissue by using dynamic contrast-enhanced MR imaging. Radiology. 2003;229:248–54.

57. van Dorsten FA, van der Graaf M, Engelbrecht MR, et al. Combined quantitative dynamic contrast-enhanced MR imaging and (1)H MR spectroscopic imaging of human prostate cancer. J Magn Reson Imaging. 2004;20:279–87.

58. Ogura K, Maekawa S, Okubo K, et al. Dynamic endorectal magnetic resonance imaging for local staging and detection of neurovascular bundle involvement of prostate cancer: correlation with histopathologic results. Urology. 2001;57:721–6.

59. Engelbrecht MR, Jager GJ, Laheij RJ, et al. Local staging of prostate cancer using magnetic resonance imaging: a meta-analysis. Eur Radiol. 2002;12:2294–302.

60. Hosseinzadeh K, Schwarz SD. Endorectal diffusion-weighted imaging in prostate cancer to differentiate malignant and benign peripheral zone tissue. J Magn Reson Imaging. 2004;20:654–61.

61. Issa B. In vivo measurement of the apparent diffusion coefficient in normal and malignant prostatic tissues using echo-planar imaging. J Magn Reson Imaging. 2002;16:196–200.

62. Schiebler ML, Schnall MD, Pollack HM, et al. Current role of MR imaging in the staging of adenocarcinoma of the prostate. Radiology. 1993;189:339–52.

63. Kurhanewicz J, Vigneron DB, Hricak H, et al. Three-dimensional H-1 MR spectroscopic imaging of the in situ human prostate with high (0.24–0.7-cm3) spatial resolution. Radiology. 1996;198:795–805.

64. Heerschap A, Jager GJ, van der Graaf M, et al. Proton MR spectroscopy of the normal human prostate with an endorectal coil and a double spin-echo pulse sequence. Magn Reson Med. 1997;37:204–13.

65. Coakley FV, Kurhanewicz J, Lu Y, et al. Prostate cancer tumor volume: measurement with endorectal MR and MR spectroscopic imaging. Radiology. 2002;223:91–7.

66. Kurhanewicz J, Vigneron DB, Males RG, et al. The prostate: MR imaging and spectroscopy. Present and future. Radiol Clin North Am. 2000;38:115–38, viii–ix.

67. Costello LC, Franklin RB. Citrate metabolism of normal and malignant prostate epithelial cells. Urology. 1997;50:3–12.

68. Kurhanewicz J, Dahiya R, Macdonald JM, et al. Citrate alterations in primary and metastatic human prostatic adenocarcinomas: 1H magnetic resonance spectroscopy and biochemical study. Magn Reson Med. 1993;29:149–57.

69. Kurhanewicz J, Vigneron DB, Nelson SJ, et al. Citrate as an in vivo marker to discriminate prostate cancer from benign prostatic hyperplasia and normal prostate peripheral zone: detection via localized proton spectroscopy. Urology. 1995;45:459–66.

70. Liney GP, Turnbull LW, Lowry M, et al. In vivo quantification of citrate concentration and water T2 relaxation time of the pathologic prostate gland using 1H MRS and MRI. Magn Reson Imaging. 1997;15:1177–86.

71. Sijens PE, Knopp MV, Brunetti A, et al. 1H MR spectroscopy in patients with metastatic brain tumors: a multicenter study. Magn Reson Med. 1995;33:818–26.

72. Koutcher JA, Ballon D, Graham M, et al. 31P NMR spectra of extremity sarcomas: diversity of metabolic profiles and changes in response to chemotherapy. Magn Reson Med. 1990;16:19–34.

73. Heerschap A, Jager GJ, van der Graaf M, et al. In vivo proton MR spectroscopy reveals altered metabolite content in malignant prostate tissue. Anticancer Res. 1997;17:1455–60.

74. Fulham MJ, Bizzi A, Dietz MJ, et al. Mapping of brain tumor metabolites with proton MR spectroscopic imaging: clinical relevance. Radiology. 1992;185:675–86.

75. Wefer AE, Hricak H, Vigneron DB, et al. Sextant localization of prostate cancer: comparison of sextant biopsy, magnetic resonance imaging and magnetic resonance spectroscopic imaging with step section histology. J Urol. 2000;164:400–4.

76. Scheidler J, Hricak H, Vigneron DB, et al. Prostate cancer: localization with three-dimensional proton MR spectroscopic imaging – clinicopathologic study. Radiology. 1999;213:473–80.

77. Zakian KL, Sircar K, Hricak H, et al. Correlation of proton MR spectroscopic imaging with gleason score based on step-section pathologic analysis after radical prostatectomy. Radiology. 2005;234:804–14.

78. Kaji Y, Kurhanewicz J, Hricak H, et al. Localizing prostate cancer in the presence of postbiopsy changes on MR images: role of proton MR spectroscopic imaging. Radiology. 1998;206: 785–90.

79. Males RG, Vigneron DB, Star-Lack J, et al. Clinical application of BASING and spectral/spatial water and lipid suppression pulses for prostate cancer staging and localization by in vivo 3D 1H magnetic resonance spectroscopic imaging. Magn Reson Med. 2000;43:17–22.

80. Swanson MG, Vigneron DB, Tabatabai ZL, et al. Proton HR-MAS spectroscopy and quantitative pathologic analysis of MRI/3D-MRSI-targeted postsurgical prostate tissues. Magn Reson Med. 2003;50:944–54.

81. Yuen JS, Thng CH, Tan PH, et al. Endorectal magnetic resonance imaging and spectroscopy for the detection of tumor foci in men

with prior negative transrectal ultrasound prostate biopsy. J Urol. 2004;171:1482–6.

82. Obek C, Louis P, Civantos F, et al. Comparison of digital rectal examination and biopsy results with the radical prostatectomy specimen. J Urol. 1999;161:494–8;discussion 8–9.

83. Salomon L, Colombel M, Patard JJ, et al. Value of ultrasound-guided systematic sextant biopsies in prostate tumor mapping. Eur Urol. 1999;35:289–93.

84. Mullerad M, Hricak H, Kuroiwa K, et al. Comparison of endorectal magnetic resonance imaging, guided prostate biopsy and digital rectal examination in the preoperative anatomical localization of prostate cancer. J Urol. 2005;174:2158–63.

85. Kattan MW, Eastham JA, Wheeler TM, et al. Counseling men with prostate cancer: a nomogram for predicting the presence of small, moderately differentiated, confined tumors. J Urol. 2003;170:1792–7.

86. Shukla-Dave A, Hricak H, Pucar D, et al. Indolent prostate cancer-prediction by magnetic resonance imaging and spectroscopy [abstract]. Proc Intl Soc Magn Reson Med. 2005; abstract no. 262.

87. Padhani AR, Gapinski CJ, Macvicar DA, et al. Dynamic contrast enhanced MRI of prostate cancer: correlation with morphology and tumour stage, histological grade and PSA. Clin Radiol. 2000;55:99–109.

88. Greene FL, Page DL, Fleming ID, et al. (editors). AJCC cancer staging manual. 6th ed. New York: Springer; 2002. pp. 309–16.

89. D'Amico AV, Whittington R, Malkowicz B, et al. Endorectal magnetic resonance imaging as a predictor of biochemical outcome after radical prostatectomy in men with clinically localized prostate cancer. J Urol. 2000;164(3 Pt 1):759–63.

90. Jager GJ, Severens JL, Thornbury JR, et al. Prostate cancer staging: should MR imaging be used? – A decision analytic approach. Radiology. 2000;215:445–51.

91. Yu KK, Scheidler J, Hricak H, et al. Prostate cancer: prediction of extracapsular extension with endorectal MR imaging and three-dimensional proton MR spectroscopic imaging. Radiology. 1999;213:481–8.

92. Huch Boni RA, Boner JA, Debatin JF, et al. Optimization of prostate carcinoma staging: comparison of imaging and clinical methods. Clin Radiol. 1995;50:593–600.

93. Wang L, Mullerad M, Chen HN, et al. Prostate cancer: incremental value of endorectal MR imaging findings for prediction of extracapsular extension. Radiology. 2004;232:133–9.

94. Yu KK, Hricak H, Alagappan R, et al. Detection of extracapsular extension of prostate carcinoma with endorectal and phased-array coil MR imaging: multivariate feature analysis. Radiology. 1997;202:697–702.

95. Mullerad M, Hricak H, Wang L, et al. Prostate cancer: detection of extracapsular extension by genitourinary and general body radiologists at MR imaging. Radiology. 2004;232:140–6.

96. Hull GW, Rabbani F, Abbas F, et al. Cancer control with radical prostatectomy alone in 1,000 consecutive patients. J Urol. 2002;167(2 Pt 1):528–34.

97. Catalona WJ, Ramos CG, Carvalhal GF. Contemporary results of anatomic radical prostatectomy. CA Cancer J Clin. 1999;49:282–96.

98. Bernstein MR, Cangiano T, D'Amico A, et al. Endorectal coil magnetic resonance imaging and clinicopathologic findings in T1c adenocarcinoma of the prostate. 2000;5:104–7.

99. Wang L, Hricak H, Eberhardt S, et al. Prostate cancer – value of 3D endorectal MR imaging in the evaluation of seminal vesicle invasion in patients treated by radical prostatectomy. AJR Am J Roentgenol. 2004;182 Suppl 4: S67.

100. Naya Y, Fritsche HA, Cheli CD, et al. Volume indexes of total, free, and complexed prostate-specific antigen enhance prediction of extraprostatic disease extension in men with nonpalpable prostate cancer. Urology. 2003;62:1058–62.

101. Wymenga LF, Boomsma JH, Groenier K, et al. Routine bone scans in patients with prostate cancer related to serum prostate-specific antigen and alkaline phosphatase. BJU Int. 2001;88:226–30.

102. Wang L, Hricak H, Kattan MW, et al. Combined Endorectal and Phased Array MRI in the Prediction of Pelvic Lymph Node Metastasis in Prostate Cancer. AJR Am J Roentgenol. 2006;186:743–8.

103. Bellin MF, Roy C, Kinkel K, et al. Lymph node metastases: safety and effectiveness of MR imaging with ultrasmall superparamagnetic iron oxide particles–initial clinical experience. Radiology. 1998;207:799–808.

104. Harisinghani MG, Barentsz J, Hahn PF, et al. Noninvasive detection of clinically occult lymph-node metastases in prostate cancer. N Engl J Med. 2003;348:2491–9.

105. Hovels AM, Heesakkers RA, Adang EM, et al. Cost-analysis of staging methods for lymph nodes in patients with prostate cancer: MRI with a lymph node-specific contrast agent compared to pelvic lymph node dissection or CT. Eur Radiol. 2004;14:1707–12.

106. Algra PR, Bloem JL, Tissing H, et al. Detection of vertebral metastases: comparison between MR imaging and bone scintigraphy. Radiographics. 1991;11:219–32.

107. Turner JW, Hawes DR, Williams RD. Magnetic resonance imaging for detection of prostate cancer metastatic to bone. J Urol. 1993;149:1482–4.

108. Barkhausen J, Quick HH, Lauenstein T, et al. Whole-body MR imaging in 30 seconds with real-time true FISP and a continuously rolling table platform: feasibility study. Radiology. 2001;220:252–6.

109. Lauenstein TC, Freudenberg LS, Goehde SC, et al. Whole-body MRI using a rolling table platform for the detection of bone metastases. Eur Radiol. 2002;12:2091–9.

110. Lauenstein TC, Goehde SC, Herborn CU, et al. Whole-body MR imaging: evaluation of patients for metastases. Radiology. 2004;233:139–48.

111. Lauenstein TC, Goehde SC, Herborn CU, et al. Three-dimensional volumetric interpolated breath-hold MR imaging for whole-body tumor staging in less than 15 minutes: a feasibility study. AJR Am J Roentgenol. 2002;179:445–9.

112. Silverman JM, Krebs TL. MR imaging evaluation with a transrectal surface coil of local recurrence of prostatic cancer in men who have undergone radical prostatectomy. AJR Am J Roentgenol. 1997;168:379–85.

113. Sella T, Schwartz LH, Swindle PW, et al. Suspected local recurrence after radical prostatectomy: endorectal coil MR imaging. Radiology. 2004;231:379–85.

114. Sella T, Schwartz LH, Hricak H. Retained seminal vesicles following radical prostatectomy – frequency, MRI characteristics and clinical relevance. AJR Am J Roentgenol. 2006;186:539–46.

115. Nudell DM, Wefer AE, Hricak H, et al. Imaging for recurrent prostate cancer. Radiol Clin North Am. 2000;38:213–29.

116. Sala E, Eberhardt SC, Akin O, et al. Endorectal MR imaging prior to salvage prostatectomy: tumor localization and staging. Radiology. 2006;238:176–83.

117. Coakley FV, Teh HS, Qayyum A, et al. Endorectal MR imaging and MR spectroscopic imaging for locally recurrent prostate cancer after external beam radiation therapy: preliminary experience. Radiology. 2004;233:441–8.

118. Pucar D, Shukla-Dave A, Hricak H, et al. Prostate cancer: correlation of MR imaging and MR spectroscopy with pathologic findings after radiation therapy: initial experience. Radiology. 2005;236:545–53.

119. Kurhanewicz J, Vigneron DB, Hricak H, et al. Prostate cancer: metabolic response to cryosurgery as detected with 3D H-1 MR spectroscopic imaging. Radiology. 1996;200:489–96.

Chapter 23

Prostate Carcinoma: Radionuclide Imaging and PET

N. Lawrentschuck, A.M. Scott, and D.M. Bolton

Nuclear medicine techniques play an important role in the diagnosis, monitoring, and in some cases treatment of prostate cancer. The earliest modality to have a large role in the staging of prostate cancer was bone scintigraphy, and this has remained an integral tool for over 30 years in the workup of newly diagnosed disease or in follow-up staging. Several radiolabeled agents such as strontium have also been used for therapeutic treatment of disseminated disease, particularly in the skeleton.

Two other developments again using radionuclides that emit gamma rays are emerging. First, radiolabeled monoclonal antibodies that are directed against specific antigens present on prostate cancer cells have emerged as a potential staging tool in prostate cancer. Second, prostate lymphoscintigraphy and intraoperative gamma probe application for the detection of sentinel lymph nodes have emerged as another useful technique of radionuclide imaging. In particular it has been a useful technique in identifying involved lymph nodes in penile cancer.

Finally, positron emission tomography (PET) that relies on the emission of positrons has become an increasingly powerful oncologic tool, with its role in testicular cancer as well as other organ malignancies now well established.

Bone Scintigraphy

Introduction

The current standard of practice for the detection of osseous metastatic disease remains radionuclide bone scintigraphy (bone scan). It remains the most widely accepted method for evaluating the skeleton for evidence of metastatic prostate cancer. Over time it has proven to be superior to clinical eval-

uation, plain radiography, and serum measurements of acid or alkaline phosphatase [1]. Bone scans have a sensitivity of up to 95% for detecting bone metastases [2].

Radiology focuses predominantly on structure while nuclear medicine provides complimentary information on function. Radionuclide bone scanning is performed using radiolabeled diphosphonates labeled with technetium such as ^{99m}Tc methylene diphosphonate (^{99m}Tc-MDP). The whole skeleton may be easily visualized in a short study. Bone scans are more sensitive than plain radiography for metastases since lesions cannot generally be seen on radiographs until 50% of the bone mineral matrix has been lost, while bone scanning needs only a relatively small increase in uptake due to increased bone turnover to be positive [3].

Radionuclide Bone Scanning

Conventional bone scanning involves assessment of the entire skeleton using the radiotracer ^{99m}Tc-MDP. After intravenous injection, the radiotracer is absorbed onto bone surfaces and its uptake depends on local blood flow and osteoblastic activity [4]. Patients are then placed under a gamma camera where radioactivity from isotope accumulation is detected, with uptake of radiotracer reflecting bone mineral turnover. Advanced skeletal metastases are readily detected using ^{99m}Tc-MDP scintigraphy (Fig 23.1), but early metastases may be missed because this technique relies on the osteoblastic reaction rather than the actual tumor being detected [4, 5]. As such, the sensitivity is compromised when attempting to detect microscopic or marrow infiltrate-only disease or osteolytic lesions (which are uncommon in prostate cancer).

Furthermore, the specificity may be compromised because increased radionuclide accumulation may develop in skeletal structures in response to malignant and benign bone diseases. In particular, trauma, infection, Paget's disease, and other arthropathies or bone marrow disorders may cause

N. Lawrentschuck (✉)
Department of Surgery, University of Melbourne, Heidelberg, Victoria, Australia

J.J.M.C.H. de la Rosette et al. (eds.), *Imaging in Oncological Urology*,
DOI 10.1007/978-1-84628-759-6_23, © Springer-Verlag London Limited 2009

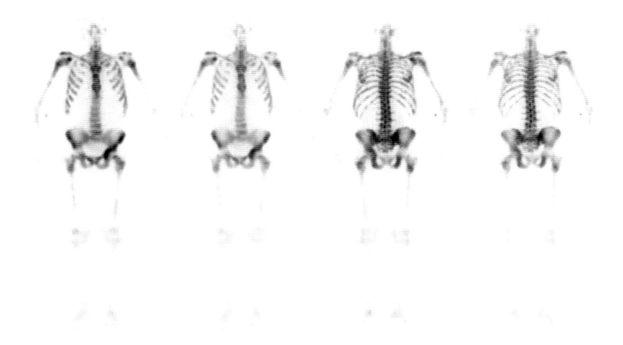

Fig. 23.1 A positive bone scan demonstrating widespread uptake in the axial skeleton ("superscan")

increased radionuclide accumulation [5]. False-positive bone scans may result (Fig. 23.2) necessitating further clinical history; plain radiography and rarely histologic biopsy may be necessary.

Bone scan accuracy appears to be maintained when patients have been administered with bisphosphonates which is becoming more common in prostate cancer with the development of newer agents [6]. One study has examined the impact of bisphosphonate therapy on bone scintigraphy results by matching bone histology at autopsy with bone scintigraphy findings in patients with hormone refractory prostate cancer. Long-term pamidronate treatment of prostate cancer bone metastases did not generally affect the ability to detect bone metastases [7].

Staging Patients with Newly Diagnosed Prostate Cancer

In a defining paper almost 30 years ago by Schaeffer and Pendergrass [8], 43% of patients with prostate cancer having an abnormal bone scan had no bone pain and a further 23% had normal serum alkaline phosphatase values. Hence bone scans were performed routinely in the evaluation of patients with newly diagnosed prostate cancer prior to the prostate-specific antigen (PSA) era to detect the presence or absence of bone metastases as serum blood tests were not reliable indicators of osseous disease [9].

However, in the PSA era, the notion of routine bone scan on diagnosis of prostate cancer has been challenged and redefined. In two landmark papers from the Mayo Clinic (Rochester, USA) involving almost 1400 patients, bone scintigraphy was consolidated as an important tool in patients newly diagnosed with prostate cancer in the PSA era. Chybowski and colleagues examined 521 randomly chosen patients with newly diagnosed prostate cancer and found that a serum PSA value less than 20 μg/L had a negative predictive value of 99.7% for bone scan findings. Clinical stage, tumor grade, serum acid phosphatase or prostatic acid phosphatase, or any combination of these had the predictive power of PSA alone [1, 10]. In the second study of 852 consecutive patients with newly diagnosed, untreated prostate cancer, with a serum PSA of 20 μg/L or less, the rate of false-negative results for PSA cut-off levels less than 20 μg/L was less than 2% [1]. Examining the figures from this study closely, the rate of false-negative results for an abnormal bone scan result was 0% with a serum value of 8 μg/L, or less, and 0.5% with a cut-off level of 10 μg/L. After these two studies it was generally considered that with a low PSA (less than 10 or 20 μg/L) a bone scan was not indicated in the absence of bone pain or a high-grade tumor (Gleason score 8 or above).

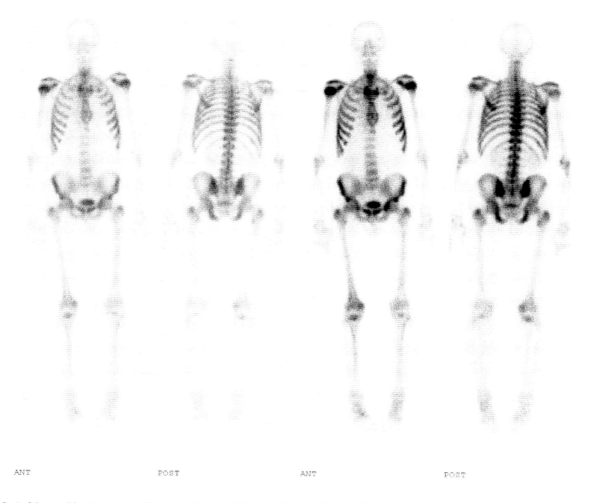

ANT   POST   ANT   POST

Fig. 23.2 A false-positive bone scan ("superscan") in a 75-year-old gentleman with prostate cancer who also had a concurrent hematologi- cal disease affecting bone marrow turnover that was responsible for the radiotracer uptake

Oesterling further emphasized that any test in medicine, including bone scans, will have false-negative results [1]. As such, patients should have a critical evaluation of their circumstance before a bone scan is denied based on PSA alone. In particular, patients having any prior treatment for prostate cancer such as radiotherapy, radical prostatectomy, or androgen deprivation therapy and those having treatment for benign prostatic hyperplasia (BPH) such as a 5-alpha-reductase inhibitor (finasteride or dutasteride) should be considered to have an unreliable serum PSA level with regard to predicting bone scan results.

The remaining controversy as to the role of bone scintigraphy in the initial assessment of prostate cancer is whether or not to perform a bone scan at first diagnosis in the absence of bone pain and a PSA in the range of 10–20 µg/L. The initial larger studies did not support a bone scan in patients with a PSA <20 µg/L. A recent study of 631 consecutive patients with newly diagnosed prostate cancer supported the initial larger studies whereby those patients with a low Gleason score, low PSA (<15 µg/L), and no bone pain could have a bone scan omitted [11]. The economics of omitting a bone scan are also important and have been highlighted in low-risk patients [1, 11]. However, recent literature suggests that there is still a demonstrable risk of bone metastases with a PSA under 10 µg/L [12] while other studies have also recommended a PSA cut-off of 10 µg/L for inclusion of bone scanning in the initial assessment [12–16]. Some have proposed bone scintigraphy where the combination of a serum alkaline phosphatase of >90 U/L together with bone pain and a PSA greater than 10 mg/ml exists but this needs further studies [17].

Patients with low-risk prostate cancer are unlikely to have metastatic disease documented by bone scan or CT. Therefore, these investigations should not be standard practice. However, symptomatic patients or those with PSA 20 ng/ml or greater, locally advanced disease, or Gleason score 8 or greater are at higher risk for bone metastases and should be considered for bone scan [18].

Assessment of Disease Activity and Treatment Response with Bone Scans

Re-staging Patients with a Rising PSA

In most cases of prostate cancer, recurrent disease presents initially as a rise in serum PSA (biochemical recurrence). Approximately one-third of patients undergoing radical prostatectomy or definitive radiation therapy will develop biochemical recurrence [19]. In many cases the rise in PSA is not accompanied by symptoms or any other signs on imaging of disease recurrence [20]. The clinical behavior of this group of patients is considered extremely heterogeneous and many patients will survive for 5–10 years with an elevated PSA as the only evidence of ongoing disease [19]. Imaging studies are frequently negative, especially in the initial stages of the rise, although there are exceptions where PSA does not reflect disease burden [21]. Patients having androgen therapy are certainly in this category [22].

The role of bone scans in the re-staging of prostate cancer depends on the clinical scenario. Early recommendations were for a routine bone scan in patients having radical prostatectomy who develop detectable PSA levels (biochemical recurrence) [20]. A survey among urologists revealed that 70% order a bone scan as part of a workup of patients with a rising PSA after radical prostatectomy [23]. Also, younger urologists are more likely to order a bone scan [24]. However, a positive bone scan in the setting of a PSA less than $10\,\mu g/L$ has been demonstrated to be only 1 or 2% [25, 26]. Other studies supported omitting a bone scan with biochemical recurrence when their PSA is less than 2 [16] or $7\,\mu g/L$ [27].

The principle use of bone scans is in patients with rising PSA values (Fig. 23.3). In a study by Cher and Bianco of 93 patients with 144 bone scans, the lowest PSA in the absence of adjuvant hormone treatment recording a positive bone scan was 46 ng/mL. They conducted an analysis revealing that stage, grade, preoperative PSA, and time to recurrence were not predictive of bone scan result. The degree of PSA recurrence and speed >5 µg/L per month were however predictive. The authors recommended that no bone scans should be performed before a significant PSA rise (greater than 40 ng/mL) in the absence of hormonal manipulation as for almost all patients the scan would be negative. Jhaveri and Klein concluded that bone scans in patients with a PSA recurrence after RP have limited usefulness until the PSA is 30 µg/L. These studies were also supported by Kane

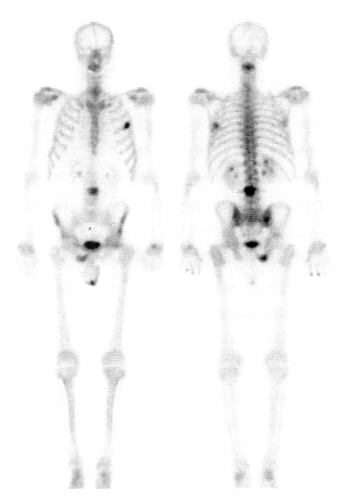

Fig. 23.3 Re-staging a 68-year-old gentleman with hormone refractory prostate carcinoma and a rising PSA to 59 µg/L. Widespread metastatic disease is apparent

et al. who followed 127 patients with biochemical recurrence with a bone scan, with 9% positive having a mean PSA of 61 ng/mL. PSA velocity was also an important determinant of scan result. A smaller study of post-radical prostatectomy patients with a biochemical recurrence also concluded the chances of finding a positive bone scan in the early stages were less than 5%.

Thus, routine bone scanning in the setting of early biochemical recurrence is probably unwarranted, especially with a PSA below 10 ng/mL, unless there is a rapid PSA rise and clinical symptoms. The published data do not clearly define a PSA threshold below which bone imaging should not be used and this could only be achieved by a large prospective study [28]. However, bone scans and possibly CT scans are often recommended in any patient with biochemical recurrence and who is being considered for additional salvage therapy [29].

Use of Serial Bone Scans in Monitoring Metastatic Prostate Cancer

In one study of 315 bone scans in 114 patients ranging from initial scan only to nine scans per patient, 17 patients had positive scans, 10 on initial scan, and 7 at follow-up. Nine patients had bone pain at the time of the first positive scan and pain developed in two patients 6 months and 2 years later, respectively. The other six patients are still asymptomatic 1–4 years later. False-positive scans were found in six other patients. No patient with bone pain had a negative scan [30]. This study and others suggest that routine bone scans in asymptomatic patients should be undertaken only where there is a high suspicion of skeletal complications based on other parameters.

The probability of positive findings in serial bone scans in untreated, localized, low to intermediate grade prostate cancer is also low when the follow-up PSA level remains $<15 \mu g/L$ [31]. Avoiding bone scans in this group of patients would translate into a significant cost saving and reduction in their psychological and physical burden [32].

The monitoring of therapeutic response of hormonal and other treatments with bone scans is also clinically useful (Fig. 23.4); however the possibility of increased uptake due to a "flare" response should always be considered. With hormone blockade approximately 3 weeks following initiation of treatment, most skeletal metastases from prostate cancer will demonstrate significantly enhanced radiotracer uptake relative to normal bone. Consequently, in the future it may be possible to improve the uptake and effectiveness of therapeutic bone-seeking radiopharmaceuticals by administering these agents following hormone therapy in patients with prostate cancer metastases [33].

Prognosis

Classifying bone scans according to the site of metastases (axial versus appendicular) had many advantages. It is easy to understand and may assist the urologist in predicting the patient prognosis. Axial metastases carry a better prognosis than appendicular metastasis [34]. In addition the percentage

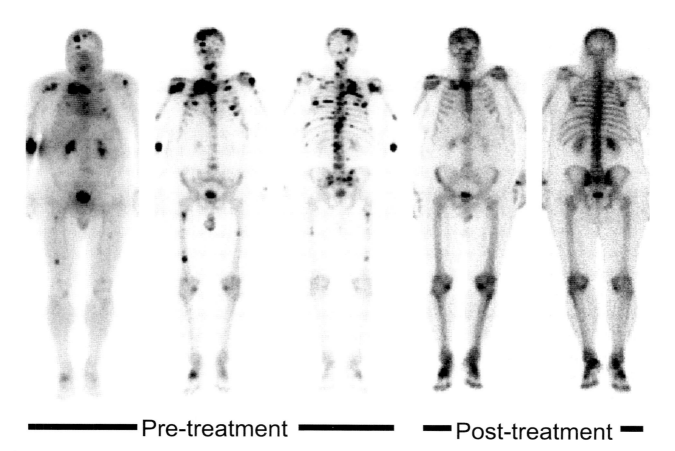

Pre-treatment   Post-treatment

Fig. 23.4 Re-staging a 76-year-old gentleman after hormonal ablation therapy. The images on the left demonstrate widespread axial metastases while those on the right display a reduced uptake after treatment

of area positive on bone scan is a novel parameter for predicting the prognosis of patients with advanced prostatic cancer [35].

Summary of Bone Scanning in Prostate Cancer

Radionuclide bone scanning is still an important tool in the diagnosis, staging, and management of prostate cancer (Table 23.1). Current guidelines still recommend a bone scan at diagnosis when a PSA is greater than 20 ng/mL, although evidence for undertaking a scan at greater than 10 ng/mL is gaining weight. For patients undergoing follow-up or re-staging, a level of 20 ng/mL or higher should necessitate a bone scan. When higher grade or stage disease occurs, or clinical symptoms of skeletal disease are present, PSA alone should not determine whether or not a bone scan is to be undertaken. Certainly, other imaging studies such as positron emission tomography will improve and may challenge radionuclide bone scanning in the future, but further studies are necessary and data still strongly favor bone scintigraphy.

Radioisotopic Treatment of Bone Pain from Metastatic Prostate Cancer

Bone metastases are the commonest cause of pain in cancer patients resulting from tumor infiltration and extension of the periosteal membranes, mechanical instability, and tumor spread from bone to contiguous neurological structures [36]. Radionuclide therapy works on the principle of internal

Table 23.1 Bone scintigraphy in asymptomatic prostate cancer patients

Disease phase	Indications for bone scan
Staging	
Initial diagnosis/ Assessment	PSA 20 μg/L or greater* Locally advanced disease Gleason score ≥8
Re-staging	
Monitoring untreated disease	PSA rise to 15 μg/L or greater Locally advanced disease Gleason score ≥8
Biochemical recurrence	PSA rise to >10 μg/L** PSA velocity >5 μg/L per month
Post-hormonal treatment	As clinically indicated Avoid flare period early in treatment as false positives

* PSA in range 10–20 μg/L remains controversial
** Low yield until PSA >30 μg/L

targeting and the systemic administration of radionuclides may be effective in treating symptomatic bony, metastases pain. The most commonly used agent is strontium-89 chloride, a calcium analogue, which is administered intravenously and preferentially localizes in tumor effectively irradiating the affected bone at a cellular level [3]. Favorable results with strontium have been reported with pain relief in 75–80% of patients, typically 1–3 weeks after treatment with the benefits often lasting many months [37, 38].

Other agents used for the treatment of bone pain include rhenium-186-hydroxyethylidine diphosphonate that is a beta-particle and gamma-photon-emitting radionuclide with a half-life of 3.7 days [39]. In a randomized controlled trial, compared with placebo, rhenium-186 resulted in a significantly longer pain response in the treatment of bone pain from metastasized prostate cancer [40]. Samarium-153-ethyleniaminetetramethylene phosphoric acid has a half-life of 1.9 days and has similar properties to rhenium-186 offering pain relief in 70% of patients [39, 41, 42]. Other agents with similar properties continue to be developed such as tin-117m stannic diethylenetriaminepentaacetic acid [43].

Patients with multifocal metastatic disease are excellent candidates for systemic therapies, whereas patients with unifocal metastatic disease may be more appropriate candidates for focal therapies such as external-beam radiation. Patients who are poorly tolerant of narcotics should be actively considered for alternative treatments such as systemic radiopharmaceuticals [44].

Contraindications to administration of current bone-seeking radioisotopes include substantial degrees of renal insufficiency or bone marrow suppression, with the most often encountered toxic side effect of treatment being thrombocytopenia that is often mild, clinically silent, requiring no specific medical intervention. Also, radioisotopes should not be used to prevent fractures or when imminent spinal cord compression is a possibility as the agents are not potent or rapid enough in their action [44, 45].

In summary, several radionuclides are available for relief of pain in prostate cancer patients with bone metastases. All provide pain relief within 2–3 weeks after a single intravenous injection, with effects typically lasting three or more months [45]. Treatment may be repeated at approximately 8- to 12-week intervals, depending on the time of return to normal leukocytes and platelet counts [46]. A temporary increase in pain is possible (flare phenomenon), similar to that with the administration of LHRH agonists, but is typically short in duration. Radionuclide treatment of painful bone metastases reduces the need for analgesics and may improve the quality of life, but we cannot accurately predict who will or will not respond [45, 46]. There are known contraindications and side effects that must be considered prior to administration.

Positron Emission Tomography

Introduction

Positron emission tomography uses radioisotopes that undergo positron emission decay. Positrons are emitted from the unstable radionuclide and interact with an electron in the surrounding tissues, resulting in an annihilation reaction with subsequent release of two 511 keV photons in opposite directions. A sophisticated ring detector surrounding the patient then detects the coincident photons and registers the interactions in the image [5].

Several different isotopes are available for use in PET scanning (Table 23.2) and a cyclotron is required to produce the radioisotopes. By tagging radioisotopes to naturally occurring substances in the human body, PET scanning is able to supply unique information on the metabolic activity of a tissue [47]. The most commonly used radionuclide in PET scanning combines the radioisotope fluorine-18 with the D-glucose analogue: 2 fluoro-2-deoxy-D-glucose (^{18}F-FDG).

Tumor imaging with ^{18}F-FDG is based on the premise that tumors are more metabolically active than their surrounding tissues and thus will metabolize more glucose. Tumor cells actively take up and shuttle ^{18}F-FDG into glycolysis [47]. Once the cycle has begun, the glucose is phosphorylated to ^{18}F-FDG-6-phosphate by hexokinase. This metabolite becomes trapped and cannot proceed along the normal pathway of glucose metabolism. Over time, increased amounts of ^{18}F-FDG accumulate within malignant cells. This abnormal concentration of ^{18}F-FDG in the tumor cells produces a detectable signal that is greater than the background, thus allowing isolation of tumor deposits [47].

Advantages of Positron Emission Tomography

Positron emission tomography (PET) offers the advantage that no allergy to FDG is known and a pacemaker or metal implants are not contraindications [48]. PET has developed as a reproducible and reliable imaging technique in a variety of malignancies, such as sarcoma, lung carcinoma, and head

Table 23.2 Commonly used isotopes in PET scanning and their half-life

Radioisotope	Half-life
Fluorine-18	110 min
Carbon-11	20 min
Bromine-75	98 min
Oxygen-15	2 min
Nitrogen-13	10 min
Indium-111	67 h

and neck tumors. This is because it is able to noninvasively measure the biochemical and/or physiological processes in vivo [49]. As outlined above the most common radiotracer used in PET imaging is ^{18}F-FDG which is able to exploit the increased rate of glycolysis in tumor compared to normal cells, leading to accumulation of this tracer in tumor foci [50]. Although the role of ^{18}F-FDG-PET in germ cell tumors and in particular diagnosing recurrence of seminoma in post-chemotherapy masses is now widely established and supported in the literature [51, 52], the place of PET in urologic oncology has not been completely defined and is fluid as technology and our understanding of tumor metabolism develops. In particular, the application of PET to prostate cancer has been difficult due to the slow rate of tumor growth that is reflected in a low rate of glycolysis [53].

Current radiographic techniques such as computerized tomography and CT are often unable to accurately stage the extent of prostatic carcinoma [54, 55]. Some promising studies with endorectal coil have offered promise in improving local staging with MRI, but offer little information as to metastatic disease MRI spectroscopy [56]. The relatively recent introduction of combined PET-CT (Fig. 23.5) has been recognized in clinical oncology as a major advance over co-registration of PET with CT data due to the ability PET-CT to combine morphological and functional imaging on the same patient simultaneously, allowing greater diagnostic accuracy [57, 58]. It has been suggested that PET-CT could even be used as a first-line investigation fore re-staging post-radical prostatectomy, although more data are required [59].

Limitations in Positron Emission Tomography of the Prostate

Perhaps the greatest limitation to PET in the urinary tract is that interpretation of uptake is often impaired by the normal urinary excretion of radioisotope. This has led to difficulties in interpretation of pathological uptake in renal tumors and bladder tumors, as well as with prostate cancer [19, 60]. It is predominantly pooling of radioisotope in the bladder combined with normal bladder activity that hampers the assessment of prostate activity. Diuretics such as frusemide as an aid may have a role, but this has not been widely used with most centers relying on hydration [60, 61]. The use of catheters with continuous bladder irrigation although time consuming but possible did not aid diagnosis of prostate cancer [62].

The low sensitivity of ^{18}F-FDG-PET for prostate cancer is also contributed by the relative indolence of the tumor in the majority of patients, especially at diagnosis. The glucose utilization of prostate carcinoma cells is not enhanced significantly enough compared to normal cells to allow delineation of the tumor on a PET study [45]. In addition to prostate cancer having a low rate of glycolysis as outlined, another issue of concern is that there is often overlap in the degree of local uptake between prostate cancer and benign prostatic hyperplasia [62, 63]. This overlap also makes interpretation of recurrence difficult as ^{18}F-FDG is not useful in distinguishing between postoperative scar and local tumor recurrence after radical prostatectomy [64].

Fluorodeoxyglucose (^{18}F-FDG) and the Prostate

^{18}F-FDG-PET imaging in prostate cancer has been problematic due to well-differentiated prostate cancer having lower glucose utilization than many other tumor types. When this is combined with the prostate's close proximity to the bladder, where there is intense accumulation of ^{18}F-FDG, there is difficulty diagnosing primary prostate cancer [65, 66]. Furthermore, Effert et al. found a low ^{18}F-FDG uptake in 81% of primary, untreated prostate tumors and no correlation with increasing tumor grade or stage [62]. Benign prostatic hyper-

trophy may also accumulate an amount of ^{18}F-FDG that is similar to that in untreated primary prostate cancer, particularly if any inflammation is present [62, 66]. Further to this, Hofer et al. confirmed it was difficult to distinguish with ^{18}F-FDG true recurrence from postoperative scarring, inflammation, and benign prostatic hyperplasia following radical prostatectomy [67]. Also, following treatment with androgen ablation, uptake may further decline in prostate cancer [68].

As far as metastatic disease is concerned, a positive predictive value of 98% was found for those metastases that were untreated (Figs. 23.5 and 23.6) [69]. However, problems were encountered in identifying pelvic lymph node metastases from reactive nodal disease (due to the small size of tumor deposits in lymph nodes), which is a key clinical differentiator of localized versus locally advanced disease and would have an impact on treatment decisions [69]. Finally, although ^{18}F-FDG-PET can provide useful information and improve the clinician's decision on further management procedures in selected patients with low PSA and bone or lymph node changes, a negative PET scan in prostate cancer should be interpreted with caution [32].

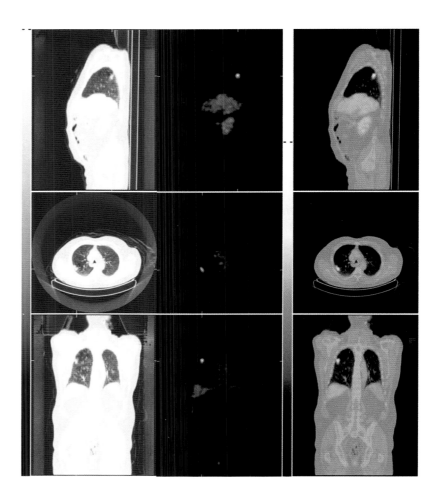

Fig. 23.5 A 60-year-old smoker with prostate cancer presents with a suspicious lesion on chest X-ray. The ^{18}F-FDG-PET/CT (left= PET; center= CT; right= fused PET/CT) study in three planes (sagittal above; axial central; coronal below) confirms uptake in the right upper lobe lesion that histology demonstrated adenocarcinoma of the prostate

Fig. 23.6 A 73-year-old smoker with known prostate cancer had an incidental left upper lobe lesion found on radiographs for osteoporosis. The ^{18}F-FDG -PET/CT was able to demonstrate uptake of radiotracer. At biopsy it was demonstrated to be non-small cell lung adenocarcinoma

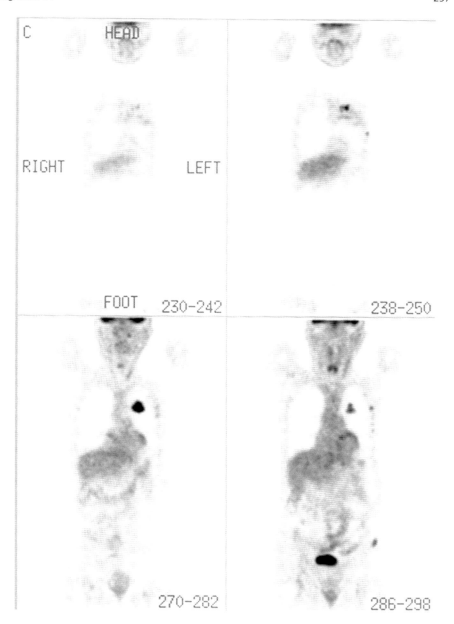

Other Radiotracers for Prostate Cancer

As imaging of glucose metabolism has not proven a dramatically useful tool to date, radiotracers able to identify cell membrane turnover, protein synthesis, DNA synthesis, and testosterone metabolism within the prostate are currently being investigated.

Choline: Fluorocholine (FCH) and Carbocholine (^{11}C-Choline)

Choline is necessary within the human body for the synthesis of phospholipids in cell membranes, methyl metabolism,

transmembrane signaling, and lipid-cholesterol metabolism and transport [70]. Magnetic resonance spectroscopy has provided evidence via in vivo studies to support the role of increased choline metabolism as a prominent feature of prostate cancer [71, 72]. Prostate cancer cells contain higher levels of choline metabolites relative to normal prostate and epithelial stromal cells on spectroscopy. Abnormal choline metabolism being a frequent feature of malignant transformation has generated substantial interest in this metabolic pathway as a tumor marker and therapeutic target [72].

Although the use of radiotracers based on choline has been studied in over 250 patients with prostate cancer, there have been mixed results using choline with two representative studies [19, 71, 73]. First, in a study of 14 patients, a high uptake of ^{11}C-choline was demonstrated to characterize not only carcinomatous but also hyperplastic prostatic tissue [73]. Again, one of the same limitations of ^{18}F-FDG. Alternatively, in a study of 17 patients, using ^{18}F-fluorocholine (^{18}F-FCH), a radiotracer based on fluorine rather than carbon, malignant tumors in the prostate may be localized based on ^{18}F-FCH uptake [71]. [18]F labeling of choline was investigated as a tracer because it was postulated that ^{18}F would be superior to ^{11}C because of its longer half-life and its shorter positron range [74]. Overall results suggest choline-based radioisotopes may be potentially useful for staging and localizing prostate cancer but more data are required.

Methionine (^{11}C-Methionine)

The uptake of ^{11}C-methionine reflects increased cellular proliferation, amino acid transport, and partially protein synthesis [75]. Biodistribution of ^{11}C-methionine over ^{18}F-FDG has been compared in a study of men with hormone refractory prostate cancer, with both demonstrating good uptake [76]. However, an advantage of ^{11}C-methionine over ^{18}F-FDG is that it is primarily metabolized in the liver and pancreas with no significant renal excretion making interpretation of tumor to background more reliable. [77].

Acetate (^{11}C-Acetate)

The uptake of acetate in malignant cells is related to lipid synthesis [78]. Acetate is converted to acetyl-coenzyme A in the mitochondria, followed by rapid clearance as carbon dioxide through the citric acid cycle [79]. ^{11}C-acetate can demonstrate areas of high metabolism and blood flow such as are found in normal renal parenchyma [66]. Increased uptake in renal malignancies without significant excretion into the urinary tract has been demonstrated [80].

Unfortunately acetate is not a cancer-specific radiotracer and accumulates in both normal and hyperplastic tissues. In one study ^{11}C-acetate uptake was greater in normal prostate tissue in men under the age of 50 years compared with benign prostatic hyperplasia or normal prostate of older patients [81]. The role of ^{11}C-acetate is yet to be defined in men with prostate cancer.

Fluorodihydrotestosterone (FDHT)

The androgen receptor has an important role in the proliferation and growth of prostate cancer. Virtually all patients with prostate cancer respond to androgen withdrawal but eventually the cancer will begin to grow, despite continued low levels of androgen [19]. Logically, a tracer based on testosterone could potentially help delineate when a tumor is androgen responsive. Fluoro-5 alpha-dihydrotestosterone (FDHT) is a new PET radiopharmaceutical that exploits the metabolism of testosterone and its derivatives in the prostate. A recent clinical trial provided the opportunity for refinement of normal-tissue radiation-absorbed dose estimates based on quantitative PET using FDHT [82]. Clinical studies are unavailable at present.

Fluorothymidine (FLT)

DNA synthesis is an obvious target for any imaging modality, given that tumor cells have a higher turnover than benign tissue. Radiotracers based on the nuclide thymidine have been developed.

[18]F-Fluorothymidine (^{18}F-FLT) has successfully imaged implanted prostate tumors (CWR22) in mice with a marked reduction of ^{18}F-FLT uptake in tumor after castration or diethylstilbestrol treatment. However, there were no differences in ^{18}F-FLT uptake in the tumor in the control group. These changes of ^{18}F-FLT uptake in tumor parallel the changes of actual tumor measurement. Their results indicate that ^{18}F-FLT is a useful tracer for detection of prostate cancer in an animal model and that it has the potential for monitoring the therapeutic effect of androgen ablation therapy in prostate cancer [83].

Applications of PET in Oncology

PET applications in cancer medicine have been focused on three clinical goals: (1) detection and diagnosis; (2) staging; and (3) treatment monitoring. Paralleling these clinical goals, basic investigations are being pursued to develop better PET methods that are specific for cancer and, more fundamentally, to use PET as a tool for achieving a better understanding of cancer biology.

Furthermore, with regard to prostate cancer and imaging an ability to delineate malignant areas within the prostate gland could potentially aid in treatment planning [57]. Although the entire prostate gland would be likely to remain the target for treatment when treating organ confined disease, knowledge of the intraprostatic distribution of tumors could potentially enable higher doses of the therapeutic agent (e.g., radiation, microwaves) to the most involved areas of the gland, the ultimate goal being more efficacious treatment with fewer side effects [71].

Diagnosis and Local Staging

There has been disappointing data in relation to the uptake of ^{18}F-FDG in primary prostatic tumors. In studies of ^{18}F-FDG uptake in diagnosis of prostate cancer, considerable overlap was found between carcinoma, which displayed low-grade FDG uptake and the uptake in BPH [62, 84].

Even if one changes to a different radiotracer such as ^{11}C-acetate; the results improve but are not acceptable as an alternative to currently used nomograms. Also, local nodal disease has not been adequately assessed in such studies [85].

In a study of 42 patients prior to definitive surgery or radiation, ^{18}F-FDG-PET appeared to have a defined prognostic value for patients with prostate cancer undergoing radical prostatectomy, and more patients need to be studied for patients undergoing endocrine therapy [86].

Re-staging

In a study of 100 patients by Picchio et al., ^{11}C-choline-PET seems to be useful for re-staging post-radical prostatectomy where there is a rising serum PSA. It was shown to be superior to ^{18}F-FDG at re-staging the disease and complimentary to other conventional imaging techniques such as bone scintigraphy, MRI, and computerized tomography but with the advantage of being undertaken in a single step. There were, however, potentially up to 53 false-negative cases, given that eight had biopsy confirming recurrence and the remaining patients were disease free at 1 year with relatively stable PSA readings [59].

Pet Versus Bone Scintigraphy for Metastatic Bone Lesions

Studies examining osseous metastases from a variety of tumors using PET found it to be a promising tool (Figs. 23.7 and 23.8) when compared to bone scan because it detects the tumor directly by metabolic activity rather than indirectly by demonstrating increased bone mineral turnover [5]. Several studies have found PET to be superior to bone scan in detecting osseous metastases [87–89]. However, it must be pointed out that although the specificity of PET may be

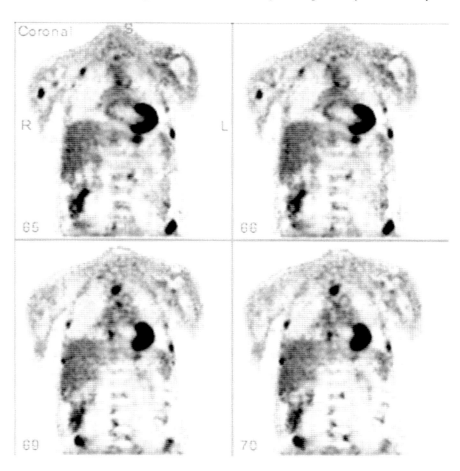

Fig. 23.7 A 68-year-old smoker with hormone refractory prostate cancer with a rising PSA to 39 µg/L and suspicious chest X-ray finings had a thoracic ^{18}F-FDG-PET study. Multiple widespread ^{18}F-FDG avid osseous metastases were demonstrated even on an old generation PET study

Fig. 23.8 A new generation ^{18}F-FDG-PET/CT (left= PET; center= CT; right= fused PET/CT) study in three planes (sagittal above; axial central; coronal below) identifying an obvious L4 bony metastasis (arrow) in a patient with metastatic prostate cancer

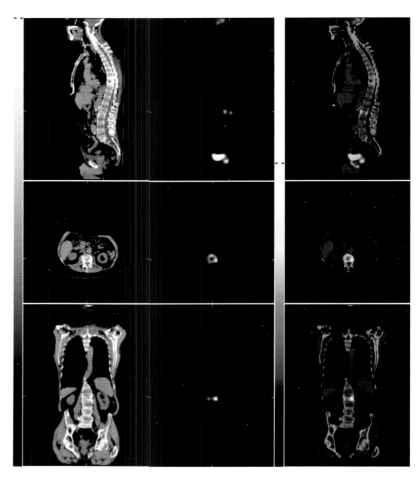

greater than bone scan for detecting metastases, PET also has false-positive results. Any tissue metabolism resulting in increased glucose utilization may be positive, in particular sarcoid and infection. Also, with regard to prostate cancer, data are limited compared to the many studies using bone scintigraphy.

Also, it is apparent that despite technological advances with imaging techniques such as computed tomography (CT), magnetic resonance imaging (MRI), and ultrasound, they have not proved to be highly accurate for staging prostate cancer [90]. This will only serve to increase research using different radioisotopes and their role in prostate cancer.

Summary

At present, the contribution that PET studies may make to the diagnosis, staging, and treatment of patients with prostate cancer is limited. However, many studies were performed using the radioisotope FDG, which is limited by the glycolic rate of tumors. Furthermore, urinary tract excretion and accumulation of tracer in the bladder make interpretation difficult. However, with the development of PET-CT providing better localization of organs and with greater understanding of newer isotopes, PET will influence prostate cancer management in the future. At present ^{18}F-FDG-PET has a role in staging and re-staging but not diagnosis while choline-PET is promising but requires further studies (Table 23.3).

Monoclonal Antibodies: Radioimmunoscintigraphy

Introduction

Labeled monoclonal antibodies directed against specific antigens on prostate cancer cells have been developed in the past decade for radioimmunoscintigraphy. The most widely studied is [111]indium-labeled monoclonal antibody or indium-111-capromab pendetide ([111]indium-CP or Prostascint, Cytigen, Princeton, NJ, USA) [91–93]. [111]Indium-CP is a whole murine antibody that is reactive with prostate-specific membrane antigen (PSMA), a glycoprotein on the surface of

Table 23.3 Summary of current PET and molecular imaging applications in prostate carcinoma

Molecular imaging modality	Disease stage	Current recommendation
^{18}F-FDG-PET	Diagnosis Staging and Re-staging	Not useful Useful for visceral, lymph node and bony disease
PET with new radiotracers e.g., ^{11}C-choline	Diagnosis, staging and re-staging	Promising but more clinical data needed
Radioimmunoscintigraphy (Immuno-PET)	Diagnosis Staging and re-staging	Not useful Promising but further clinical data needed
Sentinal node localization/lymphoscintigraphy	Preoperative node localization/node identification for excision	Promising but further clinical data needed

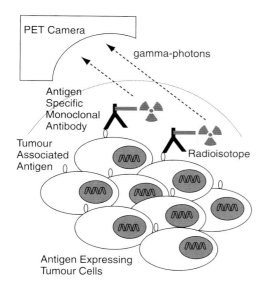

Fig. 23.9 Diagram of immuno-PET (radioimmunoscintigrapy)

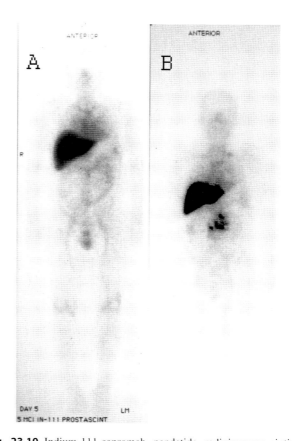

Fig. 23.10 Indium-111-capromab pendetide radioimmunoscintigraphy: a negative scan (left) and a positive scan (right) demonstrating uptake in pelvic nodal disease. Provided by Cherry T. Thomas, M.D., Digital Image Processing Lab, Department of Radiology, University of Michigan Health Systems, USA

normal and abnormal prostate epithelium [94]. Once accumulated at metastatic sites the radioactive isotope decays, resulting in the emission of gamma rays that are detected by a gamma camera (Fig. 23.9). In most instances, SPECT acquisition (single photon emission computed tomography) is utilized to detect emissions and thus construct three-dimensional images from the antibody rather than a standard gamma camera that provides only two-dimensional images (Fig. 23.10). PSMA scintigraphy using (99m)Tc-labeled MUJ591, a different antibody, has also been studied [95].

Indium-111-CP is a whole IgG antibody that clears relatively slowly from the blood stream and so imaging protocols are time consuming and must be performed over several days [45]. To speed up the process and improve accuracy, the study may be performed in conjunction with a ^{99m}Tc-labeled red blood cell procedure so that blood pool activity may be adequately evaluated [45, 96]. In future management of recurrent prostate cancer, fusion with magnetic resonance imaging or computed tomography of the pelvis can improve the specificity of the examination [97, 98].

Preoperative Staging Using Indium-111-Capromab Pendetide Radioimmunoscintigraphy

Prognostic information has also been obtained using [111]indium-CP studies. Radioimmunoscintigraphy had an impact on patient management through its detection of occult disease in more than 50% of prostate carcinoma patients studied with 80% accuracy in detecting involved nodes, thus providing information concerning the likelihood that lymph node metastases would be found during surgery [99]. Another study by Polasczik et al. [100] compared the results of radioimmunoscintigraphy in 198 patients having pelvic lymphadenectomy with high-risk cancer. Almost 40% of patients had positive scans but only 62% correlated with histopathology. In time, [111]indium-CP studies may prove beneficial, but even after a multicenter trial it was concluded that more data are required [101].

Detecting Occult Metastases in the Setting of a Rising PSA After Treatment Using Radioimmunoscintigraphy

In patients with no detectable tumor activity outside the pelvic area before salvage radiotherapy to the pelvis, there was an association with a more durable complete PSA response [45, 102, 103]. Preliminary data suggest that [111]indium-CP imaging is helpful in identifying those patients with PSA elevation after radical prostatectomy who are most likely to benefit from salvage RT [92]. This is important as it is becoming recognized that the earlier the decision to salvage radiotherapy, the better the results [104]. In two series with a population of over 100 patients having different primary modalities of treatment, indium-111-CP was used to detect recurrence in the setting of a PSA rise. All positive prostate biopsies (20 patients) correlated with [111]indium-CP scans, but only four of the seven positive lymph node biopsies correlated with scan findings. The negative biopsy results (six patients) revealed 89% sensitivity and 67% specificity for [111]indium-CP scanning. Repetition of scans appeared to be an important factor in determining occult recurrences improving the detection of regional nodes and distant nodes [105–107]. Two studies of 300 men also determined that radioimmunoscintigraphy with [111]indium-CP can assist in determining the extent of disease in patients who have increasing PSA after prostatectomy [108, 109]. These findings indicate that [111]indium-CP may be useful in some cases and in particular where scans are repeated but further studies are necessary.

The scans frequently show monoclonal antibody uptake in pelvic, abdominal, and extrapelvic retroperitoneal sites beyond the region of limited obturator node dissections and may account for the understaging and subsequent failure of radical prostatectomy in some patients. The monoclonal antibody scan seems to be a good predictor of which patients will respond to radiation therapy after radical prostatectomy, but because these patients often have nodal activity beyond the radiated field, this initial response may not be curative [110].

This agent is still under investigation and some day may aid urologists in the evaluation of prostate cancer by improving preoperative staging and demonstration of advanced disease and postoperative localization of recurrent disease. Improved staging and localization will reduce unnecessary tests and treatment that will lead to reduced morbidity, better management, earlier detection, and intervention in advanced disease and improved cost-effectiveness [111].

However, some studies have challenged the suitability of [111]indium-CP imaging for identifying patients with local prostate cancer recurrence who may achieve PSA control after salvage radiation therapy [93, 98, 112]. For example, a study of 42 patients demonstrated that although [111]indium-CP is capable of detecting recurrent prostate carcinoma at low PSA levels, it was not predictive of response to salvage radiotherapy with only 47% of men with positive scans responding [113]. A further study of 30 men also examined [111]indium-CP as a prognostic tool in patients having PSA relapse post-prostatectomy and found they were not prognostic of post-salvage radiation therapy PSA outcome [112]. Another study concluded that decision making and treatment planning can be guided, but only when co-registered studies with CT are used and the benefits are small [98].

Ultimately, some authors have concluded that current radioimmunoscintigraphy studies are not sufficiently accurate to reliably determine the presence of metastatic nodal disease from prostate cancer and have stressed the importance of rigorous clinical evaluation of future methods that are designed to detect microscopic metastatic disease of any neoplasm [93]. Certainly, a future prospective cohort study or randomized trial of [111]indium-CP radioimmunoscintigraphy may more precisely determine the suitability of this technique for identifying post-prostatectomy patients with biochemical relapse who should be spared salvage local therapy [112].

PSMA scintigraphy using (99m)Tc-labeled MUJ591 identifies prostate cancer, but is not sensitive in delineating micro-invasion of seminal vesicles, prostate capsule, or bladder neck. However, it appears to be useful in detecting prostate bed recurrence and distant micrometastasis but more studies are needed [41].

Guiding Treatment Using Indium-111-Capromab Pendetide Radioimmunoscintigraphy

The ability to guide treatment, particularly radiotherapy or brachytherapy, is a new development using [111]indium-CP radioimmunoscintigraphy [114–116]. Initially data from radioimmunoscintigraphy scans were fused with the pelvic CT scan, and this information was used to identify foci of adenocarcinoma within the prostate and this correlated well with biopsy results. This opened the possibility of escalating doses in regions containing tumor by brachytherapy, or external beam techniques such as intensity modulated radiotherapy (IMRT) [114, 116]. Eighty patients with [111]indium-CP-guided transperineal brachytherapy demonstrated progression-free survival at 4 years, but there were no other arms of comparison in this study and clearly more data with longer follow-up are required [115].

Summary

At present, it appears that [111]indium-CP imaging may be of benefit in patients who are highly suspected of having loco regional or distant spread of their prostate carcinoma in whom it is difficult to localize the extent of disease with conventional diagnostic techniques. Information obtained may help decide who will benefit from salvage radiation, especially after prostatectomy. However, it is likely that microscopic or minimal disease will not be depicted and that predictive values are not high enough to be applied to an individual patient [45]. Also, administration of the scan test is operator dependent, with nuclear medicine specialists requiring specialist training to interpret scans. Bowel and vascular structures may cause false-positive scans, and no histological confirmation of radical prostatectomy specimen recurrences have been reported to date [29].

Nevertheless, the currently available image-processing techniques are evolving rapidly and data from only a few years ago may not be relevant and so new studies must be examined fusing techniques as well as results. Furthermore, it is apparent that studies without co-registration of computed tomography images, as with recent evolution of PET-CT, may become less relevant to clinical decision making [97]. We await the publication of further studies to determine the exact clinical role of this technique in the monitoring and treatment of prostate carcinoma.

Prostate Lymphoscintigraphy and Radio-Guided Surgery for Sentinel Lymph Node Identification

Introduction

The rationale for an extended pelvic lymphadenectomy at the time of radical prostatectomy is to achieve as much reliable pathohistological staging information as possible in order to trigger postoperative adjuvant management [117]. However, some patients with minimal metastatic disease remain free of prostate-specific antigen relapse for more than 10 years after prostatectomy without any adjuvant treatment indicating that meticulous pelvic lymph node dissection seems not only to be a staging procedure, but may also have a positive impact on disease progression and long-term disease-free survival [118]. In patients with positive nodes, time to progression is significantly correlated with the number of diseased nodes. Recent evidence also suggests that current lymph node dissections of the obturator fossa alone may not be sufficient to sample all positive nodes, with up to 56% of lymph node-positive cases missed in a study of 194 patients undergoing radical prostatectomy and extensive lymph node dissection [119, 120].

Currently, the decision to undertake pelvic lymph node dissection is based on preoperative nomograms identifying high-risk patients at risk of metastatic disease [121, 122]. Against this are studies that argue that nomograms are not applicable to an individual patient and are in favor of pelvic lymphadenectomy in all patients [118, 123, 124]. This is because extended lymphadenectomy may improve survival and in a case-control study of 100 patients in an extended or normal lymphadenectomy group, those having wider dissection had PSA relapse of 8% compared to 23% in the normal group. There is also an argument that adjuvant treatment may be better guided with more information on more nodes, as those with more than one node have a significantly worse mortality even with hormonal manipulation [125, 126].

Once deciding on lymphadenectomy, evidence is accumulating that extension of pelvic lymph node dissection may be valuable for the identification of node-positive patients. Yet extended lymphadenectomy, particularly in older reported series, does carry morbidity such as lymphocoele creation [117]. Therefore, limiting the number of lymph nodes to the principal ones draining the prostate with the highest probability of bearing lymphatic spread (sentinel lymph nodes) makes histopathological study of particular nodes in great detail more feasible [119]. Conceivably an extended node sampling may be undertaken, yet by dissecting fewer nodes than conventional lymphadenectomy undertakes. There have been promising results using lymphoscintigraphy and intraoperative gamma probe application for the detection of sentinel lymph nodes (SLN) in malignant melanoma, breast, and penis cancer [127–129]. This has now been extended to prostate cancer [120, 130].

Location of Sentinel Lymph Nodes

Sentinal lymph node biopsy is traditionally a two- and occasionally three-step procedure. The day before pelvic lymphadenectomy, technetium-99m nanocolloid is transrectally injected into the prostate under ultrasound guidance. A single central application of 2–3 mL per prostate lobe is normally performed. Lymphoscintigraphy is then carried out using a gamma camera to detect increased activity in regional lymph nodes. Data are then available for the surgeon to plan for resection of particular lymph nodes prior to surgery. Intra-operatively, a gamma probe with a sterile cover may be introduced into the wound and with a sound locator and sentinel nodes from preoperative imaging may be confirmed (Fig. 23.11). Also, other nodes not demonstrated at lymphoscintigraphy with a high emission of radioactivity may be resected [131]. It is also possible to inject patent blue V dye into the organ intraoperatively and visually watch nodes take up the dye for further identification, although this is not routinely done in prostate cancer [127]. Thus, lymph nodes having been identified as sentinel nodes by means of gamma probe detection and lymphoscintigraphy or in some cases dye injection may be removed intraoperatively.

Lymph Node Involvement Using Sentinel Lymph Node Identification in Prostate Cancer

Perhaps the greatest drawback to sentinel lymph node surgery in prostate cancer is that a single node representing the primary landing zone for prostate cancer has not been identified reinforcing the existence of various lymphatic drainage systems from the prostate [117]. In a large study of 335 patients using the above techniques, patients had at least one sentinel lymph node located, with a quarter being involved by metastases on histological examination. There was only one false-negative patient [131]. A further study demonstrated that although there is diversity of lymphatic drainage of the prostate it is feasible to locate nodes and that limited pelvic lymphadenectomy alone appears to be insufficient for precise staging in patients with pretreat-

ment PSA greater than 10 ng/mL and a Gleason score greater than 6. They contend that isotope techniques could therefore improve the yield of lymphadenectomy by limiting its extent but focusing on important nodes [132]. Interestingly, in a group of lower risk patients, with PSA less than 10 ng/mL and biopsy Gleason score less than or equal to 6, positive lymph nodes were identified by radio-guided surgery in 6.8% (positive biopsies in one lobe) and 10.7% (positive biopsies in both lobes). Up to four positive sentinel lymph nodes were found. Therefore, they concluded it is not appropriate to dispense with an operative lymph node staging, even in low-risk disease [124].

Summary

In the future, the restriction of pelvic staging lymphadenectomy to scintigraphically proved sentinel lymph nodes might be possible. However, it is still an emerging technique and certainly some lymph nodes examined ex vivo have been missed on pre- and intraoperative scanning, meaning that current techniques need to be modified to ensure that accurate and complete removal of all hot nodes takes place. Therefore, currently sentinel lymph nodes can be used for prostate cancer but detailed lymph node mapping and extended dissection backup are still required until the technique improves [133]. Ultimately, if it is accepted that even modified standardized pelvic lymphadenectomy is insufficient in terms of the detection of micrometastases, then the perioperative morbidity of extensive lymph node dissection may be reduced by increasing the sensitivity of the detection of micrometastases using sentinel lymph node locating techniques [130]. Further studies of these techniques at multiple institutions are necessary before the true benefits may be identified.

Acknowledgments

We would like to acknowledge Tim Saunders, Centre for PET, Austin Hospital Heidelberg, Vic., Australia for assisting in preparing images.

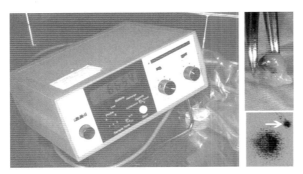

Fig. 23.11 Sentinel lymph node biopsy: The preoperative scintographic image identifying sentinel nodes (arrow) assists in surgical planning. A sentinel lymph node that has absorbed dye and recorded radioactivity on the probe (left) is removed (top right). Provided by Mr. B Mann, University of Melbourne, Department of Surgery, Melbourne, Australia

References

1. Oesterling JE, Martin SK, Bergstralh EJ, Lowe FC. The use of prostate-specific antigen in staging patients with newly diagnosed prostate cancer. Jama. 1993;269:57–60.
2. Brown ML. Bone scintigraphy in benign and malignant tumors. Radiol Clin North Am. 1993;31:731–8.

3. Prvulovich EM, Bomanji JB. The role of nuclear medicine in clinical investigation. Bmj. 1998;316:1140–6.

4. Malhotra P, Berman CG. Evaluation of bone metastases in lung cancer. Improved sensitivity and specificity of PET over bone scanning. Cancer Control. 2002;9:254, 259–60.

5. Peterson JJ, Kransdorf MJ, O'Connor MI. Diagnosis of occult bone metastases: positron emission tomography. Clin Orthop. 2003;S120–8.

6. Saad F, Gleason DM, Murray R, et al. Long-term efficacy of zoledronic acid for the prevention of skeletal complications in patients with metastatic hormone-refractory prostate cancer. J Natl Cancer Inst. 2004;96:879–82.

7. Roudier MP, Vesselle H, True LD, et al. Bone histology at autopsy and matched bone scintigraphy findings in patients with hormone refractory prostate cancer: the effect of bisphosphonate therapy on bone scintigraphy results. Clin Exp Metastasis.2003;20:171–80.

8. Schaffer DL, Pendergrass HP. Comparison of enzyme, clinical, radiographic, and radionuclide methods of detecting bone metastases from carcinoma of the prostate. Radiology. 1976;121:431–4.

9. Andriole GL, Coplen DE, Mikkelsen DJ, Catalona WJ. Sonographic and pathological staging of patients with clinically localized prostate cancer. J Urol. 1989;142:1259–61.

10. Chybowski FM, Keller JJ, Bergstralh EJ, Oesterling JE. Predicting radionuclide bone scan findings in patients with newly diagnosed, untreated prostate cancer: prostate specific antigen is superior to all other clinical parameters. J Urol. 1991;145:313–8.

11. Lee N, Fawaaz R, Olsson CA, et al. Which patients with newly diagnosed prostate cancer need a radionuclide bone scan? An analysis based on 631 patients. Int J Radiat Oncol Biol Phys. 2000;48:1443–6.

12. Wolff JM, Zimny M, Borchers H, Wildberger J, Buell U, Jakse G. Is prostate-specific antigen a reliable marker of bone metastasis in patients with newly diagnosed cancer of the prostate? Eur Urol. 1998;33:376–81.

13. Gleave ME, Coupland D, Drachenberg D, et al. Ability of serum prostate-specific antigen levels to predict normal bone scans in patients with newly diagnosed prostate cancer. Urology. 1996;47:708–12.

14. Rudoni M, Antonini G, Favro M, et al. The clinical value of prostate-specific antigen and bone scintigraphy in the staging of patients with newly diagnosed, pathologically proven prostate cancer. Eur J Nucl Med. 1995;22:207–11.

15. Haukaas S, Roervik J, Halvorsen OJ, Foelling M. When is bone scintigraphy necessary in the assessment of newly diagnosed, untreated prostate cancer? Br J Urol. 1997;79:770–6.

16. Lee CT, Oesterling JE. Using prostate-specific antigen to eliminate the staging radionuclide bone scan. Urol Clin North Am. 1997;24:389–94.

17. Wymenga LF, Boomsma JH, Groenier K, Piers DA, Mensink HJ. Routine bone scans in patients with prostate cancer related to serum prostate-specific antigen and alkaline phosphatase. BJU Int. 2001;88:226–30.

18. Abuzallouf S, Dayes I, Lukka H. Baseline staging of newly diagnosed prostate cancer: a summary of the literature. J Urol. 2004;171:2122–7.

19. Schoder H, Larson SM. Positron emission tomography for prostate, bladder, and renal cancer. Semin Nucl Med. 2004;34:274–92.

20. Terris MK, Klonecke AS, McDougall IR, Stamey TA. Utilization of bone scans in conjunction with prostate-specific antigen levels in the surveillance for recurrence of adenocarcinoma after radical prostatectomy. J Nucl Med. 1991;32:1713–7.

21. Lawrentschuk N, Webb DR, Mitchell CA. Metastatic prostate cancer to lung with normal prostate specific antigen levels. Hosp Med. 2004;65:116–7.

22. Koizumi M, Yonese J, Fukui I, Ogata E. The serum level of the amino-terminal propeptide of type I procollagen is a sensitive marker for prostate cancer metastasis to bone. BJU Int. 2001;87:348–51.

23. Ornstein DK, Colberg JW, Virgo KS, et al. Evaluation and management of men whose radical prostatectomies failed: results of an international survey. Urology. 1998;52:1047–54.

24. Tsai DY, Virgo KS, Colberg JW, et al. The age of the urologist affects the postoperative care of prostate carcinoma patients. Cancer 1999;86:1314–21.

25. Cher ML, Bianco FJ Jr, Lam JS, et al. Limited role of radionuclide bone scintigraphy in patients with prostate specific antigen elevations after radical prostatectomy. J Urol. 1998;160:1387–91.

26. Kane CJ, Amling CL, Johnstone PA, et al. Limited value of bone scintigraphy and computed tomography in assessing biochemical failure after radical prostatectomy. Urology. 2003;61:607–11.

27. Gomez P, Manoharan M, Kim SS, Soloway MS. Radionuclide bone scintigraphy in patients with biochemical recurrence after radical prostatectomy: when is it indicated? BJU Int. 2004;94:299–302.

28. Thurairaja R, McFarlane JP, Persad R. Radionuclide bone scintigraphy in patients with biochemical recurrence after radical prostatectomy: when is it indicated? BJU Int. 2005;95:189–90.

29. Seitz C, Remzi M, Djavan B. Immediate Treatment after PSA Progression. Eur Urol Supplements. 2005;4:28–42.

30. Corrie D, Timmons JH, Bauman JM, Thompson IM. Efficacy of follow-up bone scans in carcinoma of the prostate. Cancer. 1988;61:2453–4.

31. Yap BK, Choo R, Deboer G, Klotz L, Danjoux C, Morton G. Are serial bone scans useful for the follow-up of clinically localized, low to intermediate grade prostate cancer managed with watchful observation alone? BJU Int. 2003;91:613–7.

32. Freitas JE, Gilvydas R, Ferry JD, Gonzalez JA. The clinical utility of prostate-specific antigen and bone scintigraphy in prostate cancer follow-up. J Nucl Med. 1991;32:1387–90.

33. Bushnell DL, Madsen M, Kahn D, Nathan M, Williams RD. Enhanced uptake of 99Tcm-MDP in skeletal metastases from prostate cancer following initiation of hormone treatment: potential for increasing delivery of therapeutic agents. Nucl Med Commun. 1999;20:875–81.

34. Rigaud J, Tiguert R, Le Normand L, et al. Prognostic value of bone scan in patients with metastatic prostate cancer treated initially with androgen deprivation therapy. J Urol. 2002;168:1423–6.

35. Noguchi M, Kikuchi H, Ishibashi M, Noda S. Percentage of the positive area of bone metastasis is an independent predictor of disease death in advanced prostate cancer. Br J Cancer. 2003;88:195–201.

36. Campa JA III, Payne R. The management of intractable bone pain: a clinician's perspective. Semin Nucl Med. 1992;22:3–10.

37. Robinson RG, Preston DF, Spicer JA, Baxter KG. Radionuclide therapy of intractable bone pain: emphasis on strontium-89. Semin Nucl Med. 1992: 22:28–32.

38. Robinson RG, Preston DF, Schiefelbein M, Baxter KG. Strontium 89 therapy for the palliation of pain due to osseous metastases. Jama. 1995:274:420–4.

39. Maxon HR III, Thomas SR, Hertzberg VS, et al. Rhenium-186 hydroxyethylidene diphosphonate for the treatment of painful osseous metastases. Semin Nucl Med. 1992;22:33–40.

40. Han SH, de Klerk JM, Tan S, et al. The PLACORHEN study: a double-blind, placebo-controlled, randomized radionuclide study with (186)Re-etidronate in hormone-resistant prostate cancer patients with painful bone metastases. Placebo Controlled Rhenium Study. J Nucl Med. 2002;43:1150–6.

41. Collins C, Eary JF, Donaldson G, et al. Samarium-153-EDTMP in bone metastases of hormone refractory prostate carcinoma: a phase I/II trial. J Nucl Med. 1993;34:1839–44.

42. Turner JH, Martindale AA, Sorby P, et al. Samarium-153 EDTMP therapy of disseminated skeletal metastasis. Eur J Nucl Med 1989;15:784–95.

43. Srivastava SC, Atkins HL, Krishnamurthy GT, et al. Treatment of metastatic bone pain with tin-117m Stannic diethylenetriamine-pentaacetic acid: a phase I/II clinical study. Clin Cancer Res. 1998;4:61–8.

44. Sartor O. Radioisotopic treatment of bone pain from metastatic prostate cancer. Curr Oncol Rep. 2003:5:258–62.

45. Oyen WJ, Witjes JA, Corstens FH. Nuclear medicine techniques for the diagnosis and therapy of prostate carcinoma. Eur Urol. 2001;40:294–9.

46. Silberstein EB, Eugene L, Saenger SR. Painful osteoblastic metastases: the role of nuclear medicine. Oncology (Huntingt). 2001;15:157–63; discussion 167–170, 174.

47. Brush JP. Positron emission tomography in urological malignancy. Curr Opin Urol. 2001;11:175–9.

48. Bachor R, Kotzerke J, Gottfried HW, Brandle E, Reske SN, Hautmann R. Positron emission tomography in diagnosis of renal cell carcinoma. Urologe A. 1996;35:146–50.

49. Sung J, Espiritu JI, Segall GM, Terris MK. Fluorodeoxyglucose positron emission tomography studies in the diagnosis and staging of clinically advanced prostate cancer. BJU Int. 2003;92:24–7.

50. Hain SF, Maisey MN. Positron emission tomography for urological tumours. BJU Int. 2003;92:159–64.

51. Putra LJ, Lawrentschuk N, Ballok Z, et al. 18F-fluorodeoxyglucose positron emission tomography in evaluation of germ cell tumor after chemotherapy. Urology. 2004;64:1202–7.

52. De Santis M, Becherer A, Bokemeyer C, et al. 2-18 fluoro-deoxy-D-glucose positron emission tomography is a reliable predictor for viable tumor in postchemotherapy seminoma: an update of the prospective multicentric SEMPET trial. J Clin Oncol. 2004;22:1034–9.

53. Hoh CK, Seltzer MA, Franklin J, deKernion JB, Phelps ME, Belldegrun A. Positron emission tomography in urological oncology. J Urol. 1998;159:347–56.

54. Tuzel E, Sevinc M, Obuz F, Sade M, Kirkali Z. Is magnetic resonance imaging necessary in the staging of prostate cancer? Urol Int. 1998;61:227–31.

55. Barbieri A, Monica B, Sebastio N, Incarbone GP, Di Stefano C. [Value and limitations of transrectal ultrasonography and computer tomography in preoperative staging of prostate carcinoma]. Acta Biomed Ateneo Parmense. 1997;68:23–6.

56. Jung JA, Coakley FV, Vigneron DB, et al. Prostate depiction at endorectal MR spectroscopic imaging: investigation of a standardized evaluation system. Radiology. 2004;233:701–8.

57. Bujenovic S. The role of positron emission tomography in radiation treatment planning. Semin Nucl Med. 2004;34:293–9.

58. Beyer T, Townsend DW, Brun T, et al. A combined PET/CT scanner for clinical oncology. J Nucl Med. 2000;41:1369–79.

59. Picchio M, Messa C, Landoni C, et al. Value of [11C] choline-positron emission tomography for re-staging prostate cancer: a comparison with [18F]fluorodeoxyglucose-positron emission tomography. J Urol. 2003;169:1337–40.

60. Ramdave S, Thomas GW, Berlangieri SU, et al. Clinical role of F-18 fluorodeoxyglucose positron emission tomography for detection and management of renal cell carcinoma. J Urol. 2001;166:825–30.

61. Diehl M, Manolopoulou M, Risse J, et al. Urinary fluorine-18 fluorodeoxyglucose excretion with and without intravenous application of furosemide. Acta Med Austriaca. 2004;31:76–8.

62. Effert PJ, Bares R, Handt S, Wolff JM, Bull U, Jakse G. Metabolic imaging of untreated prostate cancer by positron emission tomography with 18fluorine-labeled deoxyglucose. J Urol. 1996;155:994–8.

63. Shreve PD, Anzai Y, Wahl RL. Pitfalls in oncologic diagnosis with FDG PET imaging: physiologic and benign variants. Radiographics. 1999;19:61–77; quiz 150–151.

64. Hofer C, Laubenbacher C, Block T, Breul J, Hartung R, Schwaiger M. Fluorine-18-fluorodeoxyglucose positron emission tomography is useless for the detection of local recurrence after radical prostatectomy. Eur Urol. 1999;36:31–5.

65. Seltzer MA, Barbaric Z, Belldegrun A, et al. Comparison of helical computerized tomography, positron emission tomography and monoclonal antibody scans for evaluation of lymph node metastases in patients with prostate specific antigen relapse after treatment for localized prostate cancer. J Urol. 1999;162:1322–8.

66. Mathews D, Oz OK. Positron emission tomography in prostate and renal cell carcinoma. Curr Opin Urol. 2002;12:381–5.

67. Hofer C, Kubler H, Hartung R, Breul J, Avril N. Diagnosis and monitoring of urological tumors using positron emission tomography. Eur Urol. 2001;40:481–7.

68. Oyama N, Akino H, Suzuki Y, et al. FDG PET for evaluating the change of glucose metabolism in prostate cancer after androgen ablation. Nucl Med Commun. 2001;22:963–9.

69. Shreve PD, Grossman HB, Gross MD, Wahl RL. Metastatic prostate cancer: initial findings of PET with 2-deoxy-2-[F-18] fluoro-D-glucose. Radiology. 1996;199:751–6.

70. Zeisel SH. Choline: an essential nutrient for humans. Nutrition. 2000;16:669–71.

71. Kwee SA, Coel MN, Lim J, Ko JP. Prostate cancer localization with 18fluorine fluorocholine positron emission tomography. J Urol. 2005;173:252–5.

72. Ackerstaff E, Pflug BR, Nelson JB, Bhujwalla ZM. Detection of increased choline compounds with proton nuclear magnetic resonance spectroscopy subsequent to malignant transformation of human prostatic epithelial cells. Cancer Res. 2001;61:3599–603.

73. Sutinen E, Nurmi M, Roivainen A, et al. Kinetics of [(11)C]choline uptake in prostate cancer: a PET study. Eur J Nucl Med Mol Imaging. 2004;31:317–24.

74. Hara T, Kosaka N, Kishi H. Development of (18)F-fluoroethylcholine for cancer imaging with PET: synthesis, biochemistry, and prostate cancer imaging. J Nucl Med. 2002;43:187–99.

75. Hatazawa J, Ishiwata K, Itoh M, et al. Quantitative evaluation of L-[methyl-C-11] methionine uptake in tumor using positron emission tomography. J Nucl Med. 1989;30:1809–13.

76. Macapinlac HA, Humm JL, Akhurst T, et al. Differential Metabolism and Pharmacokinetics of L-[1-(11)C]-Methionine and 2-[(18)F] Fluoro-2-deoxy-D-glucose (FDG) in Androgen Independent Prostate Cancer. Clin Positron Imaging. 1999;2:173–81.

77. Nunez R, Macapinlac HA, Yeung HW, et al. Combined 18F-FDG and 11C-methionine PET scans in patients with newly progressive metastatic prostate cancer. J Nucl Med. 2002;43:46–55.

78. Yoshimoto M, Waki A, Yonekura Y, et al. Characterization of acetate metabolism in tumor cells in relation to cell proliferation: acetate metabolism in tumor cells. Nucl Med Biol. 2001;28:117–22.

79. Oyama N, Akino H, Kanamaru H, et al. 11C-acetate PET imaging of prostate cancer. J Nucl Med. 2002;43:181–6.

80. Shreve P, Chiao PC, Humes HD, Schwaiger M, Gross MD. Carbon-11-acetate PET imaging in renal disease. J Nucl Med. 1995;36:1595–601.

81. Kato T, Tsukamoto E, Kuge Y, et al. Accumulation of [11C]acetate in normal prostate and benign prostatic hyperplasia: comparison with prostate cancer. Eur J Nucl Med Mol Imaging. 2002;29:1492–5.

82. Zanzonico PB, Finn R, Pentlow KS, et al. PET-based radiation dosimetry in man of 18F-fluorodihydrotestosterone, a new radiotracer for imaging prostate cancer. J Nucl Med. 2004;45:1966–71.

83. Oyama N, Ponde DE, Dence C, Kim J, Tai YC, Welch MJ. Monitoring of therapy in androgen-dependent prostate tumor model by measuring tumor proliferation. J Nucl Med. 2004;45:519–25.

84. Liu IJ, Zafar MB, Lai YH, Segall GM, Terris MK. Fluorodeoxyglucose positron emission tomography studies in diagnosis and staging of clinically organ-confined prostate cancer. Urology. 2001;57:108–11.

85. Oyama N, Miller TR, Dehdashti F, et al. 11C-acetate PET imaging of prostate cancer: detection of recurrent disease at PSA relapse. J Nucl Med. 2003;44:549–55.

86. Oyama N, Akino H, Suzuki Y, et al. Prognostic value of 2-deoxy-2-[F-18]fluoro-D-glucose positron emission tomography imaging for patients with prostate cancer. Mol Imaging Biol. 2002; 4:99–104.

87. Yang SN, Liang JA, Lin FJ, Kao CH, Lin CC, Lee CC. Comparing whole body (18)F-2-deoxyglucose positron emission tomography and technetium-99m methylene diphosphonate bone scan to detect bone metastases in patients with breast cancer. J Cancer Res Clin Oncol. 2002;128:325–8.

88. Cook GJ, Houston S, Rubens R, Maisey MN, Fogelman I. Detection of bone metastases in breast cancer by 18FDG PET: differing metabolic activity in osteoblastic and osteolytic lesions. J Clin Oncol. 1998;16:3375–79.

89. Nakamoto Y, Osman M, Wahl RL. Prevalence and patterns of bone metastases detected with positron emission tomography using F-18 FDG. Clin Nucl Med. 2003;28:302–7.

90. el-Gabry EA, Halpern EJ, Strup SE, Gomella LG. Imaging prostate cancer: current and future applications. Oncology (Huntingt). 2001;15:325–6; discussion 339–342.

91. Babaian RJ, Murray JL, Lamki LM, et al. Radioimmunological imaging of metastatic prostatic cancer with 111indium-labeled monoclonal antibody PAY 276. J Urol. 1987;137:439–43.

92. Haseman MK, Rosenthal SA, Polascik TJ. Capromab Pendetide imaging of prostate cancer. Cancer Biother Radiopharm. 2000;15:131–40.

93. Bermejo CE, Coursey J, Basler J, Austenfeld M, Thompson I. Histologic confirmation of lesions identified by Prostascint scan following definitive treatment. Urol Oncol. 2003;21:349–52; discussion 353.

94. Freeman LM, Krynyckyi BR, Li Y, et al. The role of (111) In Capromab Pendetide (Prosta-ScintR) immunoscintigraphy in the management of prostate cancer. Q J Nucl Med. 2002;46:131–7.

95. Nargund V, Al Hashmi D, Kumar P, et al. Imaging with radiolabelled monoclonal antibody (MUJ591) to prostate-specific membrane antigen in staging of clinically localized prostatic carcinoma: comparison with clinical, surgical and histological staging. BJU Int. 2005;95:1232–6.

96. Kelty NL, Holder LE, Khan SH. Dual-isotope protocol for indium-111 capromab pendetide monoclonal antibody imaging. J Nucl Med Technol. 1998;26:174–7.

97. Sodee DB, Faulhaber PF, Nelson AD, Bakale G. The prognostic significance of indium-111-capromab penetide. J Clin Oncol. 2004;22:379–80; author reply 380–371.

98. Schettino CJ, Kramer EL, Noz ME, Taneja S, Padmanabhan P, Lepor H. Impact of fusion of indium-111 capromab pendetide volume data sets with those from MRI or CT in patients with recurrent prostate cancer. AJR Am J Roentgenol. 2004;183: 519–24.

99. Hinkle GH, Burgers JK, Neal CE, et al. Multicenter radioimmunoscintigraphic evaluation of patients with prostate carcinoma using indium-111 capromab pendetide. Cancer. 1998;83:739–47.

100. Polascik TJ, Manyak MJ, Haseman MK, et al. Comparison of clinical staging algorithms and 111indium-capromab pendetide immunoscintigraphy in the prediction of lymph node involvement in high risk prostate carcinoma patients. Cancer. 1999;85: 1586–92.

101. Sodee DB, Malguria N, Faulhaber P, Resnick MI, Albert J, Bakale G. Multicenter ProstaScint imaging findings in 2154 patients with prostate cancer. The ProstaScint Imaging Centers. Urology. 2000;56:988–93.

102. Kahn D, Williams RD, Haseman MK, Reed NL, Miller SJ, Gerstbrein J. Radioimmunoscintigraphy with In-111-labeled capromab pendetide predicts prostate cancer response to salvage radiotherapy after failed radical prostatectomy. J Clin Oncol. 1998;16: 284–9.

103. Murphy GP, Maguire RT, Rogers B, et al. Comparison of serum PSMA, PSA levels with results of Cytogen-356 ProstaScint scanning in prostatic cancer patients. Prostate. 1997;33: 281–5.

104. Jani AB, Blend MJ, Hamilton R, et al. Radioimmunoscintigraphy for postprostatectomy radiotherapy: analysis of toxicity and biochemical control. J Nucl Med. 2004;45:1315–22.

105. Elgamal AA, Troychak MJ, Murphy GP. ProstaScint scan may enhance identification of prostate cancer recurrences after prostatectomy, radiation, or hormone therapy: analysis of 136 scans of 100 patients. Prostate. 1998;37:261–9.

106. Murphy GP, Elgamal AA, Troychak MJ, Kenny GM. Follow-up ProstaScint scans verify detection of occult soft-tissue recurrence after failure of primary prostate cancer therapy. Prostate. 2000;42:315–7.

107. Kahn D, Williams RD, Seldin DW, et al. Radioimmunoscintigraphy with 111indium labeled CYT-356 for the detection of occult prostate cancer recurrence. J Urol. 1994;152:1490–5.

108. Petronis JD, Regan F, Lin K. Indium-111 capromab pendetide (ProstaScint) imaging to detect recurrent and metastatic prostate cancer. Clin Nucl Med. 1998;23:672–7.

109. Kahn D, Williams RD, Manyak MJ, et al. 111Indium-capromab pendetide in the evaluation of patients with residual or recurrent prostate cancer after radical prostatectomy. The ProstaScint Study Group. J Urol. 1998;159:2041–6; discussion 2046–2047.

110. Levesque PE, Nieh PT, Zinman LN, Seldin DW, Libertino JA. Radiolabeled monoclonal antibody indium 111-labeled CYT-356 localizes extraprostatic recurrent carcinoma after prostatectomy. Urology. 1998;51:978–84.

111. Burgers JK, Hinkle GH, Haseman MK. Monoclonal antibody imaging of recurrent and metastatic prostate cancer. Semin Urol. 1995;13:103–12.

112. Thomas CT, Bradshaw PT, Pollock BH, et al. Indium-111-capromab pendetide radioimmunoscintigraphy and prognosis for durable biochemical response to salvage radiation therapy in men after failed prostatectomy. J Clin Oncol. 2003;21: 1715–21.

113. Wilkinson S, Chodak G. The role of 111indium-capromab pendetide imaging for assessing biochemical failure after radical prostatectomy. J Urol. 2004;172:133–6.

114. Ellis RJ, Vertocnik A, Sodee B, et al. Combination conformal radiotherapy and radioimmunoguided transperineal 103Pd implantation for patients with intermediate and unfavorable risk prostate adenocarcinoma. Brachytherapy. 2003;2:215–22.

115. Ellis RJ, Vertocnik A, Kim E, et al. Four-year biochemical outcome after radioimmunoguided transperineal brachytherapy for patients with prostate adenocarcinoma. Int J Radiat Oncol Biol Phys. 2003;57:362–70.

116. Ellis RJ, Kim EY, Conant R, et al. Radioimmunoguided imaging of prostate cancer foci with histopathological correlation. Int J Radiat Oncol Biol Phys. 2001;49:1281–6.

117. Heidenreich A, Ohlmann C, Polyakov S. Anatomical extent of pelvic lymphadenectomy in bladder and prostate cancer. Eur Urol Suppl. 2005;4:14–24.

118. Bader P, Burkhard FC, Markwalder R, Studer UE. Disease progression and survival of patients with positive lymph nodes after radical prostatectomy. Is there a chance of cure? J Urol. 2003;169:849–54.

119. Wawroschek F, Wagner T, Hamm M, et al. The influence of serial sections, immunohistochemistry, and extension of pelvic lymph node dissection on the lymph node status in clinically localized prostate cancer. Eur Urol. 2003;43:132–6; discussion 137.

120. Wawroschek F, Vogt H, Weckermann D, Wagner T, Hamm M, Harzmann R. Radioisotope guided pelvic lymph node dissection for prostate cancer. J Urol. 2001;166:1715–9.

121. Partin AW, Kattan MW, Subong EN, et al. Combination of prostate-specific antigen, clinical stage, and Gleason score to predict pathological stage of localized prostate cancer. A multi-institutional update. Jama. 1997;277:1445–51.

122. Crawford ED, Batuello JT, Snow P, et al. The use of artificial intelligence technology to predict lymph node spread in men with clinically localized prostate carcinoma. Cancer. 2000;88:2105–9.

123. Heidenreich A, Varga Z, Von Knobloch R. Extended pelvic lymphadenectomy in patients undergoing radical prostatectomy: high incidence of lymph node metastasis. J Urol. 2002;167:1681–6.

124. Weckermann D, Wawroschek F, Harzmann R. Is there a need for pelvic lymph node dissection in low risk prostate cancer patients prior to definitive local therapy? Eur Urol. 2005;47:45–50; discussion 50–41.

125. Messing EM, Manola J, Sarosdy M, Wilding G, Crawford ED, Trump D. Immediate hormonal therapy versus observation after radical prostatectomy and pelvic lymphadenectomy for node-positive prostate cancer: at 10 years results EST3886. J Clin Onc. 2004;22(14S):(Abstract 4570).

126. Messing EM, Manola J, Sarosdy M, Wilding G, Crawford ED, Trump D. Immediate hormonal therapy compared with observation after radical prostatectomy and pelvic lymphadenectomy in men with node-positive prostate cancer. N Engl J Med. 1999;341:1781–8.

127. Mann BG, Buchanan M, Collins PJ, Lichtenstein M. High incidence of micrometastases in breast cancer sentinel nodes. Aust N Z J Surg. 2000;70:786–90.

128. Kroon BK, Horenblas S, Nieweg OE. Contemporary management of penile squamous cell carcinoma. J Surg Oncol. 2005; 89:43–50.

129. Borgognoni L, Urso C, Vaggelli L, Brandani P, Gerlini G, Reali UM. Sentinel node biopsy procedures with an analysis of recurrence patterns and prognosis in melanoma patients: technical advantages using computer-assisted gamma probe with adjustable collimation. Melanoma Res. 2004;14:311–9.

130. Wawroschek F, Vogt H, Weckermann D, Wagner T, Harzmann R. The sentinel lymph node concept in prostate cancer - first results of gamma probe-guided sentinel lymph node identification. Eur Urol. 1999;36:595–600.

131. Wawroschek F, Vogt H, Wengenmair H, et al. Prostate lymphoscintigraphy and radio-guided surgery for sentinel lymph node identification in prostate cancer. Technique and results of the first 350 cases. Urol Int. 2003;70:303–10.

132. Bastide C, Brenot-Rossi I, Garcia S, et al. [Feasibility and value of the isotope sentinel node mapping technique in prostate cancer]. Prog Urol. 2004;14:501–6.

133. Takashima H, Egawa M, Imao T, Fukuda M, Yokoyama K, Namiki M. Validity of sentinel lymph node concept for patients with prostate cancer. J Urol. 2004;171:2268–71.

Chapter 24

Considerations: Imaging in Prostate Cancer

A. Heidenreich

Introduction

Prostate cancer (PCA) is the most common solid cancer among European men with a continuously increasing incidence. Adequate management and follow-up of PCA relies not only on valid pathohistology information of the prostate biopsy but also on adequate detection and diagnosis, accurate staging, and posttreatment monitoring by sensitive imaging modalities. Reliable diagnosis of early, organ-confined, or even locally advanced PCA is the first step to initiate an individualized risk-adapted therapy thereby improving therapeutic outcome.

The major goal for future PCA imaging appears to be a more accurate disease characterization by combining anatomical, functional, and (molecular) imaging information. New developments of microbubble contrast agents and color Doppler techniques for transrectal ultrasonography, innovative technical improvements of endorectal magnetic resonance imaging (MRI) with or without spectroscopy, optimization of positron emission tomography combined with computed tomography (PET/CT), and improvement to detect bone metastases by whole-body MRI resulted in a significant increase of the imaging armamentarium available to improve diagnosis, staging, and outcome of PCA patients.

Herein we review the clinical role for imaging on the detection and management of prostate cancer.

Detection and Intraprostatic Localization of Prostate Cancer

Transrectal Ultrasonography (TRUS)

TRUS with high-resolution ultrasound probes of 7.5–12 MHz represents the standard imaging modality for initial evaluation and biopsy guidance since it has been shown that the zonal anatomy of the prostate can be well distinguished by this imaging method [1, 2]. TRUS also plays an important role in therapy such as directing brachytherapy seeds or cryosurgery probes into the prostate. The greatest challenge for TRUS, however, remains the early and valid detection of PCA which is highly operator dependent. Currently, the sensitivity of TRUS as a diagnostic test to detect PCA is as low as for digital rectal examination. Current criteria being suspicious for the presence of PA are (1) bulges of the prostatic capsule especially if present in the ventral part of the apex and (2) reduced echogenicity in the peripheral zone. However, even in experienced hands sensitivity and specificity to detect PCA is only as high as 50%. Criteria for the identification of extraprostatic extension of PCA are bulging and irregularities of the capsule adjacent to a suspicious lesion. Seminal vesicle invasion is either suspected by extension of the hypoechoic mass into the seminal vesicle, echogenic cancer within the seminal vesicle, or asymmetry of the seminal vesicles.

The low reliability of TRUS to identify early, small-volume PCA has led to the recommendation to perform multiple (10–12), systemic TRUS-guided prostate biopsies of the peripheral zone to identify non-visible PCA.

Innovative sonographic techniques using microbubble contrast agents and targeted imaging have been developed to better detect early PCA and to better identify locally advanced disease [3, 4].

A. Heidenreich (✉)
Division of Oncological Urology, Department of Urology, University of Köln, Kerpener Str. 62, 50924 Köln, Germany,
axel.heidenreich@uk-koeln.de

Transrectal Color Doppler and Power Doppler Ultrasonography

Since PCA has been associated with an increased perfusion of cancer-involved areas, the idea of ultrasound color Doppler and power Doppler techniques is to better identify prostate cancer by reliable detection of intraprostatic areas of increased blood flow [1]. Doppler sonography collects information on the blood flow direction, the speed and quantity of blood perfusing the tissue due to the measurement of a frequency shift caused by the moving corpuscular components of the blood. However, Doppler sonography has its limitations to detect details of organ perfusion and microvasculature due to the small diameter of the blood vessels and the low blood flow. The power Doppler technique represents an innovative non-invasive technique with a high sensitivity to also recognize areas of small amounts of slow-velocity flow which might be missed by standard color Doppler techniques. The microvascular imaging becomes possible after intravenous injection of small gas-filled microbubbles which cause a substantial increase of the echo reflected from blood-perfused areas of the tissue thereby enabling the investigator to identify small vessels and areas of increased angiogenesis potentially marking neoplastic tissue alterations against normal healthy tissue.

Various groups have demonstrated that the PCA detection rate at first biopsy is significantly enhanced if color Doppler-targeted biopsies are taken as compared to TRUS-guided systematic biopsies [5]. Furthermore, it has been shown, that a negative power Doppler TRUS signal is able to exclude most of the patients without PCA in the PSA range of 2.5–10 ng/ml. As an additional tool at TRUS biopsy power Doppler has a high negative predictive value and may help to reduce the number of unnecessary biopsies [6]. In another large trial comprising the comparative data on 619 consecutive patients undergoing TRUS and color Doppler TRUS with directed or systematic biopsies, color Doppler imaging was compared to gray-scale TRUS and pathohistology [7]. About half of the biopsy-proven PCA had abnormalities on color Doppler TRUS as compared to normal findings on gray-scale TRUS. More interestingly, approximately three quarters of the men with color Doppler TRUS abnormalities demonstrated moderate to high-grade Gleason scores which were clearly identified as clinically significant PCA. These data have been corroborated by others making color Doppler TRUS a clinically helpful tool to identify significant PCA with a high sensitivity. Although very promising, these findings have to be validated and confirmed in the community of hospital-based and office-based urologists.

Besides improving the detection rate of PCA at initial biopsy, color Doppler TRUS might be helpful to identify local recurrences in the scenario of a rising PSA following radical prostatectomy [8, 9]. In various clinical series, the findings of gray-scale TRUS, power Doppler TRUS, and endorectal MRI were compared with TRUS-guided and power Doppler TRUS-guided biopsies of the vesicourethral anastomosis and the perianastomotic soft tissue. In all series, TRUS-related abnormalities were identified in about 75% of the patients; biopsies of areas with hypervascularities were always positive for cancer and resulted in a very high sensitivity and positive predictive value of 93 and 100%, respectively, as compared to 93 and 93% for gray-scale TRUS. However, one has to consider that the mean PSA serum level at the time of biopsy was above 1 ng/ml not necessarily reflecting the true clinical scenario where the decision-making process has to be made at much lower PSA levels.

Contrast-Enhanced Transrectal Ultrasonography

As compared to benign prostatic tissue, prostate cancer is associated with an increased microvessel density which appears to be predictors of advanced stage, metastatic disease, and cancer-specific survival. Due to the small diameter these microvessels can neither be identified by normal gray-scale TRUS nor by power Doppler TRUS. However, contrast-enhanced TRUS can visualize the microvasculature after intravenous injection of microbubble containing contrast agents due the fact that these microbubbles will stay in the vessels for several minutes and expose an enhanced acoustic reflectivity. Thereby, microvessels beyond the resolution for conventional color Doppler ultrasound can identified by the intense reflected signals resulting from intravascular microbubbles. Several reports have demonstrated that contrast-enhanced ultrasound investigations of the blood flow of the prostate allow for prostate cancer visualization and therefore, for targeted biopsies [10–12]. Comparisons between systematic and contrast-enhanced ultrasound-targeted biopsies have shown that the targeted approach detects more cancers with a lower number of biopsy cores. Furthermore, contrast-enhanced ultrasound has been shown to detect cancers with higher Gleason scores compared with the systematic approach, which seems to improve prostate cancer grading. In a comparative study of three different ultrasound techniques, the sensitivity by biopsy site was significantly greater on contrast-enhanced sonography (68%) than on gray-scale (39%) and color Doppler (41%) sonography [10]. However, one has to consider that also contrast-enhanced TRUS has its limitations in the accurate detection of PCA as has been demonstrated in a recent large series including 304 men undergoing TRUS, contrast-enhanced TRUS, and color Doppler TRUS [11]. Targeted biopsy cores were obtained from sites of greatest enhancement, followed by spatially distributed cores in a modified sextant distribution. Although carcinoma was found significantly more often in the targeted biopsies as in the sextant cores and contrast-enhanced TRUS provided a statistically significant improvement in discrimination between benign and malignant biopsy sites, the technique was not sufficient to predict which patients have benign versus malignant disease. The majority of cancers missed by the targeted approach were located at the prostatic apex so that it might be recommendable to apply a targeted biopsy strategy in the peripheral zone and a systematic biopsy at the apex. The poor discrimination rate between benign and malignant prostatic tissue might have resulted from the local hyperperfusion related to benign prostatic hyperplasia. One emerging strategy to overcome this problem is to pretreat patients with finasteride or dutasteride for up to 4 weeks to decrease blood flow and to better allow a clear distinction between cancer and benign disease [12].

Elastography

It is well known that some diseases, such as cancer, lead to a change of tissue hardness (i.e., the so-called elasticity modulus). The wide range of elastic tissue properties and the difference in elasticity of tumors and the adjacent tissues have provided motivation for developing elasticity imaging techniques [13]. These research efforts have converged with the development of a new imaging modality, the so-called elastography, with the acquired and processed images referred to as elastograms. The reconstruction of tissue elasticity provides the sonographer with important additional information which can be applied for the diagnosis of malignant diseases such as prostate cancer. The elasticity modulus, i.e., the tissue elasticity distribution, can be calculated from the exerted strain and the stress of the examined structures, e.g., from the transrectal ultrasound probe during conventional TRUS. Variation of the pressure exerted with the probe onto the prostate, results in changes of the ultrasound images. Prostate cancer is characterized by a limited elasticity and compressibility translating into a typical ultrasound image of a "dark zone" as compared to the non-malignant prostate tissue. Clinical trials and experiences are limited, however, a 20% improvement in the PCA detection rate has been demonstrated in those studies being performed [14, 15]. These data have to be confirmed in future clinical studies including a larger patient population and a multiinstitutional setting.

Magnetic Resonance Imaging (MRI)

MRI can be used for PCA detection, local and locoregional staging at initial diagnosis and during follow-up. Currently, MRI and endorectal MRI are recommended for cancer detection only in the clinical scenario of a suspected PCA but negative ultrasound-guided prostate biopsies [2]. Optimal MRI techniques for the detection and local staging of PCA require an endorectal coil in combination with a pelvic phased-array coil. PCA is best detected on T2-weighted images due to the decreased signal intensity of the cancer areas as compared to the generally increased signal intensity of the normal prostate [16, 17]. These differences cannot be depicted on T1-weigthed images where the whole prostate usually exhibits a homogenous signal intensity. In general, however, sensitivity figures for the detection and correct localization of PCA in the peripheral zone varied between 37 and 96%; detection rate is much worse in the transition zone. Since postbiopsy hemorrhage and biopsy-associated local inflammation of the prostate gland can result in difficulties to adequately interpret MRI findings, a delay of 6–8 weeks after biopsy is recommended [18].

In order to enhance the prediction patterns, dynamic contrast-enhanced MRI techniques have been developed taking advantage of the finding that PCA usually enhances earlier than the unaffected peripheral zone and associated benign prostatic hyperplasia. Various studies have demonstrated a significant improvement of sensitivity by about 10–20% using T2-weigthed sequences when correlated with whole-mount histology [19–21]. However, it also has been shown that MRI-based detection of PCA is highly dependent on tumor size with <5% of tumors ≤5 mm in diameter and 89% of those >10 mm being correctly identified [22]. Dynamic contrast-enhanced MRI only shows a minimal improvement. Nevertheless, current data demonstrate a high sensitivity and specificity of MRI to predict transrectal biopsy results at a 70–80% level. MRI is extremely helpful to detect most intraprostatic cancers and might be used for (1) scanning of intermediate- and high-risk patients, (2) targeting biopsies in suspicious areas thereby increasing the PCA detection rate, and (3) increasing the negative predictive value in men thereby eliminating the need for rebiopsy of the prostate.

Magnetic Resonance Spectroscopic Imaging (MRSI)

MRI and MRSI allow a detailed anatomic and metabolic evaluation of the prostate gland taking advantage of the excellent depiction of the prostatic zonal anatomy by T2-weigthed images and the assessment of prostate cancer metabolism characterized by high levels of choline and low levels of citrate [23]. The combined use of both MRI and MRSI has been shown to increase the detection rate of tumors in the peripheral and the transition zone [24, 25]. Recent studies also have indicated that MRSI might be able to predict the aggressiveness of PCA since there are different metabolic abnormalities associated with different

Gleason scores [26]. For Gleason score 6 PCA the depiction rate was 44% as compared to 90% for Gleason score 8–10 cancers. Today, the use of combined MRI/MRSI is limited to very few centers and the initial encouraging and promising data have to be validated in larger patient cohorts diagnosed in more institutions.

However, MRSI will be an important imaging modality for the future since it might be possible to identify specific MRSI imaging patterns associated with key molecular markers associated with biological aggressiveness of PCA such as Ki-67, Bcl-2, and PTEN [27].

Detection of Locally Advanced Disease

In general, TRUS even in combination with the most innovative techniques has a low sensitivity to accurately predict locally advanced PCA, e.g., extracapsular extension and seminal vesicle invasion [1, 2]. Indirect criteria such as bulging or irregularities of the prostatic capsule, and asymmetry or irregularity of the seminal vesicles to predict T3 disease are associated with 70% sensitivity.

MRI with or without endorectal coil significantly increases the detection rate of PCA as has been shown above. However, its sensitivity to identify extracapsular extension and seminal vesicle involvement shows a considerably high variation of 13–95% and 23–80%, respectively [28, 29]. Although a recent study demonstrated a significant improvement to predict ECE when comparing pathohistological data of radical prostatectomy specimens with findings of preoperative endorectal MRI, it became evident that the contribution of MRI was only substantial when interpretation of the films was performed by specialists in genitourinary MRI [30]. However, even among those specialists an interobserver variability ranging from 53 to 93% has been described making it currently unlikely that MRI will become the major staging tool of PCA unless MR technology will further mature, become more accurate, and observer independent [2, 17, 23]. Based on the data available it is highly unlikely that dynamic-contrast-enhanced MRI or MRSI will further improve the staging accuracy of PCA.

Therefore, it will be one of the major tasks for the future to develop imaging strategies better delineating locally advanced disease to better trigger initial management of PCA.

Detection of Lymph Node Metastases in the Small Pelvis

The identification of positive lymphonodular disease in the small pelvis is of utmost importance for the planning of adequate treatment strategies in the individual patient. Currently, none of the standard radiological techniques predicts the presence of lymph node metastases accurately when compared to extended pelvic lymphadenectomy. However, there are some innovative techniques which might overcome this clinically significant staging problem in the near future.

Reported CT sensitivity for the detection of lymph node metastases typically is in the range of about 35% [31]. This low sensitivity is basically due to the fact that a lymph node size >1 cm in diameter is required for the identification of lymph node metastases. Therefore, it is recommended to perform CT scans only in patients with intermediate- and high-risk PCA at a PSA serum level >20 ng/ml or a biopsy Gleason score >7 (Table 24.1) [32].

MR imaging, dynamic-enhanced MRI, and even MRSI have no advantage of CT to predict the presence of lymph node metastases and the same recommendation with regard to its use in pretherapeutic staging can be made.

The use of lymphotropic paramagnetic iron oxide nanoparticles with a size of 30–50 nm as contrast agent at MR imaging might improve the detection of nodal disease [33]. The lymphotropic nanoparticles extravasate from blood vessels after intravenous injection and enter the reticulo-endothelial system of lymph nodes by direct transcapillary passage or by non-selective endothelial transcytosis. The process of intralymphatic localization usually requires 24–36 hours so that two imaging studies about 48 hours apart are necessary to adequately assess lymph node morphology. Within normal or benign lymph nodes the nanoparticles are phagocytosed by macrophages resulting in a drop of signal intensity in T2-weighted MR images. Lymph nodes which are infiltrated by cancer cells lack functioning macrophages and therefore, retain their high signal intensity on T2-weighted images. However, the enhancement pattern after nanoparticle injection clearly is dependent on the nodal metastatic tumor burden and the detection of minimal cancer infiltration in smaller lymph nodes still is difficult and might contribute to false-negative results. False-positive interpretations might result from fibrosis, fatty hilum, reactive lymphoid follicular hyperplasia, and granulomatous or infectious diseases with nodal necrosis.

Initial results on a group of 30 patients with genitourinary malignancies demonstrated a significantly improved sensitivity and specificity of 100 and 80% to accurately detect pelvic lymph node metastases [34]. In a more recent trial on 80 men with clinically localized prostate cancer LNMRI was used to identify lymph node metastases in the small pelvis; MRI findings were correlated with pathohistological findings of dissected lymph nodes. LNMRI was shown to increase the sensitivity for detection of lymph node metastases from 35% when using MRI alone to 90% [35]; specificity also increased from 90 to 98% making LNMRI a potentially useful imaging technique for preoperative staging of the small pelvis. However, there are some limitations of the study which have to be addressed in the near future before LNMRI will become a routine staging method for PCA. Patients underwent a formal lymph node dissection of the obturator fossa only; in all other areas only suspicious lymph nodes were resected. As we know from anatomical mapping studies, about 60% of all lymph node metastases are located outside the obturator fossa including the external, internal, and common iliac artery [36, 37]. Therefore, the true rate of false-negative results cannot be determined adequately by the study design used. Nevertheless, LNMRI appears to be the most promising imaging modality to identify pelvic lymph node metastases and more multiinstitutional trials with a standard extended pelvic lymphadenectomy should be performed.

In the past sentinel lymphoscintigraphy (SLN) has been described as an imaging staging tool for planning of the necessity and the extent of pelvic lymphadenectomy in PCA patients undergoing radical prostatectomy [38]. Planar films are taken preoperatively and intraoperatively; the use of gamma probe facilitates dissection of all lymph nodes storing the ^{99m}Tc-nanocolloid. However, there are clear limitations of this technique such as poor sensitivity of planar lymphoscintigraphy to identify all lymph nodes involved in the primary drainage of the prostate. Furthermore, SLN is not able to identify all metastatic lymph nodes either due to the presence of micrometastases with a diameter below the resolution of SLN or due to macrometastases blocking the lymphatic drainage of ^{99m}Tc-nanocolloid into the lymph nodes. Therefore, SLN does not represent an innovative staging tool with future potentials. Single-photon emission computed tomography (SPECT) fused with computed tomography or MRI improved spatial resolution and orientation and thereby allows a more precise localization of ^{99m}Tc-containing lymph nodes. However, experiences are very limited and need some further validation by future clinical trials correlating pathohistology of all resected lymph nodes with preoperative imaging findings.

Detection of Systemic Metastases

The skeletal system is the main metastatic site of prostate cancer and bone scanning represents the mainstay of diagnosis to identify osseous metastases at initial diagnosis or during follow-up of prostate cancer patients. At initial diagnosis, a bone scan is not recommended in men with low-risk PCA (cT1c, PSA <10 ng/ml, biopsy Gleason score ≤6) due to the very low frequency of positive findings in <1% of patients (Table 24.1) [32]. However, chances to identify metastases are increasing to 10–15% in men with PSA serum levels >50 ng/ml. In early clinical studies it has been shown that bone scanning is clearly superior to identify bone metastases when compared to clinical symptoms (34% improvement, Palmer) and conventional radiographs (28% improvement, [39]). However, skeletal scintigraphy is limited by the detection of small metastatic deposits and by the identification of metastases without cortical involvement. Besides staging response assessment to treatment such as androgen deprivation, chemotherapy or palliative radiation can be performed by skeletal scintigraphy. Accurate response assessment is difficult and prone to misinterpretations since a flare-up phenomenon peaking 6–8 weeks after treatment and resulting from increased bone turnover as response to therapy has to be considered. Furthermore, it sometimes appears to be very difficult to differentiate new lesions from regressing lesions or from progression of minimal deposits at initial investigation. It is probably for these reasons that bone scanning never has been used as an imaging method of choice to evaluate response to therapy in clinical trials.

In this scenario, MRI of the axial skeleton, single-photon emission computed tomography, and positron emission tomography (PET) appear to be more sensitive in the detection and follow-up of osseous metastases in men with advanced PCA. MRI of the axial skeleton has been demonstrated to be superior to skeletal scintigraphy with regard to diagnosis and follow-up of bone metastases in men with hormone refractory prostate cancer [40]. In another clinical

Table 24.1 Use of imaging in staging prostate cancer

Guideline society	Recommendation
European Association of Urology, 2007	Bone scan, CT: PSA >20 ng/ml, any PCA with Gleason score 8–10, locally advanced disease (cT3); endorectal MRI/MR spectroscopy mentioned as still experimental staging options
American Urological Association, 2001	Bone scan: PSA >20 ng/ml, any Gleason score 8–10 PCA, locally advanced PCA (cT3). CT/MRI if PSA >25 ng/ml, endorectal MRI/MR spectroscopy not mentioned
American College of Radiology, 2000	Bone scanning, CT, or MRI: PSA >10 ng/ml, Gleason score >6
American Joint Committee on Cancer, 2002	Bone scan, CT/MRI: PSA >20 ng/ml, Gleason score >7

comparative analysis of planar bone scintigraphy, SPECT, 18F-flouride PET, and 18F-flouride PET/CT in 44 men with high-risk PCA, the superiority of 18F-flouride PET/CT over SPECT over bone scintigraphy with regard to sensitivity and specificity to detect bone metastases could be demonstrated [41, 42]. Of all 18F-flouride PET/CT lesions, 52 and 19% were overlooked by skeletal scintigraphy and SPECT, respectively. For the future, whole-body MRI or 18F-flouride PET/CT might become the imaging modality of choice for detection and assessment of osseous metastases in PCA.

Summary

As pointed numerous innovative imaging modalities for the detection, diagnosis, staging, and follow-up of prostate cancer have emerged over the recent years. Most of the imaging techniques described still have to be put into clinical perspective with regard to their general use because some of the techniques are still limited to few centers only despite initial promising being published about 10 years ago. With regard to the detection and initial diagnosis of PCA contrast-enhanced TRUS and color Doppler TRUS seem to represent the most promising tools which easily can be integrated into daily clinical routine.

In patients with multiple negative biopsies but still suspicious characteristics for the presence of PCA, contrast-enhanced MRI and 11C-choline PET/CT are the most promising imaging tools to identify cancer.

Identification of PCA with extracapsular extension and/or seminal vesicle invasion still represents a challenge to urologists and radiologists. Currently, prospectively validated nomograms are as sensitive but significantly less cost intense as sophisticated imaging techniques.

None of the routinely available imaging tools are sensitive enough to accurately predict lymph node metastases in the small pelvis. Surgical-extended pelvic lymphadenectomy represents the most reliable technique currently available. In the near future, MRI with lymphotrophic nanoparticles will improve pretherapeutic imaging modalities.

Skeletal scintigraphy still represents the imaging modality of choice to scan the entire skeleton for the presence of metastases. However, 18F-flouride SPECT/CT and whole-body MRI are more sensitive in the detection and follow-up of osseous metastases and will replace bone scanning in the near future.

Future Perspectives

For the future, imaging techniques predicting presence, localization, and local extent of PCA in combination with molecular markers predicting the biological behavior of PCA will revolutionize our current understanding and management of PCA. Recent results of clinical phase-II and phase-III trials have reinforced the view that many patients with PCA are overtreated. It will be a challenge for the near future to differentiate those men with an aggressive, but curative PCA from those with either insignificant or incurable PCA by the identification of serum, tissue, and imaging biomarkers.

Currently, a considerable amount of clinical studies is under way to correlate preoperative MRSI spectral patterns with the immunohistochemical expression of molecular markers such as Ki-67, Bcl-2, p27 on whole mount sections.

With regard to the early detection of systemic metastasis the androgen receptor (AR) has been identified as a potential target for molecular imaging of AR-positive PCA cells using radiolabeled ligands [43, 44]. Fluorine-labeled non-steroidal androgen receptor antagonists (FDHT) in combination with PET have been developed and clinically evaluated in men with biopsy-proven metastatic PCA. FDHT-PET demonstrated a higher sensitivity to detect bone lesions as compared to conventional imaging techniques; however, positive studies were associated with higher PSA serum levels and positive AR expression. Androgen deprivation therapy decreased the diagnostic accuracy so that more specific targets must be identified for men with low or no AR expression, low PSA values, and hormone refractory disease.

In another preclinical model, diffusion MRI and functional diffusion mapping have been identified as an imaging biomarker accurately assessing therapeutic response of hormone refractory prostate cancer after docetaxel-based chemotherapy [45]. Although very promising, the quantitative aspects of functional diffusion mapping MRI still have to be validated in clinical settings.

References

1. Loch T. Urologic imaging for localized prostate cancer 2007. World J Urol. 2007;25:121.
2. Hricak H, Choyke PL, Eberhardt SC, Leibel SA, Scardino PT. Imaging prostate cancer: a multidisciplinary perspective. Radiology. 2007;243:28.
3. Wijkstra H, Wink MH, de la Rosette JJ. Contrast specific imaging in the detection and localization of prostate cancer. World J Urol. 2004;22:346.
4. Halpern EJ. Contrast-enhanced ultrasound imaging of prostate cancer. Rev Urol. 2006;8 Suppl 1:S29.
5. Pelzer A, Bektic J, Berger AP, Pallwein L, Halpern EJ, Horninger W, et al. Prostate cancer detection in men with prostate specific antigen 4 to 10 ng/ml using a combined approach of contrast enhanced color Doppler targeted and systematic biopsy. J Urol. 2005;173:1926.
6. Remzi M, Dobrovits M, Reissigl A, Ravery V, Waldert M, Wiunig C, et al. European Society for Oncological Urology

(ESOU): Can power Doppler enhanced transrectal ultrasound guided biopsy improve prostate cancer detection on first and repeat prostate biopsy? Eur Urol. 2004;46:451.

7. Cheng S, Rifkin MD. Color Doppler imaging of the prostate: important adjunct to endorectal ultrasound of the prostate in the diagnosis of prostate cancer. Ultrasound Q. 2001;17:185.

8. Drudi FM, Giovagnorio F, Carbone A, Ricci P, Petta S, Cantisani V, et al. Transrectal colour Doppler contrast sonography in the diagnosis of local recurrence after radical prostatectomy–comparison with MRI. Ultraschall Med. 2006;27:146.

9. Tamsel S, Killi R, Apaydin E, Hekimgil M, Demirpolat G. The potential value of power Doppler ultrasound imaging compared with grey-scale ultrasound findings in the diagnosis of local recurrence after radical prostatectomy. Clin Radiol. 2006; 61:325.

10. Yi A, Kim JK, Park SH, Kim KW, Kim HS, Kim JH, et al. Contrast-enhanced sonography for prostate cancer detection in patients with indeterminate clinical findings. AJR. 2006;186:1431.

11. Halpern EJ, Ramey JR, Strup SE, Frauscher F, McCue P, Gomella LG. Detection of prostate carcinoma with contrast-enhanced sonography using intermittent harmonic imaging. Cancer. 2005;104:2373.

12. Yves EP, Gomella LG, Halpern EJ. Effect of dutasteride therapy on Doppler evaluation of the prostate: preliminary results. Radiology. 2005;237:197.

13. Frey H. Realtime elastography. A new ultrasound procedure for the reconstruction of tissue elasticity. Radiologe. 2003; 43(10):850–5.

14. König K, Scheipers U, Pesavento A, Lorenz A, Ermert H, Senge T. Initial experiences with real-time elastography guided biopsies of the prostate. J Urol. 2005;174(1):115–7.

15. Cochlin DL, Ganatra RH, Griffiths DF. Elastography in the detection of prostatic cancer. Clin Radiol. 2002;57(11):1014–20.

16. Cruz M, Tsuda K, Narumi Y, et al. Characterization of low-intensity lesions in the peripheral zone of prostate on pre-biopsy endorectal coil MR imaging. Eur Radiol. 2002;12:357–65.

17. Kirkham APS, Emberton M, Allen C. How good is MRI at detection and characterising cancer within the prostate? Eur Urol. 2006;50:1163–7.

18. Qayyum A, Cookley FV, Lu Y, et al. Organ confined prostate cancer: effect of prior transrectal biopsy on endorectal MRI and MR spectroscopic imaging. AJR Am J Roentgenol. 2004; 183:1079–83.

19. Schlemmer HP, Merkle J, Grobholz R, et al. Can preoperative contrast-enhanced dynamic MR imaging for prostate cancer predict microvessel density in prostatectomy specimens? Eur Radiol. 2004;14:309–14.

20. Ito H, Kamoi K, Yokoyama K, Yamada K, Nishimura T. Visualization of prostate cancer using dynamic contrast-enhanced MRI: comparison with transrectal power Doppler ultrasound. Br J Radiol. 2003;76:617–24.

21. Hara N, Okuizumi M, Koike H, Kawaguchi M, Bilim V. Dynamic contrast-enhanced magnetic resonance imaging (DCE-MRI) is a useful modality for the precise detection and staging of early prostate cancer. Prostate. 2005;62:40–7.

22. Ikonen S, Karkkainen P, Kivisaari L, et al. Magnetic resonance imaging of clinically localized prostate cancer. J Urol. 1998;159:915–9.

23. Vilanova JC, Barceló J. Prostate cancer detection: magnetic resonance (MR) spectroscopic imaging. Abdom Imaging. 2007; (Epub ahead of print).

24. Scheidler J, Hricak H, Vigneron DB, et al. Prostate cancer: localization with three-dimensional proton MR spectroscopic imaging – clinicopathologic study. Radiology. 1999;213:473–80.

25. Wefer AE, Hricak H, Vigneron DB, et al. Sextant localization of prostate cancer: comparison of prostate biopsy, magnetic resonance imaging, and magnetic resonance spectrocopic imaging with step section histology. J Urol. 2000;164:400–4.

26. Zakian KL, Sircar K, Hricak H, et al. Correlation of proton MR spectroscopic imaging with Gleason score based on step-section pathologic analysis after radical prostatectomy. Radiology. 2005;234:804–14.

27. Kurhanewicz J, Swanson MG, Nelson SJ, Vigneron DB. Combined magnetic resonance imaging and spectroscopic imaging approach to molecular imaging of prostate cancer. J Magn Reson Imaging. 2002;16:451–63.

28. Sala E, Akin O, Moskowitz CS, et al. Endorectal MR imaging in the evaluation of seminal vesicle invasion: diagnostic accuracy and multivariate feature analysis. Radiology. 2006;238:929–37.

29. Cornud F, Flam T, Chauveinc L, et al. Extraprostatic spread of clinically localized prostate cancer : factors predictive of pT3 tumor and of positive endorectal MR imaging examination results. Radiology. 2002;224:203–10.

30. Mullerad M, Hricak H, Wang L, Chen HN, Kattan MW, Scardina PT. Prostate cancer: detection of extracapsular extension by genitourinary and general body radiologists at MR imaging. Radiology. 2004;232:140–6.

31. Wolf JS JR, Cher M, Dall'era M, Presti JC, Hricak H, Carroll PR. The use and accuracy of cross-sectional imaging and fine needle aspiration cytology for detection of pelvic lymph node metastases before radical prostatectomy. J Urol. 1995; 153:993–9.

32. Aus G, Abbou CC, Bolla M, Heidenreich A, Schmid HP, van Poppel H, et al. EAU guidelines on prostate cancer. Eur Urol. 2005;48:546–51.

33. Saokar A, Braschi M, Harinsinghani MG. Lymphotrophic nanoparticle enhanced MR imaging (LNMRI) for lymph node imaging. Abdom Imaging. 2006;31:660–7.

34. Bellin MF, Roy C, Kinkel K, et al. Lymph node metastases: safety and effectiveness of MR imaging with ultrasmall superparamagnetic iron oxide particles – initial clinical experience. Radiology. 1998;207:799–808.

35. Harisinghani MG, Barentsz J, Hahn PF, et al. Noninvasive detection of clinically occult lymph node metastasis in prostate cancer. N Engl J Med. 2003;348:2491–9.

36. Heidenreich A, Varga Z, v Knobloch R. Extended pelvic lymphadenectomy in patients undergoing radical prostatectomy: high incidence of lymph node metastases. J Urol. 2002;167:1681–6.

37. Bader P, Burkhardt FC, Markwalder R, Studer UE. Is a limited lymph node dissection an adequate staging procedure for prostate cancer? J Urol. 2002;168:514–8.

38. Wawroschek F, Vogt H, Wengenmair H, et al. Prostate lymphoscintigraphy and radio-guided surgery for sentinel lymph node identification in prostate cancer. Technique and results of the first 350 cases. Urol Int. 2003;70:303–10.

39. Palmer E, Henrikson K, McKusik K, Strauss HW, Hochberg F. Pain as an indicator of bone metastasis. Acta Radiol. 1988; 29:445–9.

40. Tombal B, Rezazadeh A, Therasse P, van Cangh PJ, Vande Berg B, Lecouvet FE. Magnetic resonance imaging of the axial skeleton enables objective measurement of tumor response on prostate cancer bone metastases. Prostate. 2005;65:178–87.

41. Even-Sapir E, Metser U, Mishani E, Lievshitz G, Lerman H, Leibovitch I. The detection of bone metastases in patients with high risk prostate cancer: 99m Tc-MDP planar bone scintigraphy, single-and multi field of view SPECT, 18F-flouride PET, and 18F-flouride PET/CT. J Nucl Med. 2006;47:287–97.

42. Delpassand ES, Garcia JR, Bhadkamar V, Podoloff DA. Value of SPECT imaging of the thoracolumbar spine in cancer patients. Clin Nucl Med. 1995;20:1047–51.

43. Dehdashti F, Picus J, Michalski JM, et al. Positron tomographic assessment of androgen receptors in prostatic carcinoma. Eur J Nucl Med Mol Imaging. 2005;32:344–50.

44. Parent EE, Dence CS, Sharp TL, et al. Synthesis and biological evaluation of a flourine-18-labeled nonsteroidal androgen receptor antagonist, N-(3-[18F]flouro-4-nitronaphthyl)-cis-5-norbornene-endo-2,3-dicarboxylic imide. Nucl Med Biol. 2006;33:615–24.

45. Lee KC, Sud S, Meyer CR, et al. An imaging biomarker of early treatment response in prostate cancer that has metastasized to the bone. Cancer Res. 2007;67:3524–8.

Chapter 25

Testicular Carcinoma: Introduction

P. Albers and P. Laguna

Introduction

Testicular cancer represents between 1 and 1.5% of male neoplasms and overall 5% of urological tumors. Over the last 30 years the incidence of testicular cancer is rising, especially in northern industrialized countries in America as well as in Europe, with peak incidences of up to ten cases per 100,000 males, e.g., in Denmark [1, 2].

Up to 5% of the cases are bilateral. In 95% of the patients, the histology reveals a germ cell tumor which is characterized by a specific genetic marker (supernumerical copies of the short arm of chromosome 12, isochromosome i(12p)). Intratubular germ cell neoplasia (testicular intraepithelial neoplasia, TIN) has been shown to be a precursor lesion in the majority of germ cell tumors [3].

Epidemiological risk factors for the development of testicular tumors are a history of cryptorchidism or undescended testis, a hypotrophic (<12 ml) or atrophic testicle, Klinefelter's syndrome, familial history of testicular tumors among first-grade relatives (brothers, father), the presence of a contralateral tumor, or TIN and infertility [4].

Currently, testicular tumors show excellent cure rates in the order of 95% for all stages of disease. The main factors contributing to this are careful staging at the time of diagnosis; adequate early treatment based on an interdisciplinary management including chemotherapy, radiotherapy, and surgery; very strict follow-up and salvage therapies; and treatment at least of advanced and recurrent tumors under the guidance of a reference center.

Future aims in the management of testis cancer patients are (1) the reduction of treatment in patients with low-stage disease and a cure rate of almost 100% and (2) the intensification of treatment in advanced stages to improve on the cure rates of, e.g., "poor prognosis" patients of currently about 50–60% [5].

Therefore, initially correct staging is the cornerstone of testicular cancer management. Consequently, in addition to expert histopathology evaluation of the primary tumor and tumor marker half-life kinetics, it is mandatory to assess

- status of abdominal and supraclavicular nodes, and the liver
- presence or absence of mediastinal nodal involvement and lung metastases
- status of brain and bone if any suspicious symptoms are present.

In addition, correct imaging is crucial in treatment monitoring and assessment of final treatment response. Based on the correct re-staging during and after chemotherapy, the indication for subsequent management modalities like residual tumor resection is tailored individually. Last, the final assessment after multimodality treatment in conjunction with the initial stage is the basis for follow-up recommendations again including imaging techniques.

Computerized tomography (CT) of the chest, abdomen, and pelvis are required as initial staging investigations. Oral and intravenous contrast media are mandatory [6, 7]. For the evaluation of the lungs and the mediastinum, chest CT scans are more sensitive than chest plain X-ray films [8–10]. However, it should be noted that pulmonary/pleural nodules of <1 cm can represent false positive findings in CT scans. Furthermore, CT scans of the abdomen and pelvis might be incorrect in up to 30% of cases due to difficulties in the interpretation of lymph nodes based on morphology and size alone which make the differentiation between clinical stages I and IIA unreliable [11]. A detailed description of the location, number, and size of lymph nodes should be provided in the radiology report. Ultrasound of the retroperitoneum is less sensitive than CT. Performing magnetic resonance tomography (MRT) scans of the abdomen and pelvis does not provide additional information and should be restricted to patients in whom intravenous contrast media cannot be given [12, 13]. The sensitivity of positron emission tomography (PET) is not superior to the sensitivity of computer tomography. Outside clinical trials PET scans are therefore not

P. Albers (✉)

J.J.M.C.H. de la Rosette et al. (eds.), *Imaging in Oncological Urology*,
DOI 10.1007/978-1-84628-759-6_25, © Springer-Verlag London Limited 2009

recommended as part of the initial staging [14–19]. Recently, the first results of a large prospective multicenter trial of PET staging in low-stage disease have been presented showing no benefit of PET staging over CT staging in stage I disease [20]. The MRC trial of PET staging in low-stage disease, however, is yet ongoing and results have to be awaited for final conclusions. In metastatic seminoma, however, PET scan has proven to be of great value in predicting vital residual tumor after induction chemotherapy [21–23]. A bone scan should be obtained in a patient with elevated level of the alkaline phosphastase or if bone metastases are clinically suspected. Imaging of the brain by CT or preferably by MRT is required in patients with metastatic disease and "intermediate" or "poor" prognosis according to the IGCCCG classification as well as in all patients in whom brain metastases are clinically suspected [24, 25].

Imaging in testis cancer is a crucial diagnostic tool as well as an important method in the planning of multimodality approaches (chemotherapy and surgery). The correct performance and interpretation of imaging modalities is of utmost importance. The interdisciplinary evaluation of imaging results improves the quality of the single method. Neither surgeons nor medical oncologists should rely on an only written medical report of an imaging method. The staging by imaging is mainly improved by an interdisciplinary conference (tumor board discussion). New tracers and technical improvements may in future add to the high standard of staging which has already influenced the interdisciplinary management of testis cancer.

References

1. Huyghe E, Matsuda T, Thonneau P. Increasing incidence of testicular cancer worldwide: a review. J Urol. 2003;170:5–11. EBM III. http://www.ncbi.nlm.nih.gov/entrez/query.fcgi?cmd=Retrieve&db=PubMed&list_uids=12796635&dopt=Abstract.
2. McGlynn KA, Devesa SS, Sigurdson AJ, Brown LM, Tsao L, Tarone RE. Trends in the incidence of testicular germ cell tumors in the United States. Cancer. 2003;97:63–70. EBM III–IIb.
3. Dieckmann KP, Loy V. Prevalence of contralateral testicular intraepithelial neoplasia in patients with testicular germ cell neoplasm. J Clin Oncol. 1996;14:3126–32. EBM IIa–IIb.
4. Moller H, Prener A, Skakkebaek NE. Testicular cancer, cryptorchidism, inguinal hernia, testicular atrophy and genital malformations: case-control studies in Denmark. Cancer Causes Control. 1996;7:264–74. EBM IIa. http://www.ncbi.nlm.nih.gov/entrez/query.fcgi?cmd=Retrieve&db=PubMed&liuids=8740739&dopt=Abstract.
5. International Germ Cell Cancer Collaborative Group (IGCCCG). The International Germ Cell Consensus Classification: a prognostic factor based staging system for metastatic germ cell cancer. J Clin Oncol. 1997;15:594–603. EBM IA/IIA/IIB/III.
6. Leibovitch I, Foster RS, Kopecky KK, et al. Identification of clinical stage A nonseminomatous testis cancer patients at extremely low risk for metastatic disease: A combined approach using quantive immunohistochemical, histopathologic, and radiologic assessment. J Clin Oncol. 1998;16:261–8.
7. White PM, Howard GC, Best JJ, et al. The role of computed tomographic examination of the pelvis in the management of testicular germ cell tumours. Clin Radiol. 1997;52:124–9. EBM IIB.
8. White PM, Adamson DJA, Howard GCW, et al. Imaging of the thorax in the management of germ cell testicular tumours. Clin Radiol. 1999;54:207–11. EBM IIB+III.
9. Meyer CA, Conces DJ. Imaging of intrathoracic metastases of nonseminomatous germ cell tumors. Chest Surg Clin N Am. 2002;12:717–38.
10. See WA, Hoxie L. Chest staging in testis cancer patients: imaging modality selection based upon risk assessment as determined by abdominal computerized tomography scan results. J Urol. 1993;150:874–8.
11. Leibovitch I, Foster RS, Kopecky KK, et al. Improved accuracy of computerized tomography based clinical staging in low stage nonseminomatous germ cell tumor using size criteria of retroperitoneal lymph nodes. J Urol. 1995;154:1759–63.
12. Bellin M, Roy C, Kinkel K, Thoumas D, et al. Lymph node metastases: Safety and effectiveness of MR imaging with ultrasmall superparamagnetic iron oxide particles - initial clinical experience. Radiology. 1998;207:799–808.
13. Hogeboom WR, Hoekstra HJ, Mooyart EL, et al. Magnetic resonance imaging of retroperitoneal lymph node metastases of nonseminomatous germ cell tumors of the testis. Eur J Surg Oncol. 1993;19:429–37.
14. Albers P, Bender H, Yilmaz H, et al. Positron emission tomography in the clinical staging of patients with stage I and II germ cell tumors. Urology. 1999;53:808–11. EBM III.
15. Cremerius U, Wildberger JE, Borchers H, et al. Does positron emission tomography using 18-fluoro-2-deoxyglucose improve clinical staging of testicular cancer? - Results of a study of 50 patients. Urology. 1999;54:900–4.
16. Hoh CK, Seltzer MA, Franklin J, et al. Positron emissions tomography in urological oncology. J Urol. 1998;159:347–56.
17. Weber WA, Avril N, Schwaiger M. Relevance of positron emission tomography (PET) in oncology. Strahlenther Onkol. 1999;175:356–76.
18. Tsatalpas P, Beuthien-Baumann B, Kropp J, Manseck A, Tiepolt C, Hakenberg OW, et al. Diagnostic value of 18F-FDG positron emission tomography for detection and treatment control of malignant germ cell tumors. Urol Int. 2002;68:157–63.
19. Spermon JR, De Geus-Oei LF, Kiemeney LA, Witjes JA, Oyen WJ. The role of (18)fluoro-2-deoxyglucose positron emission tomography in initial staging and re-staging after chemotherapy for testicular germ cell tumours. BJU Int. 2002;89:549–56.
20. De Wit M for the German Testicular Cancer Study Group. 18-FDG PET staging in early stage testicular cancer. Proceedings ASCO 2005, abstract no 4504.
21. De Santis M, Bokemeyer C, Becherer A, Stoiber F, Oechsle K, Kletter K, et al. Predictive impact of 2-18fluoro-2-deoxy-D-glucose positron emission tomography for residual postchemotherapy masses in patients with bulky seminoma. J Clin Oncol. 2001;19:3740–44. EBM IIb. http://www.ncbi.nlm.nih.gov/entrez/query.fcgi?cmd=Retrieve&db=PubMed&list_uids=11533096&dopt=Abstract.
22. De Santis M, Becherer A, Bokemeyer C, Stoiber F, Oechsle K, Sellner F, et al. 2-18fluoro-deoxy-D-glucose positron emission tomography is a reliable predictor for viable tumor in postchemotherapy seminoma: an update of the prospective mulitcentric SEMPET trial. J Clin Oncol. 2004; 22:1034–9. EBM IIb.
23. Becherer A, Santis MD, Karanikas G, Szabo M, Bokemeyer C, Dohmen BM, et al. FDG PET is superior to CT in the prediction

of viable tumour in post–chemotherapy seminoma residuals. Eur J Radiol. 2005;54:284–8. EBM IIb.

24. Bokemeyer C, Nowak P, Haupt A, et al. Treatment of brain metastases in patients with testicular cancer. J Clin Oncol. 1997;15:1449–54. EBM III.

25. Fossa SD, Bokemeyer C, Gerl A, et al. Treatment outcome of patients with brain metastases from malignant germ cell tumors. Cancer. 1999;85:988–997. EBM IIA.

Chapter 26

Testicular Carcinoma – Conventional Imaging Techniques

M.A. Saksena and M.G. Harisinghani

Introduction

Although imaging does not play a significant role in the initial diagnosis of testicular cancer it is vital for the staging of this malignancy. As testicular cancer progresses it metastasizes in a predictable pattern to the retroperitoneal lymph nodes below the renal vessels [1]. Pretreatment imaging plays a significant and useful role in the evaluation of nodal metastases and the detection of distant metastatic disease.

Conventionally, bipedal lymphangiography has been the primary modality for the evaluation of nodal metastases. However, in recent times the lymphograhic studies performed for oncologic staging are being increasingly replaced by cross-sectional imaging modalities such as CT and MRI. Similarly, the chest X-ray is being replaced by chest CT scans for evaluating intrathoracic disease. This article reviews the technique and efficacy of conventional imaging techniques in the metastatic workup of patients with testicular cancer and highlights their utility in the ever-changing milieu of testicular cancer management.

Nodal Drainage Pathway in Testicular Cancer

Testicular lymphatics are unique in that they run along the spermatic vessels and bypass the pelvic nodes draining directly into the para-aortic nodes [1]. Donohue et al. evaluated 275 retroperitoneal lymphadnectomy specimens and demonstrated that right testicular tumors commonly spread first to the interaortocaval nodes just below the left renal vein while left testicular tumors usually spread to the preaortic and the left para-aortic nodes [2]. Nodal spread from right-sided tumors commonly crosses over to involve the left-sided nodes causing contralateral nodal metastases while the reverse is highly unusual [3]. Once the primary para-aortic nodes are involved the draining lymphatics get obstructed and pelvic nodes may get involved due to retrograde spread. Similarly, spread to nodes in the chest is seen only after the para-aortic nodes are affected making evaluation of chest nodes redundant in cases where the abdominal nodes are negative. Nodal drainage patterns are significantly altered in malignancy of the undescended testicle and iliac nodes may be primarily involved in these cases.

Bipedal Lymphangiography

Lymphography is unique in its ability to demonstrate derangements in the internal architecture of normal-sized lymph nodes. As conventional cross-sectional imaging techniques rely on the relatively insensitive size criteria for the characterization of lymph nodes, the ability to detect abnormality in normal-sized lymph nodes allows lymphography to detect micrometastatic disease on non-enlarged nodes [4]. Testicular cancer predictably metastasizes to the pelvic and para-aortic nodes, both of which are readily visualized on bipedal lymphangiography. The contrast injected remains in the lymphatics for a long time and repeat radiographs can be taken during follow-up studies in patients being treated with surveillance.

Technique

Bipedal lymphangiography is a minimally invasive outpatient procedure and does not require conscious sedation. The patient is placed in the supine position on an X-ray table and the skin on the dorsum of each foot is prepared with sterile precautions. Methylene blue dye is then injected in the web spaces between the first and the second toes bilaterally. This dye percolates into the lymphatics on the dorsal aspect of the feet making them visible within 5–15 min. Ideally a

M.A. Saksena (✉)
Division of Abdominal Imaging and Intervention, Department of Radiology, Massachusetts, General Hospital, 55 Fruit street, Boston MA 02114, msaksena@partners.org

J.J.M.C.H. de la Rosette et al. (eds.), *Imaging in Oncological Urology*,
DOI 10.1007/978-1-84628-759-6_26, © Springer-Verlag London Limited 2009

lymphatic channel lateral to the base of the first metatarsal is identified and the skin over the channel is anesthetized by infiltrating 1% lidocaine. An approximately 1 cm vertical incision is made over the lymphatic channel to be cannulated. Once the channel is isolated, it is obstructed distally and holding it with minimal traction a fine 27–30 gauge needle is placed within. On satisfactory cannulation of the visualized lymphatic the cannula is secured in place by a silk ligature or adhesive strips. Although the standard contrast agent used for bipedal lymphangiography is ethiodol (an iodinated ester of fatty acids of the poppy seed oil), lipiodol ultrafluid (a 48% iodinated glycerol ester) can also be used [5]. Intralymphatic injection of 6–7 ml of contrast at the rate of 4–10 ml/h is made with an appropriate injector. Close attention must be paid to the rate of injection as a high rate of injection can result in rupture of the lymphatic. Multiple radiographs can then be taken to ensure visualization of major lymphatic trunks in the leg. Rate of flow into the proximal lymphatics can be accelerated by gentle muscular contraction of the legs and thighs. On completion of injection the cannula is removed and the dorsal wounds are sutured and dressed. Once the contrast is visualized in the lymphatics, a complete series of radiographs evaluating the major nodal chains in the pelvis and para-aortic regions are obtained (dynamic phase). Follow-up radiographs are obtained after 24 h (nodal or filling phase) and interpreted. If both bipedal lymphangiography and CT scans are being performed, CT should be performed after bipedal lymphangiography so as to enhance visualization of the contrast-enhanced nodes on CT [6].

Radiographic Appearance

Normal lymphatics appear homogenous, even textured, and demonstrate fine granularity. Normal nodes are non-enlarged, well defined, smooth and demonstrate a smooth indentation at the nodal hilum. Nodes may minimally increase in size 24–48 h after the injection of contrast but revert to normal in a few days [6]. The first nodes to be opacified are the inguinal nodes followed by chains within the pelvis, external iliac and obturator. The internal iliac and presacral nodes are usually not opacified. Subsequently the common iliac nodes are visible followed by higher nodes in the para-aortic regions. The diagnostic finding in malignant lymph nodes is a focal filling defect not traversed by lymphatics representing a region of malignant infiltration. Other findings suggestive of malignant involvement are foamy lacelike appearance, increase in size, non-visualization of expected nodal groups, or presence of lymphaticovenous anastomoses [3]. Metastatic nodes may or may not be enlarged in size (Fig 26.1).

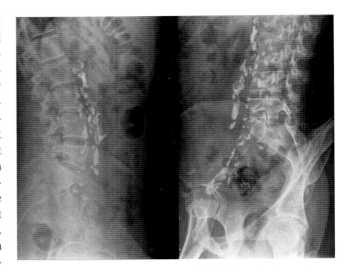

Fig. 26.1 A 32-year-old man presented with right testicular seminoma. Bilateral lymphangiogram performed demonstrates a large metastatic lymph node in the retroperitoneum with an ill-defined filling defect (*arrow*). Adjacent normal nodes appear normal in size and are smooth with no filling defects (*arrow head*)

Complications

Majority of complications encountered in bipedal lymphangiography are secondary to the dye. The complications of bipedal lymphangiography are [5]

1. Pulmonary oil embolization
2. Pulmonary infarction
3. Allergic reactions to methylene blue and ethiodized oil
4. Intraalveolar hemorrhage
5. Hypothyroidism
6. Arterial embolization to brain or kidney in patients with right to left shunts

Clinical Impact

Cross-sectional imaging techniques utilize nodal size evaluation to characterize lymph nodes. It has been established that the size criteria are both insensitive and non-specific [4]. Bipedal lymphangiography has the distinct advantage of the ability to demonstrate internal architecture in normal-sized nodes. Under ideal circumstances metastatic filling defects measuring 5–7 mm can be detected in normal-sized nodes [3]. As stated above nodal spread from testicular cancer is predictable and involves the para-aortic nodes before spreading to any other nodal groups. These primary nodal zones are well visualized and accurately characterized on bipedal lymphangiography [3] and this led to its extensive utilization before the advent of computed tomography. The accuracy of bipedal lymphangiography in detection of nodal metastases ranges from 62 to 89%, its sensitivity from 54 to 89%, and specificity from 67 to 100% [3, 7–9]. Initial studies performed in the late 1980s evaluating CT and lymphography found both modalities to be complimentary to each other, with lymphography being useful in patients with negative CT studies. CT scans were useful in better defining the extent of disease in patients with abnormal bipedal lymphangiography and in studying sites of potential relapse [10]. Other studies have consistently demonstrated better sensitivity, specificity, and accuracy of CT scans which is constantly improving in technique [11]. A study by Bussar-Maatz et al. did demonstrate bipedal lymphangiography to have higher sensitivity (71%) compared to CT (41%) but a lower specificity of 60% while CT had a specificity of (94%) [12].

False positive nodes occur in bipedal lymphangiography due to reactive changes and filling defects from other causes such as fat or sinus histiocytosis [13]. False negative bipedal lymphangiograms are more worrisome and occur secondary to non-opacification of affected nodes or presence of micrometastases too small to create a visible filling defect. Sentinel lymph node of the testes at the level of L1/2 on the left and L1/3 on the right may not be opacified [3].

However, it is an invasive procedure with associated complications, and its use should be reserved in patients with early disease and negative CT scans in whom surgical lymphadnectomy is not warranted based on tumor histology and serum markers [7, 14–16]. Although some studies have found lymphangiography to be more sensitive than CT in detecting nodal disease, other features such as tumor markers and primary tumor vascular invasion are more important for staging [17]. In the follow-up patient, CT should be the modality of choice due to unacceptably high false negative rates on lymphangiography [18]. Hence in conclusion, although some authors have indicated a continuing role of bipedal lymphangiography in the evaluation of patients with negative CT studies, it is now rarely used for the initial staging of patients with testicular cancer.

Chest Radiographs

Detection of intrathoracic metastases is a part of the pretreatment staging of patients with newly diagnosed testicular cancer and is performed by chest radiographs and chest CT scans. In early-stage testicular seminoma and non-seminomatous germ cell tumors (NSGCT), it is highly unusual to have thoracic disease if there is no metastatic spread in the abdomen. Although, chest X-ray (CXR) alone has been found to be sufficient initial chest staging in all patients who have a negative CT of the abdomen [19] these results must be interpreted with caution as CT abdomen may miss retroperitoneal disease in normal-sized nodes. Poste-

rior mediastinal nodes and retrocrural nodes which may be involved are difficult to evaluate on CXR. In higher stage tumors, chest CT must be performed as CXR alone has a high false negative rate [19]. With the advent of improved CT techniques, CT of the chest is the modality of choice for staging testicular carcinoma [7, 20].

Ultrasonography (US)

Scrotal sonography is often the initial modality used to investigate a suspicious testicular abnormality. Intra and extratesticular masses can be identified and characterized with a high degree of accuracy [21]. As described by Nachtsheim et al. there are two categories of testicular masses seen on US examination. Non-seminomatous germ cell testicular tumors are hypoechoic compared to normal testes and demonstrate cystic spaces, with acoustic shadowing and irregular margins extending into the testicular parenchyma. Seminomas and lymphomas are also hypoechoic but are homogenous and have sharply defined borders demarcating them from the normal testicular parenchyma. In patients who have already been treated for testicular cancer, the risk of metachronous contralateral tumor formation ranges from 1.5 to 3.2% [22]. Scrotal sonography can be used to evaluate the contralateral testes in following up patients with treated germ cell tumors.

Conclusion

Conventional imaging plays an important role in the initial diagnosis and post-treatment surveillance of patients with testicular tumors. Although, bipedal lymphangiography has been largely replaced by newer cross-sectional techniques, chest radiographs continue to be effective in detecting intrathoracic metastatic disease. Advances in scrotal sonography techniques are also useful in diagnosing indeterminate testicular masses and in surveillance of the contralateral normal testes. Intraabdominal spread of disease is best evaluated by newer cross-sectional modalities which will be discussed in the next chapter.

References

1. Bosl GJ, Motzer RJ. Testicular germ-cell cancer. N Engl J Med. 1997;337:242–53.
2. Donohue JP, Roth LM, Zachary JM, Rowland RG, Einhorn LH, Williams SG. Cytoreductive surgery for metastatic testis cancer: Tissue analysis of retroperitoneal masses after chemotherapy. J Urol. 1982;127:1111–4.

3. von Eschenbach AC, Jing BS, Wallace S. Lymphangiography in genitourinary cancer. Urol Clin North Am. 1985;12:715–23.

4. Jager GJ, Barentsz JO, Oosterhof GO, Witjes JA, Ruijs SJ. Pelvic adenopathy in prostatic and urinary bladder carcinoma: MR imaging with a three-dimensional TI-weighted magnetization-prepared-rapid gradient-echo sequence. AJR Am J Roentgenol. 1996;167:1503–7.

5. Guermazi A, Brice P, Hennequin C, Sarfati E. Lymphography: an old technique retains its usefulness. Radiographics. 2003;23:1541–58; discussion 1559–60.

6. Vinnicombe SJ, Norman AR, Nicolson V, Husband JE. Normal pelvic lymph nodes: Evaluation with CT after bipedal lymphangiography. Radiology. 1995;194:349–55.

7. Heiken JP, Balfe DM, McClennan BL. Testicular tumors: Oncologic imaging and diagnosis. Int J Radiat Oncol Biol Phys. 1984;10:275–87.

8. Lien HH, Fossa SD, Ous S, Stenwig AE. Lymphography in retroperitoneal metastases in non-seminoma testicular tumor patients with a normal CT scan. Acta Radiol Diagn (Stockh). 1983;24:319–22.

9. Lien HH, Kolbenstvedt A, Talle K, Fossa SD, Klepp O, Ous S. Comparison of computed tomography, lymphography, and phlebography in 200 consecutive patients with regard to retroperitoneal metastases from testicular tumor. Radiology. 1983;146:129–32.

10. Taylor RE, Duncan W, Best JJ. Influence of computed tomography scanning and lymphography on the management of testicular germ-cell tumours. Clin Radiol. 1986;37:539–42.

11. Thomas JL, Bernardino ME, Bracken RB. Staging of testicular carcinoma: comparison of CT and lymphangiography. AJR Am J Roentgenol. 1981;137:991–6.

12. Bussar-Maatz R, Weissbach L. Retroperitoneal lymph node staging of testicular tumours. TNM study group. Br J Urol. 1993;72:234–40.

13. Jing B, Wallace S, Zornoza J. Metastases to retroperitoneal and pelvic lymph nodes: computed tomography and lymphangiography. Radiol Clin North Am. 1982;20:511–30.

14. Tesoro-Tess JD, Pizzocaro G, Zanoni F, Musumeci R. Lymphangiography and computerized tomography in testicular carcinoma: How accurate in early stage disease? J Urol. 1985;133:967–70.

15. Macher MS, Steinfeld AD. Relative role of abdominal pelvic CT and lymphangiography in staging of testicular seminoma. Urology. 1985;26:193–5.

16. Marks LB, Shipley WU, Walker TG, Waltman AC. Role of lymphangiography in staging testicular seminoma. Urology. 1991;38:264–6.

17. Stephenson NJ, Sandeman TF, McKenzie AF. Has lymphography a role in early stage testicular germ cell tumours? Australas Radiol. 1995;39:54–7.

18. Williams MP, Husband JE. Computed tomography scanning and post-lymphangiogram radiography in the follow-up of patients with metastatic testicular cancer. Clin Radiol. 1989;40:47–50.

19. Moul JW. Proper staging techniques in testicular cancer patients. Tech Urol. 1995;1:126–32.

20. Williams MP, Husband JE, Heron CW. Intrathoracic manifestations of metastatic testicular seminoma: A comparison of chest radiographic and CT findings. AJR Am J Roentgenol. 1987;149:473–5.

21. Nachtsheim DA, Scheible FW, Gosink B. Ultrasonography of testis tumors. J Urol. 1983;129:978–81.

22. Bradford TJ, Montie JE, Hafez KS. The role of imaging in the surveillance of urologic malignancies. Urol Clin North Am. 2006;33:377–96.

Chapter 27

Cross-Sectional Imaging Techniques: The Use of Computed Tomography (CT) and Magnetic Resonance Imaging (MRI) in the Management of Germ Cell Tumors

M. De Santis,[†] G. Strau,* and M. Bachner[†]

Introduction and General Implications

Since germ cell tumors (GCT) have become a curable disease with the introduction of cisplatin-containing chemotherapy, sophisticated treatment strategies designed to reduce treatment morbidity without compromising the treatment outcome have been defined.

Cross-sectional imaging techniques have become an important tool in these treatment concepts for staging, restaging, post-treatment follow-up, or as part of surveillance strategies. Balancing the diagnostic benefits against the risks of additional radiation for young males is crucial. Still, the most appropriate use of cross-sectional imaging techniques in many clinical situations during the management of GCT is unclear.

In general and because GCT are rare accounting for less than 1% of all male cancers [1], radiologic staging is best performed by radiologists with specific experience and interest in the field [2, 3].

This chapter will focus on the use of these imaging techniques in common clinical situations and will highlight the standard use, advantages, limitations, risks, and future perspectives of computed tomography (CT) and magnetic resonance imaging (MRI).

Computed Tomography (CT)

Computed tomography is the most frequently used tool in the assessment of cancer. This is also true for GCT.

The main advantages of CT scanning are much better contrast resolution compared to conventional radiography, minimized superimposition of overlying structures due to the cross-sectional technique, fast examination procedure, oral and i.v. contrast application, and widespread availability. CT has an excellent reproducibility with the same system settings (collimation pitch) and provides excellent images for measuring tumor size.

Disadvantages of this imaging technique mainly revolve around concerns about the radiation risk and contraindications of iodinated contrast agents, e.g., allergic reactions and impaired renal or thyroid function [4, 5].

Magnetic Resonance Imaging (MRI)

In nearly every molecule of the body, protons and neutrons are capable of producing nuclear magnetic resonance signals, which are used to generate a magnetic resonance image. Protons, which provide the strongest signal, are used for the typical MR images.

Extracellular gadolinium is the MR contrast agent with the most general use [5]. The advantages of MRI are that it is a non-ionizing radiation method using radiofrequency pulses and providing MR images with high resolution and high soft tissue contrast in any plane. Current MRI techniques and more spacious equipment have reduced the psychological stress involved and can even be used in claustrophobic patients [4].

The main disadvantages of MRI are long acquisition times, which are significantly longer than with CT; lower patient throughput; and substantially higher cost. Pacemakers are an absolute contraindication for MRI.

MRI rarely is the first modality of choice for the primary diagnosis of tumors, even in 2006. It is usually

M. De Santis and M. Bachner (✉)
[†]3rd Medical Department – Center for Oncology and Hematology Kaiser Franz Josef – Spital der Stadt Wien and Ludwig Boltzmann-Institute for Applied Cancer Research Vienna (LBI-ACR VIEnna)
Kaiser Franz Josef – Spital der Stadt Wien and Applied Cancer Research Institution for Translational Research Vienna (ACR-ITR VIEnna), Kundratstrasse 3, A-1100 Vienna, Austria
maria.desantis@wienkav.at
*Department of Radiology, Kaiser Franz Josef - Spital der Stadt Wien, Kundratstrasse 3, A-1100 Vienna, Austria

J.J.M.C.H. de la Rosette et al. (eds.), *Imaging in Oncological Urology*,
DOI 10.1007/978-1-84628-759-6_27, © Springer-Verlag London Limited 2009

reserved for specific problems or special questions unresolved by CT scanning and/or ultrasonography. Or it is used in the first place, if CT is contraindicated by the type of radiation delivered or by the need for iodinated contrast material [6].

Imaging of Primary Tumors: Role of MRI and CT

Testicular Primary Tumors

There is no significant difference in MRI signaling between malignant and benign solid testicular germ cell tumors. Both are characterized by a mid-intense T1-weighted (fat-sensitive) signal, which compares well with normal testicular tissue, and a T2-weighted (water-sensitive) signal, which is lower than that of normal testis tissue [7]. The tunica albuginea is best defined on T2-weighted images as a low-intensity line [8]. Gadolinium enhancement does not add any information for characterizing lesions [7, 9], but helps to differentiate the epididymis from the testis on T2-weighted images by its hyperintensity relative to the testis.

Testicular GCT usually present as painless asymptomatic testicular swellings. Pain is present in about 25% of cases only and does not rule out testicular cancer [10].

The diagnostic method of first choice for examining scrotal enlargement is palpation followed by ultrasonography, which is sufficiently sensitive, in fact as sensitive as MRI, for the majority of focal testicular lesions. One exception is that, if ultrasonographic findings are suggestive of an epidermoid cyst, a tumor-like lesion, MRI provides proof by typical T1- and T2-hyperintense signals of intracystic keratin tissue [11]. Clinical examination of both testicles is of particular importance to pick up MRI-isointense testicular tumors [10].

MRI may be used if the ultrasonographic images are of suboptimal quality or if there is a discrepancy between the clinical and sonographic findings. In patients with very large testicular lesions or diffuse tumor infiltration without a capsule, MRI is of additional use [10].

MRI staging of testicular primary tumors is of academic interest only, because total removal of the tumor is the treatment of choice in any case of malignancy, in pure seminomas, as well as in non-seminomatous testicular tumors of any clinical stage. MRI provides a typical homogeneous hypo-intense T2-weighted signal without a capsule in pure seminomas, whereas non seminomatous germ cell tumor (NSGCT) are characterized by a heterogeneous T2-weighted hypo-intense signal with a capsule (see Fig. 27.1). A variety of exceptions to these typical images do not permit to differentiate benign from malignant tissue or seminoma from NSGCT with sufficient certainty. Regressive processes such

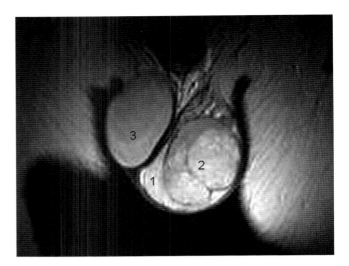

Fig. 27.1 T2-weighted testicular MRI. 1: Normal testicular tissue. 2: Inhomogeneous, mainly hyperintense tumor, histologically classical seminoma. 3: Hypointense testicular prosthesis.

as necrosis may be the cause of heterogenic areas within seminomas [7, 9, 12, 13]. Although the tunica albuginea generates a consistently low signal, differentiating tumors infiltrating it from those that just come close to it is difficult [14]. Furthermore, false-positive results have been obtained in inflammatory reactions mimicking tumor infiltration of the spermatic cord. The staging accuracy of testicular primaries with MRI turned out to be between 63 and 87% [12, 15].

For diagnosing cryptorchidism or testicular agenesis MRI is superior to palpation and ultrasonography, especially if the ectopic location is the abdominal cavity rather than the inguinal canal (see Sect. Undescended Testis, Cryptorchidism).

CT does not play a specific role in testicular primary tumors and is only used, if additional imaging, apart from palpation and ultrasonography, is needed, but MRI is not available.

Summary

Clinical examination (palpation) and ultrasonography are the diagnostic tools of choice for evaluating testicular swelling or suspect testicular changes. MRI provides additional information in equivocal cases, but cannot replace the histopathologic diagnosis of testicular tumors.

Undescended Testis, Cryptorchidism

True undescended testis, i.e., failure to descend spontaneously within the first year of life, occurs in about 0.4% of men. This circumstance may become a diagnostic challenge in adults during staging procedures of suspected extragonadal primary tumors or incidentally discovered masses, asymptomatic or symptomatic, due to hemorrhage, torsion, or acute abdomen.

The cryptorchid testis is a clear risk factor for the development of a testicular tumor. Approximately 10% of testicular neoplasms are associated with abnormal descent. The likelihood of malignant degeneration of an undescended testis is about 30–50 times greater than in a regularly descended one. Cancer occurs four times as often in abdominal or atrophic than in canalicular testes. Early orchidopexy, if possible anatomically, does not change the risk of malignancy in the cryptorchid testis. It does, however, facilitate follow-ups with, hopefully, earlier detection of cancer [16, 17]. Undescended testes are mostly palpable and detected in the inguinal canal (80%). Careful clinical examination followed by ultrasonography is the primary diagnostic step. Only when the search for the testis is unsuccessful MRI is the diagnostic method of choice to detect the organ in the pelvis or abdomen. Preoperative imaging is not routinely needed in children, but it is helpful in adults to plan surgery appropriately, no matter whether laparoscopic or open. The main advantages of MRI in the search for undescended testes are the multiplanar image acquisition and the capacity to differentiate canalicular from extracanalicular testis. In addition, MRI can differentiate between undescended testis and testicular agenesis with a high measure of certainty [18, 19]. According to the literature, agenesis is the cause of non-palpable testes in 15–63% of cases [11, 20]. Recent MRI developments have enhanced the technique's potential to differentiate agenetic and ectopic testis (gadolinium-enhanced venography) [21].

If MRI is not available, CT may be used as an alternative.

Extragonadal Primaries

Primary extragonadal GCT account for approximately 5–7% of GCT [22] and may develop at multiple sites. The most common sites are midline, e.g., the mediastinum and the retroperitoneum. The sacrococcygeal region and the pineal gland are rarely involved. The underlying cause of these extragonadal tumors is thought to be an aberrant migration of germ cell tumor cells of yolk sac origin during embryonic development [23]. Several other hypotheses have been discussed [24, 25].

Patients with extragonadal primaries carry an increased risk of metachronous testicular cancer. Therefore, careful monitoring of the testes is mandatory [26].

Primary Retroperitoneal Germ Cell Tumors, "Burned Out" Primary Tumors

The diagnosis of a primary retroperitoneal GCT should always be preceded by a thorough examination of both testicles to exclude a very small or a so-called "burned out" testicular primary tumor. This is a well-known phenomenon, although not fully understood. The pathogenetic development is thought to be based on a high metabolic rate of the tumor with loss of a sufficient vascular supply and eventual tumor regression, the so-called "burned out" tumor.

MRI of the testes may be used if sonography is unclear, even after chemotherapy or during follow-up. The majority of patients diagnosed with an extragonadal retroperitoneal primary present either with a testicular intratubular/intraepithelial neoplasia (TIN) or with other pathological changes within the testicles, e.g., scars or microcalcifications, rather suggestive of a testicular primary. Therefore, true and definitely extragonadal retroperitoneal primaries are a rare condition, accounting for less than a third of these patients [27].

Imaging and treatment of retroperitoneal primary tumors with or without metastases follow the criteria for retroperitoneal metastatic disease (see Section Staging at Presentation).

Primary Mediastinal Germ Cell Tumors

Primary mediastinal GCT are mostly found in the anterior mediastinum within or adjacent to the thymic gland. Rarely, they emerge in the posterior mediastinum. Histologically, these tumors differentiate out of one or multiple germinal layers (endo-, meso-, ectodermal). They are defined by the absence of a gonadal as well as a retroperitoneal tumor manifestation [28, 29]. CT of the chest is the tool of choice for diagnosis and for restaging. MRI has no specific role for routine staging of the mediastinum.

Benign (mature teratoma) as well as malignant histologies of germ cell origin are found in the mediastinum. The latter cannot be differentiated from lymphoma or thymoma by CT only. If tumor markers are negative, biopsies are needed to confirm the diagnosis.

Mature teratomas are found in 60–75% of cases [28, 30, 31]. They are well-defined masses with cystoid components of low density and fatty tissue in about half of the cases [31–33]. Calcifications are typical features, followed by fat/fluid levels [31, 34, 35] and soft tissue components. The latter are usually not the major components of mediastinal teratomas [36].

In summary, the three components fat, fluid, and calcifications permit a visual differentiation between teratoma and other malignant tumor entities like lymphoma, thyroid cancer, and thymoma on CT images.

It is not possible to distinguish mature/benign from malignant teratomas by CT scanning alone with a sufficient measure of certainty, although malignant tumors tend to harbor more soft tissue components. Malignant teratomas may grow

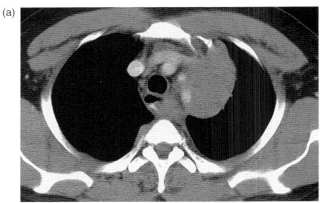

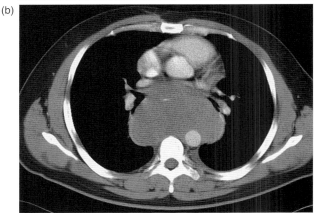

Fig. 27.2 Chest CT with i.v. and oral contrast. Primary mediastinal seminoma. (a) Mass in the anterior mediastinum. (b) Posterior mediastinal mass

aggressively with infiltration of the chest wall and metastatic spread [36–38]. Malignant non-seminomatous germ cell tumors of the mediastinum have a very poor prognosis [39].

The most common malignant GCT of the mediastinum are pure seminomas (SGCT). They are usually large homogeneous masses and may contain small low-density areas due to hemorrhage or necrosis [28, 30, 37] (see Fig. 27.2). In NSGCT hemorrhage and necrosis are more common and sometimes responsible for up to 50% of the tumor volume [36, 38].

MRI in Selected Clinical Situations

Staging at Presentation

So far, MRI has not shown any superiority compared to the staging accuracy of CT imaging [40]. Neither MRI nor FDG PET can detect microscopic disease. Just like CT, MRI only picks up enlarged lymph nodes. The only advantages of MRI for staging purposes are that it does not deliver ionizing radi-

ation with all its associated risks for the young male population (see Section CT and Radiation Risk) and that it can be used whenever CT is contraindicated.

Restaging After Chemotherapy

MRI cannot specify the effect of chemotherapy. Nor can it detect viable tumor, necrosis, or fibrosis in residual disease. However, MRI does provide better three-dimensional information than CT about the location and dimension of residual lymph node metastases for planning retroperitoneal lymph node dissection (RPLND) or residual tumor resection in the retroperitoneum, especially if the anatomy is unclear [41, 42]. Most retroperitoneal lymph nodes are inhomogeneous on T1- and T2-weighted images, maybe due to differently responding components. 2-^{18}Fluoro-2-deoxy-D-glucose positron emission tomography (FDG PET) combined with CT for evaluating pure seminoma residuals can be regarded as the standard tool for clinical decision making [43]. This does not apply to the evaluation of NSGCT residuals after chemotherapy, where FDG PET is not able to provide a restaging accuracy of more than 57% for viable tumor and teratoma [44] (see chapter 28).

Summary

To date CT remains the standard diagnostic tool for restaging. Only in residual pure seminomatous tumors FDG PET is of additional value and a standard tool for decision making. There might be an emerging role for MRI staging in the future.

MRI for Central Nervous System (CNS) Imaging

CNS metastases are rare in GCT patients. They occur in only 1% of all patients and in 10% of those with advanced disease. However, CNS imaging is recommended in patients with neurologic signs and symptoms [45] as well as in asymptomatic patients with an "intermediate" or "poor" prognosis according to the IGCCCG classification (International Germ Cell Cancer Collaborative Group) [39]. Patients with poor prognostic features and histologic evidence of chorionic carcinoma carry an increased risk of cerebral metastases [46, 47]. MRI of the CNS is the diagnostic method of choice especially for symptomatic patients. Advantages of MRI (see Fig. 27.3) for CNS imaging compared to CT (see Fig. 27.4) are the higher sensitivity [48] and, therefore, the

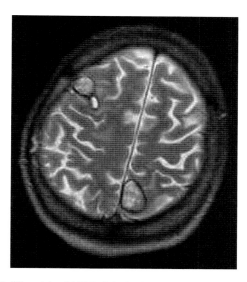

Fig. 27.3 T2-weighted MRI of the brain. Three brain metastases, surrounded by hemosiderin deposits due to hemorrhage

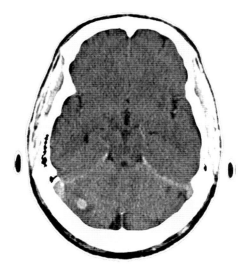

Fig. 27.4 Brain CT. Contrast-enhancing metastasis and perifocal edema (+)

chance to detect additional small lesions as well as the radioprotection of the ocular lens. Even CNS metastases should be approached with curative intent. The long-term survival rate of patients with brain metastases at initial staging is up to 30–40% [49, 50].

Liver Metastases

Of the non-pulmonary visceral pathologies, liver metastases occur in about 6% of NSGCT patients. They are known to carry a poor prognosis [39]. Patients with advanced bulky disease or poor prognostic features (see Table 27.1) should

be carefully examined to make sure that liver involvement is not missed. CT scanning of the abdomen, including liver imaging, is the standard diagnostic tool for GCT staging according to the European Guidelines [51]. In order to clarify specific questions or uncertainties, MRI has become the standard of care in the diagnosis of unclear lesions in the liver. Yet, if the picture is unclear and the lesions are accessible, the diagnosis should be established by a biopsy, especially if the liver lesion is the only poor prognostic feature and would therefore prompt a different classification and treatment strategy. Although the image quality for investigating the liver was improved by newer non-enhanced T1- and T2-weighted sequences, contrast agents still have their place for diagnosing liver lesions. Standard MRI protocols for the liver include the administration of gadolinium chelate. Liver metastases may be hypo- or hypervascular or nearly isointense to liver parenchyma on both T1- and T2-weighted images [6]. Metastases from GCT may vary in their MRI appearance even within one and the same patient due to different histologic components. In general, the main advantage of MRI imaging of the liver is that it collects many different types of data. Therefore, it is the imaging technique with the strongest likelihood of detecting liver metastases of different sizes and histologic components. In comparisons of current MRI with current CT techniques, MRI has been rated as being more accurate than CT for detecting liver metastases [52, 53].

MRI and Future Aspects

Whole-Body Magnetic Resonance Imaging

Whole-body MRI using a slow fluid-sensitive sequence (short-tau inversion recovery sequence, "STIR") is very sensitive for detecting bone metastases or bone marrow infiltration by lymphoma or myeloma [54–56]. In the management of GCT it could replace skeletal scintigraphy for detecting bone marrow metastases in the rare cases of very advanced pure seminomas.

New Contrast Agents

Research on new contrast agents like ferumoxtran-10 nanoparticles, which have a superparamagnetic iron oxide core, may help to improve the detection rate of metastases in normal-sized lymph nodes or equivocal nodes. Ultra-small-particle iron oxide agents are picked up by normal lymph nodes, which then appear black on an iron-sensitive MRI sequence [57, 58]. So far, no data for lymph node metastases of GCT are available. However, the agent has been used in a number of malignancies including abdominal and pelvic disease [59].

Summary of MRI in GCT

For routine staging of GCT, MRI is standard whenever CNS disease or liver metastases are suspected. It may be used to clarify specific uncertainties of CT imaging. Due to improved technique and shorter acquisition times as well as a lack of radiation burden, MRI might gain in importance for staging, restaging and follow-up of GCT in the near future.

CT in Selected Clinical Situations

Staging at Presentation

For clinical staging at presentation **CT of the abdomen, pelvis, and chest** is presently the imaging method of choice in NSGCT patients and provides the basis for staging according to the UICC and IGCCCG classifications [39, 60] (see Tables 27.1 and 27.2a–d). More invasive techniques like lymphography were abandoned in the mid-1980s because, compared to CT, they did not provide additional information affecting the management of testicular cancer patients [61, 62].

Oral and intravenous (i.v.) contrast should be standard, provided renal and thyroid functions permit its use. Common pitfalls with i.v. contrast omitted are the misinterpre-

tation of vessels because of anatomic variants, particularly because the expected sites of spread from testicular lesions are exactly within these regions [63–70]. Anatomic variants include

1. Variable prevalences of a circumaortic and retroaortic course of the left renal vein
2. Supernumerary left renal vein
3. Doubled vena cava
4. Normal asymmetry of common iliac veins (left common iliac vein larger with at least a twofold difference)
5. Insufficiently opacified bowel loops
6. Anatomic variant of the testicular veins

After retroperitoneal lymph node dissection (RPLND) misinterpretation of retroperitoneal changes on **abdominal CT scans** may be due to [71]

1. Hypodense postoperative seromas mimicking hypodense lymph nodes in the retroperitoneum (see Fig. 27.5a–c)
2. Blurring of contours by loss of fat tissue
3. Postoperative fibrotic changes and shrinkage
4. Change of bowel loop location (more posterior than preoperatively)

The distribution of retroperitoneal **lymph node metastases** in GCT patients follows the lymphatic drainage of the testis, which is well documented in the literature, and retracks the path of embryonic development. Left-sided testicular primaries are expected to metastasize first to the left

Table 27.1 Prognostic classification according to the IGCCCG 1997 [39]

Groups	Non-seminoma	Seminoma
Good prognosis	56% of cases	90% of cases
5-Year progression-free survival	89%	82%
5-Year survival	92%	86%
With all of	Testis/retroperitoneal primary	Any primary site
	No non-pulmonary visceral metastases	No non-pulmonary visceral metastases
	AFP < 1000 ng/ml and	Normal AFP
	hCG < 5000 mIU/l (1000 ng/ml) and	Any hCG
	LDH < 1.5x upper limit of normal	Any LDH
Intermediate prognosis	28% of cases	10% of cases
5-Year progression-free survival	75%	68%
5-Year survival	80%	73%
With all of	Testis/retroperitoneal primary	Any primary site
	No non-pulmonary visceral metastases	Non-pulmonary visceral metastases
	AFP ≥ 1000 and ≤ 10000 ng/ml or	Normal AFP
	hCG ≥ 5000 and ≤ 50000 mIU/l or	Any hCG
	LDH ≥ 1.5 and ≤ 10x upper limit of Normal	Any LDH
Poor prognosis	16% of cases	No patients classified as poor prognosis
5-year progression-free survival	41%	
5-year survival	48%	
With any of	Mediastinal primary	
	Non-pulmonary visceral metastases	
	AFP > 10000 ng/ml or	
	hCG > 50000 mIU/l or	
	LDH > 10x upper limit of normal	

Table 27.2 TNM classification of germ cell tumors [60]

a: Primary tumor (T)	
pTX	Primary tumor cannot be assessed
pT0	No evidence of primary tumor
pTis	Intratubular germ cell neoplasia (carcinoma in situ)
pT1	Tumor limited to the testis and epididymis without vascular/lymphatic invasion; tumor may invade into the tunica albuginea but not the tunica vaginalis
pT2	Tumor limited to the testis and epididymis with vascular/lymphatic invasion or tumor extending through the tunica albuginea with involvement of the tunica vaginalis
pT3	Tumor invades the spermatic cord with or without vascular/lymphatic invasion
pT4	Tumor invades the scrotum with or without vascular/lymphatic invasion
b: Regional lymph nodes (R)	
Clinical	
NX	Regional lymph nodes cannot be assessed
N0	No regional lymph node metastasis
N1	Metastasis with a lymph node mass 2 cm or less in greatest dimension; or multiple lymph nodes, none more than 2 cm in greatest dimension
N2	Metastasis with a lymph node mass more than 2 cm but not more than 5 cm in greatest dimension; or multiple lymph nodes, any one mass greater than 2 cm but not more than 5 cm in greatest dimension
N3	Metastasis with a lymph node mass more than 5 cm in greatest dimension
Pathologic (pN)	
pNX	Regional lymph nodes cannot be assessed
pN0	No regional lymph node metastasis
pN1	Metastasis with a lymph node mass 2 cm or less in greatest dimension and less than or equal to 5 nodes positive, none more than 2 cm in greatest dimension
pN2	Metastasis with a lymph node mass more than 2 cm but not more than 5 cm in greatest dimension; or more than 5 nodes positive, none more than 5 cm; or evidence of extranodal extension of tumor
pN3	Metastasis with a lymph node mass more than 5cm in greatest dimension
c: Distant metastasis (M)	
MX	Distant metastasis cannot be assessed
M0	No distant metastasis
M1	Distant metastasis
M1a	Non-regional nodal or pulmonary metastasis
M1b	Distant metastasis other than to non-regional lymph nodes and lungs
d: Serum tumor markers (S)	
SX	Marker studies not available or not performed
S0	Marker study levels within normal limits
S1	LDH < 1.5x UNL AND
	hCG (mIU/ml) < 5000 AND
	AFP (ng/ml) < 1000
S2	LDH 1.5–10x UNL OR
	hCG (mIU/ml) 5000–50000 OR
	AFP (ng/ml) 1000–10000
S3	LDH > 10 x UNL OR
	hCG (mIU/ml) > 50000 OR
	AFP (ng/ml) > 10000

renal hilar nodes, the pre- and para-aortic (upper part) and left common iliac regions, whereas pre-, para-, and interaortocaval as well as right common iliac node groups are considered to be the primary lymphatic spread of right-sided testicular tumors [45, 72–75] (see Fig. 27.6a and b). Previous inguinal or scrotal surgery is a known risk factor for the uncommon spread to the inguinal and pelvic nodes [76, 77].

Retroperitoneal hematoma following bleeding from an inappropriately ligated vessel at orchidectomy is a possible source of false-positive **abdominal CT scans** [78–80].

The accuracy of detecting metastatic disease in normal-size lymph nodes is limited, mainly because the size of normal retroperitoneal lymph nodes in healthy people varies substantially (6–20 mm) due to methodological differences and variations in size at different anatomic locations [81–83] (see Table 27.3). Even the combined measurement of long and short diameters of the largest lymph nodes in different retroperitoneal regions does not add to accuracy [84].

As a rule, the short diameter on axial sections is used, although no consensus has been defined so far for standard

(a) (b)

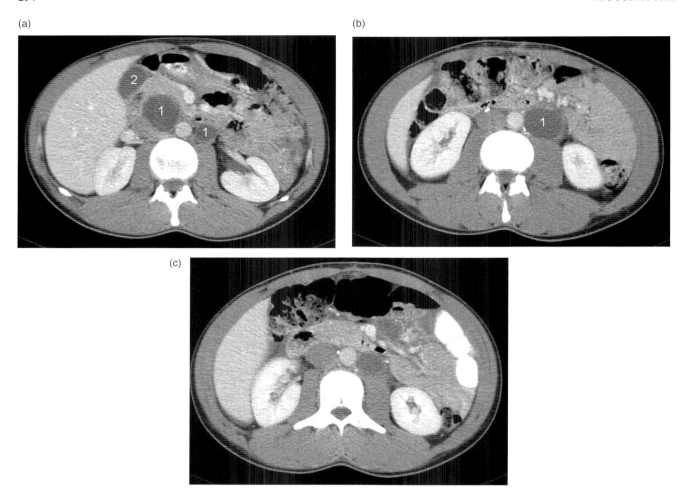

(c)

Fig. 27.5 Abdominal CTs with i.v. and oral contrast. (a) Anatomy before surgery. 1: Enlarged abdominal lymph nodes. 2: Gall bladder. (b) Same patient, first follow-up after retroperitoneal residual tumor resection. 1: Hypodense postoperative seroma mimicking a hypodense lymph node (seroma and former lymph node of same density). (c) Same patient, second follow-up after surgery. Spontaneous size reduction of seroma

measurements of retroperitoneal lymph nodes. In clinical studies different measurements have been used [85–87].

CT diagnosis is not only based on size. The shape and the potential absence of a fatty center, inhomogeneities, or additional signs like strong enhancement after contrast administration reflecting hypervascularization, which may be due to tumor or inflammation, are other important criteria. Yet, these criteria are controversially discussed in the literature [88]. The strongest correlation of CT-enlarged retroperitoneal nodes with malignancy is their location within the primary landing zone.

The staging accuracy of CT scans at presentation of stage I and II GCT is about 70% [82, 89–91]. 20–30% of clinical stage II patients turn out to be stage I pathologically, whereas 30% of clinical stage I patients are understaged by CT [90, 92].

Not surprisingly, several authors showed in retrospective analyses that the smaller the cut-off for a still normal-sized node, the higher the sensitivity, but the lower the specificity.

Para-aortic lymph nodes of >10 mm are suspect of metastatic involvement in any case of GCT. A cut-off value as low as 4 mm (short axis) has been suggested for para-aortic nodes anterior to the midportion of the aorta in patients with NSGCT [84, 93, 94] (see Table 27.4).

In **summary**, any number of nodes within the expected primary landing zone, irrespective of their size, should raise serious suspicion of occult metastases [81, 82, 89, 93, 95–97].

The prevalence of **pelvic nodes** is low (only 8%) and the additional radiation burden with pelvic CT is high with an increase of the effective dose equivalent (EDE) by 2.6 mSv (74%). For pelvic disease two mechanisms have been postulated: retrograde spread from extensive abdominal metastases and disruption of the normal lymphatic drainage of the testis. White et al. retrospectively evaluated 443 CT examina-

(a)

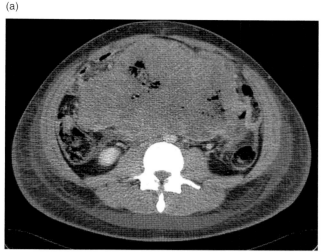

(b)

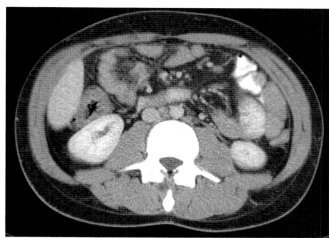

Fig. 27.6 Abdominal CTs with i.v. and oral contrast. (a) Bulky retroperitoneal disease at presentation (intermediate prognosis). High image noise due to intensive care unit conditions and distinctive anasarca of patient. (b) Same patient after four courses of cisplatin-containing chemotherapy. Very good partial remission, tumor-marker negative, histologically necrosis and mature teratoma at residual tumor resection

Table 27.3 Average diameter of normal sized lymph nodes in adults according to anatomic location: after Prokop (2003, p. 623) [83]

Location	Threshold diameter (mm)
Retrocrural nodes	6
Gastrohepatic nodes	8
Pancreaticoduodenal nodes	10
Mesenteric nodes	10
High pre-aortic and celiac nodes	10
Para-aortocaval nodes	11

Table 27.4 Abdominal CT for GCT staging according to size cut-off and relation to the abdominal aorta: after Hilton (1997) [93]

Node size: cut-off (mm)	Specificity (%)	Sensitivity (%)
> 10	37	100
> 8	47	100
> 6	67	83
> 4	93	58

tions of 167 patients to investigate the true value of pelvic CT and to analyze risk factors for pelvic disease. The strongest single risk factor was found to be bulky abdominal disease. Therefore, CT of the pelvis should be included in the primary staging procedures. **Further pelvic CT scans** for restaging and follow-up are recommended only for patients at high risk for pelvic disease [72, 74, 77, 98] (see Sections Response Evaluation and Follow-Up).

The retroperitoneum and the lungs are sites of predilection for metastases of GCT. On staging **CT scans of the chest**, which are recommended for all patients with NSGCT [51], all pulmonary nodules, regardless of their size, are suspect. Only calcified foci are a safe exception to this rule (see Fig. 27.7a and b).

Intrathoracic disease occurs in 17–25.7% of NSGCT patients [29, 99–101] (see Figs. 27.8 and 27.9) and 50% of patients with retroperitoneal lymph node metastases are expected to have concomitant pulmonary metastases; 10% are found to have isolated intrathoracic involvement [102].

In pure seminomatous germ cell tumors pulmonary involvement is rare with a rate of only 0.3–3.5% [29, 101]. Therefore, staging CT of the chest may be omitted and replaced by chest x-ray, if the retroperitoneum is clear [51, 97].

Supradiaphragmatic nodal involvement in association with pulmonary metastases is seen in 12–25% of patients [101, 102]. The most common sites are the para-esophageal, subcarinal, and posterior mediastinal areas [103, 104]. Isolated mediastinal involvement is relatively uncommon in NSGCT (9%), but more frequent in pure seminomas [29].

(a)   (b)

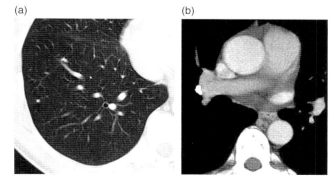

Fig. 27.7 Chest CT with i.v. and oral contrast. Patient with stage Ib NSGCT. (a) Small pulmonary lesions at follow-up. (b) Same patient. Calcified hilus lymph node, supporting the hypothesis of non-recent tuberculosis rather than pulmonary metastases

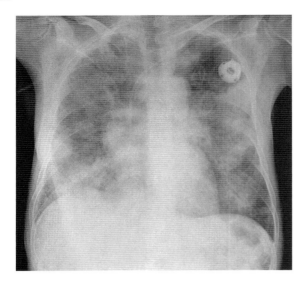

Fig. 27.8 Chest x-ray. NSGCT, high intrapulmonary tumor load, clinically severe dyspnea.

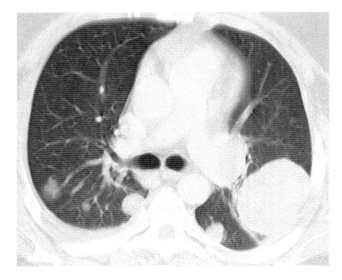

Fig. 27.9 Chest CT with i.v. and oral contrast; lung window. NSGCT with poor prognosis; multiple intrapulmonary lesions

Measurement of intrathoracic lymph nodes is usually based on the short-axis diameter. The threshold for a normal-size lymph node in all thoracic regions has been reported to be 10 mm. Subcarinal lymph nodes with a 12 mm short axis as the upper limit of normal are an exception [32].

The overall accuracy of chest CT for diagnosing metastases does not exceed 70% with excellent sensitivity but relatively poor specificity. False-positive results lead to unnecessary re-evaluations with CT scanning associated with an increase in the radiation dose delivered or the risks of invasive procedures [32, 82].

Pitfalls in staging chest CTs comprise **normal structures and variants** and different coincidental conditions:

1. Thymic hyperplasia (for thymic rebound phenomenon see Section Relapse)
2. Normal pericardial recesses mistaken for nodal metastases (both structures may be of low density) [101]
3. Large transverse sinus of the superior pericardium simulating a paratracheal lymph node [105]
4. Posterior pericardial recess and oblique sinus of the pericardium simulating a low-density subcarinal or paraesophageal node [106]
5. The cisterna chyli [107]
6. Coincidental presence of **sarcoidosis:**

Typical findings on chest CT (better still on high-resolution CT) images that are sources of potential errors in GCT imaging, but **suspicious of sarcoidosis,** are [108] (see Fig. 27.10)

- Small, well-defined nodules in relation to the pleural surfaces, interlobular septa, centrilobular structures
- Large nodules (> 1 cm) or consolidation
- Lymph node enlargement, usually symmetrical

In tumor marker negative patients with a clear retroperitoneum and isolated mediastinal node enlargement or lung nodules, biopsies should be obtained to establish the diagnosis.

Response Evaluation

Response evaluation in GCT is based on a consistent tumor marker decline measured directly before each treatment course and on CT data (see Fig. 27.6a and b). The management of GCT patients does not include interim staging

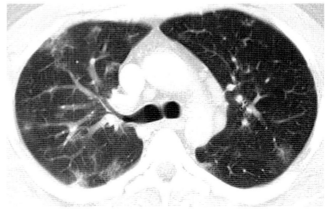

Fig. 27.10 Chest CT with i.v. and oral contrast; lung window. Multiple ill-defined, fuzzy pulmonary lesions mimicking intrapulmonary metastases. Differential diagnosis of sarcoidosis was histologically verified; improvement after corticosteroid therapy

after two or three courses of chemotherapy, as is common practice for other tumor entities. Response evaluation by CT scanning in GCT is performed only at the sites of former metastatic disease and after completion of the planned three to four courses of cisplatin-based chemotherapy, unless a clear tumor marker increase measured on day one of each chemotherapy course indicates progression. Tumor marker flare-ups between chemotherapy courses may be due to release from necrotic tumor cell tissue, especially after the first chemotherapy course, and should not prompt additional imaging or changes in treatment [51]. Metastases growing during chemotherapy are usually found to harbor mature teratoma components [42, 109]. These have to be removed after completing chemotherapy.

Up to one third of all patients with NSGCT metastases present with **residual masses**, although their tumor marker levels returned to normal ("marker-negative partial remission; PRm−"). CT, FDG PET, MRI, and predictive models based on regression analyses [44, 110] have so far not reliably predicted the histology of the residuals. Necrosis/fibrosis, mature teratoma with or without malignant transformation, and viable tumor are expected in 40, 40, and 20%, respectively [109, 111–113]. In six studies discordant pathology was reported in 25–47% of cases after multiple resections [46]. Therefore, complete resection of all residual NSGCT lesions is the only way of curing this group of patients.

Restaging in Pure Seminomatous Germ Cell Tumors (SGCT)

Residual lesions after chemotherapy of bulky SGCT are expected to be present in 50–75% of patients. Overall, less than 20% of the resected residual masses harbor viable tumor and the presence of mature teratoma is negligible. CT combined with FDG PET for evaluating pure seminoma residuals can be regarded as a standard tool for clinical decision making in this patient group (see chapter 28).

Just as in NSGCT, MRI is used in SGCT, if CT contrast is contraindicated or if the anatomy is unclear after CT imaging [41, 42]

Relapse

Relapses are expected in about 20% of all patients with germ cell cancer, depending strongly on the prognostic group at primary staging according to the IGCCCG classification [39]. A rise in tumor marker levels and/or the presence of radiological, rarely clinical, signs provides diagnostic evidence suggesting relapse. For relapsers with rising marker levels and unequivocal signs of progressive disease on CT, salvage treatment should be instituted: salvage chemotherapy, followed by salvage surgery, and primary salvage surgery are the standard treatment options.

The following situations raise diagnostic problems:

1. Rising tumor markers unmatched by clinical/radiological abnormalities
2. Radiological evidence of new lesions or an increase in the volume of a pre-existing one unassociated with rising marker levels

In the latter case, CT pitfalls at relapse mimicking pulmonary metastases or relapse are

(a) Pulmonary changes on chest CT not matching the clinical picture or without rising markers due to sarcoidosis (see Fig. 27.10)
(b) Radiologic manifestations of pulmonary drug toxicity [114–117]: bleomycin-induced manifestations with multiple discrete nodules simulating metastases and an acinar filling pattern (see Section Computed Tomography and Pulmonary Changes due to Drug Toxicity in GCT Patients)
(c) Infections or originally unrecognized residuals after infections: tuberculosis (see Fig. 27.7a and b)
(d) Thymic rebound following chemotherapy [118–122].

CT and Radiation Risk

Given the young population at risk for testicular cancer, the high cure rates and the lifelong follow-up, it is essential to minimize the radiation burden following the "ALARA" principle ("as low as reasonably achievable"). CT, the standard procedure for the diagnosis, staging, response evaluation, and follow-up, generates ionizing radiation, which is itself a potent mutagen and carcinogen. Worldwide, radiation exposure from medical procedures is continuously rising. CT accounts for 5% of all radiologic examinations, but contributes 34–70% of the collective radiation dose [123–126].

The estimated cancer risk following exposure to low levels of ionizing radiation has been discussed controversially in several reports by international organizations [123, 127, 128] and in scientific publications by individual researchers [126, 129, 130] in the past few decades. These estimates have largely been derived from data of survivors of atomic bombings [129, 131–133] and from studies of medically, occupationally, or environmentally overexposed groups [123, 128]. Unanswered questions as to the actual risk of fatal cancer induction include the legitimacy of linear extrapolation from higher to lower radiation doses as well as unknown effects of dose fractionation in this field of interest. Individual risk factors for cancer induction caused by radiation include genetic susceptibility and the age at exposure [126, 129, 130].

The quantity most relevant for assessing the risk of cancer detriment from a CT procedure is the "effective dose" measured in millisieverts (mSv). This quantity incorporates the different radiation sensitivities of the organs of the body and therefore permits to compare the risk estimates associated with partial or whole-body radiation exposures [127].

A typical CT examination of the abdomen with an effective dose of 10 mSv increases the risk of fatal cancer induction by approximately 1:2000 [127] in addition to the natural incidence of fatal cancer in the U.S. population, which is about 1:5 (see Table 27.5). In other words, for any one person the risk of radiation-induced cancer is much smaller than the natural risk of cancer. Nevertheless, this small increase in the radiation-associated risk of fatal cancer induction may become a major public health concern and is a vital individual issue for young testicular cancer survivors.

The possibilities of reducing the radiation dose are manifold and can only be optimized in an interdisciplinary approach of

1. *Manufacturers* by introducing automatic exposure controls and automatic tube current modulation, improving scanning efficiency by the use of pre-patient collimation of x-ray beams, better filters, higher gantry rotation times, better image reconstruction algorithms, and more efficient detector geometry [134]
2. *Radiologists* by strictly limiting the volume scanned to the actual area of interest, using "low-dose" protocols (reducing current and voltage, increasing pitch, adapting scanning parameters to patient attributes such as weight or circumference), shielding, selecting adequate image reconstruction parameters, and avoiding unnecessary scanning (e.g., before and after contrast enhancement) [134–141]
3. *Referring clinicians* by optimizing follow-up schedules with respect to patient- and treatment-related risk factors [77, 101, 142–148]

Table 27.5 Diagnostic procedures: summary of average effective doses and estimated lifetime cancer risks

Diagnostic procedure	Average effective dose (mSv)	Equivalent number of chest x-rays	Estimated lifetime cancer risk (mortality)
Chest x-ray	0.02	1	1:1,000,000
CT chest	8	400	1:2500
CT abdomen	10	500	1:2000
CT pelvis	10	500	1:2000

Follow-Up

Follow-up strategies depend strongly on the individual clinical situation and the risk of relapse of the individual patient. The use, frequency, and duration of CT scanning for follow-up are under debate for most clinical situations.

As for strategies to reduce radiation, a few recommendations about the use or possible omission of CT scans can be made. These are mainly based on retrospective data.

According to the data of White et al., **pelvic CT scans** for restaging and follow-up are recommended only for patients at high risk for pelvic disease [72, 74, 77, 98], i.e.,

1. Presence of unequivocal node enlargement in the abdomen/retroperitoneum (bulky disease > 5 cm)
2. Previous history of maldescent and orchidopexy
3. Other previous inguinal scrotal surgery
4. Invasion of the tumor through the tunica vaginalis of the testis

Randomized data specifically addressing the role of CT scanning for follow-up is available only for stage I NSGCT patients on surveillance.

A multicenter trial prospectively compared two CT follow-up schedules for post-orchidectomy patients with stage I testicular teratoma on surveillance. Mainly low-risk stage I patients (without vascular invasion of the primary tumor) were included. The investigators excluded a more than 1.6% difference in relapsing to a higher-risk group between 5 or 2 CT scans of chest and abdomen performed at 3, 6, 9, 12, and 24 months versus 3 and 12 months. Thus, CT scans at 3 and 12 months should be considered standard surveillance with the advantage of less cumulative radiation exposure [143].

Chest CT versus conventional chest x-ray for follow-up has long been a matter of controversy and still is.

In a prospective study Gels et al. [148] found pulmonary-only relapses in no more than 9.6% out of 154 patients on surveillance. A retrospective review by Harvey et al. [145] included 168 patients; 42 (25%) had a relapse. Only one patient (0.6%) presented with pulmonary-only relapse.

In the randomized study presented by Mead et al. [143], chest x-ray was the first to signal relapse in all pulmonary cases of the two-CT scan group, whereas chest CT reported relapse first in only 3 out of 167 patients on surveillance. In view of these summary data, the actual role of chest CT for follow-up is questionable. Chest-only relapses are very rare and chest relapses in general are most likely to be picked up by chest x-ray, although possibly later. This fact, however, does not impair the prognosis of the patients according to the IGCCCG classification [39]. Therefore, chest CT safely can be replaced by chest x-ray in GCT patients on surveillance.

Computed Tomography and Pulmonary Changes due to Drug Toxicity in GCT Patients

In order to react appropriately and quickly enough, risk factors and typical clinical and radiologic manifestations should be kept in mind, when **bleomycin**-induced toxicity might be the reason for unclear CT findings or clinical manifestations during re-staging or follow-up. The usual incidence of bleomycin-induced pulmonary toxicity is approximately 4–7% [115, 149, 150]. Of the patients affected, about 15–27% go on to die of fatal pulmonary fibrosis (about 1% of all patients treated with any dosage of bleomycin) [151]. The typical time to clinical or radiologic changes is 4–10 weeks after treatment is initiated [150, 152, 153].

Known *risk factors* in a multivariate analysis by O'Sullivan et al. were [154]

- Age > 40 years
- Impaired renal function (GFR < 80 ml/min)
- Stage IV disease (pulmonary metastases, high pulmonary tumor burden)
- Cumulative bleomycin dose > 300 IU

Whenever early pulmonary changes due to bleomycin (see Fig. 27.11) are expected or to be ruled out, CT of the chest and especially high-resolution CT (HR-CT) of the chest is more sensitive than chest x-ray. A slight reduction of the DLCO on lung function testing is usually the first sign. Early recognition of morphologic changes and their extent is crucial. Discontinuation of the drug before permanent damage occurs is the most important therapeutic step.

The first detailed description of CT changes indicating pulmonary bleomycin toxicity was published by Bellamy et al. in 1985 [155]. In 23% of patients with normal chest x-rays parenchymal lung damage was detected. The authors described three **degrees of lung damage** with the respective CT correlations:

Minor damage: pleural-based linear and nodular opacities at the lung bases

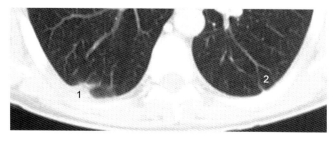

Fig. 27.11 High-resolution CT of the chest. 1: Subpleural triangular opacity (Pfeil right lung). 2: Discrete linear pleural-based opacity (Pfeil left lung)

Moderate damage: coarse reticular and nodular shadowing extending across the pulmonary parenchyma and toward the mediastinum

Severe damage: confluent, irregular opacities extending throughout the lung with the apices relatively spared

Further possible clinical and radiologic manifestations of drug-induced pulmonary toxicity, including bleomycin, described by Rossi et al. are [114] diffuse alveolar damage (DAD) and obliterating bronchiolitis, organizing pneumonia (BOOP) with hetero- and homogeneous peripheral opacities in both upper and lower lobes and on CT scans as poorly defined nodular consolidation. These can give rise to misinterpretation as malignant lesions [153].

If the clinical picture is not indicative of relapse and bleomycin-induced changes are suspected on CT scans, observation is considered sufficient including repeated chest x-rays and chest CTs. In such cases invasive procedures/biopsies can be avoided [117]. Complete resolution of bleomycin-induced CT abnormalities is expected in nearly half of the patients with mild or moderate changes over several months [155]. This is not to be expected in patients with severe CT changes due to pulmonary fibrosis.

References

1. Horwich A. In: Horwich A, editor. Testicular cancer – investigation and management: Chapman and Hall Medical; 1996. pp. 1–17.
2. Loughrey GJ, Carrington BM, Anderson H, Dobson MJ, Lo Ying Ping F. The value of specialist oncological radiology review of cross-sectional imaging. Clin Radiol. 1999;54(3):149–54; discussion 54–5.
3. Lawton AJ, Mead GM. Staging and prognostic factors in testicular cancer. Semin Surg Oncol. 1999;17(4):223–9.
4. Barentsz J, Takahashi S, Oyen W, et al. Commonly used imaging techniques for diagnosis and staging. J Clin Oncol. 2006;24(20):3234–44.
5. Schnall M, Rosen M. Primer on imaging technologies for cancer. J Clin Oncol. 2006;24(20):3225–33.
6. Semelka RC, Helmberger TK. Contrast agents for MR imaging of the liver. Radiology. 2001;218(1):27–38.
7. Hricak H, Hamm B, Bohyun K. Imaging of the scrotum: Raven Press; 1995.
8. Noone T, Huch-Böni R, Semelka RC. MRI of the abdomen and pelvis. New York: Wiley-Liss; 1997. pp. 541–69.
9. Cramer BM, Schlegel EA, Thueroff JW. MR imaging in the differential diagnosis of scrotal and testicular disease. Radiographics. 1991;11(1):9–21.
10. Kubik-Huch RA, Hailemariam S, Hamm B. CT and MRI of the male genital tract: radiologic-pathologic correlation. Eur Radiol. 1999;9(1):16–28.
11. Woodward PJ, Sohaey R, O'Donoghue MJ, Green DE. From the archives of the AFIP: tumors and tumorlike lesions of the testis: radiologic-pathologic correlation. Radiographics. 2002;22(1):189–216.

12. Johnson JO, Mattrey RF, Phillipson J. Differentiation of seminomatous from nonseminomatous testicular tumors with MR imaging. AJR Am J Roentgenol. 1990;154(3):539–43.

13. Oyen R, Verellen S, Drochmans A, Baert L, Marchal G, Moerman P, Baert AL. Value of MRI in the diagnosis and staging of testicular tumors. J Belge Radiol. 1993;76(2):84–9.

14. Baker LL, Hajek PC, Burkhard TK, et al. MR imaging of the scrotum: pathologic conditions. Radiology. 1987;163(1): 93–8.

15. Thurnher S, Hricak H, Carroll PR, Pobiel RS, Filly RA. Imaging the testis: comparison between MR imaging and US. Radiology. 1988;167(3):631–6.

16. Muttarak M, Peh WC, Chaiwun B. Malignant germ cell tumours of undescended testes: imaging features with pathological correlation. Clin Radiol. 2004;59(2):198–204.

17. Nguyen HT, Coakley F, Hricak H. Cryptorchidism: strategies in detection. Eur Radiol. 1999;9(2):336–43.

18. Fritzsche PJ, Hricak H, Kogan BA, Winkler ML, Tanagho EA. Undescended testis: value of MR imaging. Radiology. 1987;164(1):169–73.

19. Kier R, McCarthy S, Rosenfield AT, Rosenfield NS, Rapoport S, Weiss RM. Nonpalpable testes in young boys: evaluation with MR imaging. Radiology. 1988;169(2):429–33.

20. Frush DP, Sheldon CA. Diagnostic imaging for pediatric scrotal disorders. Radiographics. 1998;18(4):969–85.

21. Lam WW, Tam PK, Ai VH, Chan KL, Chan FL, Leong L. Using gadolinium-infusion MR venography to show the impalpable testis in pediatric patients. AJR Am J Roentgenol. 2001;176(5):1221–6.

22. Pottern L, Goedert J. Epidemiology of testicular cancer. In: Javadpour N, editor. Principles and management of testicular cancer. New York: Thieme; 1986. pp. 107–19.

23. Skakkebaek NE, Rajpert-De Meyts E, Jorgensen N, et al. Germ cell cancer and disorders of spermatogenesis: an environmental connection? Apmis. 1998;106(1):3–11; discussion 2.

24. Chaganti RS, Houldsworth J. The cytogenetic theory of the pathogenesis of human adult male germ cell tumors. Review article. Apmis. 1998;106(1):80–3; discussion 3–4.

25. Oliver RT. Atrophy, hormones, genes and viruses in aetiology germ cell tumours. Cancer Surv. 1990;9(2):263–86.

26. Hartmann JT, Fossa SD, Nichols CR, et al. Incidence of metachronous testicular cancer in patients with extragonadal germ cell tumors. J Natl Cancer Inst. 2001;93(22):1733–8.

27. Scholz M, Zehender M, Thalmann GN, Borner M, Thoni H, Studer UE. Extragonadal retroperitoneal germ cell tumor: evidence of origin in the testis. Ann Oncol. 2002;13(1):121–4.

28. Nichols CR. Mediastinal germ cell tumors. Clinical features and biologic correlates. Chest. 1991;99(2):472–9.

29. Williams MP, Husband JE, Heron CW. Intrathoracic manifestations of metastatic testicular seminoma: a comparison of chest radiographic and CT findings. AJR Am J Roentgenol. 1987;149(3):473–5.

30. Marchevsky A, Kaneko M. Surgical pathology of the mediastinum. New York: Raven Press; 1992.

31. Brown LR, Aughenbaugh GL. Masses of the anterior mediastinum: CT and MR imaging. AJR Am J Roentgenol. 1991;157(6):1171–80.

32. Naidich D, Webb W, Müller N, Krinsky G, Zerhouni E. computed tomography and magnetic resonance of the thorax. Lippincott Williams & Wilkins; 1998. p. 357.

33. Suzuki M, Takashima T, Itoh H, Choutoh S, Kawamura I, Watanabe Y. Computed tomography of mediastinal teratomas. J Comput Assist Tomogr. 1983;7(1):74–6.

34. Fulcher AS, Proto AV, Jolles H. Cystic teratoma of the mediastinum: demonstration of fat/fluid level. AJR Am J Roentgenol. 1990;154(2):259–60.

35. Seltzer SE, Herman PG, Sagel SS. Differential diagnosis of mediastinal fluid levels visualized on computed tomography. J Comput Assist Tomogr. 1984;8(2):244–6.

36. Rosado-de-Christenson ML, Templeton PA, Moran CA. From the archives of the AFIP. Mediastinal germ cell tumors: radiologic and pathologic correlation. Radiographics. 1992;12(5): 1013–30.

37. Lee KS, Im JG, Han CH, Han MC, Kim CW, Kim WS. Malignant primary germ cell tumors of the mediastinum: CT features. AJR Am J Roentgenol. 1989;153(5):947–51.

38. Levitt RG, Husband JE, Glazer HS. CT of primary germ-cell tumors of the mediastinum. AJR Am J Roentgenol. 1984;142(1):73–8.

39. International Germ Cell Cancer Collaborative Group. International Germ Cell Consensus Classification: a prognostic factor-based staging system for metastatic germ cell cancers. J Clin Oncol. 1997;15(2):594–603.

40. Ellis JH, Bies JR, Kopecky KK, Klatte EC, Rowland RG, Donohue JP. Comparison of NMR and CT imaging in the evaluation of metastatic retroperitoneal lymphadenopathy from testicular carcinoma. J Comput Assist Tomogr. 1984;8(4):709–19.

41. Hogeboom WR, Hoekstra HJ, Mooyaart EL, Sleijfer DT, Freling NJ, Willemse PH, Schraffordt Koops, H. The role of magnetic resonance imaging and computed tomography in the treatment evaluation of retroperitoneal lymph-node metastases of nonseminomatous testicular tumors. Eur J Radiol. 1991;13(1):31–6.

42. Hogeboom WR, Hoekstra HJ, Mooyaart EL, Sleijfer DT, Schraffordt Koops H. Magnetic resonance imaging of retroperitoneal lymph node metastases of non-seminomatous germ cell tumours of the testis. Eur J Surg Oncol. 1993;19(5):429–37.

43. De Santis M, Becherer A, Bokemeyer C, et al. 2-18fluoro-deoxy-D-glucose positron emission tomography is a reliable predictor for viable tumor in postchemotherapy seminoma: an update of the prospective multicentric SEMPET trial. J Clin Oncol. 2004;22(6):1034–9.

44. De Wit M, Hartmann M, Brenner W, et al. [18F]-FDG-PET in germ cell tumors following chemotherapy: results of the German multicenter trial. J. Clin Oncol. 2006 ASCO Annual Meeting Proceedings Part I. 2006;24, No 18S (June 20 Supplement): 4521.

45. Bosl GJ, Motzer RJ. Testicular germ-cell cancer. N Engl J Med. 1997;337(4):242–53.

46. Hartmann JT, Kanz L, Bokemeyer C. Diagnosis and treatment of patients with testicular germ cell cancer. Drugs. 1999;58(2): 257–81.

47. Kollmannsberger C, Nichols C, Bamberg M, et al. First-line high-dose chemotherapy +/− radiation therapy in patients with metastatic germ-cell cancer and brain metastases. Ann Oncol. 2000;11(5):553–9.

48. Davis PC, Hudgins PA, Peterman SB, Hoffman JC Jr. Diagnosis of cerebral metastases: double-dose delayed CT vs contrast-enhanced MR imaging. Ajnr. 1991;12(2):293–300.

49. Bokemeyer C, Nowak P, Haupt A, et al. Treatment of brain metastases in patients with testicular cancer. J Clin Oncol. 1997;15(4):1449–54.

50. Fossa SD, Bokemeyer C, Gerl A, et al. Treatment outcome of patients with brain metastases from malignant germ cell tumors. Cancer. 1999;85(4):988–97.

51. Schmoll HJ, Souchon R, Krege S, et al. European consensus on diagnosis and treatment of germ cell cancer: a report of the European Germ Cell Cancer Consensus Group (EGCCCG). Ann Oncol. 2004;15(9):1377–99.

52. Semelka RC, Schlund JF, Molina PL, et al. Malignant liver lesions: comparison of spiral CT arterial portography and MR imaging for diagnostic accuracy, cost, and effect on patient management. J Magn Reson Imaging. 1996;6(1):39–43.

53. Vassiliades VG, Foley WD, Alarcon J, et al. Hepatic metastases: CT versus MR imaging at 1.5T. Gastrointest Radiol. 1991;16(2):159–63.

54. Kellenberger CJ, Epelman M, Miller SF, Babyn PS. Fast STIR whole-body MR imaging in children. Radiographics. 2004;24(5):1317–30.

55. Walker R, Kessar P, Blanchard R, et al. Turbo STIR magnetic resonance imaging as a whole-body screening tool for metastases in patients with breast carcinoma: preliminary clinical experience. J Magn Reson Imaging. 2000;11(4):343–50.

56. Ladd SC, Zenge M, Antoch G, Forsting M. Whole-body MR diagnostic concepts. Rofo. 2006;178(8):763–70.

57. Bellin MF, Roy C, Kinkel K, et al. Lymph node metastases: safety and effectiveness of MR imaging with ultrasmall superparamagnetic iron oxide particles–initial clinical experience. Radiology. 1998;207(3):799–808.

58. Atri M. New technologies and directed agents for applications of cancer imaging. J Clin Oncol. 2006;24(20):3299–308.

59. Harisinghani MG, Barentsz J, Hahn PF, et al. Noninvasive detection of clinically occult lymph-node metastases in prostate cancer. N Engl J Med. 2003;348(25):2491–9.

60. UICC manual of clinical oncology. New Jersey: John Wiley & Sons; 2004.

61. Husband JE, Grimer DP. Staging testicular tumours: the role of CT scanning. J R Soc Med. 1985;78 Suppl 6:25–31.

62. Ehrlichman RJ, Kaufman SL, Siegelman SS, Trump DL, Walsh PC. Computerized tomography and lymphangiography in staging testis tumors. J Urol. 1981;126(2):179–81.

63. Royal SA, Callen PW. CT evaluation of anomalies of the inferior vena cava and left renal vein. AJR Am J Roentgenol. 1979;132(5):759–63.

64. Moul JW, Maggio MI, Hardy MR, Hartman DS. Retroaortic left renal vein in testicular cancer patient: potential staging and treatment pitfall. J Urol. 1992;147(2):454–6.

65. Dixon AK, Ellis M, Sikora K. Computed tomography of testicular tumours: distribution of abdominal lymphadenopathy. Clin Radiol. 1986;37(6):519–23.

66. Brener BJ, Darling RC, Frederick PL, Linton RR. Major venous anomalies complicating abdominal aortic surgery. Arch Surg. 1974;108(2):159–65.

67. Pick J, BJ. A. The renal vascular pedicle: an anatomical study of 430 body halves. J Urol. 1940;44:411–34.

68. Dubowitz DJ. Problem in diagnostic imaging. Clin Anat. 1997;10(4):279–82.

69. Bass JE, Redwine MD, Kramer LA, Huynh PT, Harris JH Jr. Spectrum of congenital anomalies of the inferior vena cava: cross-sectional imaging findings. Radiographics. 2000;20(3):639–52.

70. Meanock CI, Ward CS, Williams MP. A potential pitfall of pelvic computed tomography. Br J Radiol. 1988;61(727):584–5.

71. von Krogh J, Lien HH, Ous S, Fossa SD. Alterations in the CT image following retroperitoneal lymphadenectomy in early stage non-seminomatous testicular tumor. Acta Radiol Diagn (Stockh). 1985;26(2):187–91.

72. Ray B, Hajdu SI, Whitmore WF Jr. Proceedings: Distribution of retroperitoneal lymph node metastases in testicular germinal tumors. Cancer. 1974;33(2):340–8.

73. Donohue JP, Zachary JM, Maynard BR. Distribution of nodal metastases in nonseminomatous testis cancer. J Urol. 1982;128(2):315–20.

74. Mason MD, Featherstone T, Olliff J, Horwich A. Inguinal and iliac lymph node involvement in germ cell tumours of the testis: implications for radiological investigation and for therapy. Clin Oncol (R Coll Radiol). 1991;3(3):147–50.

75. Bradey N, Johnson RJ, Read G. Abdominal computed tomography in teratoma of the testis: its accuracy in stage I disease and an assessment of the distribution of retroperitoneal lymph-node metastases in other stages of the disease. Br J Radiol. 1987;60(713):487–91.

76. Busch FM, Sayegh ES, Chenault OW Jr. Some uses of lymphangiography in the management of testicular tumors. J Urol. 1965;93:490–5.

77. White PM, Howard GC, Best JJ, Wright AR. The role of computed tomographic examination of the pelvis in the management of testicular germ cell tumours. Clin Radiol. 1997;52(2):124–9.

78. Page JE, Prendergast CM, King DM. Retroperitoneal haematoma following orchidectomy: implications for staging computed tomography. Br J Radiol. 1990;63(750):490–2.

79. Kullmann G, Lien HH. Intraabdominal hematoma following orchiectomy: a potential pitfall in using CT for staging of testicular cancer. Radiology. 1987;163(1):129–30.

80. Tran T, Grech P, Crofton ME. Computed tomographic staging of testicular tumours: an unexpected source of error. Br J Radiol. 1989;62(742):942–4.

81. Leibovitch L, Foster RS, Kopecky KK, Donohue JP. Improved accuracy of computerized tomography based clinical staging in low stage nonseminomatous germ cell cancer using size criteria of retroperitoneal lymph nodes. J Urol. 1995;154(5):1759–63.

82. Lien HH, Stenwig AE, Ous S, Fossa SD. Influence of different criteria for abnormal lymph node size on reliability of computed tomography in patients with non-seminomatous testicular tumor. Acta Radiol Diagn (Stockh). 1986;27(2):199–203.

83. Prokop M, Galanski M. Spiral and multislice computed tomography of the body. Thieme Medical Publishers; 2003.

84. Forsberg L, Dale L, Hoiem L, et al. Computed tomography in early stages of testicular carcinoma. Size of normal retroperitoneal lymph nodes and lymph nodes in patients with metastases in stage II A. A SWENOTECA study: Swedish-Norwegian Testicular Cancer Project. Acta Radiol Diagn (Stockh). 1986;27(5):569–74.

85. World Health Organization. Handbook for reporting results of cancer treatment. 1979. WHO Offset Publication No 48.

86. Therasse P, Arbuck SG, Eisenhauer EA, et al. New guidelines to evaluate the response to treatment in solid tumors. European Organization for Research and Treatment of Cancer, National Cancer Institute of the United States, National Cancer Institute of Canada. J Natl Cancer Inst. 2000;92(3):205–16.

87. Jaffe CC. Measures of response: RECIST, WHO, and new alternatives. J Clin Oncol. 2006;24(20):3245–51.

88. Lien HH, Lindskold L, Stenwig AE, Ous S, Fossa SD. Shape of retroperitoneal lymph nodes at computed tomography does not correlate to metastatic disease in early stage non-seminomatous testicular tumors. Acta Radiol. 1987;28(3):271–3.

89. Fernandez EB, Moul JW, Foley JP, Colon E, McLeod DG. Retroperitoneal imaging with third and fourth generation computed axial tomography in clinical stage I nonseminomatous germ cell tumors. Urology. 1994;44(4):548–52.

90. Donohue JP, Thornhill JA, Foster RS, Bihrle R, Rowland RG, Einhorn LH. The role of retroperitoneal lymphadenectomy in clinical stage B testis cancer: the Indiana University experience (1965 to 1989). J Urol. 1995;153(1):85–9.

91. Stephenson AJ, Bosl GJ, Motzer RJ, et al. Retroperitoneal lymph node dissection for nonseminomatous germ cell testicular cancer: impact of patient selection factors on outcome. J Clin Oncol. 2005;23(12):2781–8.

92. Gatti JM, Stephenson RA. Staging of testis cancer. Combining serum markers, histologic parameters, and radiographic imaging. Urol Clin North Am. 1998;25(3):397–403.

93. Hilton S, Herr HW, Teitcher JB, Begg CB, Castellino RA. CT detection of retroperitoneal lymph node metastases in patients with clinical stage I testicular nonseminomatous germ cell cancer: assessment of size and distribution criteria. AJR Am J Roentgenol. 1997;169(2):521–5.

94. Dorfman RE, Alpern MB, Gross BH, Sandler MA. Upper abdominal lymph nodes: criteria for normal size determined with CT. Radiology. 1991;180(2):319–22.

95. Donohue JP, Thornhill JA, Foster RS, Rowland RG, Bihrle R. Primary retroperitoneal lymph node dissection in clinical stage A non-seminomatous germ cell testis cancer. Review of the Indiana University experience 1965–1989. Br J Urol. 1993;71(3): 326–35.

96. Stomper PC, Fung CY, Socinski MA, Jochelson MS, Garnick MB, Richie JP. Detection of retroperitoneal metastases in early-stage nonseminomatous testicular cancer: analysis of different CT criteria. AJR Am J Roentgenol. 1987;149(6):1187–90.

97. Moul JW. Proper staging techniques in testicular cancer patients. Tech Urol. 1995;1(3):126–32.

98. MacVicar D. Staging of testicular germ cell tumours. Clin Radiol. 1993;47(3):149–58.

99. Lien HH, Lindskold L, Fossa SD, Aass N. Computed tomography and conventional radiography in intrathoracic metastases from non-seminomatous testicular tumor. Acta Radiol. 1988;29(5):547–9.

100. See WA, Hoxie L. Chest staging in testis cancer patients: imaging modality selection based upon risk assessment as determined by abdominal computerized tomography scan results. J Urol. 1993;150(3):874–8.

101. White PM, Adamson DJ, Howard GC, Wright AR. Imaging of the thorax in the management of germ cell testicular tumours. Clin Radiol. 1999;54(4):207–11.

102. Cagini L, Nicholson AG, Horwich A, Goldstraw P, Pastorino U. Thoracic metastasectomy for germ cell tumours: long term survival and prognostic factors. Ann Oncol. 1998;9(11):1185–91.

103. Meyer CA, Conces DJ. Imaging of intrathoracic metastases of nonseminomatous germ cell tumors. Chest Surg Clin N Am. 2002;12(4):717–38.

104. Wood A, Robson N, Tung K, Mead G. Patterns of supradiaphragmatic metastases in testicular germ cell tumours. Clin Radiol. 1996;51(4):273–6.

105. Choi YW, McAdams HP, Jeon SC, Seo HS, Hahm CK. The "High-Riding" superior pericardial recess: CT findings. AJR Am J Roentgenol. 2000;175(4):1025–8.

106. Budoff MJ, Lu B, Mao S, et al. Evaluation of fluid collection in the pericardial sinuses and recesses: noncontrast-enhanced electron beam tomography. Invest Radiol. 2000;35(6): 359–65.

107. Gollub MJ, Castellino RA. The cisterna chyli: a potential mimic of retrocrural lymphadenopathy on CT scans. Radiology. 1996;199(2):477–80.

108. Webb W, Müller N, Naidich D. High-resolution CT of the lung. 3rd ed. Lippincott Williams & Wilkins; 2000.

109. Donohue JP, Rowland RG, Kopecky K, et al. Correlation of computerized tomographic changes and histological findings in 80 patients having radical retroperitoneal lymph node dissection after chemotherapy for testis cancer. J Urol. 1987;137(6): 1176–9.

110. Steyerberg EW, Gerl A, Fossa SD, et al. Validity of predictions of residual retroperitoneal mass histology in nonseminomatous testicular cancer. J Clin Oncol. 1998;16(1):269–74.

111. Toner GC, Panicek DM, Heelan RT, et al. Adjunctive surgery after chemotherapy for nonseminomatous germ cell tumors: recommendations for patient selection. J Clin Oncol. 1990;8(10): 1683–94.

112. Fizazi K, Tjulandin S, Salvioni R, et al. Viable malignant cells after primary chemotherapy for disseminated nonseminomatous germ cell tumors: prognostic factors and role of postsurgery chemotherapy–results from an international study group. J Clin Oncol. 2001;19(10):2647–57.

113. Loehrer PJ Sr, Hui S, Clark S, et al. Teratoma following cisplatin-based combination chemotherapy for nonseminomatous germ cell tumors: a clinicopathological correlation. J Urol. 1986;135(6):1183–9.

114. Rossi SE, Erasmus JJ, McAdams HP, Sporn TA, Goodman PC. Pulmonary drug toxicity: radiologic and pathologic manifestations. Radiographics. 2000;20(5):1245–59.

115. White DA, Stover DE. Severe bleomycin-induced pneumonitis. Clinical features and response to corticosteroids. Chest. 1984;86(5):723–8.

116. Glasier CM, Siegel MJ. Multiple pulmonary nodules: unusual manifestation of bleomycin toxicity. AJR Am J Roentgenol. 1981;137(1):155–6.

117. Lien HH, Brodahl U, Telhaug R, Holthe H, Fossa SD. Pulmonary changes at computed tomography in patients with testicular carcinoma treated with cis-platinum, vinblastine and bleomycin. Acta Radiol Diagn (Stockh). 1985;26(5):507–10.

118. Tait DM, Goldstraw P, Husband JE. Thymic rebound in an adult following chemotherapy for testicular cancer. Eur J Surg Oncol. 1986;12(4):385–7.

119. Carmosino L, DiBenedetto A, Feffer S. Thymic hyperplasia following successful chemotherapy. A report of two cases and review of the literature. Cancer. 1985;56(7):1526–8.

120. Due W, Dieckmann KP, Stein H. Thymic hyperplasia following chemotherapy of a testicular germ cell tumor. Immunohistological evidence for a simple rebound phenomenon. Cancer. 1989;63(3):446–9.

121. Kissin CM, Husband JE, Nicholas D, Eversman W. Benign thymic enlargement in adults after chemotherapy: CT demonstration. Radiology. 1987;163(1):67–70.

122. Murphy BR, Conces DJ Jr, Nichols CR. Thymic hyperplasia after chemotherapy: two case reports and a literature review. Indiana Med. 1991;84(9):624–7.

123. UNSCEAR: United Nations Scientific Committee on the Effects of Atomic Radiation. 2000 Report to the General Assembly, Annex D: medical radiation exposures. New York, United Nations, 2000.

124. Shrimpton PC, Edyvean S. CT scanner dosimetry. Br J Radiol. 1998;71(841):1–3.

125. IAEA Annual Report: Nuclear Safety Review for the Year 2005.

126. Mayo JR, Aldrich J, Muller NL. Radiation exposure at chest CT: a statement of the Fleischner Society. Radiology. 2003;228(1): 15–21.

127. ICRP. International Commission on Radiological Protection. 1990 Recommendations of the International Commission on Radiological Protection. Publication 60. 1991.

128. BEIR V. Health effects of exposure to low-levels of ionizing radiation. Committee on the biological effects of ionizing radiations. Washington DC: National Academic Press; 1990.

129. Brenner DJ, Elliston CD. Estimated radiation risks potentially associated with full-body CT screening. Radiology. 2004;232(3): 735–8.

130. Brenner D, Elliston C, Hall E, Berdon W. Estimated risks of radiation-induced fatal cancer from pediatric CT. AJR Am J Roentgenol. 2001;176(2):289–96.

131. Pierce DA, Preston DL. Radiation-related cancer risks at low doses among atomic bomb survivors. Radiat Res. 2000;154(2): 178–86.

132. Pierce DA, Shimizu Y, Preston DL, Vaeth M, Mabuchi K. Studies of the mortality of atomic bomb survivors. Report 12, Part I. Cancer: 1950–1990. Radiat Res. 1996;146(1):1–27.

133. Preston DL, Shimizu Y, Pierce DA, Suyama A, Mabuchi K. Studies of mortality of atomic bomb survivors. Report 13: Solid cancer and noncancer disease mortality: 1950–1997. Radiat Res. 2003;160(4):381–407.

134. Kalra MK, Maher MM, Toth TL, et al. Strategies for CT radiation dose optimization. Radiology. 2004;230(3):619–28.

135. Ravenel JG, Scalzetti EM, Huda W, Garrisi W. Radiation exposure and image quality in chest CT examinations. AJR Am J Roentgenol. 2001;177(2):279–84.

136. Haaga JR. Radiation dose management: weighing risk versus benefit. AJR Am J Roentgenol. 2001;177(2):289–91.

137. Prasad SR, Wittram C, Shepard JA, McLoud T, Rhea J. Standard-dose and 50%-reduced-dose chest CT: comparing the effect on image quality. AJR Am J Roentgenol. 2002;179(2):461–5.

138. Slovis TL. CT and computed radiography: the pictures are great, but is the radiation dose greater than required? AJR Am J Roentgenol. 2002;179(1):39–41.

139. Zhu X, Yu J, Huang Z. Low-dose chest CT: optimizing radiation protection for patients. AJR Am J Roentgenol. 2004;183(3):809–16.

140. Nickoloff EL, Alderson PO. Radiation exposures to patients from CT: reality, public perception, and policy. AJR Am J Roentgenol. 2001;177(2):285–7.

141. Fitzgerald R, Twiss D, Mehra R, Evans M, Qaiyum M, Collins M. Low-dose computed tomography surveillance of patients with testicular tumours. Clin Oncol (R Coll Radiol). 2004;16(2):158.

142. Wright AR, Collie DA, Williams JR, Hashemi-Malayeri B, Stevenson AJ, Turnbull CM. Pulmonary nodules: effect on detection of spiral CT pitch. Radiology. 1996;199(3):837–41.

143. Rustin GJ, Mead GM, Stenning SP, et al. Randomized trial of two or five computed tomography scans in the surveillance of patients with stage I nonseminomatous germ cell tumors of the testis: Medical Research Council Trial TE08, ISRCTN56475197—the National Cancer Research Institute Testis Cancer Clinical Studies Group. J Clin Oncol. 2007;25:1310–5.

144. Fernandez EB, Colon E, McLeod DG, Moul JW. Efficacy of radiographic chest imaging in patients with testicular cancer. Urology. 1994;44(2):243–8; discussion 8–9.

145. Harvey ML, Geldart TR, Duell R, Mead GM, Tung K. Routine computerised tomographic scans of the thorax in surveillance of stage I testicular non-seminomatous germ-cell cancer–a necessary risk? Ann Oncol. 2002;13(2):237–42.

146. Segal R, Lukka H, Klotz LH, Eady A, Bestic N, Johnston M. Surveillance programs for early stage non-seminomatous testicular cancer: a practice guideline. Can J Urol. 2001;8(1):1184–92.

147. Sharir S, Foster RS, Donohue JP, Jewett MA. What is the appropriate follow-up after treatment? Semin Urol Oncol. 1996;14(1):45–53.

148. Gels ME, Hoekstra HJ, Sleijfer DT, et al. Detection of recurrence in patients with clinical stage I nonseminomatous testicular germ cell tumors and consequences for further follow-up: a single-center 10-year experience. J Clin Oncol. 1995;13(5):1188–94.

149. Cooper JA Jr, White DA, Matthay RA. Drug-induced pulmonary disease. Part 1: Cytotoxic drugs. Am Rev Respir Dis. 1986;133(2):321–40.

150. Aronchick JM, Gefter WB. Drug-induced pulmonary disorders. Semin Roentgenol. 1995;30(1):18–34.

151. Lee-Chiong T. Drug-induced pulmonary disorders. In: Sperber M, editor. Diffuse lung disorders: a comprehensive clinical-radiological overview. Springer; 1999. pp. 403–36.

152. Balikian JP, Jochelson MS, Bauer KA, et al. Pulmonary complications of chemotherapy regimens containing bleomycin. AJR Am J Roentgenol. 1982;139(3):455–61.

153. Webb W, Higgins C. Thoracic imaging: pulmonary and cardiovascular radiology. Lippincott Williams & Wilkins; 2004. pp. 463–74.

154. O'Sullivan JM, Huddart RA, Norman AR, Nicholls J, Dearnaley DP, Horwich A. Predicting the risk of bleomycin lung toxicity in patients with germ-cell tumours. Ann Oncol. 2003;14(1):91–6.

155. Bellamy EA, Husband JE, Blaquiere RM, Law MR. Bleomycin-related lung damage: CT evidence. Radiology. 1985;156(1):155–8.

Chapter 28

Positron Emission Tomography (PET) in Germ Cell Tumors (GCT)

M. De Santis, A. Maj-Hes, and M. Bachner

Introduction

Both the treatment and outcome of germ cell tumors (GCT) have changed with the implementation of cisplatin-based chemotherapy. High cure rates even in advanced tumor stages provide a unique scenario for young cancer survivors who look for optimal patient management with minimal acute and long-term morbidity and toxicity. Non-invasive staging tools like serum tumor marker assays and imaging studies such as computed tomography (CT) both made substantial contributions to this goal. Improved staging and response evaluation help to avoid unnecessary overtreatment by risk-adapted approaches precisely tailored to the individual patient.

However, conventional staging techniques still are prone to considerable over- and understaging attributable to their sensitivity and specificity [1–3].

Positron emission tomography (PET) is a more recent addition to the battery of clinical diagnostic tools. With this imaging technique, a non-invasive method for determining regional metabolic processes has become available. The use of PET in oncology is based on the well-founded assumption that the visualization of metabolic changes often precedes measurable morphologic alterations in neoplastic tissue [4–7]. Thus PET has added a new dimension, i.e., metabolic imaging, to current anatomy-derived imaging techniques.

Physics

The principle underlying positron emission tomography (PET) is that when binding to electrons, positrons from positron-emitting radioisotopes release annihilation gamma rays. These consist of two photons of 511 keV each separating in diametrical directions and are detected by a ring of detectors with opposed scintillation crystals, which recognize coincident radiation events. PET produces both dynamic data like the movements in time of the injected tracer and its distribution in a circumscribed area and static data such as those obtained by whole body scans, which image the structures of interest in three dimensions (coronal, transverse, and sagittal) and are generally used for evaluating cancer patients. Standard tracer *uptake values* (SUVs) are being calculated in an attempt to quantify the intensity of local tracer uptake in the region of interest and to obtain results, which are easily compared with the results at another point in the course of the disease:

SUV = decay corrected maximal region of interest activity/injected dose / body weight

However, the usefulness and the reproducibility of SUVs compared to visual interpretation by an experienced nuclear physicist have repeatedly been questioned [8, 9].

Currently, the most sophisticated standard scanners, i.e., full-ring tomograph scanners [10], have a resolution of 4–5 mm. They detect volumes with positive tracer uptake down to 8–10 mL. The technology involved is complex and the costs incurred are high.

Tracers in GCT

In oncology, $2-^{18}$fluoro-2-deoxy-D-glucose (FDG) is currently the most widely used tracer, because it selectively accumulates in cancer cells. On account of the regionally increased blood flow and the elevated activity of glucose transporters (GluT1) and intracellular hexokinase, cancer cells are avid glucose seekers. ^{18}F substitution at the C2

M. De Santis (✉)
3rd Medical Department - Center for Oncology and Hematology
Ludwig Boltzmann-Institute for Applied Cancer Research Vienna
(LBI-ACR VIEnna)
Kaiser Franz Josef - Spital der Stadt Wien and
Applied Cancer Research Institution for Translational Research Vienna
(ACR-ITR VIEnna)/CEADDP
Kundratstrasse 3, A-1100 Vienna, Austria
maria.desantis@wienkav.at

J.J.M.C.H. de la Rosette et al. (eds.), *Imaging in Oncological Urology*,
DOI 10.1007/978-1-84628-759-6_28, © Springer-Verlag London Limited 2009

of the glucose structure turns ^{18}FDG-6-phosphate into a polar molecule, which cannot be further metabolized and, as cancer cells contain little glucose-6-phosphatase, is trapped in them. These mechanisms contribute to distinguishing active tumor from non-neoplastic cells by its increased tracer uptake [11–13].

A few other tracers have been under investigation for GCTs, among them L-(1-carbon-11)tyrosine [14], which has, however, not been found to be suited for evaluating residual masses in GCT.

The following physiologic issues and limitations of FDG PET should be considered before clinical decision-making with the help of FDG PET:

Physiologic FDG Uptake

FDG also actively accumulates in normal tissues of the brain, the myocardium, the liver, the smooth muscles, and the bone marrow and is eliminated along renal and urinary pathways. Three-dimensional imaging and iterative reconstruction help to differentiate these superimposed structures from neoplastic tissue [15].

False Positive FDG PET Results

High FDG uptake is not totally tumor specific. It is well known that inflammatory and granulomatous tissue such as sarcoidosis show extensive tracer uptake caused by elevated macrophage activity [16–18]. This is also true for inflammatory reactions up to several months after irradiation [19, 20]. Active [^{18}F]FDG uptake by phagocytes within abscesses or by granulation tissue surrounding abscesses causes false positive results, whereas chemically sterile abscesses do not accumulate FDG [4]. Macrophage accumulation due to resorption of necrotic post-treatment tumor tissue will cause false positive FDG PET studies. Most importantly, there may be a metabolic flare within the first days after chemotherapy. Therefore, PET should not be performed too early in germ cell residual tumors after chemotherapy, i.e., within 2–4 weeks post-chemotherapy [17, 21, 22].

False Negative FDG PET Results

The timing of PET studies is of utmost importance. FDG uptake by neoplastic tissue may be reduced within 2 weeks of exposure to cytostatics [16]. This phenomenon is tumor- and treatment specific. In gastrointestinal stroma tumors (GIST), for instance, reduced uptake (true negative result) after exposure to imatinib mesylate has been described after only 24 h [23].

The size of the lesions to be evaluated is important as well. Due to the limited resolution we do not expect FDG PET to be positive in low-volume disease, e.g., lesions < 5 mm. But PET may detect extremely active lesions between 5 and 10 mm in size [5, 24–30].

PET for Non-invasive Tumor Staging

Consistent prospective data have established the clinical role of FDG PET in oncology particularly for staging non-small-cell lung cancer, colorectal cancer, and melanoma, for evaluating single pulmonary lesions, for detecting liver metastases, and for staging cancers with unknown primaries [11, 13, 31–35]. In Non-Hodgkin's lymphoma and Hodgkin's disease PET has become crucial for staging, treatment evaluation, early detection of relapse, and most recently for distinguishing aggressive and indolent disease [36–41].

FDG PET in Germ Cell Tumors (GCT)

Germ cell tumors as well as their secondaries are generally characterized by a high FDG uptake. Pure seminomas accumulate even more FDG than non-seminomatous lesions [5, 16, 42]. This very fact led numerous research teams to investigate the clinical role of FDG PET in GCT.

The following chapter will summarize the current state-of-the-art knowledge about the use of PET in different clinical situations during the treatment of germ cell tumors. Evidence derived from published trials and its consequences will be discussed. The pros and cons of PET scanning will be put into the context of crucial points in clinical decision-making. These include

- Staging at presentation
- Response evaluation
- Management of relapse

Staging at Presentation

Non-seminomatous and Seminomatous Germ Cell Tumors (NSGCT and SGCT)

Staging of GCT at presentation in clinical stages I and II with CT scans has a limited accuracy of about 70% [2, 30, 43, 44]. After staging by CT 20–30% of clinical stage II patients turn out to be stage I pathologically. On the other hand, CT underestimates the pathologic stage in up to 30% of patients

[43, 45]. The smaller the lymph nodes the higher the sensitivity, but the lower the specificity [2, 46, 47].

The role of FDG PET for initial staging in unselected NSGCT and SGCT patients was the subject of investigation in several trials [5, 16, 22, 24–29], two of which [22, 29] reported a higher sensitivity and a higher negative predictive value (NPV) for PET versus CT. The specificities of the two methods were comparable. No clinical consequences were drawn. Recently, a German group investigated the sensitivity, specificity, and accuracy of FDG PET in stage I/II NSGCT patients scheduled for primary retroperitoneal lymph node dissection (RPLND). There was no difference between CT and FDG PET in terms of false negative results, especially in small lesions [30].

In most of the studies PET failed to detect small (< 1 or < 0.5 cm) retroperitoneal lymph nodes [5, 24–30] and mature teratomas [24, 28]. One of the positive PET scans in one trial was attributable to sarcoidosis [16]. None of the trials unequivocally established a benefit of PET versus conventional staging with tumor markers and CT at presentation.

Summary

To date there is no proof of a benefit of PET for staging at presentation.

Clinical Stage I Non-seminomatous Germ Cell Tumors (NSGCT)

After orchiectomy about 30% of clinical stage I NSGCT patients staged with conventional techniques like (spiral-) CT scans will relapse within the first 2 years after the diagnosis.

The most accurate staging technique for the retroperitoneum, i.e., retroperitoneal lymphadenectomy, is very invasive for just a staging procedure, and its cure rate is no better than 10–15% [1, 47]. Systematic adjuvant short-term chemotherapy of high-risk clinical stage I patients in terms of risk-adapted treatment [48] is tantamount to overtreatment in as many as 50% of cases. Therefore, improved staging tools would be of utmost importance in clinical stage I GCT.

Three of four trials examining FDG PET for staging clinical stage I NSGCT patients with no more than a total of 27 patients correlated PET data with histopathology data obtained from subsequent (RPLND) [24, 27, 28]. In all three trials PET failed to improve clinical staging. Of 22 negative PET scans, seven proved to be false negative (NPV 68%): in six patients the histologically positive lymph nodes were smaller than 0.5 cm and in the remaining patient PET failed to detect a mature teratoma. PET (sensitivity 42%) correctly identified no more than 5 out of 12 metastasizing patients [24, 27, 28]. In the fourth study by Lassen et al. [49], PET

data of 46 patients were compared to clinical follow-up data collected during surveillance. In this prospective trial, by contrast, 7 out of 10 relapses were correctly predicted (sensitivity 70%) and no more than 3 out of 39 negative PET scans proved to be false negative (NPV 92%). This prompted the authors to conclude that FDG PET had improved clinical staging in their patients. A CT review later on classified two patients to be stage II, who finally had to be removed from the analysis. After all, the sensitivity of FDG PET in this study fell to 50% [50]. Based on the initial results of this trial [49], the Medical Research Council initiated a prospective large-scale trial to investigate the role of FDG PET in high-risk clinical stage I NSGCT. PET-positive patients enrolled in this trial were subjected to adjuvant chemotherapy, while those with negative PET scans were put on surveillance. The study was closed early in 2005, after 33 out of 88 PET-negative patients had relapsed, with a 1 year relapse-free rate of 63.3% instead of the expected 2-year relapse-free rate of > 90% [51].

Summary

FDG PET has no role for staging or early detection of micrometastases in clinical stage I NSGCT.

Clinical Stage I Seminoma

Clinical stage I seminoma patients overall run a relapse risk of 18% [52] without further adjuvant treatment. Patients are usually offered adjuvant standard radiation therapy or are put on a surveillance protocol. Adjuvant chemotherapy with carboplatin has become a third option [53, 54], because randomized data still lack sufficient follow-up time and peer-reviewed publication. Any kind of adjuvant treatment in clinical stage I seminoma causes an overtreatment rate of about 80%.

So far, no scientific evidence is available for a positive role of PET in this clinical setting. Albers and Müller-Matheis [24, 27] described 31 clinical stage I seminoma patients, all of them with negative PET scans. But as all of them had undergone adjuvant radiotherapy, there is no way of telling whether the PET data was correct or not.

The role of PET in an adjuvant setting should be analyzed in patients under surveillance.

Summary

FDG PET has no advantage over CT in staging clinical stage I SGCT.

Clinical Stage II Disease/NSGCT

In clinical stage II, particularly in stage IIa disease, pathologic staging with RPLND shows that in up to 25% of cases patients are overstaged by CT [43]. FDG PET data for this clinical situation are contradictory: in a study by Albers et al. [24] CT staging was false positive in four out of nine clinical stage II NSGCT patients, while PET correctly staged all nine patients. Of the seven patients with clinical stage II disease contributed by Spermon et al. [28], all were correctly staged by CT, while PET failed to detect metastatic embryonic carcinoma in a retroperitoneal lymph node 1.2 cm in size and metastatic mature teratoma in another.

Summary

There is no evidence-based support for the use of FDG PET in stage II NSCGT.

Response Evaluation

Post-chemotherapy Residual Masses in NSGCT

After completion of cisplatin-based chemotherapy, one quarter to one third of all patients with metastases of NSGCT present with residual masses, although their tumor marker levels have returned to normal (marker-negative partial remissions; PRm-). These patients are candidates for residual tumor surgery. Multiple series of histological studies after RPLND show that only 40–45% of these residuals consist of necrotic/fibrotic tissue, while 10–20% harbor viable tumor and 30–45% mature teratoma [55, 56]. The latter two, viable tumor and mature teratoma, are the source of recurrences and therefore have to be removed. Complete resection of all residual NSGCT lesions is the only way of curing this group of patients [57, 58].

However, resection of mere necrosis/fibrosis only does not offer any therapeutic benefits. Neither retrospective trials nor predictive models [59] based on regression analyses have so far reliably predicted the histology of the residual masses. Therefore, several authors [16, 17, 27–29, 42, 60–63] evaluated FDG PET for its predictive potential in this clinical setting. Four of them were prospective trials [17, 27, 42, 61].

The authors unequivocally found that PET predicted viable tumor within the residual lesions with a high measure of diagnostic accuracy, except in very small residuals. Unfortunately, FDG PET failed to distinguish between mature teratoma and necrosis/fibrosis, because both accumulate very little or no FDG. Therefore, FDG PET does not help in deciding for or against surgery. Based on kinetic modeling, only Sugawara et al. [63] reported differences in the kinetic rate constants of FDG uptake between mature teratoma and necrosis/fibrosis, albeit in no more than six patients.

The German multicenter trial, first presented as an abstract in 2006, showed an accuracy of only 57% for FDG PET for predicting vital tumor and teratoma in 141 patients with post-chemotherapy residual tumors. There was also a high rate of false positive results. Interestingly, the PET scans had been performed at an average of only 8.5 days after chemotherapy [30].

The studies quoted provided two important messages for the proper use and interpretation of PET in post-chemotherapy patients: (1) In some of them [16, 17, 27–29] inflammatory reactions with abundant macrophages accompanying tumor necrosis seen histologically were the most common cause of false positive PET scans. (2) FDG PET studies done shortly after chemotherapy (within less than 2 weeks) may be false negative because of a putative suppression of tumor cell metabolic activity regardless of their final treatment response [16]. Both of these observations suggest that an interval of several weeks post-chemotherapy should be allowed for PET scans.

Summary

Current evidence does not support the use of FDG PET for post-chemotherapy evaluation of NSGCT lesions.

Post-chemotherapy Residual Masses in SGCT

Residual lesions after chemotherapy of bulky SGCT are expected to be present in 50–75% of patients. Overall, less than 20% of the resected residual masses harbor viable tumor. Therefore, the management of seminoma residuals is controversial. Trying to find risk factors for the presence of viable tumor within the residual lesions, some authors found that the likelihood rose with the residual tumor size [64, 65]. The cut-off was drawn at a size of 3 cm.

The pronounced desmoplastic reaction of the tissue surrounding residual seminoma masses makes their resection technically demanding. Consequently, some authors prefer surveillance and reserve surgery for patients with progressive lesions [66], while others only resect lesions larger than 3 cm in diameter [65]. The advantage of FDG PET in SGCT compared to its use in NSGCT is that the presence of mature teratoma is extremely rare in SGCTs [65]. FDG PET, on the other hand, reliably differentiates viable tumor from necrosis/fibrosis in residual NSGCT. Therefore, two research groups examined seminoma residuals with FDG

PET in prospective trials comparing the results with histologic data or the clinical outcome.

In the single-center Indiana University study [67], only 1 out of 29 patients undergoing PET scanning at arbitrary intervals post-chemotherapy was PET-positive. The authors concluded that FDG PET was not helpful in distinguishing necrosis from viable seminoma, because it was false positive in one and false negative in five cases. In the Austrian–German prospective multicenter trial, by contrast, an interval of at least 4 weeks post-chemotherapy was mandatory for PET scanning. Preliminary data from the first 37 PET scans showed the specificity and the positive predictive value (PPV) to be 100% at a sensitivity of 89% and a NPV of 97% [64]. The discrepancies between these data and those found in the Indiana University study prompted the Austrian–German researchers to continue the trial and to expand it to 51 patients with post-chemotherapy residual masses and 56 FDG PET scans: All residual lesions > 3 cm and 95% of those ≤ 3 cm were correctly predicted by FDG PET. The specificity, sensitivity, PPV, and NPV of FDG PET was 100, 80, 100, and 96%, respectively (Fig. 28.1). This is clearly superior to CT. The authors concluded that FDG PET was the best predictor of viable residual tumor in post-chemotherapy seminoma residuals and should be used

as a standard tool for clinical decision-making in this patient group. The main advantage of using FDG PET in this clinical setting is that, in patients with residual lesions > 3 cm, even in very large lesions, surgery can be omitted safely, if PET scans are negative. PET-positive residual lesions, according to this data set, must be regarded as harboring viable tumor and should be resected, if technically possible [68].

Summary

FDG PET combined with CT studies for the evaluation of pure seminoma residuals can be regarded as a standard tool for clinical decision-making.

Early Prediction of Treatment Response to Salvage Chemotherapy

In some tumor entities FDG PET proved to be valuable for predicting treatment response non-invasively at an early point in time [23, 41, 69–71]. For first-line chemotherapy of germ cell tumors with a clear standard treatment and excellent cure rates, early response evaluation has no benefit. In patients with poor-prognosis GCT or germ cell tumors in relapse, however, strategies for a better and earlier response evaluation in order to modify ineffective but toxic chemotherapy regimens are warranted. Bokemeyer et al. [72] addressed this problem in 23 patients with relapsed germ cell cancer enrolled in a high-dose salvage chemotherapy program. FDG PET scans were recorded before conventional-dose induction and before high-dose treatment together with the usual tumor marker profiles and CT scans. The results were compared with the histologic response and/or the clinical course over 6 months following high-dose treatment (relapse versus freedom from progression). FDG PET showed a sensitivity, specificity, PPV, and NPV of 100, 78, 88 and 100%, respectively, and was superior to tumor marker assays, CT and both of them (Fig. 28.2). It therefore seemed to be a valuable addition to the established prognostic model for high-dose chemotherapy of germ cell tumors [73]. However, the authors cautioned that, at this point in time, it was not justified to derive treatment decisions from PET results alone. Larger studies are necessary to confirm this approach.

Summary

To date FDG PET has not been proven to be a reliable tool for changing treatment decisions in poor-risk or relapsed germ cell tumor patients.

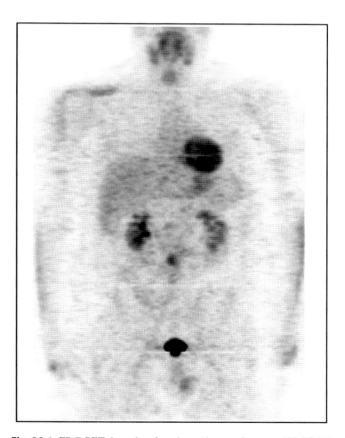

Fig. 28.1 FDG PET 6 weeks after chemotherapy for stage IIC SGCT. Histologically proven true positive residual lesion

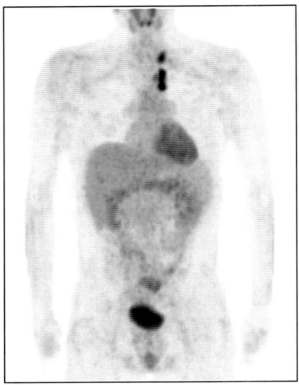

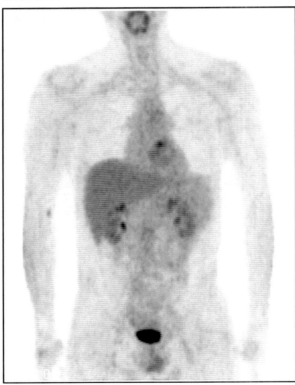

Fig. 28.2 a) Residual mediastinal lymph nodes, SGCT; true positive PET scan after completion of first line chemotherapy with clinical relapse 2 months later. b) True negative FDG PET in the same patient after first cycle of high dose chemotherapy. No residual tumor resection. Clinical follow-up and shrinkage of mediastinal residuals for >3 years

Relapse

Diagnosis of Relapse

About 20% of all patients with germ cell cancer relapse. Diagnostic evidence for this clinical situation is a rise in tumor marker levels and radiologic (rarely clinical) signs. For those who relapse with rising marker levels and unequivocal radiologic/clinical signs of progressive disease the guidelines for management are clear and well established: salvage chemotherapy, standard or high dose, followed by salvage surgery, or primary salvage surgery are the standard treatment options. For all other relapses FDG PET might be a valuable diagnostic tool. The key situations include

1. Rising tumor markers unmatched by clinical/radiologic abnormalities
2. Radiologic evidence of a new lesion or an increase in the volume of a pre-existing one unassociated with rising marker levels
3. Rising tumor marker levels in the presence of multiple residual lesions unchanged in size.

Although FDG PET appears to hold promise for answering these questions, only few reports on relapsing germ cell cancer patients, all of them retrospective or just case reports, are available [60, 62, 74].

Hain et al. [60] reported all 12 positive PET scans of 23 patients in marker-only relapse to be truly positive. PET clearly identified the site of the disease. However, 4 out of 11 scans were false negative. Subsequently, three of these PET scans turned positive and were the only imaging investigation to identify the site of the disease. In a report from France [74] FDG PET also was the only imaging study to identify the site of the disease in five out of seven patients with elevated markers. Sanchez et al. [62] found three true positive and two true negative FDG PET scans in patients with elevated markers and non-contributory CT scans and patients with normal marker levels and increasing lesions on CT, respectively, the latter mature teratoma by histologic evidence.

A patient reported by Reinhardt et al. [75] presented with negative markers and a negative FDG PET scan of a growing retroperitoneal bulk. Not surprisingly, this bulky disease proved to be a mature "growing teratoma" on histology and therefore was true negative. In another case report FDG PET showed a contralateral testicular lesion in a clinically and sonographically normal testicle to be the underlying cause of an AFP rise [76].

Summary

FDG PET can be expected to be helpful for planning elective salvage surgery in chemoresistant patients and in those with multiple residual lesions to be removed. However, evidence from pertinent studies is not available.

Conclusions

In GCT, FDG PET is not superior to conventional staging tools for staging at presentation. It is not safe for detecting lesions less than 1 cm in size and mature teratoma.

FDG PET should be used as a standard diagnostic tool in patients with pure seminomatous residual lesions. It predicts the persistence of viable tumor in this clinical situation with a high diagnostic accuracy. FDG PET-negative SGCT residual lesions may be observed safely.

NSGCT patients with residual masses do not benefit from FDG PET. Residual mature teratoma, which is PET-negative, will be missed, and has to be resected at any rate, just like PET-positive residual lesions.

In relapsing patients with a mismatch between tumor marker levels and imaging data, FDG PET may be helpful in selected cases, particularly if salvage surgery is considered.

References

1. Carlsson-Farrelly E, Boquist L, Ljungberg B. Accuracy of clinical staging in non-seminomatous testicular cancer – a single centre experience of retroperitoneal lymph node dissection. Scand J Urol Nephrol. 1995;29(4):501–6.
2. Fernandez EB, et al. Retroperitoneal imaging with third and fourth generation computed axial tomography in clinical stage I nonseminomatous germ cell tumors. Urology. 1994;44(4):548–52.
3. Rustin GJ, et al. Consensus statement on circulating tumour markers and staging patients with germ cell tumours. Prog Clin Biol Res. 1990;357:277–84.
4. Kubota R, et al. Intratumoral distribution of fluorine-18-fluorodeoxyglucose in vivo: high accumulation in macrophages and granulation tissues studied by microautoradiography. J Nucl Med. 1992;33(11):1972–80.
5. Wilson CB, et al. Imaging metastatic testicular germ cell tumours with 18FDG positron emission tomography: prospects for detection and management. Eur J Nucl Med. 1995;22(6):508–13.
6. Hoekstra OS, et al. Early treatment response in malignant lymphoma, as determined by planar fluorine-18-fluorodeoxyglucose scintigraphy. J Nucl Med. 1993;34(10):1706–10.
7. Wahl RL, et al. Metabolic monitoring of breast cancer chemohormonotherapy using positron emission tomography: initial evaluation. J Clin Oncol. 1993;11(11):2101–11.
8. Engel H, et al. Whole-body PET: physiological and artifactual fluorodeoxyglucose accumulations. J Nucl Med. 1996;37(3):441–6.
9. Keyes JW Jr. SUV: standard uptake or silly useless value? J Nucl Med. 1995;36(10):1836–9.
10. Landoni C, et al. Comparison of dual-head coincidence PET versus ring PET in tumor patients. J Nucl Med. 1999;40(10):1617–22.
11. Bomanji JB, Costa DC, Ell PJ. Clinical role of positron emission tomography in oncology. Lancet Oncol. 2001;2(3):157–64.
12. Lienhard GE, et al. How cells absorb glucose. Sci Am. 1992;266(1):86–91.
13. Nabi HA, Zubeldia JM. Clinical applications of (18)F-FDG in oncology. J Nucl Med Technol. 2002;30(1):3–9; quiz 10–1.
14. Kole AC, et al. L-[1-carbon-11]tyrosine imaging of metastatic testicular nonseminoma germ-cell tumors. J Nucl Med.1998;39(6):1027–9.
15. Vesselle HJ, Miraldi FD. FDG PET of the retroperitoneum: normal anatomy, variants, pathologic conditions, and strategies to avoid diagnostic pitfalls. Radiographics. 1998;18(4):805–23; discussion 823–4.
16. Cremerius U, et al. FDG PET for detection and therapy control of metastatic germ cell tumor. J Nucl Med. 1998;39(5):815–22.
17. Nuutinen JM, et al. Detection of residual tumours in postchemotherapy testicular cancer by FDG-PET. Eur J Cancer. 1997;33(8):1234–41.
18. Strauss LG. Fluorine-18 deoxyglucose and false-positive results: a major problem in the diagnostics of oncological patients. Eur J Nucl Med. 1996;23(10):1409–15.
19. Engenhart R, et al. Therapy monitoring of presacral recurrences after high-dose irradiation: value of PET, CT, CEA and pain score. Strahlenther Onkol. 1992;168(4):203–12.
20. Haberkorn U, et al. PET studies of fluorodeoxyglucose metabolism in patients with recurrent colorectal tumors receiving radiotherapy. J Nucl Med. 1991;32(8):1485–90.
21. Cohade C, Wahl RL. PET scanning and measuring the impact of treatment. Cancer J. 2002;8(2):119–34.
22. Hain SF, et al. Fluorodeoxyglucose PET in the initial staging of germ cell tumours. Eur J Nucl Med. 2000;27(5):590–4.
23. Stroobants S, et al. 18FDG-Positron emission tomography for the early prediction of response in advanced soft tissue sarcoma treated with imatinib mesylate (Glivec). Eur J Cancer. 2003;39(14):2012–20.
24. Albers P, et al. Positron emission tomography in the clinical staging of patients with stage I and II testicular germ cell tumors. Urology. 1999;53(4):808–11.
25. Cremerius U, et al. Does positron emission tomography using 18-fluoro-2-deoxyglucose improve clinical staging of testicular cancer? – Results of a study in 50 patients. Urology. 1999;54(5):900–4.
26. Hofer C, et al. Diagnosis and monitoring of urological tumors using positron emission tomography. Eur Urol. 2001;40(5):481–7.
27. Muller-Mattheis V, et al. Positron emission tomography with [18 F]-2-fluoro-2-deoxy-D-glucose (18FDG-PET) in diagnosis of retroperitoneal lymph node metastases of testicular tumors. Urologe A. 1998;37(6):609–20.
28. Spermon JR, et al. The role of (18)fluoro-2-deoxyglucose positron emission tomography in initial staging and re-staging after chemotherapy for testicular germ cell tumours. BJU Int. 2002;89(6):549–56.
29. Tsatalpas P, et al. Diagnostic value of 18F-FDG positron emission tomography for detection and treatment control of malignant germ cell tumors. Urol Int. 2002;68(3):157–63.
30. De Wit M, Hartmann M, Brenner W, Weißbach L, Amthauer H, Franzius C, et al. [18F]-FDG-PET in germ cell tumors following chemotherapy: Results of the German multicenter trial. J Clin Oncol, 2006 ASCO Annual Meeting Proceedings Part I. 24(18S) (June 20 Suppl) 2006:4521.
31. Eary JF. Nuclear medicine in cancer diagnosis. Lancet. 1999;354(9181):853–7.

32. Hustinx R, et al. Clinical evaluation of whole-body 18F-fluorodeoxyglucose positron emission tomography in the detection of liver metastases. Ann Oncol. 1998;9(4):397–401.

33. Lowe VJ, et al. Prospective investigation of positron emission tomography in lung nodules. J Clin Oncol. 1998;16(3):1075–84.

34. Moog F, et al. 18-F-fluorodeoxyglucose-positron emission tomography as a new approach to detect lymphomatous bone marrow. J Clin Oncol. 1998;16(2):603–9.

35. Regelink G, et al. Detection of unknown primary tumours and distant metastases in patients with cervical metastases: value of FDG-PET versus conventional modalities. Eur J Nucl Med Mol Imaging. 2002;29(8):1024–30.

36. Spaepen K, et al. Early restaging positron emission tomography with (18)F-fluorodeoxyglucose predicts outcome in patients with aggressive non-Hodgkin's lymphoma. Ann Oncol. 2002;13(9):1356–63.

37. Jerusalem G, et al. Early detection of relapse by whole-body positron emission tomography in the follow-up of patients with Hodgkin's disease. Ann Oncol. 2003;14(1):123–30.

38. Jerusalem G, et al. Whole-body positron emission tomography using 18F-fluorodeoxyglucose for posttreatment evaluation in Hodgkin's disease and non-Hodgkin's lymphoma has higher diagnostic and prognostic value than classical computed tomography scan imaging. Blood. 1999;94(2):429–33.

39. Kostakoglu L, et al. PET predicts prognosis after 1 cycle of chemotherapy in aggressive lymphoma and Hodgkin's disease. J Nucl Med. 2002;43(8):1018–27.

40. Schoder H, et al. Intensity of 18fluorodeoxyglucose uptake in positron emission tomography distinguishes between indolent and aggressive non-Hodgkin's lymphoma. J Clin Oncol. 2005;23(21):4643–51.

41. Juweid ME, et al. Response assessment of aggressive non-Hodgkin's lymphoma by integrated International Workshop Criteria and fluorine-18-fluorodeoxyglucose positron emission tomography. J Clin Oncol. 2005;23(21):4652–61.

42. Stephens AW, et al. Positron emission tomography evaluation of residual radiographic abnormalities in postchemotherapy germ cell tumor patients. J Clin Oncol. 1996;14(5):1637–41.

43. Donohue JP, et al. The role of retroperitoneal lymphadenectomy in clinical stage B testis cancer: the Indiana University experience (1965 to 1989). J Urol. 1995;153(1):85–9.

44. Stephenson AJ, et al. Retroperitoneal lymph node dissection for nonseminomatous germ cell testicular cancer: impact of patient selection factors on outcome. J Clin Oncol. 2005;23(12):2781–8.

45. Gatti JM, Stephenson RA. Staging of testis cancer. Combining serum markers, histologic parameters, and radiographic imaging. Urol Clin North Am. 1998;25(3):397–403.

46. Hilton S, et al. CT detection of retroperitoneal lymph node metastases in patients with clinical stage I testicular nonseminomatous germ cell cancer: assessment of size and distribution criteria. AJR Am J Roentgenol. 1997;169(2):521–5.

47. Donohue JP, et al. Retroperitoneal lymphadenectomy for clinical stage A testis cancer (1965 to 1989): modifications of technique and impact on ejaculation. J Urol. 1993;149(2):237–43.

48. Pont J, et al. Adjuvant chemotherapy for high-risk clinical stage I nonseminomatous testicular germ cell cancer: long-term results of a prospective trial. J Clin Oncol. 1996;14(2):441–8.

49. Lassen U, et al. Positron emission tomography with 18F-Fluoro-Deoxyglucose in clinical stage I non-seminomatous germ cell tumors. ASCO Annual Meeting. 2000:1337.

50. Lassen U, et al. Whole-body FDG-PET in patients with stage I non-seminomatous germ cell tumours. Eur J Nucl Med Mol Imaging. 2003;30(3):396–402.

51. Huddart RA, O'Doherty MJ, Padhani A, Rustin GJS, Mead GM, Joffe JK, et al. 18Fluorodeoxyglucose positron emission tomography in the prediction of relapse in patients with high-risk, clinical stage I nonseminomatous germ cell tumors: Preliminary Report of MRC Trial TE22—The NCRI Testis Tumour Clinical Study Group. J Clin Oncol. 2007;3090–5.

52. Warde P, et al. Prognostic factors for relapse in stage I seminoma managed by surveillance: a pooled analysis. J Clin Oncol. 2002;20(22):4448–52.

53. Oliver RT, Mason MD, Mead GM, von der Maase H, Rustin GJ, Joffe JK, et al. MRC TE19 collaborators and the EORTC 30982 collaborators. Radiotherapy versus single-dose carboplatin in adjuvant treatment of stage I seminoma: a randomised trial. Lancet. 2005;366(9482):293–300.

54. Oliver RT, Mead GM, Fogarty PJ, et al. Radiotherapy versus carboplatin for stage I seminoma: Updated analysis of the MRC/EORTC randomized trial (ISRCTN27163214). J Clin Oncol 2008;26 (May 20 suppl; abstr 1).

55. Donohue JP, et al. Correlation of computerized tomographic changes and histological findings in 80 patients having radical retroperitoneal lymph node dissection after chemotherapy for testis cancer. J Urol. 1987;137(6):1176–9.

56. Toner GC, et al. Adjunctive surgery after chemotherapy for nonseminomatous germ cell tumors: recommendations for patient selection. J Clin Oncol. 1990;8(10):1683–94.

57. Fizazi K, et al. Viable malignant cells after primary chemotherapy for disseminated nonseminomatous germ cell tumors: prognostic factors and role of postsurgery chemotherapy – results from an international study group. J Clin Oncol. 2001;19(10):2647–57.

58. Loehrer PJ Sr, et al. Teratoma following cisplatin-based combination chemotherapy for nonseminomatous germ cell tumors: a clinicopathological correlation. J Urol. 1986;135(6):1183–9.

59. Steyerberg EW, et al. Validity of predictions of residual retroperitoneal mass histology in nonseminomatous testicular cancer. J Clin Oncol. 1998;16(1):269–74.

60. Hain SF, et al. Fluorodeoxyglucose positron emission tomography in the evaluation of germ cell tumours at relapse. Br J Cancer. 2000;83(7):863–9.

61. Kollmannsberger C, et al. Prospective comparison of [18F] fluorodeoxyglucose positron emission tomography with conventional assessment by computed tomography scans and serum tumor markers for the evaluation of residual masses in patients with nonseminomatous germ cell carcinoma. Cancer. 2002;94(9):2353–62.

62. Sanchez D, et al. 18F-fluoro-2-deoxyglucose-positron emission tomography in the evaluation of nonseminomatous germ cell tumours at relapse. BJU Int. 2002;89(9):912–6.

63. Sugawara Y, et al. Germ cell tumor: differentiation of viable tumor, mature teratoma, and necrotic tissue with FDG PET and kinetic modeling. Radiology. 1999;211(1):249–56.

64. De Santis M, et al. Predictive impact of 2-18fluoro-2-deoxy-D-glucose positron emission tomography for residual postchemotherapy masses in patients with bulky seminoma. J Clin Oncol. 2001;19(17):3740–4.

65. Puc HS, et al. Management of residual mass in advanced seminoma: results and recommendations from the Memorial Sloan-Kettering Cancer Center. J Clin Oncol. 1996;14(2):454–60.

66. Schultz SM, et al. Management of postchemotherapy residual mass in patients with advanced seminoma: Indiana University experience. J Clin Oncol. 1989;7(10):1497–503.

67. Ganjoo KN, et al. Positron emission tomography scans in the evaluation of postchemotherapy residual masses in patients with seminoma. J Clin Oncol. 1999;17(11):3457–60.

68. De Santis M, et al. 2-18fluoro-deoxy-D-glucose positron emission tomography is a reliable predictor for viable tumor

in postchemotherapy seminoma: an update of the prospective multicentric SEMPET trial. J Clin Oncol. 2004;22(6): 1034–9.

69. Findlay M, et al. Noninvasive monitoring of tumor metabolism using fluorodeoxyglucose and positron emission tomography in colorectal cancer liver metastases: correlation with tumor response to fluorouracil. J Clin Oncol. 1996;14(3):700–8.

70. Schelling M, et al. Positron emission tomography using [(18)F]Fluorodeoxyglucose for monitoring primary chemotherapy in breast cancer. J Clin Oncol. 2000;18(8): 1689–95.

71. Smith IC, et al. Positron emission tomography using [(18)F]-fluorodeoxy-D-glucose to predict the pathologic response of breast cancer to primary chemotherapy. J Clin Oncol. 2000;18(8): 1676–88.

72. Bokemeyer C, et al. Early prediction of treatment response to high-dose salvage chemotherapy in patients with relapsed germ cell cancer using [(18)F]FDG PET. Br J Cancer. 2002;86(4): 506–11.

73. Beyer J, et al. High-dose chemotherapy as salvage treatment in germ cell tumors: a multivariate analysis of prognostic variables. J Clin Oncol. 1996;14(10):2638–45.

74. Maszelin P, et al. Fluorodeoxyglucose (FDO) positron emission tomography (PET) in testicular germ cell tumors in adults: preliminary French clinical evaluation, development of the technique and its clinical applications. Prog Urol. 2000;10(6):1190–9.

75. Reinhardt MJ, et al. FDG-PET evaluation of retroperitoneal metastases of testicular cancer before and after chemotherapy. J Nucl Med. 1997;38(1):99–101.

76. Wolf G, et al. Diagnosis of a contralateral second testicular carcinoma by F18-FDG PET. Onkologie. 2003;26(2):155–7.

Chapter 29

Considerations: Imaging in Testis Carcinoma

M.A.S. Jewett

Since the introduction of cisplatinum-based combination chemotherapy more than 30 years ago, there have been many changes in the management of germ cell cancer of the testis. The most significant changes have been driven by advances in medical imaging. Coupled with better understanding of the patterns of disease progression, of prognostic factors including the use of tumor markers and improved surgery, imaging advances have resulted in stage migration at diagnosis, earlier detection of relapse, better characterization of residual masses, and has led to reduced therapeutic radiation exposure. More patients can be spared treatment and those that need treatment can be treated earlier. CT scanning was being introduced at the same time as the discovery that cisplatinum was the most active chemotherapeutic agent. The improved outcomes are therefore multifactorial.

The excellent introductory overview by Professor Peter Albers has been expanded by both Dr. Harisinghani and Dr. De Santis (with an exhaustive reference list of new imaging techniques). They have discussed conventional imaging techniques, cross-sectional imaging techniques, nuclear scanning, and PET in detail. I will provide an overview with comments organized by the steps and problems in the clinic based on my clinical experience managing these patients in a multidisciplinary setting for many years at the Princess Margaret Hospital at the University of Toronto. I will not reference comments if the relevant reference has been included in the above contributions.

Diagnosis

Testicular germ cell tumors (TGCT) are suspected by clinical examination and history with supporting evidence from scrotal ultrasonography. The final diagnosis is made by partial or radical orchiectomy with occasional needle core biopsy or fine needle aspiration (FNA) for cytology of larger retroperitoneal or other nodal metastases in the face of advanced disease. Scrotal imaging is useful but not diagnostic alone and is rarely a reason not to operate. The imaging entity of testicular microlithiasis has received attention and testis size and location can be assessed with various imaging modalities [1]. If partial orchiectomy is more widely adopted, sonography will help to select appropriate patients. Extragonadal GCTs are usually suspected by exclusion when there are normal testes to palpation and on imaging. Various testicular abnormalities are seen after chemotherapy or in patients with extragonadal retroperitoneal GCT that raise the possibility of a "burned out" primary. This may predict a better prognosis than the usual extragonadal primary.

Initial Staging

If we assume that the incidence of seminomas and non-seminomas are about the same and that 80% of seminomas and 40% of non-seminomas present without clinical evidence of metastases, six out of ten new patients will have negative imaging after orchiectomy and five of these will remain relapse free without further treatment. These estimates are based on observations made with patients managed by initial surveillance. Therefore, at the present time, fully 50% of all new patients could be treated by orchiectomy alone. This proportion may also increase with improved imaging techniques and definition of other prognostic factors. Most metastases occur through lymphatics with well-understood drainage patterns to the retroperitoneal nodes. It is convenient to think of the aorta as the midline so that left tumors metastasize primarily to the ipsilateral para-aortic nodes. Conversely, right tumors metastasize to the interaortocaval nodes. These largely predictable patterns have made interpretation of staging CT scans more accurate. When nodal metastases occur, retrograde and antegrade spread may occur so that nodal areas such as in the root of the

M.A.S. Jewett (✉)
Division of Urology, University of Toronto, 610 University Avenue,
3-124, Toronto, Ontario, Canada M5G 2C4, m.jewett@utoronto.ca

mesentery may become involved. These areas may be difficult to appreciate as surrounding bowel may obscure the margins. A minor but important point is that the course of the ipsilateral vas deferens should be followed on staging imaging to exclude nodal disease in the pelvis, particularly in aggressive tumours. Metastases in this site may not be detected at initial staging so all restaging imaging should be reviewed, particularly after chemotherapy, when growing teratoma may make metastases visible. Lymphatic drainage from the retroperitoneal nodes is thought to occur via the cisterna chyla to the posterior mediastinal nodes and sometimes to the left supraclavicular nodes before becoming hematogenous. Occasionally, direct hematogenous spread appears to occur with or without lymphatic spread resulting in visceral metastases to lung, brain, liver, and bone. Direct extension from nodal masses can also occur to involve the spine. Local spread is rare, even with scrotal violation at the time of orchiectomy or biopsy.

Bipedal lymphography is of historical interest for all practical purposes. We have not performed this procedure for testicular cancer for more than 20 years. CT scans have replaced it.

The impact of digital PACS systems has been tremendous. Images can be accessed remotely and most importantly, manipulated by the clinician or imager to produce coronal reconstructions (more and more appreciated by all observers) as well as axial images. Intravenous and oral contrast use has reduced the false-positive rate by better identification of loops of bowel and anomalous vessels. Venous anatomy is variable and in the past, retrocaval veins, large lumbar veins, incomplete involution of left hemiazygous veins, etc., led to overstaging the retroperitoneum.

Finally the role of a plain chest X-ray in staging and follow-up is somewhat controversial and may be replaced by multidetector CT scanners. The latter innovation may allow us to eliminate contrast and reduce diagnostic radiation exposure in the abdomen and pelvis as well.

Imaging for Relapse on Surveillance

We know that currently 15–20% of all stage I patients managed by initial active surveillance will relapse and were therefore understaged. Most relapses will occur in the retroperitoneum and a few may not be detected for years. Therefore the frequency and type of imaging used is somewhat controversial. Most occur early so imaging frequency is more intense earlier. CT is the workhorse as MRI and PET have not proven themselves to be more sensitive or specific in this role. Chest imaging is relatively unrewarding and might even be eliminated [2].

Treatment of Residual Disease

Assessing the presence and location of residual retroperitoneal disease after induction chemotherapy is critical. A CT scan of abdomen and pelvis about a month after the last cycle of chemotherapy is used to decide if further surgical treatment is indicated. Most centers would observe patients with normal or near-normal retroperitoneums after chemotherapy for nodal disease. Concern for the presence of microscopic or small-volume teratoma which could contribute to late relapse has led Dr. Sheinfeld of Memorial Sloan Kettering Cancer Center to recommend surgery in most patients who had any RP disease pre-chemotherapy [3]. The pathology of RP residual disease cannot be predicted by imaging with sufficient accuracy to omit surgery. However, teratoma or necrosis/fibrosis can be suspected with sufficient certainty that organ sparing can be attempted intraoperatively. For example, it is increasingly rare to perform a left nephrectomy because the vessels cannot be dissected out of the mass. PET has been recognized as a very useful method of detecting active tumor in residual masses in patients with seminoma.

Pelvic CT should always be done to rule out the appearance of masses along the vas which may not have been noted post-orchiectomy and prechemotherapy. Residual teratoma in nodes along the cord or the spermatic vessels can be overlooked at surgery and can lead to late relapse if not removed.

It is our practice to perform a CT of the abdomen and pelvis 3–4 months after RPL to establish a new baseline after removal of RP residual masses. Interpretation can be difficult if there are lymphoceles or loops of small bowel adherent to the great vessels. Often the surgeon is in a better position to interpret these images. We do not repeat these scans again unless there are symptoms, rising markers, or some other reason to suspect recurrent disease. The rate of relapse in the RP after surgery by an experienced surgeon is extremely rare and the radiation exposure from further diagnostic imaging should be avoided. We do not have experience with PET or MRI in this situation.

Medical Imager Experience and Knowledge of Testicular Cancer

In the era of digital imaging, it is now common for clinicians to assess images of their patients at the point of care in addition to reviewing the consultation reports provided by medical imagers. Ready availability of images that can be manipulated to create multiplanar reconstructions in the operating room is a great help for surgical navigation and planning. It is critical to have a consultant medical imager who is familiar with all aspects of testis cancer.

References

1. Peterson AC, Bauman JM, Light DE, et al. The prevalence of testicular microlithiasis in an asymptomatic population of men 18 to 35 years old. J Urol. 2001;6:2061.
2. Sharir S, Warde P, Jewett MAS. Optimising the surveillance protocol for stage I nonseminoma results in significant cost savings. In: Jones WG, Appleyard I, Harnden P, et al. editors. Germ cell tumours IV. London: John Libby & Co. Ltd; 1998. pp. 381–2.
3. Eggener SE, Carver BS, Sharp DS, et al. Incidence of disease outside modified retroperitoneal lymph node dissection templates in clinical stage I or IIA nonseminomatous germ cell testicular cancer. J Urol. 2007;177:937.

Chapter 30

Penis Carcinoma: Introduction

D. M. Rodin, S. Tabatabaei, and W. S. McDougal

Epidemiology

The American Cancer Society predicted that in 2005, 1470 new cases of penile cancer would be diagnosed and that 270 men would die of the disease [1]. Carcinoma of the penis is an uncommon malignancy in the United States constituting 0.2% of all malignancies and 0.1% of cancer deaths in men. This translates into 1–2 cases per 100,000 population per annum. Carcinoma of the penis is a more common disease in other areas of the world, particularly in Asia, Africa, and South America. It can account for up to 10% of malignancies in men in this part of the world [1]. Race does not appear to play a role. The peak incidence is in the sixth and seventh decades of life.

Etiology

While the exact etiology of penile carcinoma is not entirely clear, certain factors have been associated with the disease. The presence of a foreskin, phimosis, chronic inflammatory conditions, treatment with psoralen and ultraviolet A photochemotherapy (PUVA), exposure to human papillomavirus (HPV), and history of smoking appear to have evidence implicating a role in the development of this malignancy (Table 30.1).

Table 30.1 Etiologies

Lack of circumcision / presence of foreskin
Phimosis
Chronic inflammatory conditions
Smoking
Ultraviolet light irradiation
Cervical cancer in the partner
Human papillomavirus (HPV) infection

D.M. Rodin (✉)
Massachusetts General Hospital, Harvard Medical School, 55 Fruit Street, GRB-1102, Boston, MA 02114–2696, daverodin@gmail.com

Lack of Circumcision/Presence of Foreskin

Circumcision has been established as a prophylactic measure that reduces the risk of penile cancer [2–5]. Penile squamous cell carcinoma is rare among Jews and Muslims, who practice circumcision during the neonatal period and childhood, respectively. While penile cancer is common in Africa, it is rare among the Ibos of Nigeria, who practice ritual male circumcision soon after birth [6]. The presence of cancer of the penis in a patient who has been circumcised at birth is quite rare. In a case control study, neonatal circumcision was associated with a three-fold decreased risk of cancer [6, 7]. Furthermore, it has been demonstrated that neonatal circumcision has a protective effect for invasive carcinoma while no protective effect has been noted for CIS [8].

Phimosis

Phimosis is one of the strongest predictors of invasive carcinoma [7–9]. A history of phimosis is found in approximately one-half of patients with penile carcinoma. It is hypothesized that men with phimosis are more likely to retain smegma. Smegma can cause epithelial hyperplasia and mild to moderate atypia of the squamous epithelium of the preputial sac in men with phimosis [10]. Hellberg et al. found a 65-fold increased relative risk for penile squamous cell carcinoma among males with phimosis in a Swedish case control study [9].

Chronic Inflammatory Conditions

As is true for other parts of the body, inflammation and irritation, burned areas, preexisting scars, and draining sinuses are predisposing factors for squamous cell carcinoma [11]. Hellberg et al. reported that 45% of patients with penile cancer had at least one episode of balanitis, while 8% of controls were affected by balanitis [9].

J.J.M.C.H. de la Rosette et al. (eds.), *Imaging in Oncological Urology*,
DOI 10.1007/978-1-84628-759-6_30, © Springer-Verlag London Limited 2009

Lichen sclerosis et atrophicus (LSA) is a chronic inflammatory skin condition of unknown etiology. The autoimmune response that is triggered by trauma, injury, or infection has been suggested as its predisposing factor [6, 12]. Approximately 6% of patients with LSA developed penile cancer in a 10-year follow-up study [13].

Smoking

A history of smoking is an independent risk factor for the development of penile cancer [7–9, 14, 15]. Among those who have ever smoked cigarettes, the incidence of carcinoma of the penis was 2.4 times that of men who had never smoked [7]. Daling et al. found that men diagnosed with invasive penile cancer were more likely to be smokers (OR = 4.5) than men with in situ tumors (OR=1.5) which is in contrast to Tseng et al. who found a similar increased risk in smokers for both invasive and in situ tumors [8, 16]. Although the exact etiology is not known, the accumulation of nitrosamines in genital secretions has been suggested [9].

Ultraviolet Light Irradiation

Treatment with psoralen and ultraviolet A photochemotherapy (PUVA) has been considered as a strong risk factor for penile cancer. In a 12.3-year prospective study of 892 men in a cohort of patients with psoriasis, who had been treated with oral methotrexate and PUVA, Stern et al. identified 14 patients (1.6%) with 30 genital neoplasms [17]. Recently it has been suggested that the carcinogenesis is likely to be dose dependent [18].

Cervical Cancer in the Partner

An association of penile cancer and cervical cancer in partners of patients with penile cancer has been suggested by several authors [19–22]. Hellberg, however, has clearly explained that these studies had methodological flaws, and his review of 1064 penile cancer cases in Sweden did not reveal any association with cervical cancer in their partners [23]. Other recent studies also found either weak or no-risk elevation of penile cancer in men who had partners with cervical cancer [24–26]. Thus, further studies are needed prior to making a more decisive conclusion.

Human Papillomavirus (HPV) Infection

HPV infection is a highly infective, sexually transmitted disease characterized by a high rate of spontaneous clearance.

At least 84 different types of human papillomavirus have been identified [27, 28].

Different HPV types have been associated with different genital lesions. The causal role of certain types of HPV in the development of intraepithelial neoplasia and carcinoma of the female cervix is well supported by experimental and epidemiologic data. The relative risk patterns of the 15 most common HPV types implicated in cervical neoplasm are assessed and categorized into low-risk, intermediate-risk, and high-risk groups. The DNA of high-risk HPV types has been detected in a substantial subset of penile squamous cell carcinomas as well. Dillner et al. quoted that up to 40% of penile cancer lesions were positive for HPV detected by the PCR method in two large series, with the majority of cases positive only for HPV 16 or 18 [6]. Daling et al. found that of 94 tumor specimens tested for HPV DNA, approximately 80% were HPV DNA positive with the most common subtype being HPV 16 (86.7%) [16]. The HPV positive rates were similar among those who were circumcised in childhood and those that were not. So far, a few sero-epidemiological studies indicate that exposure to HPV is indeed a major risk factor for penile cancer. We could not find any study to confirm the causal effect of this association. In addition, while several studies implicate the role of HPV, there is evidence that HPV may not necessarily be involved in all cases of penile carcinogenesis [29].

In terms of tumor characteristics, HPV DNA positive tumors were found to have less lymphatic embolization than HPV negative tumors; however no difference in lymph node metastases was detected [30].

Pre-malignant Lesions

Pre-malignant lesions of the penis may be categorized into two groups – (1) lesions that are sporadically associated with squamous cell carcinoma of the penis: Bowenoid papulosis of the penis, balanitis xerotica obliterans, and cutaneous horn of the penis; Buschke-Löwenstein tumor (Verrucous carcinoma, Giant condyloma acuminatum) and (2) lesions that are at risk for developing into invasive squamous cell carcinoma of the penis: carcinoma in situ of the penis (erythroplasia of Queyrat and Bowen's disease) (Table 30.2). The terminology of pre-malignant penile lesions is one of the major areas of confusion in the nomenclature of penile lesions.

Bowenoid Papulosis

Bowenoid papulosis, although histologically similar to carcinoma in situ, usually has a benign course [31, 32]. The lesion usually occurs in young men (mean age 29.5 years),

Table 30.2 Pre-malignant lesions

Lesions sporadically associated with squamous cell carcinoma of the penis
Bowenoid papulosis of the penis
Balanitis xerotica obliterans
Cutaneous horn of the penis
Buschke-Löwenstein tumor (Verrucous Carcinoma, Giant condyloma acuminatum)
Lesions at risk for developing into invasive squamous cell carcinoma of the penis
Carcinoma in situ of the penis
Erythroplasia of Queyrat
Bowen's disease

most commonly on the penile shaft, and usually consists of multicentric, pigmented papules ranging from 2 to 30 mm. Smaller lesions may coalesce into larger ones [31].

The etiology of Bowenoid papulosis is unknown, although viral (particularly HPV), chemical, and immunologic causes have been suggested [31, 33]. The diagnosis is confirmed by excisional biopsy.

Treatment includes surgical excision or elimination of the lesion by electrodessication, cryotherapy, laser fulguration, or topical 5-fluorouracil cream. Spontaneous regression has been reported [31].

Balanitis Xerotica Obliterans

Balanitis xerotica obliterans (BXO) is the term applied to lichen sclerosis et atrophicus of the glans penis and prepuce. This disorder most often occurs in uncircumcised, middle-aged men and may precede, coexist with, or progress to penile squamous cell carcinoma [34–37].

Although initially asymptomatic, most patients complain of penile discomfort and/or pain, difficult urination secondary to meatal stricture, and painful erection. On examination, BXO presents as a well-defined marginated white patch on the glans penis or prepuce that may involve the urethral meatus. In chronic cases, the lesion is firm due to a thick underlying fibrosis. Diagnosis is made by biopsy.

Treatment is usually difficult, and depending on the severity, consists of surgical excision, topical steroid cream, and/or laser therapy. Meatal stenosis may need repeated dilatations or even formal meatoplasty.

Cutaneous Horn

A cutaneous horn is an overgrowth and cornification of the epithelium that forms a solid protuberance. Penile horn is a rare form of cutaneous horn, with only 18 reported in North America [38]. These lesions are considered pre-malignant and one-third of the cases reported have been malignant at presentation [39, 40].

Surgical excision with a margin of normal tissue around the base of the lesion has been very successful in treating this disorder. Most malignant penile horns are of low grade, but metastasis has been reported. Therefore, wide local excision and close follow up to detect early metastasis is suggested for malignant forms [40–42].

Buschke–Löwenstein Tumor, Verrucous Carcinoma, Giant Condyloma Accuminatum

Whether the Buschke-Löwenstein tumor or giant condyloma and verrucous carcinoma are the same or different lesions is controversial. These lesions are locally invasive and may be quite aggressive. They destroy adjacent structures by local invasion. Rarely, if ever, do they metastasize. Treatment is directed at eradicating the local disease by local excision of the tumor and avoiding extensive excision of normal penile tissue. In rare cases of large, infiltrative lesions, total penectomy is indicated. Intra-aortic infusion with methotrexate has been shown to result in complete remission in three of four patients in one small study [43]. This may prove to be an effective, noninvasive treatment for this subset of penile carcinoma.

Carcinoma In Situ (CIS), Bowen's Disease, Erythroplasia of Queyrat

Although Bowen's disease and erythroplasia of Queyrat are the same histologically, they differ in their location. Erythroplasia of Queyrat is CIS of the mucocutaneous regions of the penis, namely the penile glans and prepuce. Bowen's disease is CIS of the follicle bearing remainder of the genitalia and perineal area. CIS of the penis is a velvety red, well-circumscribed lesion that usually involves the glans, or less frequently, the prepuce or shaft of the penis. Up to one-third of patients with CIS of the penis may also have invasive carcinoma of the penis [44].

Diagnosis is based on adequate biopsies of the lesion with sufficient depth to rule out invasion. These lesions respond well to limited local excision with minimal interference with penile anatomy. Circumcision is usually an adequate treatment for CIS of the prepuce. It seems that local fulguration with electrocautery is not able to adequately eradicate the tumor. Radiation therapy has been successfully used for this tumor [45].

Topical use of 5-fluorouracil at 5% concentration has shown excellent results [46, 47]. Topical imiquimod 5% cream and liquid nitrogen have also been reported with excellent cosmetic results [48, 49]. Successful use of the CO_2 or Nd:YAG laser has been reported for initial therapy as well as for recurrence [50–52]. However, due to a high incidence of recurrence, close follow-up is required. Further studies to determine the recurrence rate with varying laser power settings to achieve various margins are needed.

Invasive Carcinoma of the Penis

Squamous cell carcinoma comprises 95% of cancers of the penis. The remaining 5% of malignancies involving the penis include the sarcomas (angiosarcoma, fibrosarcoma, myelosarcoma, Kaposi's sarcoma) [53–56], melanoma [57, 58], basal cell carcinoma [59, 60], and lymphoma. Other tumors, which have been reported on very rare occasions, include rhabdomyosarcoma [61], epithelial sarcoma, malignant schwanoma, myxosarcoma, and neurofibrosarcoma.

Ninety-two percent of squamous cell carcinomas of the penis involve the glans and/or prepuce: 9% of lesions are found on the glans and prepuce, 21% on the prepuce, 48% on the glans, and 14% on the prepuce, glans, and shaft. Approximately 6% involve the coronal sulcus, and only 2% of squamous cell carcinomas are found on the shaft with no lesions elsewhere.

Natural History

Carcinoma of the penis usually presents as a small papillary, exophytic, or flat ulcerative lesion that does not resolve spontaneously. This ulcer extends gradually and may ultimately involve the entire glans or penis. It seems that flat, ulcerative tumors are usually less differentiated and are overall associated with earlier nodal metastases.

The lymphatic system is the primary route for metastases for this loco-regional malignancy. The disease first spreads to the superficial and deep inguinal nodes, followed by the pelvic nodes, long before distant metastases occur. At presentation, 30–60% of patients have enlarged inguinal lymph nodes [62–65]. Of these patients with enlarged lymph nodes, approximately 50% will have cancer in the nodes. Lymph node involvement with the cancer may also be present in 20% of patients with non-palpable nodes [66–68]. Up to 60% of patients may have tumor metastasis to the contralateral inguinal nodes [69].

The most important prognostic factors in men with squamous cell carcinoma of the penis are the presence and extent of inguinal lymph node metastases [62, 70–73]. Lymph node involvement may cause chronic infection and skin necrosis. Untreated, the majority of patients die within 1 year of diagnosis from sepsis, hemorrhage secondary to tumor erosion into the femoral vessels, and/or inanition [74]. Distant metastases to the lung, liver, bone, or brain are uncommon [66, 68, 75].

Presentation

The presence of a penile lesion is the first presentation. This could range from a subtle small papule or pustule that does not heal to a large exophytic, fungating lesion. It can occasionally present as a superficial, erythematous erosion. These lesions occur most commonly on the glans and prepuce and

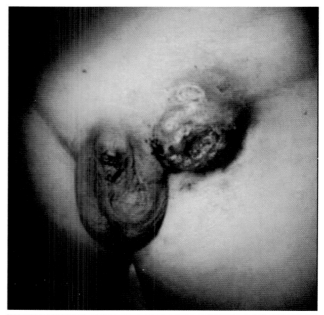

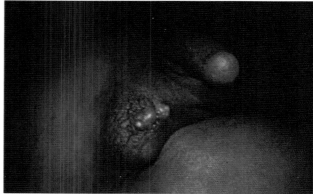

Fig. 30.1 Inguinal lymph node metastases

less commonly on the coronal sulcus and penile shaft. The initial lesions are usually painless.

The patient may present with a mass in the inguinal area, if the primary lesion was ignored due to its location under a phimotic foreskin (Fig. 30.1). The mass may be due to lymph node enlargement secondary to an inflammatory response or metastases, and it may become ulcerative, suppurative, or hemorrhagic. In the later stages of the disease, the patient may experience systemic symptoms such as weakness, weight loss, anorexia, fever, and malaise.

Diagnosis

Patient and/or physician factors often contribute to a significant delay in diagnosis. The patient's delay is usually attributable to embarrassment, guilt, fear, or ignorance. Delay in seeking medical care may be as long as one year and may include up to 50% of the patients [76]. A delay in diagnosis and treatment by the physician is usually owing to prolongation of a conservative approach (long course of antibiotics, antifungal, or topical steroid therapy) or misdiagnosis.

Physical Examination

A thorough physical examination is crucial for the diagnosis and accurate staging. The location, appearance, size, depth of involvement, and presence of tumor fixation of the penile lesion should be evaluated. The scrotum, base of the penis, and perineum should be examined for any possible tumor extension. Rectal examination rules out gross involvement of the perineal body or the presence of a pelvic mass. The inguinal area needs to be inspected and palpated thoroughly for any possible lymph node enlargement.

Biopsy

Histological confirmation of penile cancer should be obtained by a biopsy from the penile lesion in order to evaluate the depth of invasion, tumor differentiation (grade), and the presence of vascular invasion. The Broders classification histologically separates squamous cell carcinoma into three grades: well, moderate, and poorly differentiated [77]. This classification was recently confirmed by Maiche, who proposed four grades, but with similar prognostic significance [78]. Approximately 50% of squamous cell carcinomas are well differentiated, 30% are moderately differentiated, and 20% are poorly differentiated [79]. Cubilla studied a whole-organ section of 66 patients with squamous cell carcinoma

of the penis and identified four types of growth: superficially spreading squamous carcinoma (42%), vertical invasive carcinoma (32%), verrucous carcinoma (18%), and multicentric carcinoma (8%) [80]. He found that 82% of patients with vertical growth vs. 42% of patients with superficially spreading growth have inguinal lymph node metastasis.

The distinction as to degree of differentiation is particularly important as a potential predictor for metastatic disease to the groin [79, 81, 82]. It is even more powerful when combined with tumor depth of invasion [79]. This information is necessary to accurately stage the tumor and allows the surgeon to discuss the therapeutic options with the patient. Loss of the phallus is psychologically devastating to the patient, and most patients need time to cope with the diagnosis. Therefore, while it is possible to perform the biopsy (with frozen section diagnosis) and partial or total penectomy in one session, we do not advocate this approach due primarily to psychological reasons. The interval between the biopsy and the definitive radical surgery will allow the patient and his physician the opportunity to establish their relationship and address the psychological aspects of the treatment in an effort to decrease the enormous tension and stress that ensues following ablative surgery.

Imaging

Awareness of the extent and depth of the primary tumor and the involvement of inguinal lymph nodes prior to any surgical intervention is crucial in patients with penile cancer. Although this decision is usually based on physical examination, various imaging modalities, including ultrasonography, computed tomography (CT), and magnetic resonance imaging (MRI), have been used for this purpose.

CT has poor soft tissue resolution therefore rendering ultrasound and MRI superior in the evaluation of primary tumor extension. While ultrasound cannot precisely detect tumor extension in the glans penis area, it has shown adequate resolution to detect corpus cavernosum invasion. This is due to the thick tunica albuginea that is readily visible with 7.5 MHz linear array small parts transducer [83–86]. In extensive infiltrating tumors, ultrasound's ability to delineate corporal invasion is compromised significantly [87].

MRI has been tested in several studies, and it appears to be the most sensitive method for determining corpus cavernosal infiltration, but at the cost of lower specificity [87–91]. Lont has recently compared the accuracy of physical exam to MRI or ultrasound in the evaluation of primary tumor extension and concluded that physical examination alone is a reliable method for predicting corporal involvement. MRI and ultrasound may be reserved only to examine tumors in which the physical examination is equivocal [87].

CT relies on lymph node size for detecting metastasis. MRI evaluates the lymph node size and its signal intensity. Unfortunately, neither of these image modalities is able to differentiate benign vs. malignant lymph node enlargement. Furthermore, their sensitivity and specificity drop remarkably in normal-sized lymph nodes. Presently, CT and MRI do not add additional information over thorough physical examination, especially in patients with no palpable inguinal lymph nodes.

Recently we reported the use of lymphotropic superparamagnetic nanoparticles, as an MRI contrast agent, in evaluating lymph node metastasis in penile cancer patients (Fig. 30.2). Our early experience of applying this noninvasive technique in penile cancer patients is encouraging with sensitivity, specificity, and positive and negative predictive values of 100, 97, 81.2, and 100%, respectively [92]. More studies are required to establish the role of this technique in patients with penile cancer.

Staging

Unfortunately, the staging system of carcinoma of the penis is not universally accepted, and each system carries its own flaws. The original Jackson system (see Table 30.3) is not particularly helpful clinically in selecting who is most likely to have groin disease [93]. The TNM system is a bit better (Table 30.4), but again suffers from inability to predict the incidence of positive regional lymph nodes. With the TNM system, it is difficult to assign nodal status before definitive therapy. Combining the TNM system with tumor differentiation (grade) improves the prognostic ability for

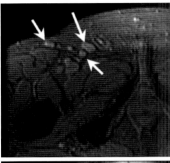
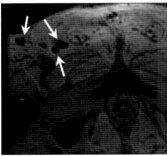
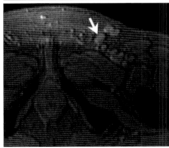
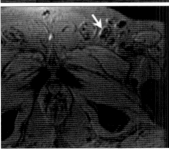

Fig. 30.2 Lymphotropic superparamagnetic nanoparticle MRI lymphangiography: (a) pre-contrast MRI in patient with benign nodes – note all nodes appear white (b) post-contrast MRI in patient with benign nodes – note all nodes appear dark due to uptake of contrast material by lymph nodes (c) pre-contrast MRI in patient with nodes containing cancer – note all nodes appear white (d) post-contrast MRI in patient with nodes containing cancer – note heterogeneous uptake of contrast; nodal tissue which contains tumor does not take up contrast and remains white while normal nodal tissue does take up contrast and appears black

Table 30.3 Jackson staging system

Stage I Tumor confined to glans or prepuce.
Stage II Tumor invasive into the shaft or corpora. No palpable adenopathy.
Stage III Palpable metastases to the groin that are resectable.
Stage IV Inoperable groin nodes or distant metastases.

Table 30.4 American Joint Committee on Cancer (AJCC) staging system for penile cancer

Primary tumor (T)	
Tx	Primary tumor cannot be assessed
T0	No primary tumor
TIS	Carcinoma in situ
Ta	Noninvasive verrucous carcinoma
T1	Tumor invades subepithelial connective tissue
T2	Tumor invades corpus spongiosum or cavernosum
T3	Tumor invades urethra or prostate
T4	Tumor invades other adjacent structures
Lymph nodes (N)	
Nx	Regional nodes cannot be assessed
N0	No regional node metastases
N1	Metastasis in a single regional lymph node
N2	Metastases in multiple or bilateral superficial inguinal lymph nodes
N3	Metastases in deep inguinal or pelvic lymph nodes; unilateral or bilateral
Distant metastasis (M)	
Mx	Distant metastasis cannot be assessed
M0	No regional lymph node metastases
M1	Distant metastasis

Table 30.5 Depth of invasive/grade staging system

		T Stage
Stage I	The tumor is superficial with no extension into the subcutaneous tissue	T0, TIS, Ta, N0
Stage 2A	Locally invasive tumor without involvement of the corpora, well or moderately differentiated	T1, N0
Stage 2B	The tumor invades the corpora or it is poorly differentiated	T1, T2, N0
Stage 3	Persistent palpable inguinal nodes	N1, N2
Stage 4	Bulky groin nodes with invasion extending outside the node, pelvic node involvement, distant metastases	N3, N4

regional nodal involvement as suggested in our modified staging system [79](Table 30.5). Thus, poorly differentiated tumors have an 80–100% incidence of metastatic disease, moderately differentiated tumors a 46% incidence, and well-differentiated tumors a 24% incidence of groin metastasis. In tumors that have not invaded into the corpora, there is only a 5–11% incidence of metastatic disease, whereas if the corpora are invaded, there is a 61–75% incidence of groin metastases [79].

The accurate evaluation of the regional lymph nodes plays a major role in staging given that carcinoma of the penis is a loco-regional disease. Considering the low incidence of penile cancer, multicenter prospective studies are needed to validate and improve the staging system.

Treatment

Local Treatment of the Primary Lesion

Mohs micrographic surgery, which involves serial local excisions of the primary tumor in thin layers, with thorough microscopic examination of each layer, may be appropriate for small lesions involving only the dermis (< 1 cm in diameter) [94–96]. This technique has the advantage of preserving the penis but is limited to very superficial lesions and is generally not particularly applicable for most cancers of the penis.

Proponents of cryotherapy [97] and laser therapy suggest that the local lesions can be destroyed with preservation of the part. While this may be successful for dermal lesions, successful eradication is less likely and the local recurrence rate is significant for lesions involving the subcutaneous tissue and/or corpora. With the use of the Nd:YAG laser as primary therapy for patients with carcinoma in situ, the local recurrence rate is 6%, for lesions that invade the subcuta-

neous tissue, the recurrence rate is between 10 and 20%, and for lesions that invade the corpora, the recurrence rate ranges between 50 and 100% [98].

A 61% recurrence rate is observed with external beam radiation therapy [99] along with an unacceptably high stricture rate. Brachytherapy has been employed for local lesions with considerable success, particularly in patients with T1 to T2 penile cancer, who insist upon preserving the penis [100, 101]. In a series of 49 men, the majority with T1 (51%) and T2 (33%) tumors, treated with primary penile interstitial brachytherapy found a local failure rate of approximately 15%. The soft-tissue necrosis rate was 16%, and the urethral stenosis rate was 12% [102].

The most effective local therapy remains surgical excision, although the cosmetic defects can be major. Circumcision is appropriate if the lesion is contained within the foreskin. However, this approach is associated with a 30% local recurrence rate. Partial penectomy is the most effective method of dealing with the disorder, provided one can establish a traditional 2 cm proximal margin. This carries with it a 6% recurrence rate. More recent data suggest smaller margins may be adequate [103]. Total penectomy has the least risk of local recurrence and is only employed when the tumor replaces the entire penis or when it is located at the base of the shaft. It results in a significant cosmetic defect, and many patients have considerable psychological issues in the postoperative period [71, 104–107]. Organ-sparing surgery, in the form of partial or total glansectomy, has recently been reported for distal invasive penile cancer with the goals of oncologic control, decreased psychological and cosmetic impact, and potential preservation of sexual function. Early follow-up reveals encouraging results in terms of recurrence, but longer follow-up in larger studies is needed [108–110].

Treatment of the Inguinal Lymph Nodes

The most important prognostic factor in men with invasive squamous cell carcinoma of the penis is the status of the inguinal lymph nodes [62, 70–73]. Squamous cell carcinoma of the penis tends to spread locally to regional lymph nodes, and distant metastasis is rare. Therefore, even in patients with local lymph node metastases, regional lymphadenectomy alone can be curative and should be performed [66, 71, 111, 112]. Studies suggest that inguinal lymphadenectomy offers 30–60% cure rate to patients with inguinal node metastases. If the tumor extends to the pelvic lymph nodes, the success rate drops to less than a 10%. Unfortunately, there is currently no effective chemotherapeutic and/or radiotherapeutic option available for cure in patients with disease extending beyond the inguinal lymph nodes. Most of these patients will succumb to disease within one to two years [68, 113].

In terms of lymphatic drainage, the prepuce drains with the shaft skin to the superficial inguinal nodes. The glans drains with the corporal bodies to the deep inguinal nodes, which drain to the pelvic nodes. Rarely, deeply invasive tumors, particularly those at the base of the penis, may bypass the groin and drain directly to the pelvic nodes. Due to multiple cross-communications, lesions on one side of the penis may metastasize to the contralateral groin.

Approximately 50% of patients have palpable nodes. In many cases, these nodes are inflammatory due to infection of the primary lesion. Therefore, a patient should be re-staged after the primary lesion has been eradicated, the wound has been closed, and the patient is infection free following a six-week course of antibiotics. If patients are re-evaluated, those with non-palpable groin nodes will have a 20% incidence of metastatic disease, if all patients are subjected to a groin dissection.

Tumor grade and depth of invasion (stage) have significant prognostic value in predicting lymph node involvement [71, 79, 112, 114]. While almost 30% of patients with grade I penile squamous cell carcinoma have inguinal lymph node involvement, about 80% of grade III tumors have positive inguinal lymph nodes [79, 115]. In patients whose primary lesion involves the corpora (T2) and the tumor is poorly differentiated, approximately 80% of such patients will in fact have positive groin nodes [79, 112]. If there are discrete palpable lymph nodes, approximately 86% of patients with high-grade tumors will have pathologically positive nodes on dissection.

Pre-emptive lymphadenectomy is a point of contention due to its morbidity and the defined number of patients who would unnecessarily undergo lymphadenectomy if all patients were subjected to regional groin dissection. Therefore, a watch and wait approach has been adopted over the years. Unfortunately, this relegates patients with non-palpable microscopic disease to a much worse survival. Those with non-palpable microscopic disease, who undergo groin dissections, have a markedly improved survival over those in whom the microscopic disease is allowed to develop into palpable disease at which point a groin dissection is performed [68, 70, 71, 79, 116].

In an effort to avoid unnecessary groin dissections, it has been suggested that a sentinel lymph node biopsy would be predictive of the status of the groin [117–119]. Unfortunately, the location of the sentinel node is variable, yielding its clinical use unreliable by many [120–123].

Intraoperative lymph node mapping (IOLM) has been proposed in an effort to circumvent the problem with anatomic variability of the sentinel node [124]. There has been significant experience using this technique with breast and melanoma malignancies [124]. Injection of a vital blue dye and/or technetium-labeled colloid around the primary lesion allows the surgeon to follow its drainage to a single or

a few lymph nodes in the inguinal region [125–127]. Selective biopsies of these nodes assist to outline the extent of the lymph node dissection. In the absence of any sentinel node involvement, some would argue that there is no need for radical inguinal lymph node dissection (high negative predictive value). In a recent report by Horenblas, 55 patients were scanned and biopsied. One-third was found not to have surgical findings that correlated with scintigraphy. Twenty percent had positive nodes and 6% of patients, who were found to have negative nodes, within a 3-year period, were found to develop evidence of positive groin nodes [128]. The number of false negatives is at least 6% as the follow-up in the current contemporary series is too short to determine the true false-negative rate. Horenblas published two subsequent updated series and found an approximately 80% sensitivity with this technique [129, 130]. Thus, this methodology does eliminate a number of patients who would needlessly undergo a groin dissection at the expense of subjecting all patients to groin sentinel node biopsies. Unfortunately, at this time, the combination of tumor differentiation and tumor stage combined are as predictive as sentinel node biopsies either with or without blue dye.

One study suggested performing ultrasound-guided fine needle aspiration cytology as the initial diagnostic test in clinically node negative patients [131]. Upon examining 34 groins in 27 patients, they achieved a sensitivity of 39% and specificity of 100%. They found that the number of dynamic sentinel node biopsies required in their protocol was reduced by 11%. Methods to improve the accuracy of sentinel node biopsy should be sought prior to its becoming a reliable staging tool in patients with clinical node negative disease.

Other prognostic factors have been investigated in attempt to avoid surgical morbidity. One factor with encouraging preliminary results is p53 protein expression. p53 overexpression was significantly positively correlated with cell differentiation, depth of primary lesion, and nodal metastases. Multivariate analysis revealed p53 immunostaining – at a cutoff value of 10%, was the predominant factor predicting lymph node metastases, and cause specific death [132]. Lopes et al. also found that the immunoreactivity of p53 was significantly related to lymph node metastases on both univariate and multivariate analyses. Patients with p53 immunoreactivity were at a 4.8-fold increased risk for metastases. When they examined survival rates, they found a significantly decreased survival rate in those patients with p53 positivity on univariate analysis, but this did not reach statistical significance on multivariate analysis [133].

Ki-67 is a non-histone nuclear matrix protein expressed in all cell-cycle phases, except G0. Given that Ki-67 has been correlated with tumor differentiation, nodal involvement, and disease progression in squamous cell carcinoma of the head and neck, it has been evaluated as a marker in penile cancer.

While it was correlated with tumor differentiation, only an associated trend was noted in terms of advanced stage, nodal metastases, and clinical disease progression [134].

There has been some investigation of squamous cell carcinoma antigen as a potential serum marker to aid in the early detection of nodal metastases in men with squamous cell carcinoma of the penis. While preliminary results show promise, limited numbers of study patients limit the study power.

Although the statistical power of these studies was weakened by their small numbers and controversy remains over detection methods as well as the definition of p53 positivity, these results are an encouraging base for which to build further research. However, newer imaging techniques may leave these markers as unnecessary in the future [135].

New modalities for lymph node imaging, particularly with lymphotropic contrast agents used with MRI, are extremely exciting. Based on our early experience with this technology at Massachusetts General Hospital, MR lymphangiogram, in all likelihood, will have a diagnostic efficacy sufficient to predict who should and who should not receive a groin dissection.

Based on our proposed modified staging system [79](Table 30.5), stages I and IIA disease have an extremely low likelihood of metastatic groin disease (0–12%), and their survival in our experience approximates 100%. Patients with IIB disease have a 78–88% incidence of groin metastases. Of these patients, there is a 17% 5-year survival in those who undergo watchful waiting versus a 92% 5-year survival for those who have an immediate lymphadenectomy versus a 33% 5-year survival for those who have their lymphadenectomy delayed until nodes become palpable. Patients with stage III disease who undergo an immediate lymphadenectomy have a 75% survival, whereas if no lymphadenectomy is performed, there is a 33% survival [79]. This was confirmed by Horenblas [136]. Thus, it is clear that patients who have non-palpable microscopic metastases to the groin and an immediate groin dissection have a much better prognosis than do those in whom the lymphadenectomy is delayed until nodal disease becomes palpable. The challenge is to differentiate who is most likely to have microscopic metastases without subjecting a large group of patients to an unnecessary operation with potential considerable morbidity [113, 114, 137–139].

Complications resulting from inguinal lymphadenectomy have been reported as skin edge necrosis (7.5–50%), major flap necrosis (2.5–5%), wound infection (7.5–15%), lymphedema (10–50%), seroma formation (6–16%), and death (0–1%) [137, 139–142]. In addition, a second operation is required in approximately 15% of patients [141].

However, if the lymph node dissection is performed for microscopic non-palpable disease, the complication rate is much less. In our experience, the complications include small wound seroma (15%), minor skin edge necrosis not requiring a secondary procedure (20%), minor, self-limited lymphedema (20%), prolonged lymphedema (5%). None have required secondary operations. The group at MD Anderson has also reported similar results [141].

In our opinion, currently, the most predictive method of determining the probability of microscopic nodal metastases is grade of primary tumor combined with depth of invasion. For the present, patients who have clinically negative groins and have a Grade III lesion invasive to the corpora should have bilateral groin dissections. If the groin dissection is positive, a pelvic lymphadenectomy should subsequently be performed on the ipsilateral side. It is our preference to do the bilateral groin dissection in patients with any Grade III tumor or any tumor whose primary lesion invades the corpora. Perhaps the sentinel node biopsy may be useful in these latter patients, as only about 60% of them will harbor microscopic metastatic disease. Of course, patients with persistently palpable groin nodes should undergo a groin dissection. In this group, approximately 86% of patients will have metastatic disease. It is our preference to perform the bilateral superficial and deep node dissections in one setting. When the permanent pathology has returned, a pelvic lymphadenectomy is performed on the positive side. Our technique is described in Glenn's Textbook of Urologic Surgery [143]. Although some would suggest that a pelvic lymphadenectomy is not likely to impact survival, on occasion we have found an isolated positive node in the pelvis that resulted in long-term survival. In addition, the knowledge of pelvic node status has prognostic significance and allows us to consider adjuvant chemotherapy in positive cases.

On occasion, a groin dissection must be performed for palliative reasons. Under these circumstances, large tissue defects may be created in the process of removing all visible tumor. These defects can be closed with an abdominal advancement flap as we have previously described [144]. Following closure of the wound, radiation therapy may be given to the pelvis for palliation; however, invariably these patients will suffer significant external genitalia lymphedema, which can be quite disabling in the final stages of life.

The Role of Radiation and Chemotherapy in Squamous Cell Carcinoma of the Penis

The role of radiation and topical chemotherapy for the primary lesion has been discussed previously. Several non-randomized studies have reviewed the role of radiation therapy for the treatment of metastatic inguinal nodes [69, 145]. The results are overall dismal and indicate the role of radiation therapy merely as a palliative measure at the present time [146].

Due to the limited number of cases and lack of prospective studies, an optimal chemotherapy protocol has not yet been developed. Most of the chemotherapy regimens are based on the results of chemotherapy trials in squamous cell carcinoma of the head and neck. Cisplatin, methotrexate, bleomycin, and vincristine have been used alone or in combination. It appears that adjuvant or neoadjuvant use of chemotherapy agents may be beneficial and result in partial response in many cases [147–150]. Newer agents, such as epidermal growth factor receptor tyrosine kinases, have shown some response when used in combination with platinum- or taxane-based therapies, and are currently being studied [151]. Recent work has shown increased amounts of COX-2 and mPGES-1 detected in penile intraepithelial neoplasia and carcinoma. This asks whether COX-2 inhibition will be a mechanism by which to prevent or treat penile cancer [152]. The optimal chemotherapy regimen remains to be determined.

Future Challenges

In the future, the optimum treatment of penile cancer will need to be developed. This requires additional knowledge of the tumor biology. Furthermore, the staging system needs to be revised to allow more accurate prediction of tumor extension prior to surgery. New imaging technologies, including lymphotropic agents, need to be applied to improve the staging accuracy. A multidisciplinary approach incorporating surgical ablation, applying various energy modalities (i.e. radiation, laser, cryotherapy, thermotherapy, high intensity focused ultrasound, etc.) and chemotherapy protocols needs to be developed to optimize disease-free status.

References

1. American cancer society detailed guide: penile cancer. What are the key statistics about penile cancer? http://www.cancer.org/docroot/CRI/content/CRI_2_4_1X_What_are_the_key_statistics_for_penile_cancer. Accessed August 2005.
2. Schoen EJ. The status of circumcision of newborns. N Engl J Med. 1990;322(18):1308–12.
3. Brinton LA, Li JY, Rong SD, et al. Risk factors for penile cancer: results from a case-control study in China. Int J Cancer. 1991;47(4):504–9.
4. Melmed EP, Pyne JR. Carcinoma of the penis in a Jew circumcised in infancy. Br J Surg. 1967;54(8):729–31.
5. Kochen M, McCurdy S. Circumcision and the risk of cancer of the penis. A life-table analysis. Am J Dis Child. 1980;134(5):484–6.
6. Dillner J, von Krogh G, Horenblas S, et al. Etiology of squamous cell carcinoma of the penis. Scand J Urol Nephrol. 2000;205 Suppl:189–93.
7. Maden C, Sherman KJ, Beckmann AM, et al. History of circumcision, medical conditions, and sexual activity and risk of penile cancer. J Natl Cancer Inst. 1993;85(1):19–24.
8. Tseng HF, Morgenstern H, Mack T, et al. Risk factors for penile cancer: results of a population-based case-control study in Los Angeles County (United States). Cancer Causes Control. 2001;12:267–77.
9. Hellberg D, Valentin J, Eklund T, et al. Penile cancer: is there an epidemiological role for smoking and sexual behaviour? Br Med J (Clin Res Ed). 1987;295(6609):1306–8.
10. Reddy CR, Devendranath V, Pratap S. Carcinoma of the penis-role of phimosis. Urology. 1984;24(1):85–8.
11. Bain L, Geronemus R. The association of lichen planus of the penis with squamous cell carcinoma in situ and with verrucous squamous carcinoma. J Dermatol Surg Oncol. 1989;15(4):413–7.
12. Powell JJ, Wojnarowska F. Lichen sclerosus. Lancet. 1999;353(9166):1777–83.
13. Bissada NK, Morcos RR, el-Senoussi M. Post-circumcision carcinoma of the penis. I. Clinical aspects. J Urol. 1986;135(2):283–5.
14. Daling JR, Sherman KJ, Hislop TG, et al. Cigarette smoking and the risk of anogenital cancer. Am J Epidemiol. 1992;135(2):180–9.
15. Harish K, Ravi R. The role of tobacco in penile carcinoma. Br J Urol. 1995;75(3):375–7.
16. Daling JR, Madeleine MM, Johnson LG, et al. Penile cancer: importance of circumcision, human papillomavirus and smoking in in situ and invasive disease. Int J Cancer. 2005;116:606–16.
17. Stern RS. Genital tumors among men with psoriasis exposed to psoralens and ultraviolet A radiation (PUVA) and ultraviolet B radiation. The photochemotherapy follow-up study. N Engl J Med. 1990;322(16):1093–7.
18. Aubin F, Puzenat E, Arveux P, et al. Genital squamous cell carcinoma in men treated by photochemotherapy. A cancer registry-based study from 1978 to 1998. Br J Dermatol. 2001;144(6):1204–6.
19. Martinez I. Relationship of squamous cell carcinoma of the cervix uteri to squamous cell carcinoma of the penis among Puerto Rican women married to men with penile carcinoma. Cancer. 1969;24(4):777–80.
20. Graham S, Priore R, Graham M, et al. Genital cancer in wives of penile cancer patients. Cancer. 1979;44(5):1870–4.
21. Cocks PS, Peel KR, Cartwright RA, et al. Carcinoma of penis and cervix. Lancet. 1980;2(8199):855–6.
22. Cocks PS, Adib RS, Hunt KM. Concurrent carcinoma of penis and carcinoma-in situ of the cervix in a married couple. Case report. Br J Obstet Gynaecol. 1982;89(5):408–9.
23. Hellberg D, Nilsson S. Genital cancer among wives of men with penile cancer. A study between 1958 and 1982. Br J Obstet Gynaecol. 1989;96(2):221–5.
24. Maiche AG, Pyrhonen S. Risk of cervical cancer among wives of men with carcinoma of the penis. Acta Oncol. 1990;29(5):569–71.
25. Iversen T, Tretli S, Johansen A, et al. Squamous cell carcinoma of the penis and of the cervix, vulva and vagina in spouses: is there any relationship? An epidemiological study from Norway, 1960–92. Br J Cancer. 1997;76(5):658–60.
26. Hemminki K, Dong C. Cancer in husbands of cervical cancer patients. Epidemiology. 2000;11(3):347–9.
27. Zderic SA, Carpiniello VL, Malloy TR, et al., Urological applications of human papillomavirus typing using deoxyribonucleic

acid probes for the diagnosis and treatment of genital condyloma. J Urol. 1989;141(1):63–5.

28. Mandell GL, Bennett JE, Dolin R. Mandell, Douglas, and Bennett's principles and practice of infectious diseases; Churchill Livingstone. 2000.

29. Ferreux E, Lont AP, Horenblas S, et al. Evidence for at least three alternative mechanisms targeting the p16^{INK4A}/cyclin D/Rb pathway in penile carcinoma, one of which is mediated by high-risk human papillomavirus. J Pathol. 2003;201:109–18.

30. Bezerra ALR, Lopes A, Santiagao GH, et al. Human papillomavirus as a prognostic factor in carcinoma of the penis: analysis of 82 patients treated with amputation and bilateral lymphadenectomy. Cancer. 2001;91:2315–21.

31. Patterson JW, Kao GF, Graham JH, et al. Bowenoid papulosis. A clinicopathologic study with ultrastructural observations. Cancer. 1986;57(4):823–36.

32. Su CK, Shipley WU. Bowenoid papulosis: a benign lesion of the shaft of the penis misdiagnosed as squamous carcinoma. J Urol. 1997;157(4):1361–2.

33. Zelickson AS, Prawer SE. Bowenoid papulosis of the penis. Demonstration of intranuclear viral-like particles. Am J Dermatopathol. 1980;2(4):305–8.

34. Dore B, Grange P, Irani J, et al. Atrophicus sclerosis lichen and cancer of the glans. J Urol. 1989;95(7):415–8.

35. Campus GV, Alia F, Bosincu L. Squamous cell carcinoma and lichen sclerosus et atrophicus of the prepuce. Plast Reconstr Surg. 1992;89(5):962–4.

36. Pride HB, Miller OF III, Tyler WB. Penile squamous cell carcinoma arising from balanitis xerotica obliterans. J Am Acad Dermatol. 1993;29(3):469–73.

37. Simonart T, Noel JC, De Dobbeleer G, et al. Carcinoma of the glans penis arising 20 years after lichen sclerosus. Dermatology. 1998;196(3):337–8.

38. Lowe FC, McCullough AR. Cutaneous horns of the penis: an approach to management. Case report and review of the literature. J Am Acad Dermatol. 1985;13(2 Pt 2):369–73.

39. Raghavaiah NV, Soloway MS, Murphy WM. Malignant penile horn. J Urol. 1977;118(6):1068–9.

40. Fields T, Drylie D, Wilson J. Malignant evolution of penile horn. Urology. 1987;30(1):65–6.

41. Goldstein HH. Cutaneous horns of the penis. J Urol. 1933;30:367–74.

42. Winterhoff E, Sparks JA. Penile horn. J Urol. 1951;66(5):704–7.

43. Sheen MC, Sheu HM, Huang CH, et al. Penile verrucous carcinoma successfully treated by intra-aortic infusion with methotrexate. Urology. 2003;61:1216–20.

44. Mikhail GR. Cancers, precancers, and pseudocancers on the male genitalia. A review of clinical appearances, histopathology, and management. J Dermatol Surg Oncol. 1980;6(12):1027–35.

45. Grabstald H, Kelley CD. Radiation therapy of penile cancer: six to ten-year follow-up. Urology. 1980;15(6):575–6.

46. Goette DK, Elgart M, DeVillez RL. Erythroplasia of Queyrat. Treatment with topically applied fluorouracil. JAMA. 1975;232(9):934–7.

47. Goette DK, Carson TE. Erythroplasia of Queyrat: treatment with topical 5-fluorouracil. Cancer. 1976;38(4):1498–502.

48. Schroeder TL, Sengelmann R. Squamous cell carcinoma in situ of the penis successfully treated with imiquimod 5% cream. J Am Acad Dermatol. 2002;46:545–8.

49. Madej G, Meyza J. Cryosurgery of penile carcinoma. Short report on preliminary results. Oncology. 1982;39(6):350–2.

50. Rosemberg SK, Fuller TA. Carbon dioxide rapid superpulsed laser treatment of erythroplasia of Queyrat. Urology. 1980;16(2):181–2.

51. Rosemberg SK. Carbon dioxide laser treatment of external genital lesions. Urology. 1985;25(6):555–8.

52. Landthaler M, Haina D, Brunner R, et al. Laser therapy of Bowenoid papulosis and Bowen's disease. J Dermatol Surg Oncol. 1986;12(12):253–1257.

53. Moore SW, Wheeler JE, Hefter LG. Epitheloid sarcoma masquerading as Peyronie's disease. Cancer. 1975;35(6):1706–10.

54. Mabogunje O. Kaposi sarcoma of glans penis. Urology. 1981;17(5):476–8.

55. Parsons MA, Fox M. Malignant fibrous histiocytoma of the penis. Eur Urol. 1988;14(1):75–6.

56. Rasbridge SA, Parry JR. Angiosarcoma of the penis. Br J Urol. 1989;63(4):440–1.

57. Manivel JC, Fraley EE. Malignant melanoma of the penis and male urethra: 4 case reports and literature review. J Urol. 1988;139(4):813–6.

58. de Bree E, Sanidas E, Tzardi M, et al. Malignant melanoma of the penis. Eur J Surg Oncol. 1997;23(3):277–9.

59. Goldminz D, Scott G, Klaus S. Penile basal cell carcinoma. Report of a case and review of the literature. J Am Acad Dermatol. 1989;20(6):1094–7.

60. Ladocsi LT, Siebert CF Jr, Rickert RR, et al. Basal cell carcinoma of the penis. Cutis. 1998;61(1):25–7.

61. Dalkin B, Zaontz MR. Rhabdomyosarcoma of the penis in children. J Urol. 1989;141(4):908–9.

62. Srinivas V, Morse MJ, Herr HW, et al. Penile cancer: relation of extent of nodal metastasis to survival. J Urol. 1987;137(5):880–2.

63. Solsona E, Iborra I, Ricos JV, et al. Corpus cavernosum invasion and tumor grade in the prediction of lymph node condition in penile carcinoma. Eur Urol. 1992;22(2):115–8.

64. Ayyappan K, Ananthakrishnan N, Sankaran V. Can regional lymph node involvement be predicted in patients with carcinoma of the penis? Br J Urol. 1994;73(5):549–53.

65. Lopes A, Rossi BM, Fonseca FP, et al. Unreliability of modified inguinal lymphadenectomy for clinical staging of penile carcinoma. Cancer. 1996;77(10):2099–102.

66. Beggs JH, Spratt JS Jr. Epidermoid carcinoma of the penis. J Urol. 1964; 91(2):166–72.

67. Hardner GJ, Bhanalaph T, Murphy GP, et al. Carcinoma of the penis: analysis of therapy in 100 consecutive cases. J Urol. 1972;108(3):428–30.

68. Kossow JH, Hotchkiss RS, Morales PA. Carcinoma of penis treated surgically. Analysis of 100 cases. Urology. 1973;2(2):169–72.

69. Ekstrom T, Edsmyr F. Cancer of the penis: a clinical study of 229 cases. Acta Chir Scand. 1958;115:25–9.

70. Johnson DE, Lo RK. Management of regional lymph nodes in penile carcinoma. Five-year results following therapeutic groin dissections. Urology. 1984;24(4):308–11.

71. McDougal WS, Kirchner FK Jr, Edwards RH, et al. Treatment of carcinoma of the penis: the case for primary lymphadenectomy. J Urol. 1986;136(1):38–41.

72. Ravi R. Prophylactic Lymphadenectomy vs observation vs inguinal biopsy in node-negative patients with invasive carcinoma of the penis. Jpn J Clin Oncol. 1993;23(1):53–8.

73. Ornellas AA, Seixas AL, Marota A, et al. Surgical treatment of invasive squamous cell carcinoma of the penis: retrospective analysis of 350 cases. J Urol. 1994;151(5):1244–9.

74. Staubitz WJ, Lent MH, Mack FG, et al. Carcinoma of the penis. Cancer. 1955;8:371.

75. Johnson DE, Fuerst DE, Ayala AG. Carcinoma of the penis. Experience with 153 cases. Urology. 1973;1(5):404–8.

76. Gursel EO, Georgountzos C, Uson AC, et al. Penile cancer. Urology. 1973;1(6):569–78.

77. Broders AC. Squamous cell epithelium of the skin. Ann Surg. 1921;73:141–3.

78. Maiche AG, Pyrhonen S, Karkinen M. Histological grading of squamous cell carcinoma of the penis: a new scoring system. Br J Urol. 1991;67(5):522–6.

79. McDougal WS. Carcinoma of the penis: improved survival by early regional lymphadenectomy based on the histological grade and depth of invasion of the primary lesion. J Urol. 1995;154(4):1364–6.

80. Cubilla AL, Barreto J, Caballero C, et al. Pathologic features of epidermoid carcinoma of the penis. A prospective study of 66 cases. Am J Surg Pathol. 1993;17(8):753–63.

81. Theodorescu D, Russo P, Zhang ZF, et al. Outcomes of initial surveillance of invasive squamous cell carcinoma of the penis and negative nodes. J Urol. 1996;155(5):1626–31.

82. Heyns CF, Vollenhoven PV, Steenkamp JW, et al. Carcinoma of the penis-appraisal of a modified tumour-staging system. Br J Urol. 1997;80(2):307–12.

83. Yamashita T, Ogawa A. Ultrasound in penile cancer. Urol Radiol. 1989;11(3):174–7.

84. Dorak AC, Ozkan GA, Tamac NI, et al. Ultrasonography in the recognition of penile cancer. J Clin Ultrasound. 1992;20(9):624–6.

85. Herbener TE, Seftel AD, Nehra A, et al. Penile ultrasound. Semin Urol. 1994;12(4):320–32.

86. Horenblas S, Kroger R, Gallee MP, et al. Ultrasound in squamous cell carcinoma of the penis; a useful addition to clinical staging? A comparison of ultrasound with histopathology. Urology. 1994;43(5):702–7.

87. Lont AP, Besnard AP, Gallee MP, et al. A comparison of physical examination and imaging in determining the extent of primary penile carcinoma. BJU Int. 2003;91(6):493–5.

88. Hricak H, Marotti M, Gilbert TJ, et al. Normal penile anatomy and abnormal penile conditions: evaluation with MR imaging. Radiology. 1988;169(3):683–90.

89. Kawada T, Hashimoto K, Tokunaga T, et al. Two cases of penile cancer: magnetic resonance imaging in the evaluation of tumor extension. J Urol. 1994; 152(3):963–5.

90. de Kerviler E, Ollier P, Desgrandchamps F, et al. Magnetic resonance imaging in patients with penile carcinoma. Br J Radiol. 1995;68(811):704–11.

91. Kageyama S, Ueda T, Kushima R, et al. Primary adenosquamous cell carcinoma of the male distal urethra: magnetic resonance imaging using a circular surface coil. J Urol. 1997;158(5):1913–4.

92. Tabatabaei S, Harisinghani M, McDougal WS. Regional lymph node staging using lymphotropic nanoparticle enhanced magnetic resonance imaging with ferumoxtran-10 in patients with penile cancer. J Urol. 2005;174(3):923–7.

93. Jackson SM. The treatment of carcinoma of the penis. Br J Surg. 1966;53(1):33–5.

94. Mohs FE. Chemosurgery: microscopically controlled surgery for skin cancer-past, present and future. J Dermatol Surg Oncol. 1978;4(1):41–54.

95. Mohs FE, Snow SN, Messing EM, et al. Microscopically controlled surgery in the treatment of carcinoma of the penis. J Urol. 1985;133(6):961–6.

96. Mohs FE, Snow SN, Larson PO. Mohs micrographic surgery for penile tumors. Urol Clin North Am. 1992;19(2):291–304.

97. Farrell AM, Dawber RP. Squamous cell carcinoma of the penis. J Am Acad Dermatol. 1998;38(3):504–5.

98. Frimberger D, Hungerhuber E, Zaak D, et al. Penile carcinoma. Is Nd:YAG laser therapy radical enough? J Urol. 2002;168(6):2418–21.

99. Zouhair A, Coucke PA, Jeanneret W, et al. Radiation therapy alone or combined surgery and radiation therapy in squamous-cell carcinoma of the penis? Eur J Cancer. 2001;37(2):198–203.

100. Kiltie AE, Elwell C, Close HJ, et al. Iridium-192 implantation for node-negative carcinoma of the penis: the Cookridge Hospital experience. Clin Oncol. 2000;12(1):25–31.

101. Crook J, Grimard L, Tsihlias J, et al. Interstitial brachytherapy for penile cancer: an alternative to amputation. J Urol. 2002;167(2 Pt 1):506–11.

102. Crook JM, Jezioranski J, Math M, et al. Penile brachytherapy: results for 49 patients. Int J Radiat Oncol Biol Phys. 2005;62(2):460–7.

103. Agrawal A, Pai D, Ananthakrishnan N, et al. The histological extent of the local spread of carcinoma of the penis and its therapeutic implications. BJU Int. 2000;85:299–301.

104. Hanash KA, Furlow WL, Utz DC, et al. Carcinoma of the penis: a clinicopathologic study. J Urol. 1970;104(2):291–7.

105. Jensen MO. Cancer of the penis in Denmark 1942 to 1962(511 cases). Dan Med Bull. 1977;24(2):66–72.

106. Opjordsmoen S, Fossa SD. Quality of life in patients treated for penile cancer. A follow-up study. Br J Urol. 1994;74(5):652–7.

107. Opjordsmoen S, Waehre H, Aass N, et al. Sexuality in patients treated for penile cancer: patients' experience and doctors judgement. Br J Urol. 1994;73(5):554–60.

108. Bissada NK, Yakout HH, Fahmy WE, et al. Multi-institutional long-term experience with conservative surgery for invasive penile carcinoma. J Urol. 2003;169:500–2.

109. Pietrzak P, Corbishley C, Watkin N. Ogran-sparing surgery for invasive penile cancer: early follow-up data. BJU Int. 2004;94:1253–7.

110. McDougal WS. Phallic preserving surgery in patients with invasive squamous cell carcinoma of the penis. J Urol. 2005;174(6):2218–20.

111. Fraley EE, Zhang G, Manivel C, et al. The role of ilioinguinal lymphadenectomy and significance of histological differentiation in treatment of carcinoma of the penis. J Urol. 1989;142(6):1478–82.

112. Horenblas S, van Tinteren H. Squamous cell carcinoma of the penis. IV. Prognostic factors of survival: analysis of tumor, nodes and metastasis classification system. J Urol. 1994;151(5):1239–43.

113. Skinner DG, Leadbetter WF, Kelley SB. The surgical management of squamous cell carcinoma of the penis. J Urol. 1972;107(2):273–7.

114. Lopes A, Hidalgo GS, Kowalski LP, et al. Prognostic factors in carcinoma of the penis: multivariate analysis of 145 patients treated with amputation and lymphadenectomy. J Urol. 1996;156(5):1637–42.

115. Horenblas S, van Tinteren H, Delemarre JF, et al. Squamous cell carcinoma of the penis. III. Treatment of regional lymph nodes. J Urol. 1993;149(3):492–7.

116. Fegen P, Persky L. Squamous cell carcinoma of the penis: its treatment, with special reference to radical node dissection. Arch Surg. 1969;99(1):117–20.

117. Cabanas RM. An approach for the treatment of penile carcinoma. Cancer. 1977;39(2):456–66.

118. Cabanas RM. Anatomy and biopsy of sentinel lymph nodes. Urol Clin North Am. 1992;19(2):267–76.

119. Cabanas RM. Application of the sentinel node concept in urogenital cancer. Recent Results Cancer Res. 2000;157:141–9.

120. Perinetti E, Crane DB, Catalona WJ. Unreliability of sentinel lymph node biopsy for staging penile carcinoma. J Urol. 1980;124(5):734–5.

121. Wespes E, Simon J, Schulman CC. Cabanas approach: is sentinel node biopsy reliable for staging penile carcinoma? Urology. 1986;28(4):278–9.

122. Srinivas V, Joshi A, Agarwal B, et al. Penile cancer-the sentinel lymph node controversy. Urol Int. 1991;47(2):108–9.

123. Pettaway CA, Pisters LL, Dinney CP, et al. Sentinel lymph node dissection for penile carcinoma: the M.D. Anderson Cancer Center experience. J Urol. 1995;154(6):1999–2003.

124. Morton DL, Wen DR, Wong JH, et al. Technical details of intraoperative lymphatic mapping for early stage melanoma. Arch Surg. 1992;127(4):392–9.

125. Han KR, Brogle BN, Goydos J, et al. Lymphatic mapping and intraoperative lymphoscintigraphy for identifying the sentinel node in penile tumors. Urology. 2000;55(4):582–5.

126. Valdes Olmos RA, Tanis PJ, Hoefnagel CA, et al. Penile lymphoscintigraphy for sentinel node identification. Eur J Nucl Med. 2001;28(5):581–5.

127. Tanis PJ, Lont AP, Meinhardt W, et al. Dynamic sentinel node biopsy for penile cancer: reliability of a staging technique. J Urol. 2002;168(1):76–80.

128. Horenblas S, Jansen L, Meinhardt W, et al. Detection of occult metastasis in squamous cell carcinoma of the penis using a dynamic sentinel node procedure. J Urol. 2000;163(1):100–4.

129. Tanis PJ, Lont AP, Meinhardt W, et al. Dynamic sentinel node biopsy for penile cancer: reliability of a staging technique. J Urol. 2002;168:76–80.

130. Lont AP, Horenblas S, Tanis PJ, et al. Management of clinically node negative penile carcinoma: improved survival after the introduction of dynamic sentinel node biopsy. J Urol. 2003;170:783–6.

131. Kroon BK, Horenblas S, Deurloo EE, et al. Ultrasonography-guided fine-needle aspiration cytology before sentinel node biopsy in patients with penile carcinoma. BJU Int. 2005;95:517–21.

132. Martins ACP, Faria SM, Cologna AJ, et al. Immunoexpression of p53 protein and proliferating cell nuclear antigen in penile carcinoma. J Urol. 2002;167:89–93.

133. Lopes A, Bezerra ALR, Pinto CAL, et al. p53 as a new prognostic factor for lymph node metastasis in penile carcinoma: analysis of 82 patients treated with amputation and bilateral lymphadenectomy. J Urol. 2002;168:81–6.

134. Berdjis N, Meye A, Nippgen J, et al. Expression of Ki-67 in squamous cell carcinoma of the penis. BJU Int.2005;96:146–8.

135. Laniado ME, Lowdell C, Mitchell H, et al. Squamous cell carcinoma antigen: a role in the early identification of nodal metastases in men with squamous cell carcinoma of the penis. BJU Int. 2003;92:248–50.

136. Kroon BK, Horenblas S, Lont AP, et al. Patients with penile carcinoma benefit from immediate resection of clinically occult lymph node metastases. J Urol. 2005;173(3):816–9.

137. Ornellas AA, Seixas AL, de Moraes JR. Analyses of 200 lymphadenectomies in patients with penile carcinoma. J Urol. 1991;146(2):330–2.

138. Kamat MR, Kulkarni JN, Tongaonkar HB. Carcinoma of the penis: the Indian experience. J Surg Oncol. 1993;52(1):50–5.

139. Ravi R. Morbidity following groin dissection for penile carcinoma. Br J Urol. 1993;72(6):941–5.

140. Johnson DE, Lo RK. Complications of groin dissection in penile cancer. Experience with 101 lymphadenectomies. Urology. 1984;24(4):312–4.

141. Bevan-Thomas R, Slaton JW, Pettaway CA. Contemporary morbidity from lymphadenectomy for penile squamous cell carcinoma: the M.D. Anderson Cancer Center Experience. J Urol. 2002;167(4):1638–42.

142. Nelson BA, Cookson MS, Smith JA, et al. Complications of inguinal and pelvic lymphadenectomy for squamous cell carcinoma of the penis: a contemporary series. J Urol. 2004;172: 494–7.

143. Graham SD, Kean TE, Glenn JF. Glenns Urologic Surgery. 6th ed. Philadelphia: Lippincott Williams & Wilkins; 2004.

144. Tabatabaei S, McDougal WS. Primary skin closure of large groin defects after inguinal lymphadenectomy for penile cancer using an abdominal cutaneous advancement flap. J Urol. 2003;169(1): 118–20.

145. el-Demiry MI, Oliver RT, Hope-Stone HF, et al. Reappraisal of the role of radiotherapy and surgery in the management of carcinoma of the penis. Br J Urol. 1984;56(6):724–8.

146. Vaeth JM, Green JP, Lowy RO. Radiation therapy of carcinoma of the penis. Am J Roentgenol Radium Ther Nucl Med. 1970;108(1):130–5.

147. Pizzocaro G, Piva L. Adjuvant and neoadjuvant vincristine, bleomycin, and methotrexate for inguinal metastases from squamous cell carcinoma of the penis. Acta Oncol. 1988;27(6b): 823–4.

148. Hussein AM, Benedetto P, Sridhar KS. Chemotherapy with cisplatin and 5-fluorouracil for penile and urethral squamous cell carcinomas. Cancer. 1990;65(3):433–8.

149. Dexeus FH, Logothetis CJ, Sella A, et al. Combination chemotherapy with methotrexate, bleomycin and cisplatin for advanced squamous cell carcinoma of the male genital tract. J Urol. 1991;146(5):1284–7.

150. Shammas FV, Ous S, Fossa SD. Cisplatin and 5-fluorouracil in advanced cancer. J Urol. 1992;147(3):630–2.

151. Forero L, Patnaik A, Hammond LA, et al. Phase I, pharmacokinetic (PK) and biologic study of OSI-774, a selective epidermal growth factor receptor (EGFR) tyrosine kinase (TK) inhibitor in combination with paclitaxel and carboplatin. 2002 ASCO Annual Meeting, abstract no.1908.

152. Golijanin D, Tan JY, Kazior A, et al. Cyclooxygenase-2 and microsomal prostaglandin E synthase-1 are overexpressed in squamous cell carcinoma of the penis. Clin Cancer Res. 2004;10: 1024–31.

Chapter 31

Conventional Imaging in Penis Cancer

M.G. Harisinghani and M.A. Saksena

Introduction

Accurate pretreatment staging implications and includes evaluation of the size and extent of the primary tumor, assessment of regional lymph nodes for nodal metastasis, and detection of distant metastatic disease. Assessment of the primary tumor is commonly performed by physical palpation performed to evaluate invasion into the corpus spongiosum, corpora cavernosa, and the skin. This method frequently results in understaging, and accurate assessment of local invasion is ideally performed by pathological analysis [1]. Similarly, ilioinguinal lymph node dissection is performed to assess the local nodes and has been shown to provide a significant benefit in patients who have nodal metastases. But this invasive procedure is associated with significant morbidity and mortality even with modern surgical techniques. Hence, pretreatment imaging plays a significant role in the staging of penile cancer.

This chapter reviews the conventional imaging methods utilized for staging penile cancer.

Cavernosography

Before the advent of modern imaging modalities cavernosography was used to evaluate patients with penile cancer. It involves injection of contrast directly into the corpora cavernosa and has been shown to be safe and simple method preoperative staging of penile cancers and aids in determining the level of penectomy [2]. In a study of 10 patients, a corpus cavernosogram was used to assess the involvement of the corpora cavernosa, and findings were correlated with histopathology. It led to disease upstaging in one patient and two patients had disease extension more proximally than that

apparent by physical palpation [2]. However, this is an invasive method and in the current milieu of non-invasive cross-sectional imaging it is of historic significance only.

Follow-Up of Penile Carcinoma

Although penectomy with surgical lymphadenectomy provides high cure rates even in patients with nodal metastatic disease, routine follow-up is recommended to evaluate both local recurrence and development of nodal metastases. Follow-up is usually performed by physical examination as the penis and inguinal nodes are amenable to direct clinical evaluation. Chest radiographs can help to evaluate for distant metastases particularly in patients with known nodal metastatic involvement. Pelvic nodes can be assessed by cross-sectional imaging methods such as computed tomography (CT). Cross-sectional imaging in penile cancer is discussed in the following chapter.

References

1. Vapnek JM, Hricak H, Carroll PR. Recent advances in imaging studies for staging of penile and urethral carcinoma. Urol Clin North Am. 1992;19:257–266.
2. Raghavaiah NV. Corpus cavernosogram in the evaluation of carcinoma of the penis. J Urol. 1978;120:423–424.

M. G. Harisinghani (✉)
White 270, Massachusetts General Hospital, Boston, MA 02114, USA

Chapter 32

Cross-Sectional Imaging in Penis Cancer

M.A. Saksena and M.G. Harisinghani

Introduction

When diagnosed early (stages I and II), penile cancer is highly curable, whereas curability decreases sharply for stages III and IV. Hence, assessment of the clinical stage and depth of invasion are vital for both therapeutic decision-making and prognosis. Although, physical examination has long been utilized to predict primary tumor size and cavernosal infiltration it is not as sensitive as MRI in making these evaluations. Awareness of local or distant metastatic lymph node disease is also crucial in deciding the surgical technique and predicting survival. Physical palpation to detect nodal metastases has high-incidence false-negative and false-positive results; 10-20% of non-palpable normal-sized nodes may harbor micrometastatic disease while palpable nodes are metastatic only 40–60% of the time [1–3]. Pelvic nodes, which may also be a site of metastatic disease, are not amenable to clinical evaluation. Ilioinguinal lymph node dissection used to assess inguinal lymph nodes has been shown to be therapeutic and may be associated with improved long-term survival. However, it can be complicated by scrotal and leg edema, infection, flap necrosis, and seroma formation [4–6]. Therefore, reliable non-invasive imaging methods utilized to assess inguinal nodal disease may prevent surgery in patients with uninvolved inguinal nodes. Hence, pretreatment imaging has a significant role to play in both staging the primary tumor and nodal evaluation. This chapter elucidates the various cross-sectional modalities used in staging penile cancer and illustrates their specific applications.

Anatomy

The shaft of the penis is formed by the paired corpora cavernosa lying dorsolaterally and the single ventral corpora spongiosum. The corpora spongiosum contains the urethra and extends anteriorly to form the glans penis. Its proximal portion is connected to the urogenital diaphragm and is surrounded by the bulbospongiosus muscle. The corpora cavernosa are the primary erectile structures of the penis and are attached to the pubic symphysis and the linea alba via the suspensory ligament of the penis. Tunica albuginea is the deepest thick fibrous layer that surrounds all three penile corpora and separates the cavernosa from the spongiosum. The two cavernosa are separated by a thin septum. Tunica albuginea normally measures 2–3 mm and thins down to about 0.5 mm during erection. The Buck's fascia is a thick penile fascia, which lies external to the tunica. It is surrounded by a continuation of the scarpa's fascia in the abdomen and pelvis known as the Colles' fascia. Colles' fascia is the loose superficial fascia of the penis and is in turn covered by skin. They are of intermediate signal on T1 and high signal on T2-weighted sequence. It is hypointense on all pulse sequences and appears thicker around the corpora cavernosa due to fusion with Buck fascia. Tunica dartos is located just deep to the skin. Gadolinium enhancement of the cavernosa proceeds centrifugally, extending from cavernosal arteries to the periphery [7] (Fig. 32.1).

Paired internal pudendal branches of the internal iliac artery supply the penis, and the venous drainage is through the deep and superficial dorsal penile veins which connect to the pudendal plexus and drain into the internal pudendal veins. Lymphatic drainage of the penis and hence nodal metastatic spread of cancer differs by location. The glans drains into the deep inguinal and external iliac nodes while the shaft drains first to the superficial inguinal nodes. Lymphatic drainage from the urethra is directly into the internal iliac nodes bypassing the inguinal nodes. Bilateral lymphatics communicate with each other resulting in bilateral nodal involvement in unilateral tumors.

M.A. Saksena (✉)
Division of Abdominal Imaging and Intervention, Department of Radiology. Massachusetts General Hospital, 55 Fruit street, Boston MA 02114, msaksena@partners.org

J.J.M.C.H. de la Rosette et al. (eds.), *Imaging in Oncological Urology*,
DOI 10.1007/978-1-84628-759-6_32, © Springer-Verlag London Limited 2009

Penile Cancer Pathology

Penile cancer predominantly presents in the sixth and seventh decades of life and is rare under 40 years of age. Squamous cell carcinoma accounts for 95% of all primary neoplasms of the penis. It is most commonly located in the glans penis (48%), prepuce (21%), glans and prepuce (9%), coronal sulcus (6%), and shaft (2%).

The risk of penile cancer is three times higher in uncircumcised men and increases with poor hygiene through accumulation of smegma and other irritants and phimosis. Chronic inflammatory conditions, smoking, treatment with psoralen or ultraviolet A photo chemotherapy, and infection from human papilloma virus 16 and 18 are all risk factors for the development of penile cancer.

Non-squamous penile neoplasms include sarcoma, melanoma, basal cell carcinoma, and lymphoma. Penile metastases are rare with primary tumors being primarily in the urogenital tract.

Staging the Primary Tumor

The TNM classification (Table 32.1) is a commonly used staging system for penile neoplasms. An alternative older classification system is the Jackson classification system (Table 32.2). Irrespective of the classification used imaging plays a significant role in the staging of penile cancer.

MRI is the primary imaging modality used in the evaluation of the primary tumor of the penis. Other cross-Sectional

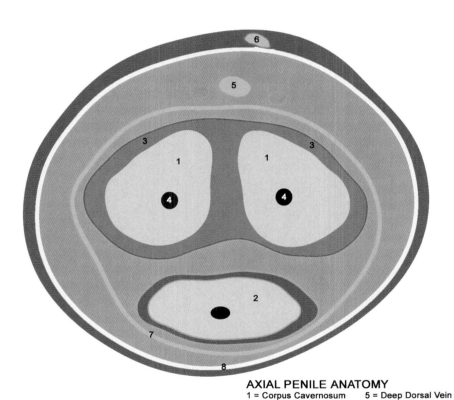

AXIAL PENILE ANATOMY

1 = Corpus Cavernosum	5 = Deep Dorsal Vein
2 = Corpus Spongiosum	6 = Superficial Dorsal Vein
3 = Tunica Albuginea	7 = Buck's Fascia
4 = Cavernosal Arteries	8 = Dartos Tunica

Fig. 32.1 Normal penile anatomy (reprinted with permission from Singh et al. [7]). (a) Drawing (axial view) illustrates the normal penile anatomy. *1* = corpora cavernosa, *2* = corpus spongiosum, *3* = tunica albuginea, *4* = cavernosal arteries, *5* = deep dorsal vein, *6* = superficial dorsal vein, *7* = Buck fascia, *8* = dartos tunica. (b) Axial T2-weighted MR image shows the two corpora cavernosa and the ventral corpus spongiosum. The tunica albuginea surrounds the corpora cavernosa. (c) Drawing (*sagittal view*) illustrates the normal penile anatomy. *1* = corpus cavernosum, *2* = corpus spongiosum, *3* = urethra, *4* = glans penis, *5* = tunica albuginea. (d) Sagittal MR image shows the corpus spongiosum flaring posteriorly into bulbous spongiosum. (e) Axial T2-weighted MR image shows the base of the penis and the attachment of the posterior portion of the corpora cavernosa, known as the crura to the pubic arch. (f) Sagittal contrast material-enhanced T1-weighted MR image shows the corpus cavernosum and the corpus spongiosum

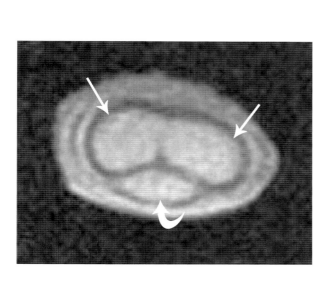

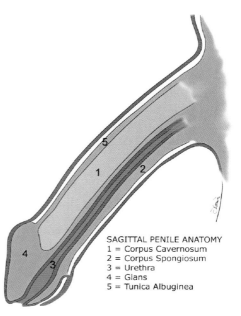

SAGITTAL PENILE ANATOMY
1 = Corpus Cavernosum
2 = Corpus Spongiosum
3 = Urethra
4 = Glans
5 = Tunica Albuginea

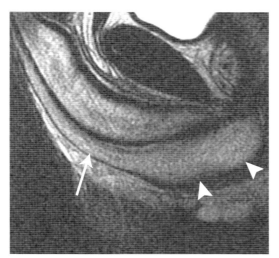

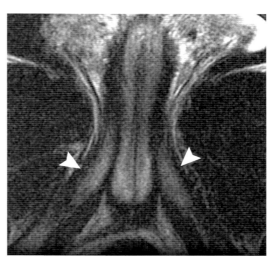

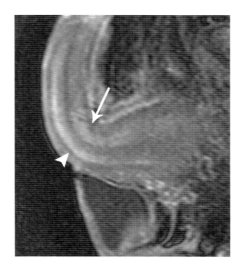

Table 32.1 TNM classification of penile carcinoma (reprinted with permission from Singh et al. [7])

Stage	Description
Tumor (T)	
Tx	Primary tumor cannot be assessed
T0	No evidence of primary tumor
Tis	Carcinoma in situ
T1	Invasion of subepithelial connective tissue
T2	Invasion of one or more corpora
T3	Invasion of urethra or prostate gland
T4	Invasion of other adjacent structures
Lymph node (N)	
Nx	Regional lymph node cannot be assessed
N0	No regional lymph node metastasis
N1	Metastasis in a single superficial inguinal lymph node
N2	Metastases in multiple or bilateral superficial inguinal lymph nodes
N3	Unilateral or bilateral metastases in deep inguinal or pelvic lymph nodes
Metastasis (M)	
Mx	Distant metastasis cannot be assessed
M0	No evidence of distant metastasis
M1	Distant metastasis

Table 32.2 The Jackson classification of staging penile cancer

Extent of tumor involvement	Stage of malignancy
Lesion confined to the glans	Stage I
Lesion invading into the shaft or corpora	Stage II
Inguinal node metastases amenable to surgery	Stage III
Tumor invades adjacent structures (extending of the shaft), inoperable inguinal node metastases, and/or distant metastases	Stage IV

modalities such as computed tomography (CT) and ultrasound (US) lack the required soft tissue resolution to adequately stage primary penile neoplasms. However, CT does have a role in nodal evaluation, detection of distant metastatic disease, and diagnosis of postoperative complications.

MR Imaging Technique

The patient is placed supine with a towel between his legs inferior to the perineum, in order to elevate the penis and scrotum. The penis is then dorsiflexed over the lower abdomen and taped in position so as to decrease organ motion during the study. If imaging in the flaccid state is inadequate pharmacological tumescence may be achieved by intracavernosal alprostadil (prostaglandin E1 analogue) injection. [8, 9]. However, this technique should only be utilized if images in the flaccid state do not provide enough information as a risk of priapism exists in a small number of patients [9]. Although most penile prostheses are consid-

ered safe for MRI examination information about a particular implant must be obtained before a patient with a penile prostheses is cleared for an MR.

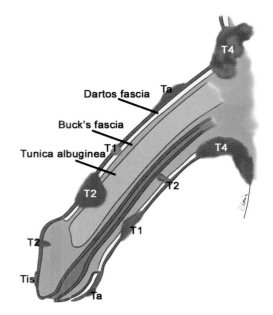

Fig. 32.2 Drawing illustrates local staging of penile neoplasms: T1, invasion of subepithelial connective tissue; T2, invasion of one or more corpora; T3, invasion of urethra or prostate gland; T4, invasion of other adjacent structures; and *Tis*, carcinoma in situ (reprinted with permission from Singh et al. [7])

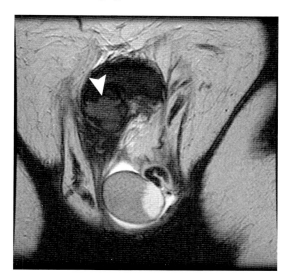

Fig. 32.3 Squamous cell carcinoma of the penis. Coronal T2-weighted MR image shows a mass with heterogeneous signal intensity (*arrowhead*) involving the corpora cavernosa. Hydrocele is seen incidentally (reprinted with permission from Singh et al. [7])

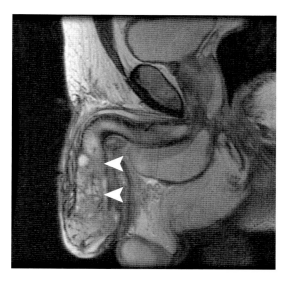

Fig. 32.5 Verrucous carcinoma of the penis. Sagittal T2-weighted MR image demonstrates a mass with heterogeneous signal intensity (*arrowheads*) involving the glans penis and the corpora cavernosa (reprinted with permission from Singh et al. [7])

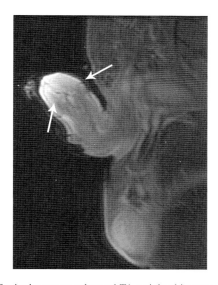

Fig. 32.4 Sagittal contrast enhanced T1-weighted images demonstrate a 2.5 cm squamous cell carcinoma (arrows) demonstrating invasion of the glans

MR Imaging Protocol

A 3- or 5 inch surface coil is placed on the penis. Images are obtained with a small field of view (12–16), high matrix, and thin slices. Typical sequences performed include axial spin echo T1-weighted images, triplane fast spin echo T2-weighted images, and three-dimensional fat- saturated T1-weighted gradient echo images obtained before, during, and after the administration of intravenous gadolinium. A body coil may be used to obtain images of the entire pelvis to evaluate for nodal metastases.

Normal MR Appearance

The corpora are of intermediate signal intensity on T1-weighted images, hyperintense on T2-weighted images, and demonstrate contrast enhancement on post-gadolinium images [10]. The corpora cavernosum maybe of a different signal intensity than corpora spongiosum. Corpora cavernosa enhance after the spongiosum in a centrifugal manner probably due to the presence of a central cavernosal artery [11]. The urethral walls are hypointense compared to the corpus spongiosum within which it lies. A T1 and T2 hypointense rim surrounds the corpora representing the tunica albuginea.

MR Staging of Penile Cancer

The local extent of a primary penile tumor has significant therapeutic implications. Lesions limited to the glans or the prepuce are classified as T1 disease and are amenable to minimal surgery with good 5-year survival rates. In contrast infiltrative tumors with invasion of the corpus may undergo penile amputation and have poorer survival rates, which decrease further in the presence of nodal metastases. Table 32.1 elucidates the TNM classification used to stage penile cancers.

The traditional approach of the assessment of a primary penile tumor by physical examination alone is ineffective in accurate primary tumor staging while CT does not have the soft tissue resolution needed for complete evaluation of primary penile tumors. Although ultrasound has been utilized

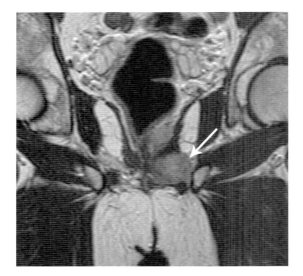

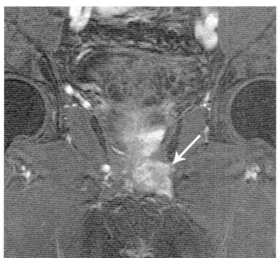

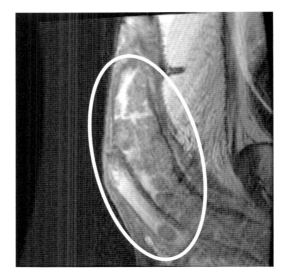

Fig. 32.7 Penile metastases from a prostatic primary neoplasm. Sagittal contrast-enhanced T1-weighted MR image shows extensive multiple low-signal-intensity lesions (*circled*) involving the corpora cavernosa and the corpus spongiosum (reprinted with permission from Singh et al. [7])

Fig. 32.6 Adenoid cystic carcinoma arising from the Cowper gland. Coronal T2-weighted (a) and gadolinium-enhanced T1-weighted (b) MR images show a mass (*arrow*) centered at the bulbous urethra and infiltrating the left obturator internus muscle (reprinted with permission from Singh et al. [7])

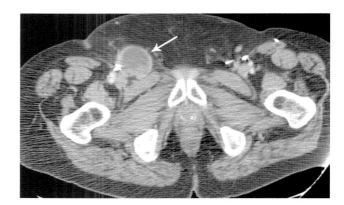

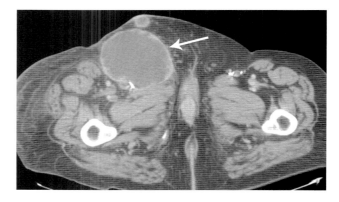

for penile tumor staging it is ineffective in nodal evaluation and lacks the superior tissue resolution provided by MRI.

The much-needed accurate staging of the primary tumor can be effectively performed with an MR examination, which also serves to evaluate regional nodes. T2-weighted and gadolinium-enhanced T1-weighted MR images are the primary sequences used to define the extent of the primary tumor. The primary neoplasm usually presents as a solitary, infiltrative tumor, which is hypointense compared to normal penile tissue on both T1- and T2-weighted images and demonstrates enhancement on post-gadolinium T1-weighted images. The tunica albuginea is normally well visualized as a hypointense rim surrounding the corpora. Disruption

Fig. 32.8 Inguinal nodal metastases from penile cancer post-inguinal lymphadenectomy. (a) Axial CT scans demonstrate enlarged right inguinal lymph node (arrow) consistent with nodal metastases from the patient's primary penile cancer. (b) Repeat CT scan performed 4 weeks later demonstrates an increase in nodal size (arrow) with a necrotic center and a thick enhancing rim

of this rim by the hypointense tumor suggests invasion into the tunica. The depth of tumor invasion, degree of corporal involvement, and urethral invasion can be evaluated on MRI and provide vital information for primary tumor staging.

The presence of multiple satellite nodules within the penile shaft, which are similar in signal characteristics to a primary squamous cell penile cancer, raise the suspicion for a epitheloid sarcoma [12]. Epitheloid sarcoma is a malignant soft tissue neoplasm, which is rarely seen involving the penis.

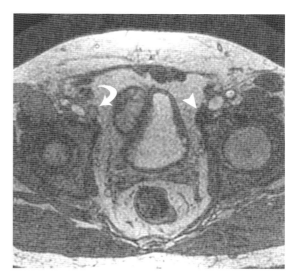

Fig. 32.9 (continued)

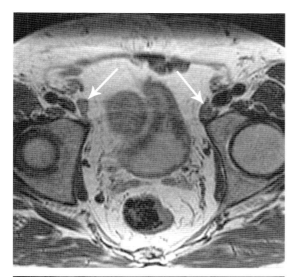

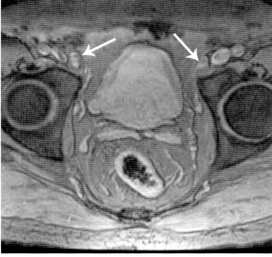

Fig. 32.9 Metastatic external iliac lymphadenopathy from penile carcinoma. (a) T2-weighted MR image and (b) axial T2∗ image obtained before the administration of ultrasmall superparamagnetic iron oxide particles shows bilateral external iliac lymphadenopathy (*arrows*). (c) T2-weighted MR image obtained after the administration of the iron oxide particles, the right external iliac lymph node (*arrow*) appears bright due to lack of particle uptake, a finding that indicates replacement of the lymph node parenchyma by metastatic tissue. The left external iliac lymph node (*arrowhead*) shows normal particle uptake and is hypointense owing to susceptibility effect

Rare non-squamous penile tumors may differ in MR appearance. Melanomas are hyperintense on both T1- and T2-weighted images and demonstrate intense contrast enhancement. Rhabdomyosarcomas are similar to the surrounding muscle in signal intensity and enhance heterogeneously following gadolinium administration. Metastatic lesions present as multiple discrete masses in the corpora cavernosa and spongiosum. They are typically hypointense on T1- and T2-weighted sequences. Irrespective of tumor histology contrast-enhanced MR imaging is effective and accurate in defining the tumor limits and hence in determining extent of excision.

Nodal Staging

The presence and extent of inguinal nodal metastases is the most important prognostic factor in invasive squamous cell carcinoma of the penis [13, 14]. In patients with nodal disease confined to the inguinal nodes, inguinal lymphadenectomy is curative with 30–90% disease-free rates while patients with pelvic nodal disease have a 5-year survival rate of less than 10% [15, 16]. The incidence of nodal metastatic disease has been associated with the grade and stage of the primary tumor. Patients with well-differentiated tumors have a 24% chance of nodal spread while those with poorly differentiated tumors have a 33% chance of nodal metastatic disease. [17]. As described before the location of nodal disease depends on the site of the primary tumor.

Physical palpation to detect nodal metastases has high-incidence false-negative and false-positive results; 10–20% of non-palpable normal-sized nodes may harbor micrometastatic disease while palpable nodes are metastatic only 40–60% of the time [1–3]. Although inguinal lymphadenectomy is curative it is associated with significant mortality and morbidity. If all patients with penile cancer underwent bilateral groin dissection a significant number would be subjected to a needless operation. Hence, non-invasive imaging has a significant role in identifying patients who would benefit from a groin dissection. Although depth of invasion and the grade of the primary lesion have been proposed as markers of nodal disease these even when combined have a positive predictive value of about 80% [18]. Therefore there is a significant role for a diagnostic test, which can evaluate regional lymph nodes with a high predictive value.

Lymphotropic Nanoparticle-Enhanced MRI

Lymphotropic nanoparticle-enhanced MRI (LNMRI) has emerged as a promising new technique for non-invasive nodal evaluation in patients undergoing staging for various malignancies [19–21]. It utilizes a novel contrast agent consisting of ultrasmall superparamagnetic iron oxide (ferumoxtran-10; AMI-227; Combidex®, Advanced Magnetics Inc, Cambridge, MA; Sinerem®, Laboratoire Guerbet, Aulnay-sous-Bois, France) particles which are small enough in size to migrate across the capillary walls and localize within lymph nodes allowing robust characterization of nodes independent of the size criterion [22, 23]. On intravenous administration these particles extravasate from the vessels into the interstitial space, from where they are transported to lymph nodes. Within a normal lymph node, nodal macrophages (which comprise the reticuloendothelial system [RES]) phagocytose these nanoparticles causing them to accumulate within the node. Intranodal accumulation of the contrast agent causes normal nodes to take up agent and turn dark on post-contrast T2- and T2∗-weighted imaging. Metastatic nodes lack functional macrophages and retain high signal intensity on post-contrast imaging. Tabatabaei et al. reported a sensitivity of 100%, a specificity of 97%, and a negative predictive value of 100% for nodal evaluation with LNMRI in patients with penile cancer. This is higher than those achieved by either clinical evaluation or other cross-sectional modalities. In the future as these contrast agents become readily available LNMRI promises to play a significant role in the nodal evaluation of all patients with malignancy including those with penile cancer.

Distant Metastases

About 2.3% of patients with penile cancer present with distant metastases [24]. The commonest sites of distant metastatic disease are the lung, liver, and retroperitoneum. CT is the modality of choice for detection of distant metastatic disease. It allows for efficient screening of the chest and abdomen for metastatic disease and can be used for both initial evaluation and follow-up imaging.

Role of Imaging in Follow-Up of Penile Cancer

Post-treatment evaluation of patients with penile cancer is primarily based on clinical evaluation as both the penile and inguinal regions are accessible to physical examination. As per the EAU guidelines patients treated with conservative therapy such as laser surgery, brachytherapy, or local resection should undergo clinical evaluation every 2 months for 2 years and every 3 months in the third year [25]. Long-term follow-up every 6 months should be performed to detect late recurrences. For patient's treated with surgery a follow-up visit every 4 months for 2 years, every 6 months for a year, and annually thereafter is recommended. In patients under surveillance after removal of the primary tumor, groin evaluation can be performed clinically every 2 months for 2 years, every 3 months for another year, and biannually for another 2 years [25]. Patients who develop new palpable lymph nodes almost always have metastatic nodal involvement. Patients who have undergone inguinal lymphadenectomy and had negative nodes should be followed up clinically every 4 months for 2 years and biannually for another year [25].

No radiological studies are usually performed in patients who do not demonstrate clinical signs of recurrence. Abdominal pelvic CT scans and LNMRI studies can be used to evaluate suspicious nodal involvement. Other imaging such as bone scan and chest radiographs is performed to evaluate specific symptoms such as back pain. No routine imaging follow-up is recommended in these patients.

Follow-up in patients with positive nodes after surgery (pN1–3) depends on the number of nodes involved and the type of adjuvant therapy used. Frequency of CT scans and chest radiographs is not defined and is often established by the institution [25]. Bone scans can be used to evaluate for specific symptoms.

Conclusions

Pre-treatment staging based on clinical evaluation alone can often lead to inaccurate staging in patients with penile cancer. Contrast-enhanced MRI provides the soft tissue detail necessary for the assessment of the local extent of the tumor. Palpable groin nodes do not always signify metastatic nodal involvement, and non-invasive imaging techniques of CT and LNMRI help distinguish inflammatory nodal enlargement from metastatic nodal disease. Hence, groin dissection can be avoided in patients who do not have malignant nodal disease. Additionally, identification of micrometastatic disease in unenlarged nodes leads to adequate management and helps improve patient outcomes. Imaging plays a significant role in clinical decision-making in patients with penile cancer in any stage and its judicious use aids in making treatment decision and predicting prognosis.

References

1. Hoppmann HJ, Fraley EE. Squamous cell carcinoma of the penis. J Urol. 1978;120:393–8.
2. Catalona WJ. Role of lymphadenectomy in carcinoma of the penis. Urol Clin North Am. 1980;7:785–92.
3. Abi-Aad AS, deKernion JB. Controversies in ilioinguinal lymphadenectomy for cancer of the penis. Urol Clin North Am. 1992;19:319–24.
4. Ornellas AA, Seixas AL, Marota A, Wisnescky A, Campos F, de Moraes JR. Surgical treatment of invasive squamous cell carcinoma of the penis: Retrospective analysis of 350 cases. J Urol. 1994;151:1244–9.
5. Johnson DE, Lo RK. Complications of groin dissection in penile cancer. experience with 101 lymphadenectomies. Urology. 1984;24:312–4.
6. Solsona E, Iborra I, Rubio J, Casanova JL, Ricos JV, Calabuig C. Prospective validation of the association of local tumor stage and grade as a predictive factor for occult lymph node micrometastasis in patients with penile carcinoma and clinically negative inguinal lymph nodes. J Urol. 2001;165:1506–9.
7. Singh AK, Saokar A, Hahn PF, Harisinghani MG. Imaging of penile neoplasms. Radiographics. 2005;25:1629–38.
8. Vossough A, Pretorius ES, Siegelman ES, Ramchandani P, Banner MP. Magnetic resonance imaging of the penis. Abdom Imaging. 2002;27:640–59.
9. Scardino E, Villa G, Bonomo G, et al. Magnetic resonance imaging combined with artificial erection for local staging of penile cancer. Urology. 2004;63:1158–62.
10. Hricak H, Marotti M, Gilbert TJ, et al. Normal penile anatomy and abnormal penile conditions: Evaluation with MR imaging. Radiology. 1988;169:683–90.
11. Kaneko K, De Mouy EH, Lee BE. Sequential contrast-enhanced MR imaging of the penis. Radiology. 1994;191:75–7.
12. Oto A, Meyer J. MR appearance of penile epithelioid sarcoma. AJR Am J Roentgenol. 1999;172:555–6.
13. McDougal WS, Kirchner FK Jr, Edwards RH, Killion LT. Treatment of carcinoma of the penis: the case for primary lymphadenectomy. J Urol. 1986;136:38–41.
14. Ravi R. Correlation between the extent of nodal involvement and survival following groin dissection for carcinoma of the penis. Br J Urol. 1993;72:817–9.
15. Kossow JH, Hotchkiss RS, Morales PA. Carcinoma of penis treated surgically. analysis of 100 cases. Urology. 1973;2:169–72.
16. McDougal WS. Carcinoma of the penis: Improved survival by early regional lymphadenectomy based on the histological grade and depth of invasion of the primary lesion. J Urol. 1995;154:1364–6.
17. Ekstrom T, Edsmyr F. Cancer of the penis; a clinical study of 229 cases. Acta Chir Scand. 1958;115:25–45.
18. McDougal WS. Carcinoma of the penis. J Urol. 1994;151:1250.
19. Tabatabaei S, Harisinghani M, McDougal WS. Regional lymph node staging using lymphotropic nanoparticle enhanced magnetic resonance imaging with ferumoxtran-10 in patients with penile cancer. J Urol. 2005;174:923–7; discussion 927.
20. Anzai Y, Piccoli CW, Outwater EK, et al. Evaluation of neck and body metastases to nodes with ferumoxtran 10-enhanced MR imaging: Phase III safety and efficacy study. Radiology. 2003;228:777–88.
21. Harisinghani MG, Barentsz J, Hahn PF, et al. Noninvasive detection of clinically occult lymph-node metastases in prostate cancer. N Engl J Med. 2003;348:2491–9.
22. Weissleder R, Elizondo G, Wittenberg J, Rabito CA, Bengele HH, Josephson L. Ultrasmall superparamagnetic iron oxide: characterization of a new class of contrast agents for MR imaging. Radiology. 1990;175:489–93.
23. Weissleder R, Heautot JF, Schaffer BK, et al. MR lymphography: study of a high-efficiency lymphotrophic agent. Radiology. 1994;191:225–30.
24. Rippentrop JM, Joslyn SA, Konety BR. Squamous cell carcinoma of the penis: evaluation of data from the surveillance, epidemiology, and end results program. Cancer. 2004;101:1357–63.
25. Solsona E, Algaba F, Horenblas S, Pizzocaro G, Windahl T, European Association of Urology. EAU guidelines on penile cancer. Eur Urol. 2004;46:1–8.

Chapter 33

Penis Carcinoma – Radionuclide Imaging and PET

R.A. Valdés Olmos, B.K. Kroon, C.A. Hoefnagel, and S. Horenblas

The most important radionuclide imaging modality for penile carcinoma is sentinel node lymphoscintigraphy. Experience with 18F-FDG PET and radionuclide imaging with other tracers has been limited to a few patients.

Sentinel Node Lymphoscintigraphy

Concerning the sentinel node procedure in penile carcinoma, lymphoscintigraphy is oriented to identify the lymph nodes receiving direct drainage from the primary tumor. In this context tracer characteristic, route of administration and image acquisition are determinant factors to obtain optimal results.

Radiopharmaceuticals

Numerous radiopharmaceuticals have been used for sentinel node lymphoscintigraphy including ^{99m}Tc-labeled dextran, ^{99m}Tc human serum albumin, and various labeled colloids [1]. Most used labeled colloids are ^{99m}Tc antimony trisulfide colloid with a particle size of 3–40 nm and a wide application in Australia, ^{99m}Tc sulfur colloid with particles between 100 and 400 nm and mostly used in North America, and ^{99m}Tc nanocolloidal albumin with particles under 80 nm (95% smaller than 25 nm) and predominantly used in Europe. Also ^{99m}Tc colloidal rhenium sulfide, filtered ^{99m}Tc sulfur colloid, ^{99m}Tc stannous phytate, and ^{99m}Tc microcolloidal albumin have been used for sentinel node imaging. An overview of the radiopharmaceuticals for lymphoscintigraphy ranked according to the particle size is given in Table 33.1. For penile carcinoma, the most extensive validation has been using ^{99m}Tc nanocolloid.

Table 33.1 Radiopharmaceuticals for lymphoscintigraphy and particle size

Radiopharmaceutical	Particle range (nm)
[99m]Tc human serum albumin	2–3
[99m]Tc dextran	2–3
[99m]Tc DTPA-mannosyl-dextran	6–8
[99m]Tc antimony sulfide	3–30
[198]Au colloid	5–30
[99m]Tc-filtered sulfur colloid	15–50
[99m]Tc nanocolloidal albumin	5–80
[99m]Tc sulfur colloid	100–400
[99m]Tc stannous fluoride	50–600
[99m]Tc stannous phytate	200–1000
[99m]Tc microcolloidal albumin	200 −>1000

The visualization of the sentinel node depends on the transport of the tracer particles through lymphatic pathways from the injection site [2]. When radiolabeled particles reach the sentinel node they are trapped and subsequently absorbed through phagocytosis by the macrophages in the lymph node. At least three aspects may be of importance in this respect.

Particle Size

Very small particles travel so quickly that only a fraction is retained in the first draining lymph node. Particles smaller than 5 nm may also penetrate the capillary membranes with incorporation in blood; this may lead to an intense uptake in liver and spleen as may be observed on scintigraphy. Particles larger than 100 nm may become trapped in interstitial space and never enter the lymphatic system [1]; this decreased migration from the injection site may result in non- or faint lymph node visualization and may lead to underestimation of the number of sentinel nodes. Particle sizes between 10 and 50 nm have been associated with optimal lymph channel visualization and lymph node uptake [3]. However, due to spill, more second-echelon lymph nodes may be observed, which may lead to a certain overestimation of the number of sentinel nodes. To solve this limitation,

R.A. Valdés Olmos (✉)
Department of Nuclear Medicine, Netherlands Cancer Institute, Amsterdam, The Netherlands

J.J.M.C.H. de la Rosette et al. (eds.), *Imaging in Oncological Urology*,
DOI 10.1007/978-1-84628-759-6_33, © Springer-Verlag London Limited 2009

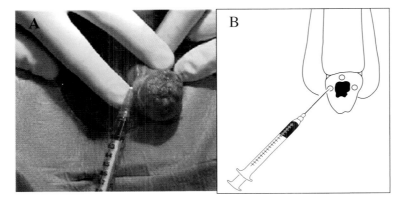

Fig. 33.1 (a) Intradermal administration of the tracer around the primary lesion in a patient with a T2 squamous cell carcinoma of the penis. (b) Schematic illustration of the intradermal tracer administration at three sites around the primary tumor

recently, ^{99m}Tc-DTPA-manosyl-dextran with an average particle size of 7 nm, ultrahigh receptor affinity and high lymph node extraction as well as fast migration rate from injection site has been proposed for sentinel node detection [4].

Particle Number

Lymphoscintigraphy by intradermal tracer administration, as applied in penile carcinoma, is associated with a high and fast migration rate of colloid particles from the injection site. Lymph node uptake is based on the ingestion of particles by the macrophages and this receptor-mediated phagocytosis may be improved by the activation of an increased number of receptors [5]. In accordance with this observation, the tracer dosage and the particle concentration must be optimized using adequate dilution volumes to prepare radiopharmaceuticals. For ^{99m}Tc nanocolloid, dilution volumes of 2–4 ml with injection volumes of 0.3–0.4 ml lead to the adequate visualization of lymphatic channels during the dynamic phase of the study and subsequently the early static images. This is mostly accompanied by intense lymph node uptake.

Radiopharmaceutical Dosage

A dosage of 60–80 MBq is associated with both sentinel node and lymph channel visualization in almost all patients investigated for penile carcinoma [6]. These dosages are mostly employed when the operation takes place the day after scintigraphy. When surgical procedure is performed the same day as scintigraphy, lower dosages are recommended in order to reduce radiation exposure of the surgeon. However, the use of lower dosages may be accompanied by less optimal visualization of lymphatic ducts at scintigraphy.

Tracer Administration

For penile carcinoma the tracer is injected intradermally. Subcutaneous administration is easier to accomplish but may not delineate the route of drainage from an overlying cutaneous site. Additionally, drainage from the dermis is a lot faster than drainage from subcutaneous tissue. Application of a spray containing xylocaine 10% 30 min before tracer administration is recommended. Alternatively a lidocaine/prilocaine-based cream may be used. This local anesthesia ensures that subsequent tracer injections are well tolerated and relatively easy to perform. A volume of 0.3 ml containing the tracer is subsequently administered intradermally around the tumor. Injection is divided into three depots of 0.1 ml as illustrated in Fig. 33.1. Each depot is injected raising a wheal. The tracer is injected proximally from the tumor. For large tumors not restricted to the glans, the tracer can be administered in the prepuce. Injection margins within 1 cm from the primary tumor are recommended. In patients with excision biopsy scar, injections may also be administered using similar margins. However, whether lymphatic drainage can be altered by tumor excision is still not established. Taking an injection distance of 5 mm a reproducibility of 100% for penile lymphoscintigraphy has been reported [7]. Expanding the injection distance from the site of the primary lesion may increase the ambiguous zone of drainage, cross a lymphatic watershed, and visualize additional basins not really related to drainage of the tumor site.

Gamma Camera Imaging and Skin Marking

There are various reasons to perform lymphoscintigraphy in the sentinel node procedure:

- To point out the draining lymph node field at risk for metastatic disease
- To indicate the number of sentinel nodes
- To help distinguish first-tier lymph nodes from second-echelon lymph nodes
- To identify lymph nodes in unpredictable locations
- To mark the location of the sentinel node on the skin
- To accomplish these purposes gamma camera acquisition must meet the highest standard of quality concerning methodology and image interpretation

There is consensus that sentinel node lymphoscintigraphy must be sequential, with images obtained at various time intervals. Low-energy, high-resolution collimators and camera set for the 140 KeV photon energy peak of ^{99m}Tc are necessary. Lymphoscintigraphy must match the sentinel concept and therefore must be able to visualize the lymphatic channels and identify the lymph nodes receiving direct drainage from the tumor. To detect these sentinel nodes, gamma camera acquisition recognizes two parts

(a) Dynamic scintigraphy, on the basis of 20 s images in a matrix of $128 \times 128 \times 16$, performed during the first 15–20 min after tracer injection, preferably in both the anterior and lateral projection with a dual-head gamma camera, if available. The dynamic study is helpful to identify lymphatic ducts when a rapid drainage from the injection site is expected as occurs in penile lymphoscintigraphy. In some cases the computer-assisted summation of all dynamic images in a 20-min image may help to differentiate first-echelon from second-echelon lymph nodes (Fig. 33.2).

(b) Static images using a $256 \times 256 \times 16$ matrix in both the anterior and lateral projections with an acquisition time of 5 min at 20–30 min and 2 h are recommended. Additional images at 4–6 h are strongly recommended when no sentinel nodes are visualized or when a slow migration from the injection is observed. To improve image interpretation and sentinel node identification, the use of simultaneous transmission scanning by means of a flood source of cobalt-57 of ^{99m}Tc gives excellent information about the body contour. Also some reference points can be indicated to identify anatomical structures such as the inguinal ligament. Static images are important to differentiate the further lymphatic drainage, which may enable to identify both additional sentinel nodes with delayed filling located in unexpected locations and secondary lymph nodes.

Sentinel node identification on lymphoscintigraphy is followed by localization and marking on skin in order to enable intraoperative localization using the hand-held gamma probe, usually the day after scintigraphy. With the gamma camera in real-time view mode and the sentinel node within the field of

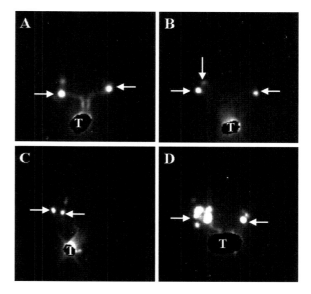

Fig. 33.2 Anterior images showing different patterns of lymphatic drainage of ^{99m}Tc nanocolloid from injection site to sentinel nodes (*arrows*). (a) Bilateral drainage with visualization of lymphatic ducts leading to one sentinel in each groin. (b) Bilateral drainage with two lymphatic ducts leading to two sentinel nodes in the right groin and one sentinel node in the left groin. (c) Unilateral drainage with two lymphatic channels and two sentinel nodes in the right groin. (d) Drainage to the right groin with a cluster of lymphatic nodes whereas in the left groin one sentinel node and two second-echelon nodes are visualized

view, a marker source or pen is moved over the skin. When the signal of this radioactive marker coincides with the hot spot of the sentinel node this point is marked on the skin. Subsequently, the site of the sentinel node is marked with non-erasable ink. To avoid pitfalls due to skin or lymph node mobility, sentinel node marking must be performed in the position in which the patient will be operated.

Drainage Patterns and Image Interpretation

There are two major criteria to identify sentinel nodes on lymphoscintigraphy:

- The visualization of lymphatic ducts, leading to the identification of lymph nodes with direct drainage from the injection site
- The visualization of the first draining lymph nodes in each lymph node group

In penile lymphoscintigraphy, after peritumoral injection, the dorsal lymph channels of the penis are first observed. The most frequent pattern of visualization (80%) is the bilateral drainage to both groins. This pattern is, however, asynchronous in two thirds of the cases and frequently late lymph node filling of the contralateral side is only visualized on

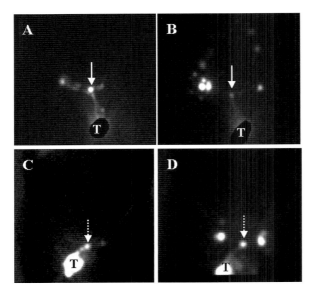

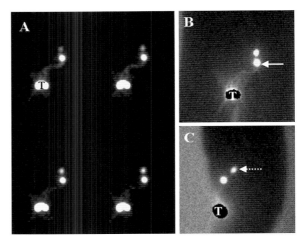

Fig. 33.3 (a) Anterior early images showing intense accumulation of ⁹⁹ᵐTc nanocolloid at the level of the prepubic bifurcation of the penile lymphatic channel (*arrow*). Note that this lymphatic duct activity decreases at the 2 h image (b). By contrast, in another patient intense prepubic activity seen on early image (c) persists on delayed images (*dotted arrow*). (d) At surgery a prepubic sentinel node was removed

Fig. 33.4 (a) Dynamic phase of lymphoscintigraphy showing drainage to the left groin with visualization of one duct leading to an inguinal sentinel node (*arrow*). A second-echelon lymph node is observed just above the sentinel node. Note that in contrast to anterior image (b), lateral image (c) can differentiate inguinal from iliac lymph nodes (*dotted arrow*)

delayed images. Drainage from the injection site mostly occurs through one or two afferent lymphatic vessels leading to visualization of one or two sentinel nodes in each groin. In some cases a cluster of inguinal lymph nodes may be visualized (Fig. 33.2). During the dynamic phase of the study as well as on early static images an intense accumulation of radioactivity may be observed in the pubic area at the site of the bifurcation of the penile dorsal common lymphatic vessel (Fig. 33.3). This accumulation decreases or disappears on delayed images. When a persistent accumulation is observed at the pubic area with increase of radioactivity on delayed images, a prepubic sentinel node may be considered. Inguinal second-echelon lymph nodes are usually seen on the early static images whereas iliac second-echelon lymph nodes are often observed on delayed images. Lateral images can differentiate inguinal from iliac lymph nodes (Fig. 33.4).

Although overall sentinel node visualization rate may reach 99% in experienced hands, interpretation of lymphoscintigraphy may be complicated by non-visualization of the sentinel node. In 10% of the groins sentinel nodes are not visualized, mostly concerning patients with unilateral drainage [8]. Various reasons may explain the absent or faint sentinel node uptake:

– Low tracer dosage
– Tumor involvement of the sentinel node
– Patient age with less visualization in older patients
– Unsatisfactory tracer quality
– Insufficient particle number

– Too short or too long intervals between tracer injection and lymphoscintigraphy

Recently, pre-operative ultrasonography of the groin combined with fine-needle aspiration cytology was introduced to detect impalpable grossly involved tumor-positive nodes. Detection of these nodes may indirectly reduce non-visualization on scintigraphy [9].

Beside these factors it is necessary to recognize some pitfalls such as injection of part of the radiopharmaceutical in blood vessels or into the corpus cavernosum (Fig. 33.5). Also during tracer injection the high pressure of the intradermal bleb can result in spreading of some of the radioactivity on needle removal with subsequent skin contamination which can be confused with lymph node uptake.

Clinical Relevance

The sentinel node procedure in penile carcinoma is of important diagnostic, prognostic, and therapeutic value at the cost of only minor morbidity. In an evaluation of 10 years experience, Kroon et al. [10] found a sentinel node visualization rate of 99% by lymphoscintigraphy and sentinel node metastases in 22% of the patients after intraoperative sentinel node localization. The sentinel node was the only tumor-positive node in 78% of the dissection specimens. The 5–year disease-specific survival was 96% for patients with a tumor-negative sentinel node and 66% for patients with a tumor-positive sentinel node. Most of the false-negative cases were found in the learning phase of the experience.

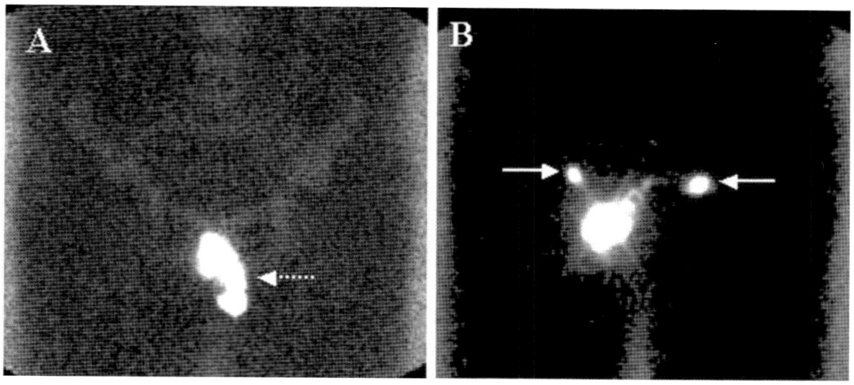

Fig. 33.5 Pitfall in lymphoscintigraphy. (a) Anterior image showing penile accumulation (*dotted arrow*) after administration of the tracer into the corpus cavernosum without lymphatic drainage. (b) After a second injection the day after, lymphatic drainage is observed with visualization of sentinel nodes in both groins (*arrows*)

This aspect was recently evaluated [11]. The false-negative rate decreased from 19 to 5% after optimization of the procedure. Also the groin complication rate dropped from 10.2 to 5.7%.

Positron Emission Tomography (PET) with ^{18}F-FDG

Some malignancies such as malignant melanoma, lymphoma, lung, and colorectal cancer are characterized by increased glycolytic activity, enhanced glucose utilization, and intense tumor uptake of ^{18}F-FDG on PET. Also in squamous cell carcinoma of the penis, intense uptake of ^{18}F-FDG may be observed in lymph node metastases (Fig. 33.6). However there is no extensive validation of the modality. In a series including 13 patients both sensitivity and specificity reached 75% with respect to the primary lesions. In the detection of lymph node metastases the sensitivity of PET was 80% and the specificity 100%. Sensitivity was 89% for superficial inguinal lymph node metastases and 100% for deep inguinal and obturator lymph node basins [12]. At the Netherlands Cancer Institute ^{18}F-FDG PET was evaluated on the basis of 30 procedures in 26 patients with clinical T3/T4 penile carcinoma. In 30 tumor-positive groins the sensitivity of PET was 93% and the specificity 96%. In 26 tumor-negative groins the sensitivity was 60% and the specificity 95%. With respect to the iliac lymph node basins, the sensitivity of PET was 92% and the specificity 93%. Metastases at distance were found in five patients. It can be concluded that ^{18}F-FDG PET appears to be a sensitive modality to detect regional and distant metastases in patients with intermediate and high T stage as well as in recurrences. Additionally, in patients with advanced disease scheduled to receive chemotherapy, ^{18}F-FDG PET may contribute to the monitoring of therapy response [13]. Finally the introduction of

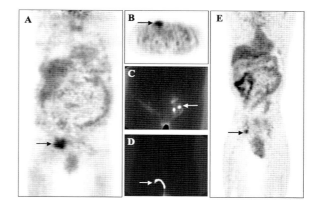

Fig. 33.6 Coronal (a) and transaxial (b) PET images showing intense accumulation of ^{18}F-FDG in lymph node metastases of the right groin (*black arrows*). Note that on lymphoscintigraphy (d) of the same patient there is an abnormal drainage to the right groin without lymph node filling. By contrast, there is normal drainage to the left groin with depiction of two sentinel nodes (*white arrows*). In another patient (d) there is prolonged visualization of the radioactivity in lymph vessel (*white arrow*) without filling of the sentinel node of the right groin. Coronal FDG-PET (e) shows abnormal uptake in lymph node metastasis of the right groin (*black arrow*)

PET/CT systems with improved PET signal will lead to a further application of this diagnostic modality in penile cancer by improving localization of metastases (Fig. 33.7).

Radionuclide Imaging with other Tracers

Both ^{67}Ga-citrate and ^{99m}Tc-MIBI may be helpful for the diagnostic imaging of lymph node metastases of penile carcinoma. Intense uptake of ^{67}Ga-citrate may be observed in metastatic inguinal lymph nodes and the decrease in abnormal groin uptake appears to correlate with clinical improvement [14]. Also scintigraphy with ^{99m}Tc-MIBI may lead to the detection of occult regional metastases [15].

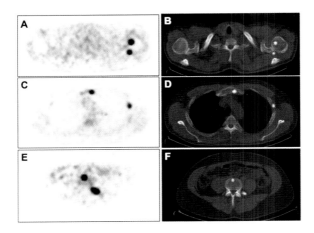

Fig. 33.7 Coronal FDG-PET images (a, c, e) showing various metastases in a patient with recurrent penile cancer. Note that PET/CT fused images are able to precise the anatomical location of the metastases in bone and soft tissue by displaying the increased PET signal of the metastases in color (b, d, f)

Conclusions

In patients with penile cancer and clinically negative groins, sentinel node biopsy is the procedure of election to stage the groin. Lymphoscintigraphy is widely validated and can guide intraoperative probe sentinel node detection in almost all patients.

^{18}F-FDG PET appears to be a sensitive modality to detect regional and distant metastases in patients with intermediate and high T stage as well as in recurrences. However, further validation of this modality using PET/CT hybrid systems is necessary.

References

1. Wilhem AJ, Mijnhout GS, Franssen EJF. Radiopharmaceuticals in sentinel lymph-node detection – an overview. Eur J Nucl Med. 1999;26 Suppl:S36–42.

2. Alazraki NP, Eshima D, Eshima LA, Herda SC, Murray DR, Vansant JP. Lymphoscintigraphy, the sentinel node concept, and the intraoperative gamma probe in melanoma, breast cancer and other potential cancers. Semin Nucl Med. 1997;27:55–67.

3. Strand SE, Bergqvist L. Radiolabeled colloids and macromolecules in lymphatic system. Crit Rev Ther Drug Carrier Sys. 1989;6: 211–38.

4. Vera DR, Wallace AM, Hoh CK, Mattrey RF. A synthetic macromolecule for sentinel node detection: 99mTc-DTPA-manosyl-dextran. J Nucl Med. 2001;42:951–9.

5. Griffin FM, Griffin JA, Leider JE, Silverstein SC. Studies on the mechanism of phagocytosis I. Requirements of circumferential attachment of particle-bound ligands to specific receptors on the macrophage plasma membrane. J Exp Med. 1975;142: 1263–82.

6. Valdés Olmos RA, Tanis PJ, Hoefnagel CA, Jansen L, Nieweg OE, Meinhardt W, et al. Penile lymphoscintigraphy for sentinel node identification. Eur J Nucl Med. 2001;28:581–5.

7. Kroon BK, Valdés Olmos RA, Nieweg OE, Horenblas S. Reproducibility of lymphoscintigraphy for lymphatic mapping in patients with penile carcinoma. J Urol. 2005;174:2214–7.

8. Kroon BK, Valdés Olmos RA, Nieweg OE, Horenblas S. Nonvisualization of sentinel lymph nodes in penile carcinoma. Eur J Nucl Med Mol Imaging. 2005;32:1096–9.

9. Kroon BK, Horenblas S, Deurloo EE, Nieweg OE, Teertstra HJ Ultrasonography-guided fine-needle aspiration cytology before sentinel node biopsy in patients with penile carcinoma. BJU Int. 2005;95:517–21.

10. Kroon BK, Horenblas S, Meinhardt W, van der Poel HG, Bex A, van Tinteren H, et al. Dynamic sentinel node biopsy in penile carcinoma: evaluation of 10 years experience. Eur Urol. 2005;47: 601–6.

11. Leijte JA, Kroon BK, Valdés Olmos RA, Nieweg OE, Horenblas S. Reliability and safety of current dynamic sentinel node biopsy for penile carcinoma. Eur Urol. 2007;52:170–7.

12. Scher B, Seitz M, Reiser M, Hungerhuber E, Hahn K, Tiling R, et al. 18F-FDG PET/CT for staging of penile cancer. J Nucl Med. 2005;46:1460–5.

13. Joerger M, Warzinek T, Klaeser B, Kluckert JT, Schmid HP, Gillesen S. Major tumor regression after paclitaxel and carboplatin polychemotherapy in a patient with advanced penile cancer. Urology. 2004;63:778–80.

14. Abello R, Lamki LM. Ga-67 uptake by metastatic carcinoma of the penis. Clin Nucl Med. 1992;17:23–26.

15. Alonso O, Lago G, Lopes de Amorim MC, Gelvalisi ME, Andruskevicius P, Rodriguez S, et al. Examination of regional lymph nodes in penile carcinoma by 99mTc-MIBI scintigraphy. Rev Esp Med Nucl. 2003;22:250–2.

Chapter 34

Considerations: Imaging in Penis Carcinoma

S. Horenblas, B.K. Kroon, R.A. Valdés Olmos, and C.A. Hoefnagel

Introduction

Malignant tumors of the penis consist of 95% of the cases of squamous cell carcinoma. The other 5% comprises of other tumors originating in the skin, like melanoma and basal cell cancer, or tumors arising from elements of cavernous tissue like soft tissue tumors [1–3]. Ideally, imaging modalities should help the clinician in deciding on the appropriate therapy of the primary tumor by exactly delineating the extent of the tumor and invasion in various structures of the penis, like the cavernous tissues and the urethra. Squamous cell carcinoma shows a very strong tendency for lymphatic spread first, with hematogenic spread in very advanced cases only [4]. Timely management of lymph node metastasis is of utmost importance [5, 6]. Imaging should also inform the clinician on the absence or presence of regional metastases in the groin area. In more advanced cases knowledge of spread to second echelon lymph nodes in the pelvic region and further spread to retroperitoneal lymph nodes is essential for a rational approach.

Imaging of the Primary Tumor

The extent of the primary tumor in squamous cell carcinoma of the penis has important prognostic and therapeutic implications. The prognostic difference between deeply infiltrating tumors and superficially growing tumors has been recognized for a long time and is expressed already in the first TNM classification system for squamous cell carcinoma of the penis [7]. Size of the tumor was surpassed by depth of infiltration as a classification criterion in the most recent classification [8]. A distinction was made between tumors infiltrating into the deeper structures of the penis and tumors

Table 34.1 1987 TNM Classification [8]

T-Primary tumor
T X Primary tumor cannot be assessed
TO No evidence of primary tumor
Tis Carcinoma in situ
Ta Non-invasive verrucous carcinoma
TI Tumor invades subepithelial connective tissue
T2 Tumor invades corpus spongiosum or cavernosum
T3 Tumor invades urethra or prostate
T4 Tumor invades other adjacent structures
N-Regional lymph nodes
NX Regional lymph nodes cannot be assessed
NO No regional lymph node metastasis
NI Metastasis in a single superficial inguinal lymph node
N2 Metastasis in multiple or bilateral superficial inguinal lymph nodes
N3 Metastasis in deep inguinal or pelvic Iymph node(s), unilateral or bilateral
M-Distant metastasis
MX Distant metastasis cannot be assessed
MO No distant metastasis
MI Distant metastasis
Stage grouping
Stage O   Tis NO MO Ta NO MO
Stage I   TI NO MO
Stage II   TI NI MO T2 NO, NI MO
Stage III   TI N2 MO T2 N2 MO T3 NO, NI, N2 MO
Stage IV   T4 Any N MO Any T N3 MO Any T Any N MI

invading the superficial layers only (Table 34.1) This distinction, how important this may be, is not easily made on clinical grounds only.

The main issue in the management of the primary tumor is the decision whether to amputate or not. Standard partial penile amputation as a treatment for localized squamous cell carcinoma is increasingly being replaced by methods that conserve the penis [9, 10]. Main danger is the risk for local recurrence, which increases proportionally with size and depth of infiltration of the tumor. Therefore, the extension of the primary carcinoma must be assessed with great care. Staging on clinical grounds only is not always easy, as the often accompanying infection can give the impression of deep infiltration while microscopic invasion can easily be missed. Comparing clinical and pathological staging in a series with almost 100 patients with squamous cell cancer

S. Horenblas (✉)
Netherlands Cancer Institute/Antoni van Leeuwenhoek Hospital, Plesmanlaan 121, 1066 CX, Amsterdam, s.horenblas@nki.nl

J.J.M.C.H. de la Rosette et al. (eds.), *Imaging in Oncological Urology*,
DOI 10.1007/978-1-84628-759-6_34, © Springer-Verlag London Limited 2009

showed the following differences: in 10% of the cases the clinical stage was higher compared to the pathological stage ("overstaging"), in 16% of the tumors the pathological stage was higher than the clinical one ("understaging"). Overall a 26% difference between clinical and pathological stage was found, almost similar to a 23% difference in a study from Maiche et al. [11, 12]. Reasons for these discrepancies were clinically undetected infiltration in the subepithelial tissue or corpus spongiosum, infection, and edema masking the real size of the tumor and giving a false impression of infiltration.

Can imaging contribute to more accurate staging? Various imaging techniques have been evaluated for this purpose [13–18].

Cross-Sectional Imaging Techniques

Ultrasound

Various distinctive structures of the penis can be depicted on ultrasound investigation and used for staging penile carcinoma. The tumor itself is mostly shown as a hypoechoic lesion (Fig. 34.1). It can be distinguished from the urethra. Introducing a urethral catheter can aid in delineating the tumor. The tunica albuginea surrounding both corpora cavernosa is seen as a hyperechoic structure (Fig. 34.2). Ultrasound was shown to reliably give the extent of infiltration into the corpora cavernosa, but was not reliable enough in discerning the true extent of infiltration into the corpus spongiosum of the glans [19].

CT Scanning

Computerized tomography is limited by its ability to image in one plane only and the poor soft tissue contrast. While it has been used extensively for the detection of nodal metastases, it has been used rarely for imaging the primary tumor, as the tumor and surrounding corporal bodies are poorly differentiated [18, 20, 21]. One can conclude that CT scanning does not play a role in the imaging of the primary tumor.

Magnetic Resonance Imaging (MRI)

In contrast to CT scan, MRI imaging is not limited by imaging in one plane. Moreover, soft tissue contrast is much better than with CT scan. Lont et al. analyzed the accuracy of MRI staging of the primary tumor [17]. MR images were obtained in the axial plane using T1-weighted spin echo (T1-SE) and T2-weighted turbo-spin echo (T2-TSE) sequences. Sagittal images were acquired using a short inversion recov-

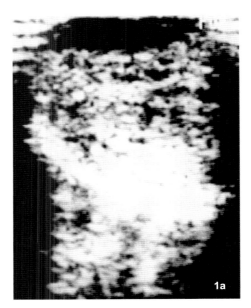

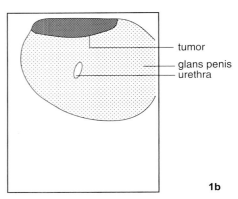

Fig. 34.1 Ultrasound examination of penile carcinoma (a) with schematic representation of distinct structures (b), showing a hypoechoic lesion

ery sequence and T1-SE sequences, before and after administering an intravenous contrast agent (gadolinium based). Tumor identification was mainly based on the presence of lesions with low signal intensity relative to the corporal bodies on the T1- or the T2-weighted images (Figs. 34.3 and 34.4). It was concluded that because of the possibility of imaging in various planes and because of the ability to visualize other structures of the penis, MRI can be useful in doubt of the true proximal extent of the tumor.

In order to improve imaging of the primary tumor, MRI was combined with artificial erection and compared with pathologic staging in nine cases of penile cancer. T1-weighted and T2-weighted MRI with and without contrast was obtained using a phased array coil. The MRI and pathologic staging coincided in eight of nine patients. In one patient no tumor was detected at MRI. Despite the differences between clinical staging and MRI staging, this had no therapeutic consequences [22].

Accuracy of Physical Examination, Ultrasound, and MRI

The accuracy of physical examination, ultrasound investigation, and magnetic resonance imaging (MRI) was compared in 33 patients [17]. All patients underwent a radiological evaluation with ultrasonography and MRI, the former using an SDD 280 LS scanner (Aloka Corp., Tokyo, Japan) with a 7.5 MHz linear-array small-parts transducer, and the latter using a 1.5 T Magnetom scanner (Siemens GmbH, Germany) with a small surface coil. An ultrasonography gel pad was used to avoid artifacts, and a urethral catheter was introduced for identification. The tumor was identified by the presence of hypoechoic lesions on the ultrasonograms that were not consistent with normal penile anatomy. Tumor size was determined in two directions using standard calipers on the ultrasonogram and in three planes on MRI. Invasion by tumor of the subepithelial stroma, corpus spongiosum, corpora cavernosa, and urethra was assessed. Infiltration depth was measured. After comparing the findings of the various investigations with histopathology, physical examination was more reliable for assessing tumor size than were ultrasonography and MRI. Furthermore physical examination predicted corpus cavernosum infiltration with the highest positive predictive value and was accurate for determining the presence of deep infiltration, missing substantial infiltration in only 2 of 33 patients (Table 34.2). For infiltration into the corpus spongiosum of the glans, the following values for positive predictive value and sensitivity were found: 94, 92, and 91% and 68, 92, and 80%, respectively, for physical examination, ultrasonography, and MRI. There were no false-positive findings of infiltration. MRI was the most sensitive method for determining cavernosal infiltration but at the cost of some false-positive results.

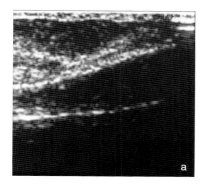

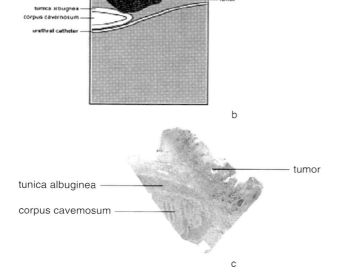

Fig. 34.2 Ultrasound examination of penile carcinoma (a) with schematic representation of distinct structures (b), showing the tumor abutting the tunica albuginea, without invading it. Histology (c) confirms the ultrasound observation (tumor not invading the tunica albuginea)

Imaging of Lymph Nodes

Squamous cell carcinoma of the penis metastasizes first to the inguinal lymph nodes and from there to the pelvic nodes. Metastases to the pelvic nodes without inguinal involvement (skip metastases) have hardly been observed, except an occasional case. By definition clinically occult metastasis are not detected by physical examination. These clinically node-negative patients present a challenge for additional imaging as approximately 20% will harbor clinically undetectable metastases. Non-invasive methods to detect these metastases are unreliable, but there is a clinical need to find occult metastases at the earliest possible stage, because survival is related to presence and extent of nodal involvement [5, 6, 23]. The optimum management of patients with clinically node-negative groins is controversial. A surveillance

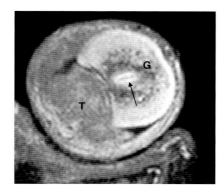

Fig. 34.3 MRI (T1 SPIR) with contrast in the transversal plane at a distal level of the penis in a patient with a T2 tumor. The tumor is seen as a low signal mass, clearly distinguished from the glans penis (T = tumor, G = glans penis, arrow indicates urethra)

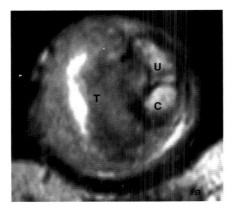 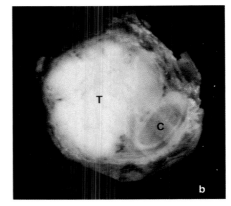

Fig. 34.4 (a) MRI (T1 TSE) without contrast in the transversal plane at a more proximal level of the penis in another patient with a T2 tumor. The tumor is seen as a mass with increased signal involving the corpus cavernosum. Some fluid collection between the preputium and the tumor is visible (T = tumor, C = corpus cavernosum, U = urethra). (b) Cross-section of the corresponding macroscopic specimen illustrates the findings on MRI, with macroscopic involvement of the corpus cavernosum (T = tumor, C = corpus cavernosum). The urethra was dissected during surgery

Table 34.2 The positive predictive value, sensitivity, and specificity of infiltration of the corpus cavernosum, as determined by physical examination, ultrasound, and MRI

Cavernosum infiltration	Positive predictive value	Sensitivity	Specificity
Physical examination	100%	71%	100%
Ultrasound	67%	57%	97%
MRI	75%	100%	91%

policy risks the patients presenting with metastasis at a stage where cure is no longer possible. On the other hand, early inguinal lymphadenectomy in all clinically node-negative patients is unnecessary in up to 80% and associated with substantial morbidity [24]. Thus better staging procedures are mandatory to improve the detection of occult metastasis and to decrease the number of unnecessary lymph node dissections. Detection of lymph node metastases in the groin and pelvis on CT scan or MRI is detected mainly by change of size. Lymph nodes smaller than 1 cm are usually considered normal. A distortion of the internal architecture by a small metastatic deposit without change of size was only visible by lymphangiography until recently [11]. Promising techniques, like modern ultrasound and MRI, using ultrasmall particles of iron oxide (USPIO), are underway to detect these occult metastases more reliably.

Patients presenting with inguinal lymph node enlargement are easily detected by physical examination. However, on average only half of them harbor lymph node metastasis, the other half is due to benign enlargement because of the often concomitant inflammation [25]. A distinction between absence and presence of lymph node metastases can be made on the basis of fine-needle aspiration biopsy guided by ultrasound or CT scanning. Understandably only a tumor-positive outcome is reliable. In patients with proven inguinal lymph node metastasis, imaging with CT scan or MRI is useful for the determination of the extent of metastatic spread.

Cross-Sectional Imaging Techniques

Ultrasound

Thanks to the high-resolution probes, ultrasound scanning is increasingly reliable in detecting occult metastases. Modern ultrasound not only visualizes alteration in size, shape, and contour of lymph nodes but also depicts changes in the cortical and hilar morphology and texture that can reflect the presence of underlying metastasis [26]. Changes in the architecture of the node occur before the node enlarges and these are identified by the radiologist. Currently the spatial resolution limit is around 2 mm. Due to overlap of sonographic features of benign and suspicious lymph nodes, fine-needle aspiration cytology (FNAC) of sonographically suspicious nodes provides a more definitive diagnosis than ultrasound alone. Potential applications have been demonstrated in a number of malignancies [27–30]. In 2001, ultrasound-guided FNAC was introduced as standard staging procedure at the Netherlands Cancer Institute-Antoni van Leeuwenhoek Hospital to improve staging of clinically node-negative penile SCC patients (Figs. 34.5 and 34.6).

The sensitivity of ultrasound-guided FNAC to reveal clinically occult lymph node metastases was 39%, with a 100% specificity. In contrast to penile cancer, ultrasound-guided FNAC has been used extensively in assessing lymph nodes in other malignancies such as breast cancer and melanoma. Sensitivity and specificity rates are about the same as reported for these tumors. With a sensitivity of 39% there is a false-negative rate of 61%, necessitating other means to

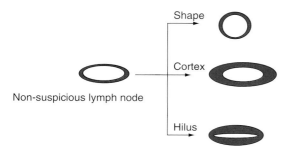

Fig. 34.5 Sonomorphologic lymph node features according to Vassallo et al. lymph node shape, cortex (normal or wide), and hilus (normal, narrow, or absent). Suspicious features for nodal involvement are a round shape, a wide cortex, and a narrow to absent hilus

assess the regional lymph nodes. At our institute we favor a so-called dynamic sentinel node biopsy (DNSB). So far ultrasound-guided FNAC cannot replace DSNB. However, it is a useful tool for preoperative screening of the clinically node-negative groins in patients with penile cancer scheduled to undergo DSNB. The commonest cause of a false-negative DSNB procedure is gross involvement of the sentinel node by tumor cells which prohibits tracer uptake with a false-negative procedure as a result [31]. These nodes in particular might be detected by ultrasound-guided FNAC. Moreover, nodal recurrences, which can occur after a false-negative DSNB procedure, might be detected earlier when compared to physical examination.

What are the causes of false-negative ultrasound results? First, the lymph node may appear abnormal and indeed contain metastatic disease, but the aspirate may fail to extract abnormal cells. This relates to erroneous sampling and can be difficult to overcome in a node with a small metastasis where placement of the needle is crucial. Second, microscopic small foci of metastases might be beyond the resolution of the transducer and therefore not show up on the images [28]. In order to improve the efficiency of ultrasound

scanning, the future effort should focus on the reduction of false-negative results. To this end, at least two strategies might be useful. First, the introduction of echogenic contrast has been advocated to increase ultrasound diagnostic power by allowing the identification of indirect features of lymph node metastases. Second, increasing the ultrasound probe ultrafrequency might ameliorate the resolution power, thus allowing the detection of lesions smaller than 2 mm [30]. In addition, a learning phase of the radiologist performing ultrasound-guided FNAC cannot be denied.

CT Scanning

Only one study exists in which the value of CT scanning in detecting regional lymph node metastases is assessed. Regional lymph node invasion that escaped clinical examination was not detected by CT [11]. Positive findings were found only in patients with clinically suspected nodes. Clinical decisions with respect to the management of regional lymph nodes should therefore not be based on negative CT findings. In patients with proved metastasis additional imaging may be of some help in the detection of pelvic node invasion and the determination of the extent of involvement (Fig. 34.7).

MR Imaging

Like in CT scanning, clinically occult metastases will not be detected by conventional MR imaging. MR imaging may be of some help in the detection of pelvic node invasion and the determination of the extent of involvement in patients with proved metastasis.

Recently, however, a promising technique has emerged with the potential to identity occult lymph node metastasis: MRI and ultrasmall particles of iron oxide (USPIO). This novel technique makes use of a lymph node-specific contrast

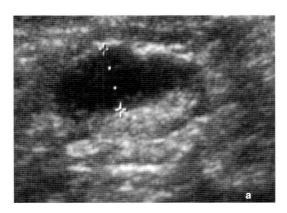
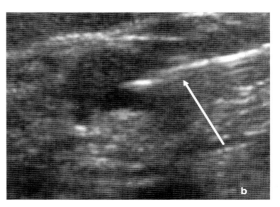

Fig. 34.6 (a) Ultrasound image of suspicious node with a wide cortex. (b) Ultrasound image of FNAC of the same node (arrow indicates needle)

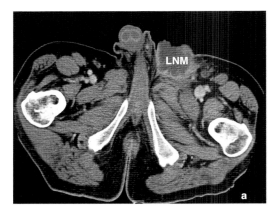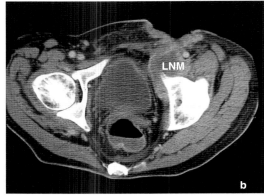

Fig. 34.7 (a) CT image in the transversal plane in a patient with a massive lymph node metastases in the left groin (LNM = lymph node metastasis). (b) Same patient at a more caudal level (LNM = lymph node metastasis)

agent that allows the identification of clinically occult metastasis. This contrast agent, known as ultrasmall particles of iron oxide (USPIO), is injected intravenously and is taken up primarily by macrophages in the lymph nodes. Presence of USPIO in the node results in signal intensity loss (darkening) on T2-weighed sequences. Metastatic growth will displace the macrophages filled with USPIO, and the metastatic part of the node therefore is high in signal intensity (whitening). Thus, metastasis within the lymph node will show as white filling defect. Metastases as small as 1 mm have been detected by using this technique [32]. In a mouse model even as few as 1,000 tumor cells could be depicted [33]. A pilot study in penile carcinoma showed a 100% sensitivity, 97% specificity, and 100% negative predictive value. Improvement of this technique could possibly replace dynamic sentinel node biopsy in the future [34].

Considerations

Primary Tumor

Small superficial tumors can be accurately staged by physical examination only. Imaging can be of help in patients in whom the extent of infiltration into the corpora cannot be determined properly by a physical examination, usually only in patients with locally extensive disease. Because of the high sensitivity for cavernosal infiltration and its precision in determining infiltration depth, MRI is the imaging method of choice. Images in the sagittal plane are particularly useful for detecting the proximal extent of the tumor. In conclusion no imaging modality is more reliable than physical examination for the assessment of the true extent of the tumor. Imaging has no important role in routine clinical management, except

where doubt exists about the proximal extent of the primary tumor.

Lymph Node Metastases

Penile carcinoma primarily metastasizes to the inguinal lymph nodes. Even in case of lymphatic metastasis many patients can still be cured. Patients presenting with inguinal lymph node enlargement are easily detected by physical examination. The diagnosis can be proven by fine-needle aspiration cytology, if possible under ultrasonographic guidance. In these patients additional CT or MRI imaging may be of some help in the detection of pelvic node invasion and the determination of the extent of involvement.

Most penile carcinoma patients, however, have no suspicious lymph nodes in their groins. This observation does not exclude the presence of disease. Approximately 25% of the patients harbor occult metastases in these lymph nodes. An important issue in the management of penile carcinoma patients is how to identify these metastases. Elective lymph node dissection is an option but will lead to overtreatment in about 75% of the patients. Moreover, inguinal lymphadenectomy is associated with major morbidity. On the other hand, a wait-and-see policy may have a negative impact on survival. Dynamic sentinel node biopsy is a minimally invasive procedure that enables detection of occult metastasis in clinically node-negative groins. To localize the sentinel node preoperatively, lymphoscintigraphy is performed after peritumoral injections of ^{99m}Tc-labeled nanocolloid tracers. Intraoperatively, the sentinel node can be identified with the aid of a blue dye and a hand-held gamma-ray detection probe. The sensitivity of dynamic sentinel node biopsy in our hands is 84%. Although minimally invasive dynamic sentinel node biopsy is burdened by an 8% complication rate. Moreover, it requires a patient to be hospitalized. Obviously, the implementation of non-invasive staging methods, i.e., imaging modalities, might improve the quality of life of penile carcinoma patients. The main problem of imaging modalities to detect occult metastases, however, is a low sensitivity. Computerized tomography and magnetic resonance imaging have a very low sensitivity and specificity in the detection of occult lymph node metastases in the groin. Ultrasound with fine-needle aspiration cytology is more accurate. However, as a staging tool, it is inadequate with a sensitivity and specificity of 39 and 100%, respectively, as reported in this chapter. The main problem is the detection of small metastases, i.e., smaller than approximately 3 mm. Positron emission tomography with ^{18}F-fluorodeoxyglucose (FDG-PET) has been advocated to detect occult lymph node metastases in several types of cancer. This technique relies not solely on anatomic identification but largely on physiological characterization of cells. However, the visualization by FDG-PET requires a minimum diameter of about 3 mm, and this technique is therefore not a good alternative for dynamic sentinel node biopsy in staging patients with clinically node-negative penile carcinoma. Magnetic resonance lymphangiography is a promising technique in the detection of occult lymph node metastases. Metastases as small as 1 mm have been detected by using this technique. Preliminary results of this technique in penile carcinoma are promising. Improvement of this technique could possibly replace dynamic sentinel node biopsy in the future.

References

1. Liegl B, Regauer S. Penile clear cell carcinoma. a report of 5 cases of a distinct entity. Am J Surg Pathol. 2004;28:1513.
2. Sanchez-Ortiz R, Huang SF, Tamboli P, et al. Melanoma of the penis, scrotum and male urethra. a 40-year single institution experience. J Urol. 2005;173:1958.
3. Stancik I, Holtl W. Penile cancer. review of the recent literature. Curr Opin Urol. 2003;13:467.
4. Horenblas S, van Tinteren H, Delemarre JF, et al. Squamous cell carcinoma of the penis. III. Treatment of regional lymph nodes. J Urol. 1993;149:492.
5. Ornellas AA, Seixas AL, Marota A, et al. Surgical treatment of invasive squamous cell carcinoma of the penis. retrospective analysis of 350 cases. J Urol. 1994;151:1244.
6. Kroon BK, Horenblas S, Lont AP, et al. Patients with penile carcinoma benefit from immediate resection of clinically occult lymph node metastases. J Urol. 2005;173:816.
7. Harmer MH. TNM classification of malignant tumors. UICC. 3rd ed. Geneva; 1978.
8. International Union Against Cancer. Penis. In: Hermanek P, Sobin LH, editors. TNM classification of malignant tumours. 4th ed. Berlin Heidelberg: Springer Verlag; 1987.
9. Mohs FE, Snow SN, Messing EM, et al. Microscopically controlled surgery in the treatment of carcinoma of the penis. J Urol. 1985;133:961.
10. Windahl T, Hellsten S. Laser treatment of localized squamous cell carcinoma of the penis. J Urol. 1995;154:1020.
11. Horenblas S, van Tinteren H, Delemarre JF, et al. Squamous cell carcinoma of the penis: accuracy of tumor, nodes and metastasis classification system, and role of lymphangiography, computerized tomography scan and fine needle aspiration cytology. J Urol. 1991;146:1279.
12. Maiche AG, Pyrhonen S. Clinical staging of cancer of the penis. By size? By localization? or By depth of infiltration? Eur Urol. 1990;18:16.
13. de Kerviler E, Ollier P, Desgrandchamps F, et al. Magnetic resonance imaging in patients with penile carcinoma. Br J Radiol. 1990;68:704.
14. Hricak H, Marotti M, Gilbert TJ, et al. Normal penile anatomy and abnormal penile conditions. evaluation with MR imaging. Radiology. 1988;169:683.
15. Kageyama S, Ueda T, Kushima R, et al. Primary adenosquamous cell carcinoma of the male distal urethra. magnetic resonance imaging using a circular surface coil. J Urol. 1997;158:1913.
16. Kawada T, Hashimoto K, Tokunaga T, et al. Two cases of penile cancer. magnetic resonance imaging in the evaluation of tumor extension. J Urol. 1994;152:963.
17. Lont AP, Besnard AP, Gallee MP, et al. A comparison of physical examination and imaging in determining the extent of primary penile carcinoma. BJU Int. 2003;91:493.
18. Horenblas S, van Tinteren H. Squamous cell carcinoma of the penis. IV. Prognostic factors of survival: analysis of tumor, nodes and metastasis classification system. J Urol. 1994;151:1239.
19. Horenblas S, Kroger R, Gallee MP, et al. Ultrasound in squamous cell carcinoma of the penis; a useful addition to clinical staging? A comparison of ultrasound with histopathology. Urology. 1994;43. 702.
20. Maiche AG. Computer tomography (CT) in the diagnosis and staging of cancer of the penis. Eur J Cancer. 1993;29A:779.
21. Vapnek JM, Hricak H, Carroll PR. Recent advances in imaging studies for staging of penile and urethral carcinoma. Urol Clin North Am. 1992;19:257.
22. Scardino E, Villa G, Bonomo G, et al. Magnetic resonance imaging combined with artificial erection for local staging of penile cancer. Urology. 2004;63:1158.
23. McDougal WS. Carcinoma of the penis. improved survival by early regional lymphadenectomy based on the histological grade and depth of invasion of the primary lesion. J Urol. 1995; 154:1364.
24. Bevan-Thomas R, Slaton JW, Pettaway CA. Contemporary morbidity from lymphadenectomy for penile squamous cell carcinoma. the M.D. Anderson Cancer Center Experience. J Urol. 2002;167:1638.
25. Horenblas S. Lymphadenectomy for squamous cell carcinoma of the penis. Part 1. diagnosis of lymph node metastasis. BJU Int. 2001;88:467.
26. Vassallo P, Wernecke K, Roos N, et al. Differentiation of benign from malignant superficial lymphadenopathy. the role of high-resolution US. Radiology. 1992;183:215.
27. Deurloo EE, Tanis PJ, Gilhuijs KG, et al. Reduction in the number of sentinel lymph node procedures by preoperative ultrasonography of the axilla in breast cancer. Eur J Cancer. 2003;39:1068.
28. Hall TB, Barton DP, Trott PA, et al. The role of ultrasound-guided cytology of groin lymph nodes in the management of squamous cell carcinoma of the vulva. Five-year experience in 44 patients. Clin Radiol. 2003;58:367.
29. Kuenen-Boumeester V, Menke-Pluymers M, de Kanter AY, et al. Ultrasound-guided fine needle aspiration cytology of axillary lymph nodes in breast cancer patients. A preoperative staging procedure. Eur J Cancer. 2003;39:170.
30. Rossi CR, Mocellin S, Scagnet B, et al. The role of preoperative ultrasound scan in detecting lymph node metastasis before sentinel node biopsy in melanoma patients. J Surg Oncol. 2003;83:80.

31. Kroon BK, Horenblas S, Estourgie SH, et al. How to avoid false-negative dynamic sentinel node procedures in penile carcinoma. J Urol. 2004;171:2191.

32. Harisinghani MG, Barentsz J, Hahn PF, et al. Noninvasive detection of clinically occult lymph-node metastases in prostate cancer. N Engl J Med. 2003;348:2491.

33. Wunderbaldinger P, Josephson L, Bremer C, et al. Detection of lymph node metastases by contrast-enhanced MRI in an experimental model. Magn Reson Med. 2002;47:292.

34. Tabatabaei S, Harisinghani M, McDougal WS. Regional lymph node staging using lymphotropic nanoparticle enhanced magnetic resonance imaging with ferumoxtran-10 in patients with penile cancer. J Urol. 2005;174:923.

Chapter 35

Future Directions in Urological Imaging

H. Wijkstra

Introduction

Imaging is a clinical tool used for diagnosis, treatment, and follow-up of most urological diseases. In uro-oncology, especially, imaging plays an important role. In most countries one or more of these urological imaging techniques are conducted and interpreted by urologists, while in other countries all imaging is performed by radiologists only. Because imaging plays such a significant role in clinical decision-making, it is of utmost importance that urologists are aware of new developments in this field.

This chapter will present some of the techniques that are now under development, and we made a selection of some of the promising techniques and this introduction presents a short overview of what will be described.

Robots, from simple camera holders to complex telesurgery systems, have been introduced in urology. An increasing number of different robotic systems are currently under development, and nowadays these robots in most cases use imaging data sets for planning procedures as for example radical prostatectomies or prostate biopsies. The use of imaging and imaging processing during the procedure to guide the robot is a development that certainly will further improve the clinical use of robots. CT, MRI, and ultrasound can be used for this purpose. The paper from John Hopkins describes in detail imaging-guided robotic-assisted interventions and presents a view for future clinical use.

Ultrasound is in most countries performed by urologists. It is indeed an important tool for diagnostic and therapeutic decisions. New developments in ultrasound and the use of contrast agents are discussed in "New developments in Ultrasound." The improved technology of hardware, and especially transducers and the increasing processing power of modern computers that makes advanced signals processing

possible, already resulted in enhanced imaging with reduction of artifacts. Using contrast agents, sensitive perfusion imaging of tissue became available during the last decade. In oncology, especially, these techniques have the potential to play an important role in diagnosis and treatment. Nowadays these techniques are so sensitive that even ultrasound imaging of the microvasculature became possible. These latter techniques are now under clinical evaluation, and it is expected that they will become available for routine clinical use in short time. Modern ultrasound contrast agents consist of small-encapsulated gas bubbles, and they can also be targeted to molecular processes, for example angiogenesis receptors, that could make sensitive molecular imaging possible. Furthermore, local drug delivery is another new development in contrast ultrasound that is discussed in this paper.

Detailed information regarding contrast agents for CT, MR, and ultrasound is presented in "Future Directions – Contrast Agents." The field of contrast has also undergone an important progress during the last decade and detailed knowledge about the chemical and physiological behavior of these agents and new developments and research in molecular imaging will result in more and more sensitive imaging techniques. Ultrasound contrast has the advantage that the contrast acts as a blood pool enhancer and therefore could make quantification of perfusion possible. Also for the other imaging modalities blood pool enhancers are now introduced. New effort is made in further quantifying these contrast studies, and this could result in more reliable and an increased sensitivity of functional imaging.

Virtual imaging and virtual reality have become available, also for clinicians, because of the availability of high-speed computers and advanced 3D/4D rendering software. The use of, for example, virtual colonoscopy is now developed from research to a screening method. Techniques and clinical applications in urology are described in detail in "Virtual Imaging." These noninvasive endoscopic techniques are nowadays available but are still underutilized in urology. The authors describe the use for urology, e.g., for diagnosis of bladder neoplasms, ureteroscopy, urethroscopy, and

H. Wijkstra (✉)
Department of Urology, Academic Medical Center, University of Amsterdam, Amsterdam, the Netherlands, h.wijkstra@amc.uva.nl

J.J.M.C.H. de la Rosette et al. (eds.), *Imaging in Oncological Urology*,
DOI 10.1007/978-1-84628-759-6_35, © Springer-Verlag London Limited 2009

363

the upper urinary tract with some cases. Next to the use as a replacement for invasive endoscopic procedures, virtual imaging provides additional views that are not available with the traditional visualization techniques. Furthermore the use of virtual imaging and especially virtual reality for teaching, training, and pre-procedure planning is described.

Optical imaging is another promising imaging technique. The working mechanisms and the potential use for bladder cancer diagnosis are presented in great detail in the section "Optical Imaging and Diagnosis in Bladder Cancer." Some of the described techniques are still experimental and others are already advancing to in vivo use. A few are now already commercially available to the urologist.

The last section of this chapter describes the use of elasticity imaging. These imaging techniques are based on the fact that many pathological conditions are associated with a change in elastic properties of the tissue. This changed elasticity can be assessed by palpation; however the diagnostic accuracy of palpation is low. In the last decade several elasticity-imaging methods for, e.g., ultrasound and MR imaging, have been proposed, and are under in vitro and in vivo evaluation. Some of these methods are nowadays already available on commercial systems. This section describes in detail all new developments in this field.

In conclusion, this chapter presents to the reader some new advances in imaging techniques that could play an important role in the diagnoses, therapy, and follow-up of urological diseases. Most of the presented imaging methods are now under investigation in in vitro and/or in vivo studies, and it is expected that some of them will become available for the clinic in the near future. Prof. Cosgrove, an expert in the field of (experimental) imaging, concludes this chapter with his considerations regarding all these new emerging imaging techniques.

Chapter 36

Image-Guided Robotic Assisted Interventions

A. Patriciu, M. Muntener, L. Kavossi, and D. Stoianovici

Introduction

The field of medical robotics emerged in the early 1980s. According to their functionality, surgical robots can be classified into two main categories [1]: surgical assistants and surgical CAD/CAM systems (as for the computer aided design and manufacturing paradigms).

Surgical assistants augment surgeon's motion capabilities from simple tasks such as camera holders to complex remote manipulation such as telesurgical systems. The early AESOP robot (formerly developed by Computer Motion, Inc.), for example, can passively hold and orient a laparoscopy camera [2] using a foot or voice control. On the other side of the spectrum are Zeus (former Computer Motion Inc.) and daVinci (Intuitive Surgical Inc.), which is perhaps the most successful surgical robot today. Both systems have three manipulators controlled from a surgeon console [3].

Surgical assistants rely on the surgeon's guidance to manipulate the instruments. These systems are currently less complex than image-guided systems. This does not mean that surgical robots such as daVinci are simple, but they are independent and self-contained, thus allowing for their isolated development and testing, which perhaps explains the head start of this category.

The second category is of the more complex surgical CAD/CAM systems. In a typical CAD/CAM workflow, images of the patient are acquired before the procedure, and a preoperative plan is developed. The target is defined in a set of images acquired intraoperatively. An instrument (usually a needle) is inserted into the body using image feedback. Image-guided operations require registration of the robot with respect to the image. This is the building of a transformation from the image to the robot space, which is specific for each type of imager and system used.

The general workflow of a minimally invasive robotic assisted procedure is shown in Fig. 36.1. Several systems use preoperative images to define the clinical target and plan and the intraoperative images for online robot guidance. This pre-post imaging approach, however, requires an additional registration of the two sets of images. The research on image-to-image registration methods is rich and well beyond the scope of this chapter. The interested reader is referred to the excellent review articles published by Vandenelsen et al. [4], Hill et al. [5] and Pluim et al. [6].

The layout of the following sections is structured according to the imaging modality used for intraoperative feedback, as these have a great influence on the structure of minimally invasive robotic system. It can be argued that the imaging modality dictates the algorithms used for robot registration and positioning and, up to a certain degree, it influences the robotic design. Also, the quantity of the image information determines the required accuracy of the system. For example, a 3D set of computed tomography (CT) slices is much easier to use and interpret than a projective X-ray image. It is this reason perhaps that made the computed tomography the favourite modality for image-guided robotic assisted intervention.

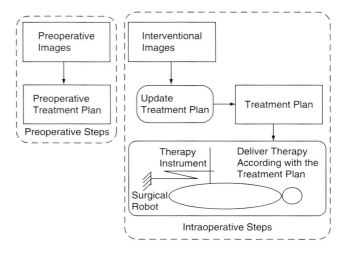

Fig. 36.1 Procedural steps in a CAD/CAM system

A. Patriciu (✉)
URobotics Laboratory, Urology Department, Johns Hopkins Medicine, Baltimore, MD, USA, http://urology.jhu.edu/urobotics

J.J.M.C.H. de la Rosette et al. (eds.), *Imaging in Oncological Urology*,
DOI 10.1007/978-1-84628-759-6_36, © Springer-Verlag London Limited 2009

CT Guided Robotic Assisted Interventions

While some systems have been developed to work with a specific imaging device, others can interface with a large array of systems. To date, CT is likely the favourite imaging modality for robotic assisted procedures.

The output of a CT is a collection of image slices of a 3D volume [7]. The 3D position of an individual image pixel is specified in a coordinate frame attached to the image. The problem of placing an instrument at a specified CT target is decomposed in two subtasks. First, the robot is registered with the CT image space; in other words, a 6 degrees of freedom (DOF) transformation from the image to the robot space is constructed. With this transformation, the target specified in the image can be interpreted to the space of the robot for the instrument positioning task.

Initial CT registration methods were developed for stereotactic neurosurgery and radiosurgery. The first methods were developed in early 1980s using three of N-shape fiducial rods [8]. The nine points resulting from the intersection of a CT image with the frame are used to compute the 6DOF registration transformation. The method exhibits high redundancy giving robustness. The transformation can be computed using a closed form formula (does not require numerical estimation methods, has fast solutions).

The Brown–Roberts–Wells (BRW) frame was employed for CT-robot registration providing excellent registration accuracy [9] in ex vivo tests. The method was generalized by Lee et al. [10] to a general registration method between a fiducial line pattern and an intersection plane. While the initial BRW frame requires for the image to intersect all 9 bars, the later method works with only six intersecting fiducials. While the accuracy of the previous described methods makes them suitable for CT guided percutaneous interventions, they require additional hardware on the robot end-effector which may be cumbersome in some clinical applications.

One of the first systems for minimally invasive surgery, Minerva, was developed for stereotactic neurosurgery. Since the skull provides a stable reference frame, neurosurgery is well suited for the application. Minerva was developed at the Micro-engineering Laboratory of the Swiss Federal Institute of Technology Centre and operates under surgeon control in conjunction with a CT scanner [11, 12].

Masamune et al. developed a minimally invasive surgical system for neurosurgery [13]. The system operates with a CT, is more compact than the previous systems and presents three stages. The first is a Cartesian (translational) stage. The second module has 2DOF and implements a virtual sphere; the instrument is pivoted around a remote centre. The last stage is the instrument translation. Also, the system design allows for the sterilization of the parts that are close to the patient. The electric parts are covered by a sterile drape.

Our URobotics group at Johns Hopkins has developed a miniature robot, PAKY-RCM, for image-guided percutaneous interventions [14]. The system has 3DOF, two rotations and one translation. The two rotations implement a remote centre of motion (RCM) concept, allowing for the orientation of a needle while maintaining the location of the needle tip. The third degree of freedom is a needle translation. The entire PAKY-RCM ensemble is attached to a passive arm allowing for the positioning of the robot.

This robot evolved into a more complex interventional system, AcuBot (Fig. 36.2), by augmenting a Cartesian stage and a "bridge" mount over the table. This was added for facilitating the fine adjustment of the initial robot placement. The system was designed to work in conjunction with a CT scanner. The target is defined by the physician in intraoperative CT images. The registration transformation from the CT image coordinate system to the robot coordinate system is computed using a laser-based registration technique [15]. The CT target coordinates are converted in robot space coordinates using the registration transformation. Then, the robot can accurately place an instrument (biopsy needle, radiofrequency (RF) probe, etc.) at the specified anatomical target. The system was successfully used clinically for kidney and liver radio-frequency ablations and biopsies under CT guidance [16].

Another approach in performing CT guided interventions was proposed by Loser et al. [17]. The method uses a visual-servoing algorithm to align the needle to a desired target. The image feedback is constructed using the fluoroscopy feature of special CT scanners. This method uses only the needle for the registration procedure but involves a significant amount of radiation since the X-ray is on during the alignment process. The method was tested ex vivo with good accuracy but clinical tests were yet not reported.

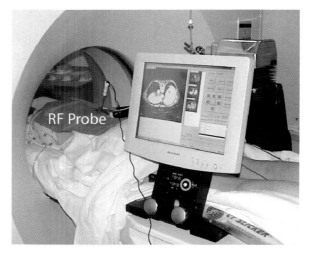

Fig. 36.2 AcuBot robot used in a liver tumour RF ablation

X-ray Guided Robotic Assisted Interventions

A widely available medical imager is the X-ray fluoroscopic unit, the C-Arm. This device provides real-time X-ray projective images. Sometimes two C-Arms are built into the same unit for bi-planar fluoroscopy providing two different (normally orthogonal) projections of the same 3D space.

The methods used in C-Arm guided robotic interventions can be classified into complete, full registration methods and asymptotic methods. In full registration methods, the 6DOF transformation from the robot space to the C-Arm space is computed and used to specify the desired target. This requires additional hardware for removing image distortion, C-Arm calibration and registration. During the calibration, the mathematical parameters of the perspective transformation are computed and can be used afterwards to calculate the target position.

The first full-registration method for C-Arm guided interventions was developed for bi-planar fluoroscopy [18]. The first two steps of the algorithm are the distortion correction and the fluoroscope calibration. Then, the registration is built by moving a marker attached to the robot in several workspace positions. The marker is imaged in each position, and the robot position is mapped to its image. Then, when a target is given, the previously constructed map is used to find the desired robot position. As an alternative to the tedious process of building the registration map by sequentially moving the robot in several points, others proposed a special registration device with multiple markers attached to the robot end-effector [19].

Another system – Neuromate – was developed for neurosurgery by Lavallee et al. [20]. The system uses preoperative magnetic resonance imaging and intraoperative orthogonal X-ray pictures to orient an interventional instrument. The system was clinically used with good results for placing electrodes in the brain.

Another medical robot was developed for hip joint replacement by Taylor et al. [21, 22]. In these procedures, the femur needs to be cut out in order to receive the implant. The robot performs bone cutting based on a preoperative plan. The robot is registered to the actual position of the femur using implanted markers or by touching the femur in several places. The system was initially tested on dogs and then clinically used.

In short, full registration methods are mathematically intensive algorithmic procedures. On the other hand, asymptotic methods use special techniques to interactively find out part of the required transformations or to directly estimate the motion required for the instrument to achieve its target. These operate somewhat similar to the way that experienced physicians intuitively handle the instruments under image feedback.

Asymptotic methods are normally based on visual servoing, which is a method originally employed in industrial robotics to increase robot performances. The first use of visual servoing in medical interventions was made by Loser and Navab [17]. The authors used visual servoing in two different C-Arm orientations to align a needle to the target. One C-Arm position was used to find a plane in the robot space that contains the target and the needle tip and is projected as a line. In order to do so, the needle is rotated in two arbitrary but dissimilar planes until it is aligned with the target. The two positions computed at the first step define a plane. With the needle restricted to move in this plane, a second C-Arm view is used to complete the alignment and to compute the insertion depth using cross-ratios. This approach does not require any C-Arm calibration or registration. However, the errors are dependent on the relative orientation of the arbitrary planes.

Two different methods for robotic assisted C-Arm guided interventions were developed by Patriciu et al. [23, 24]. Both methods are based on real-time image feedback. The first method requires two dissimilar C-Arm orientations for performing the needle alignment, while the other method was derived from the needle-superimposing technique.

The first C-Arm servoing method [23] uses a conical motion of the needle around its tip in order to find two different needle positions that projected collinear with the target. These two needle positions define a plane containing the target and the tip of the needle. Full target alignment is achieved by moving the needle in the plane found in the first C-Arm orientation and observing the image feedback from a second C-Arm's view. The second C-Arm view is also used for needle insertion feedback.

The automatic needle superimposition technique [24] starts with a needle and C-Arm positioned in a way that the needle point is at the desired entry point, and the tip of the needle is over the target in the C-Arm image. Then, the needle is automatically rotated around its tip under C-Arm feedback until the distal end of the needle is superimposed over its head and over the target. At this point, the needle is fully aligned with the target. A lateral C-Arm view is used to observe the needle insertion. The method was successfully implemented on the AcuBot robot and tested using a Percutaneous Kidney Slab (Limbs and Things Inc.) as shown in Fig. 36.3.

Ultrasound Guided Robotic Assisted Interventions

For its accessibility and markedly improved image quality in the recent years, ultrasound has become the instrument of choice for a number of minimally invasive procedures.

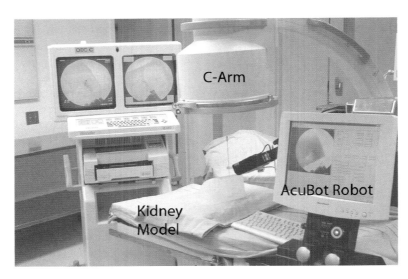

Fig. 36.3 Automatic needle alignment under C-Arm guidance – kidney mock-up tests

The advantages of ultrasound are its lack of radiation, low cost, and the real-time imaging. Disadvantages are its impermeability through air pockets (i.e. lungs) and, especially important for image-guided robotic control, its the low signal-to-noise ratio. This makes target identification tasks more difficult to achieve automatically. Another possible drawback is the fact that an ultrasound provides only localized image with a relatively low depth of penetration.

The ultrasound however is the most common imaging modality for some organs, such as the prostate. The first surgical robot to use ultrasound images was developed by Davies et al. [25]. This robot (PROBOT) was designed to perform transurethral resection of the prostate (TURP). In a TURP, the instrument is introduced through the urethra and advanced to the level of the prostate which encompasses the innermost part of the urethra. The prostate is then resected in small pieces using a cutting sling that is moved in and out of the instrument's shaft. PROBOT was devised as a small robot with goniometric arcs attached to a bigger positioning frame. PROBOT can perform the prostate resection using a preoperative plan based on ultrasound images. The ultrasound is attached to the robot, thus, the image and the robot have the same coordinate system. PROBOT was used on patients during the initial stage of the procedure and completed manually afterwards.

MR Guided Robotic Assisted Interventions

In recent years, a growing effort was devoted to build robots that can work with magnetic resonance imaging (MRI). This is particularly challenging due to the strong magnetic field present in the MR which can reach 4 T [7] in human imagers and exceed 10 T experimentally.

Massamune et al. designed, perhaps, the first MRI-compatible needle driver [26] for neurological interventions. The robot was built from non-ferromagnetic materials and actuated with ultrasonic motors (using piezoelectric effects, without magnetism). However, further applications of the system were not reported to date.

Chinzei et al. [27] developed an MR-compatible robot that can work in open MR. The system also uses ultrasonic motors that can actively orient and provide a guide for a biopsy probe or other instruments. The system was tested with good results on ex vivo models, but thus far no patient studies have been reported.

Kaiser et al. developed a system for breast biopsy [28]. The system uses ultrasonic motors for actuation and a combination of laser range sensors, as well as custom built optical rotation code transducers for position feedback. The system was tested with promising results on a body mock-up but clinical tests are still to be made.

A needle guide built within a transrectal MR coil was developed by Krieger et al. [29, 30] at the Johns Hopkins University. The device presented in Fig. 36.4 was designed for transrectal prostate biopsy. The position of the guide in MR coordinates is computed using specially designed position coils which give its real-time position directly in imager coordinates. Thus device is manually positioned and adjusted until the desired trajectory is achieved. The system was initially used on animal experiments. The system is presently undergoing clinical trials at the National Institutes of Health (NIH).

Several versions of MR-compatible robots were developed at the Institute for Medical Engineering and Biophysics, Forschungszentrum Karlsruhe, Germany [31]. Over the years, the systems used ultrasonic or hybrid ultrasonic-pneumatic actuation. Recently, a commercial version was

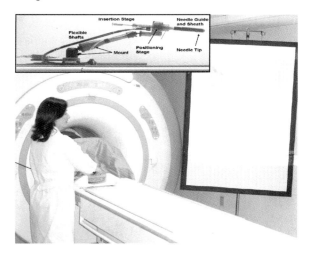

Fig. 36.4 MR-compatible device for transrectal prostate biopsy. Courtesy by Axel Krieger and Louis L. Whitcomb, Johns Hopkins University, Mech. Eng. Department

developed by INNOMEDIC Inc. (Germany) and received limited clearance for clinical use in the European Union.

Systems using ultrasonic actuation are a compromise for MR compatibility, because even though magnetism is eliminated, piezoelectric actuation requires the use of high-frequency electricity which typically interferes with the functionality of the imager. As such, the systems need to be deactivated during imaging and located distally (>0.5 m) from the imaging field.

The first fully MRI-compatible robot to be reported [32] was recently developed in our URobotics lab. In fact, this robot is designed for multi-imager compatibility [33], so that it may be used in all classes of imaging equipment. This includes uncompromised compatibility with MRI of the highest field strength, size accessibility within closed-bore

tunnel-shaped scanners and clinical intervention safety. For MRI compatibility, the robot is exclusively built of nonmagnetic and dielectric materials such as plastics, ceramics and rubbers and is electricity free. The system utilizes a new type of pneumatic stepper motors (PneuStep) specifically designed for this application [34]. These motors uniquely provide easily controllable precise and safe pneumatic actuation. Fibre optical encoding is used for feedback, so that all electric components are distally located outside the imager's room (Fig. 36.5).

The robot is designed to accommodate various end-effectors for different percutaneous interventions such as biopsy, serum injections or brachytherapy. The first end-effector developed is customized for fully-automated brachytherapy seed placement. Initial in vitro tests showed outstanding motion accuracy (<0.1 mm), and seed placement in gelatin models show that very uniform (<0.5 mm), computer controlled patters can be easily achieved Fig. 36.6. Present experiments are concentrated on brachytherapy animal trials, and new injectors for biopsy and serum injections will be developed next.

Future Directions and Discussion

A major source of errors and limitation of robotic assisted image-guided minimally invasive procedures thus far has been related to respiratory motion and soft tissue deflections. Current needle placement algorithms assume that the target does not move between the time instance when the image was acquired and the time when the needle/instrument is inserted. While this is a reasonable assumption for relatively immobile organs such as the brain, it does not hold for most organs located close to the diaphragm. These organs are known to significantly shift with breathing. While several

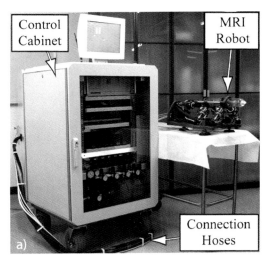

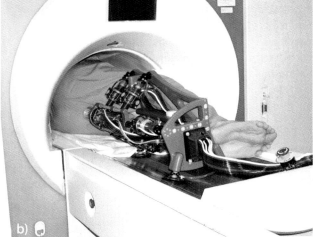

Fig. 36.5 URobotics MRI-compatible robot; (a) robot system, (b) robot in MRI scanner

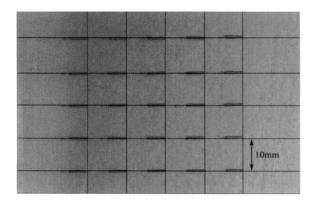

Fig. 36.6 Brachytherapy seeds automatically deployed with MR robot

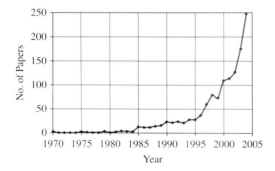

Fig. 36.7 The number of robotic publications in medical literature

practical solutions such as breath hold and respiratory gating have been employed to deal with this problem, no widely acceptable solution has yet been reached.

A count of robotics publications in the medical literature (Fig. 36.7) reveals that the impact of medical robotics has exponentially grown since its inception in late 1980s. Robots do not only augment physician's manipulation capabilities but also establish a digital platform for integrating medical information. Medical imaging data, in particular, gives robots abilities unattainable to humans, because, unlike humans, robots and imagers are digital devices.

Image-guided interventions expand clinical practice above and beyond traditional diagnosis, and do so with the use of modern tools. The initial success of surgeon–assistant systems is expected to be followed by the more promising field of image-guided systems for real-time interventions.

References

1. Taylor RH, Stoianovici D. Medical robotics in computer-integrated surgery. IEEE Trans Rob Autom. 2003;19(5):765–81. http://urology.jhu.edu/urobotics/pub/2003-taylor-ieeetra.pdf.
2. Sackier JM, Wang Y. Robotically assisted laparoscopic surgery – from concept to development. Surg Endosc Ultrasound Interv Tech. 1994;8(1):63–6.
3. Guthart GS, Salisbury JK. The intuitive telesurgery system: overview and application. Proceedings of the IEEE International Conference on Robotics and Automation (ICRA 2000). 2000.
4. Vandenelsen PA, Pol EJD, Viergever MA. Medical image matching – a review with classification. IEEE Eng Med Biol Mag. 1993;12(1):26–39.
5. Hill DLG, Batchelor PG, Holden M, Hawkes DJ. Medical image registration. Phys Med Biol. 2001;46(3):R1–45.
6. Pluim JPW, Maintz JBA, Viergever MA. Mutual-information-based registration of medical images: A survey. IEEE Trans Med Imaging. 2003;22(8):986–1004.
7. Shung KK, Smith MB, Tsui BMW. Principles of medical imaging. San Diego, CA: Academic Press, Inc; 1992.
8. Brown RA, Roberts TS, Osborn AG. Stereotaxic frame and computer software for CT-directed neurosurgical localization. Invest Radiol. 1980;15(5):444.
9. Susil RC, Anderson JH, Taylor RH. A single image registration method for CT guided interventions. Med Image Comput Comput Assist Interv – Miccai'99, Proc. 1999;1679:798–808.
10. Lee S, Fichtinger G, Chirikjian GS. Numerical algorithms for spatial registration of line fiducials from cross-sectional images. Med Phys. 2002;29(8):1881–91.
11. Glauser D, Flury P, Villotte N, Burckhardt C. Mechanical concept of the neurosurgical robot Minerva. Robotics. 1993;11:567–75.
12. Glauser D, Fankhauser H, Epitaux M, Hefti JL, Jaccottet A. Neurosurgical robot Minerva: first results and current developments J Image Guided Surg. 1995;1(5):266–72.
13. Masamune K, Ji LH, Suzuki M, Dohi T, Iseki H, Takakura K. A newly developed stereotactic robot with detachable drive for neurosurgery. Med Image Comput Comput Assist Interv – Miccai'98. 1998;1496:215–22.
14. Cleary K, Zigmundb B, Banovaca F, Whitec C, Stoianovici D. Robotically assisted lung biopsy under CT fluoroscopy: lung cancer screening and phantom study. Comput Assist Radiol Surg. 2005;740–5.http://urology.jhu.edu/urobotics/pub/2005-cleary-CARS.pdf.
15. Patriciu A, Solomon S, Kavoussi LR, Stoianovici D. Robotic kidney and spine percutaneous procedures using a new laser-based CT registration method. Lect Notes Comput Sci. 2001;2208:249–58. http://urology.jhu.edu/urobotics/pub/2001-patriciu-miccai.pdf.
16. Awad MM, Solomon SB, Patriciu A, Stoianovici D, Chou MA. Robotically-assisted radiofrequency ablation of liver tumors: comparison with standard manual techniques. Gastroenterology. 2004;126(4):A801–A801.
17. Loser M, Navab N, Bascle B, Taylor R. Visual servoing for automatic and uncalibrated percutaneous procedures. Proc. SPIE Med Imaging. 2000;3976:270–81.
18. Bzostek A, Schreiner S, Barnes AC, Cadeddu JA, Roberts WW, Anderson JH, et al. An automated system for precise percutaneous access of the renal collecting system. Cvrmed – Mrcas'97. 1997;1205:299–308.
19. Yao JH, Taylor RH, Goldberg RP. Kumar R, Bzostek A, Van Vorhis R, et al. A progressive cut refinement scheme for revision total hip replacement surgery using C-arm fluoroscopy. Med Image Comput Comput Assist Interv – Miccai'99, Proc. 1999;1679:1010–19.
20. Lavallee S, Troccaz J, Gaborit L, Cinquin P, Benabid AL, Hoffmann D. Image guided operating robot: a clinical application in stereotactic neurosurgery. IEEE International Conference on Robotics and Automation (ICRA). 1992:618–24.
21. Kazanzides P, Mittelstadt BD, Musits BL, Bargar WL, Zuhars JF, Williamson B, Cain PW, Carbone EJ. An integrated system for cementless hip replacement. IEEE Eng Medicine Biol. 1995;14(3):307–13.
22. Taylor RH, Paul HA, Kazandzides P, Mittelstadt BD, Hanson W, Zuhars JF, et al. An image-directed robotic system for

precise orthopaedic surgery. IEEE Trans Rob Autom. 1994;10(3): 261–75.

23. Patriciu A, Stoianovici D, Whitcomb LL, Jarrett T, Mazilu D, Stanimir A, et al. Motion-based robotic instrument targeting under C-Arm fluoroscopy. Lect Notes Comput Sci. 2000;1935:988–98. http://urology.jhu.edu/urobotics/pub/2000-patriciu-miccai.pdf.

24. Patriciu A, Mazilu D, Petrisor D, Kavoussi LR, Stoianovici D. Automatic targeting method and accuracy study in robot assisted needle procedures. Lect Notes Comput Sci. 2003;1:124–31. http://urology.jhu.edu/urobotics/pub/2003-patriciu-miccai.pdf.

25. Davies BL, Hibberd RD, Timoney AG, Wickham JEA. A clinically applied robot for prostatectomies. Computer integrated surgery: technology and clinical applications. MIT Press; Cambridge, Masachusetts 1996. pp. 593–601.

26. Masamune K, Kobayashi E, Masutani Y, Suzuki M, Dohi T, Iseki H, et al. Development of an MRI-compatible needle insertion manipulator for stereotactic neurosurgery. J Image Guid Surg. 1995;1:242–8.

27. Chinzei K, Hata N, Jolesz FA, Kikinis R. MR compatible surgical assist robot: System integration and preliminary feasibility study. Medical Image Computing and Computer-Assisted Intervention – Miccai 2000, LNCS – 1935;921–30.

28. Kaiser WA, Fischer H, Vagner J, Selig M. Robotic system for biopsy and therapy of breast lesions in a high-field whole-body magnetic resonance tomography unit. J. Invest Radiol. 2000;35(8): 513–9.

29. Krieger A, Susil RC, Menard C, Coleman JA, Fichtinger G, Atalar E, et al. Design of a novel MRI compatible manipulator for image guided prostate interventions. Biomed Eng, IEEE Trans. 2005;52(2):306–13.

30. Susil RC, Krieger A, Derbyshire JA, Tanacs A, Whitcomb LL, Fichtinger G, et al. System for MR image-guided prostate interventions: Canine study. Radiology. 2003;228(3):886–94.

31. Hempel E, Fischer H, Gumb L, Hohn T, Krause H, Voges U, et al. An MRI-compatible surgical robot for precise radiological interventions. Comput Aided Surg. 2003;8(4):180–91.

32. Muntener M, Patriciu A, Petrisor D, Mazilu D, Kavoussi L, Cleary K, et al. Magnetic resonance imaging compatible robotic system for fully automated brachytherapy seed placement. *Urology.* 2006;68(6):1313–7.

33. Stoianovici D. Multi-imager compatible actuation principles in surgical robotics. Int J Med Rob Comput Assist Surg. 2005;1(2):86–100. http://urology.jhu.edu/urobotics/pub/2005-stoianovici-MRCASJ.pdf.

34. Stoianovici D, Patriciu A, Mazilu D, Petrisor D, Kavoussi L. A New Type of Motor: pneumatic Step Motor. IEEE/ASME Trans Mechatronics. 2007;12:98–106.

Chapter 37

Future Directions – New Developments in Ultrasound

G.A. Schwartz and M.A. Averkiou

Overview

Medical diagnostic ultrasound has been an important imaging tool for the urologist for the last two or three decades. Its well-known advantages are the relatively low cost, lack of ionizing radiation, real-time imaging, and wide variety of special-application transducers. Moreover, in recent years, developments in technology and urologic practice point the way to increased utility and utilization of medical ultrasound.

Medical ultrasound imaging in oncologic practice and urology in particular has grown beyond diagnostics to contribute more broadly to the care cycle. With the push to detect neoplastic disease at ever earlier stages, and the widespread use of screening tests, imaging plays an essential role in screening follow-up and with the arrival of more specific indicators may take a significant role in screening itself.

At the therapeutic end of the care cycle, imaging has been a key enabler in the development and expansion of minimally invasive urologic procedures. Image-guided therapy complements the hands and instruments of the interventionalist with vision. Further developments promise to provide image guidance based not only on anatomic images but physiologic, functional images.

Ultrasound imaging technology is evolving to provide greater access, better image quality, real-time three-dimensional images, and perfusion imaging with the aid of contrast agents. These advances have come as a result of miniaturization, electronic beam control, image processing, microbubble development, and contrast imaging techniques. The combination of these developments has contributed a variety of emerging applications of particular importance in urologic oncology.

This review will look at the recent technology trends with a particular focus on perfusion imaging and quantification, perhaps the most important capability that is enabled by the convergence of these trends.

Technology Trends

Transducers

Modern ultrasonic imaging is implemented with transducers composed of arrays of piezoelectric elements, each of which can convert electrical signals into acoustic signals, and back again. Very small, uniform elements are driven with carefully timed signals in order to form and steer the resulting acoustic beam. For the first two to three decades these electronic arrays were utilized; they were one dimensional, thus the term "linear arrays." While this simplicity meant they were easy to manufacture, it also meant that the beam was electronically controlled in only one dimension, providing a single plane of imaging.

Miniaturization of the arrays has provided endo-cavity imaging for endorectal and endovaginal imaging and led to transducers integrated into catheters for intravascular and intracardiac use. These have also been shown to be useful for imaging from within the urethra, the bladder, and the ureters. Ultimately these may be combined with therapy delivery systems to provide image-guided therapy at the end of the catheter.

The one-dimensional arrays have been integrated into mechanical assemblies that sweep the single plane through a volume. This technique yields a volume scan which can be used for three-dimensional imaging, or reconstruction of image planes with any orientation in the volume. More recently, two-dimensional arrays have been developed, initially for cardiac imaging, that can provide real-time volumetric images [1]. Real-time three-dimensional imaging is helpful since it can present dynamic views that are more useful for the surgeon, yet unattainable under typical interventional conditions. The biplane mode with two real-time

M.A. Averkiou (✉)
Marie Curie Chair of Excellence, Biomedical Engineering Program
Department of Mechanical Engineering, University of Cyprus
75 Kallipoleos Str., 1678 Nicosia, CYPRUS
maverk@ucy.ac.cy

J.J.M.C.H. de la Rosette et al. (eds.), *Imaging in Oncological Urology*,
DOI 10.1007/978-1-84628-759-6_37, © Springer-Verlag London Limited 2009

orthogonal planes is showing particular value in image-guided therapy. Since the acoustic beams are electronically controlled in two dimensions, these systems are capable of much better resolution and higher rate imaging than the earlier mechanical designs.

Image Quality Improvements

Better acoustic beam control has yielded great advances in the spatial resolution of ultrasound systems, but the increased processing power of modern computers has enabled signal processing that can address two other limitations of ultrasound imaging, limited contrast resolution, and acoustic artifacts.

The coherent nature of ultrasound imaging means that it exhibits a noise pattern termed speckle, which limits the contrast resolution and dynamic range of the image. This means that subtle changes in tissue state might be obscured by speckle noise. By employing a wide range of acoustic frequencies simultaneously (termed "frequency compounding"), and combining the result, the noise can be reduced, and better lesion conspicuity can be achieved.

The compounding concept also has a spatial version, with electronic steering providing a multiplicity of look angles that are combined to produce an image that exhibits less acoustic artifacts, such as speckle and shadowing, and provides increased contrast resolution and tissue uniformity (Fig. 37.1).

Once the image has been formed, image processing techniques can be employed to further enhance detail and reduce artifact. Adaptive filters look at the image content and vary the processing characteristics based on local features in the image.

Elastography

The digital examination has been an important tool in screening and assessment of prostate tumors. Ultrasound elastography has the potential to measure the mechanical properties of tissue by imaging the displacement (strain) while under stress [2]. This "strain imaging" may be a means to locate and characterize prostate lesions [3].

Image Fusion

As minimally invasive procedures grow in practice, the importance of image guidance is growing. Combinations of imaging modalities as in "fusion" imaging have the potential to provide more complete, integrated anatomic and physiologic information [4]. By registering anatomic features, or by sensing the position of the ultrasound transducer, ultrasound images can be embedded or overlaid other imaging modalities such as CT or MR. Since real-time imaging is so important in procedure guidance, ultrasound has a particular advantage.

Perfusion Imaging with Ultrasound Contrast Agents

Introduction

While the recent advances in diagnostic ultrasound have improved the quality, accessibility, and range of application of ultrasonic imaging, the challenge of lesion detection and characterization can only be met with the use of ultrasound

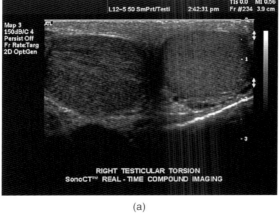
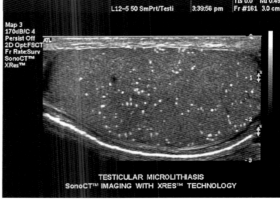

(a)   (b)

Fig. 37.1 (a) The improved contrast resolution from spatial compounding helps present the subtle texture changes due to testicular torsion. (b) Adaptive filtering further enhances both the contrast resolution and the detail resolution for improved tissue uniformity and depiction of small structures

contrast agents. Contrast agents are gas-filled microbubbles with diameters in the low-micron range. After intravenous injection they enhance the backscattered signals from blood and make possible the detection of blood flow in both the macro- (larger vessels) and microvasculature (capillaries). It is noted that blood flow in the capillaries is well below the detection threshold of Doppler techniques and may not be measured with conventional ultrasound without contrast agents. The development of neoplastic disease is usually associated with neovascularization, also referred to as angio-genesis, and may be imaged and quantified with ultrasound only with the use of contrast agents.

Microbubble Properties: Nonlinearity and Bubble Destruction

Imaging techniques have been developed to best utilize microbubble contrast agents. These techniques are based on two main properties of the microbubbles: nonlinear oscilla-tion [5] and destruction due to the ultrasound field. When an acoustic wave encounters a microbubble, it alternately com-presses the microbubble on the positive pressure and expands it on the negative pressure. On the positive portion of the wave, the microbubbles are compressed in a different fashion than the way they expand in the negative portion. This results in an asymmetric, nonlinear bubble oscillation. Instead of producing a sinusoidal echo with a clean frequency spectrum like the transmitted signal in Fig. 37.2a, it produces an odd-looking echo with asymmetric top and bottom as shown in Fig. 37.2b. It is this asymmetry that produces harmonics and can be utilized to enhance the signals from the bubbles. In Fig. 37.2c the frequency spectrum of the bubble echo (b) is shown. The first major hump is the fundamental, and the sub-sequent ones are the second, third, and fourth harmonics.

Bubbles in a liquid tend to diffuse and disappear unless they are stabilized by some form of a shell. Once the shell is disrupted the gas inside will diffuse into the surrounding fluid. The mechanical index (MI), originally defined to pre-

dict the onset of cavitation in fluids, also gives an indication of the likelihood of bubble destruction. The MI is defined as

MI = peak negative pressure/SQRT (ultrasound fre-quency)

or equivalently

MI = peak negative pressure * SQRT (period of ultra-sound wavelength)

The harder you try to expand the bubble (peak negative pressure) and the longer you expand it (period of ultrasound wavelength), the more likely it is to break. It has been well established that the acoustic power level used during routine examinations destroys the contrast microbubbles.

Harmonic Imaging

The bubbles' nonlinear behavior can be utilized to enhance the contrast relative to tissue. Harmonic imaging relies on transmitting at a fundamental frequency f_0 and forming an image from the second harmonic component $2f_0$ of the backscattered echoes by the use of filters to remove the fundamental component. Originally it was believed that harmonic imaging would allow complete separation of contrast from tissue, as it was assumed that tissue was completely linear. However, it was soon found that tissue did produce significant harmonic energy and the high sensitivity and bandwidth of modern ultrasound equipment could detect it [6]. In fact, the harmonic image produced by tissue alone has beneficial qualities such as reduced clutter in the image and improved resolution. Therefore, a tissue image is present even in the absence of a contrast agent, so that perfect separation was not achieved at the normal tissue imaging conditions (MI~1.0).

Agent Detection Imaging (ADI)

When microbubbles are interrogated and destroyed with high MI ultrasound, the backscattered signal is very large and has a broad bandwidth (many harmonic components). Studies have shown that the destruction of the bubbles allows for a great separation between tissue and contrast sig-nals. The contrast signal during bubble destruction changes rapidly from pulse to pulse and Doppler techniques are well suited for detecting these changes. Power harmonics (power Doppler at the harmonic frequency) was developed for con-trast agents to detect pulse to pulse changes in the signal returned from microbubbles. It is effectively a topographic image of the destruction of microbubbles, thus indicating the regions where bubbles were present. In recent years the high MI/destruction imaging technique has been referred to as agent detection imaging (ADI). ADI is displayed as a color

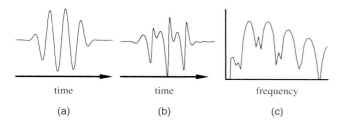

time   time   frequency

(a)   (b)   (c)

Fig. 37.2 (a) Incident acoustic wave; (b) nonlinear bubble echoes; (c) frequency spectrum of bubble echoes

overlay over a grayscale tissue image. One clinical application that uses ADI is liver metastasis detection. Contrast agents tend to stick in the liver parenchyma after the vascular phase and collect in the normal liver but not in the metastases [7]. A region in the liver may only be scanned once (just one frame) because once the bubbles are destroyed ADI images will have no signals at all. ADI is performed by sweeping the whole liver and then freezing the system and going back frame by frame to find any possible lesions.

Nonlinear Pulsing Schemes

One widely used approach of imaging contrast agents is to use a low mechanical index (MI) nonlinear imaging technique to avoid bubble destruction, and image both the macro- and micro-circulation in real time. Another important advantage of low MI imaging is that tissue is eliminated as it does not produce a nonlinear component at low acoustic power. Various pulsing schemes have been developed for the detection of nonlinear echoes from contrast microbubbles. These are pulse inversion [8], power modulation, and their combination. For a discussion of nonlinear pulsing schemes see [9, 10]. Figure 37.3 shows the behavior of a splenic hemangioma with pulse inversion (PI) at a low MI.

Microvascular Imaging (MVI)

It has been known for some time that malignant tumors force the host to grow new blood vessels to supply nutrients to support the rapid growth and spread of the tumor [11]. This process of angiogenesis starts with very small microvasculature, growing larger feeding vessels over time as the tumor grows. The ability to image angiogenesis is important in cancer diagnosis, as well as therapy assessment research. In some of

these micro-vessels the flow rate is so low that a bubble may pass through only every few seconds. It might be visible for several frames, but still gives only a fleeting glimpse of the vasculature as shown in Fig. 37.4a. Microvascular imaging (MVI) has recently been developed to capture and track the bubbles as they go through these small vessels. MVI measures changes in the image from frame to frame, suppressing any background tissue signal and capturing the bubbles as they pass through the vasculature. It enhances vessel conspicuity showing tracks of single bubbles flowing through the microvasculature as shown in Fig. 37.4b.

Clinical Applications in Contrast Radiology

The largest application for contrast agents in radiology at present is liver lesion detection and characterization. [12, 13] Certain lesions may be seen with ultrasound before injection of contrast agents, but often lesions are not seen at all without them. A more difficult task is to characterize lesions (benign or malignant), and it requires the use of contrast agents. The characterization process requires observation of the different vascular phases [arterial, portal venous, and late phase (parenchymal uptake)], the nature of vessels inside the lesion, and rate of filling. With ultrasound contrast agents, hepatocellular carcinoma (HCC), metastasis from a primary tumor at some other location, hemangioma, and focal nodular hyperplasia (FNH) are detected and characterized in the liver. This is only possible because with contrast agents it is possible to image the perfusion bed. Tumor detection with contrast agents is also possible for other organs like kidney, breast, prostate, and ovaries. Figure 37.5 shows an example of liver metastasis with Levovist and the ADI technique, which is based on bubble destruction. In Fig. 37.6 an example of an FNH scanned with low MI PI is shown.

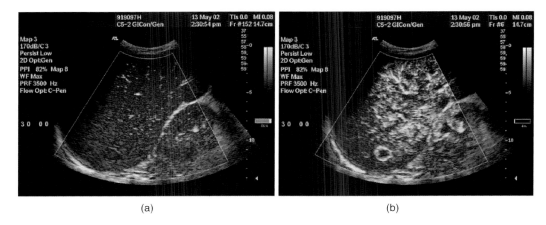

(a)   (b)

Fig. 37.3 A splenic hemangioma (indicated by the arrow) shown in power pulse inversion. (a) Initial bubble arrival and (b) peripheral filling

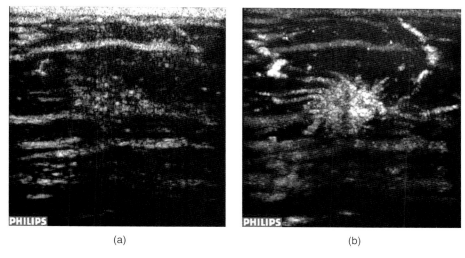

(a)   (b)

Fig. 37.4 Breast ductal carcinoma showing (a) individual bubbles in still frame of live loop and (b) processed MVI image capturing tracks of many bubbles

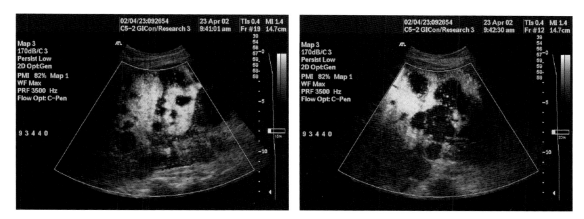

Fig. 37.5 Examples of metastases with Levovist in ADI. The black holes in the image indicate metastases

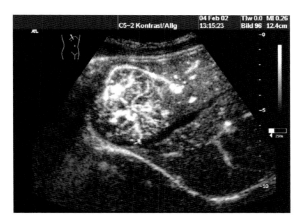

Fig. 37.6 Example of focal nodular hyperplasia with SonoVue in pulse inversion

Quantification: Kidney Transplant Perfusion

By destroying the contrast within the scan plane (once it is fully perfused with contrast microbubbles), a "negative bolus" of contrast is created locally. Then, the time it takes for contrast to refill the scan plane is an indicator of the local blood flow velocity. This has been proposed as a method for quantification of myocardial perfusion [14] and is under investigation for general imaging applications such as kidney transplant perfusion and angiogenesis quantification and monitoring. This process is illustrated in Fig. 37.7 and a replenishment curve is shown in Fig. 37.8. The smooth line shown in Fig. 37.8 is the best fit to the equation $A*(1 - \exp(-\beta t))$, in which A is related to contrast blood volume, and the time constant β is related to blood flow velocity.

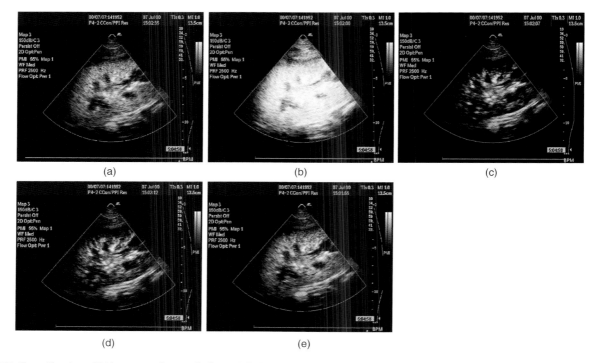

Fig. 37.7 Quantification of kidney transplant perfusion. (a) Stable perfusion prior to flash. (b) High MI flash to destroy agent. (c, d) Contrast is re-entering the region of interest. (e) Seconds later contrast has been replenished in the kidney

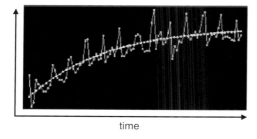

time

Fig. 37.8 Replenishment curves showing image intensity versus time from the image sequence of Fig. 37.7 and curve fit to $C(t) = A^*(1 - \exp(-\beta t))$

New Opportunities: Targeted Agents and Therapeutic Agents

With microbubble ultrasound contrast agents new opportunities open for further developments in the areas of molecular imaging and therapy. Microbubbles provide the vehicle to targeting molecular events and thus combining imaging with pathophysiology and ultimately therapy. New therapeutic strategies for the treatment of cardiovascular and neoplastic diseases are being developed [15]. Methods of microbubble targeting include targeting by intrinsic properties of the shell or by ligand conjugation. One clinical application will be targeted imaging of inflammation. Microbubble agents have been targeted to selectins (P-selectin) and to immunoglobulin-family receptors [15] and thus adhering to inflammation sites. Ultrasound-mediated gene transfection is another new area of research in the recent years. Ultrasound-mediated destruction of microbubbles directs plasmid transgene expression to the heart and is a promising method for cardiac gene therapy [16]. Efforts for the development of viral and non-viral vectors, giving efficient gene transfer and sustained expression to targeted tissues, are underway. The use of ultrasound for various forms of drug delivery has also been suggested recently [17]. The local blood–brain barrier opening is an advantageous approach for targeted drug delivery to the brain and has been shown to be possible with the use of ultrasound and microbubble contrast agents [18]. The above *is* a small example of some of the new opportunities that are opening today in the area of ultrasound, and they have the potential to dramatically change today's medical practice.

References

1. Suematsu Y, Marx GR, Stoll JA, DuPont PE, Cleveland RO, Howe RD, et al. Three-dimensional echocardiography-guided beating-heart surgery without cardiopulmonary bypass: a feasibility study. J Thorac Cardiovasc Surg. 2004;128(4):579–87.
2. Ophir J, Cespedes I, Ponnekanti H, Yazdi Y, Li X. Elastography: a quantitative method for imaging the elasticity of biological tissues. Ultrason Imaging. 1991;13:111.

3. Konig K, Scheipers U, Pesavento A, Lorenz A, Ermert H, Senge T. Initial experiences with real-time elastography guided biopsies of the prostate. J Urol. 2005;174(1):115–7.

4. Steggerda M, Schneider C, van Herk M, Zijp L, Moonen L, van der Poel H. The applicability of simultaneous TRUS-CT imaging for the evaluation of prostate seed implants. Med Phys. 2005;32(7):2262–70.

5. Leighton TG. The acoustic bubble. London, UK: Academic Press; 1994.

6. Averkiou MA, Roundhill DN, Powers JE. New imaging technique based on the nonlinear properties of tissues. Proc IEEE Ultrason Symp. 1997;2:1561–6.

7. Albrecht T, Blomley MJ, Burns PN, Wilson S, Harvey CJ, Leen E, et al. Improved detection of hepatic metastases with pulse-inversion US during the liver-specific phase of SHU 508A: multicenter study. Radiology. 2003;227(2):361–70.

8. Hope Simpson D, Chin CT, Burns PN. Pulse inversion Doppler: a new method for detecting nonlinear echoes from microbubble contrast agents. IEEE Trans Ultrason Ferroelectr Freq Control. 1999;46(2):372–82.

9. Averkiou M, Powers J, Skyba D, Bruce M, Jensen S. Ultrasound contrast imaging research. Ultrasound Q. 2003;19(1):27–37.

10. Averkiou MA, Bruce M, Jensen S, Rafter P, Brock-Fisher T, Powers J. Pulsing schemes for the detection of nonlinear echoes from contrast microbubbles. 9th European Symposium on Ultrasound Contrast Imaging, Rotterdam, The Netherlands, Jan 2004.

11. Folkman J, Beckner K. Angiogenesis imaging. Acad Radiol. 2000;7(10):783–5.

12. Leen E. The role of contrast-enhanced ultrasound in the characterisation of focal liver lesions. Eur Radiol. 2001;11 Suppl 3: E27–34.

13. Harvey CJ, Blomley MJ, Eckersley RJ, Cosgrove DO, Patel N, Heckemann RA, et al. Hepatic malignancies: improved detection with pulse-inversion US in late phase of enhancement with SH U 508A-early experience. Radiology. 2000;216(3): 903–8.

14. Wei K, Jayaweera AR, Firoozan S, Linka A, Skyba DM, Kaul S. Quantification of myocardial blood flow with ultrasound-induced destruction of microbubbles administered as a constant venous infusion. Circulation. 1998;97(5):473–83.

15. Lindner JR. Microbubbles in medical imaging: current applications and future directions. Nat Rev Drug Discov. 2004;3:527–32.

16. Bekeredjian R, Shuyuan C, Frenkel P, Grayburn PA, Shohet RV. Ultrasound-targeted microbubble destruction can repeatedly direct highly specific plasmid expression to the heart. Circulation. 2003;108:1022–6.

17. Tachibana K, Tachibana S. The use of ultrasound for drug delivery. Echocardiography. 2001;18(4):323–8.

18. Sheikov N, McDonald N, Vykhodtseva N, Jolesz F, Hynynen K. Cellular mechanisms of the blood-brain barrier opening induced by ultrasound in presence of microbubbles. Ultrasound Med Biol. 2004;30(7):979–89.

Chapter 38

Future Directions – Contrast Media

S.D. Allen, C.J. Harvey, M. Blomley, and P. Dawson

Introduction

The field of contrast agents in all three imaging modalities of computed tomography, magnetic resonance, and ultrasound has undergone dramatic developments, with huge advances being achieved in the understanding of the chemical properties of these agents, their physiological effects, and their place in the technological developments in each modality. This chapter describes these advances along with future directions.

CT Contrast Media

Over the last decade, low-osmolality iodinated contrast agents have largely replaced the high-osmolality variety due to their better safety and tolerance [1]. The original "low-osmolality" contrast agents were categorized as non-ionic monomeric (three iodine atoms per molecule) (Fig. 38.1) and ionic dimeric (ioxaglate) (six iodine atoms per molecule) (Fig. 38.2). The former has an iodine to particle number ratio of 3:1 and the latter one of 6:2 (=3:1), twice that of the classical or conventional ionic agents. Although osmolality is relatively low in these agents, it remains more than twice that of plasma. There are now several representatives of the low-osmolar non-ionic monomeric agent class, including iohexol, iopamidol, and ioversol (Fig. 38.3). Clinical trials have shown that if administered in equivalent administration protocols and iodine concentrations, then there is no significant difference of opacification efficacy or in regard to safety [2].

Over the last few years, iso-osmolar non-ionic dimeric agents such as iodixanol (Fig. 38.4) have become widely available and are now competing with the monomeric ionic compounds that have been the "workhorses" for the majority of CT investigations in many departments. These molecules like the *ionic* dimeric variety carry six iodine atoms but they do not dissociate in solution and hence maintain an iodine to particle ratio of 6:1. They are naturally hypo-osmolar with respect to plasma but are formulated with extra ions to render them iso-osmolar [3, 4].

The iso-osmolality confers a number of advantages on this type of contrast agent, many of which are relevant to urographic imaging. They induce a lesser osmotic diuresis, resulting in greater urinary concentrations and denser pyelograms [5, 6].

CT angiography and venography examinations are increasingly utilized in the assessment of urological cancer and have benefited from this iso-osmolality since there is osmotically driven self-dilution in the circulation (1,3) and since the larger molecules diffuse more slowly across the vessel walls and hence remain in the vascular space for longer, the result being better vessel opacification [7]. A similar vessel opacification to that produced by the "low-osmolar" agents can thus be obtained with a lower iodine load with some cost saving [8]. This is advantageous in patients with impaired renal function. Nephrotoxicity in patients at risk has been claimed in any case to be lower in patients receiving this group of agents [9, 10], though other studies contradict this finding [11, 12].

The superior opacification of the excretory pathway has considerable application in dedicated CT urographic examinations. In particular, better filling and density of the calyces, more frequent detection of a papillary blush, and better opacification of the renal pelvis have been shown [13].

The higher associated viscosity of these agents may be minimized by preheating to $37°C$ when it approaches the viscosity of the "low-osmolality" agents. This is an important consideration with regard to CT angiography and venography examinations, particularly with respect to the homogeneity of vascular enhancement. At lower viscosities there is a more turbulent flow pattern which allows for a greater mixing of fluids and hence a more uniform vessel opacification.

C.J. Harvey (✉)
Dept of Imaging, Imaging Sciences Department, Hammersmith Hospital, Imperial College Faculty of Medicine, Du Cane Road, London W12 ONN, UK, chris.harvey@imperial.nhs.uk

J.J.M.C.H. de la Rosette et al. (eds.), *Imaging in Oncological Urology*,
DOI 10.1007/978-1-84628-759-6_38, © Springer-Verlag London Limited 2009

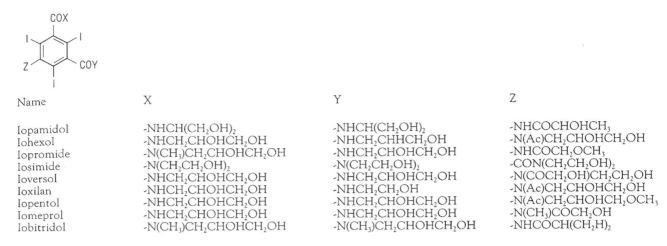

Fig. 38.1 Monomeric non-ionic agents. Reproduced with permission from Dawson P, Cosgrove DO, Grainger RG. Textbook of contrast media. Oxford: ISIS Medical Media; 1999

Fig. 38.2 Ioxaglic acid (ionic dimer). Reproduced with permission from Dawson P, Cosgrove DO, Grainger RG. Textbook of contrast media. Oxford: ISIS Medical Media; 1999

Iso-osmolar agents have also been shown to be better tolerated by patients compared to monomeric non-ionic agents, with a reduced incidence of pain and heat on administration [16, 17]. There is also a lower incidence of cardiac side effects, particularly a reduced incidence of tachycardia [18, 19].

With the evolution of multidetector CT, and its increasing application in urological oncological imaging, further demands are being placed upon the capabilities of contrast agents. Scanning times have been dramatically decreased, with a renal CT study commonly now possible in less than 10 s (collimation and slice number depending), and this is likely to fall to less than 5 s as flat panel technology is implemented (128 and 256 slice) [20]. In order to obtain

Studies have shown that the effect of the slightly higher viscosity associated with the warmed iso-osmolar agents is small relative to the effect of the osmolality and not significant in determining vessel opacification [14, 15].

Iopamidol

Iohexol

Iopromide

Fig. 38.3 Structures of non-ionic monomers: iopramidol, iohexol, and iopromide. Reproduced with permission from Dawson P, Cosgrove DO, Grainger RG. Textbook of contrast media. Oxford: ISIS Medical Media; 1999

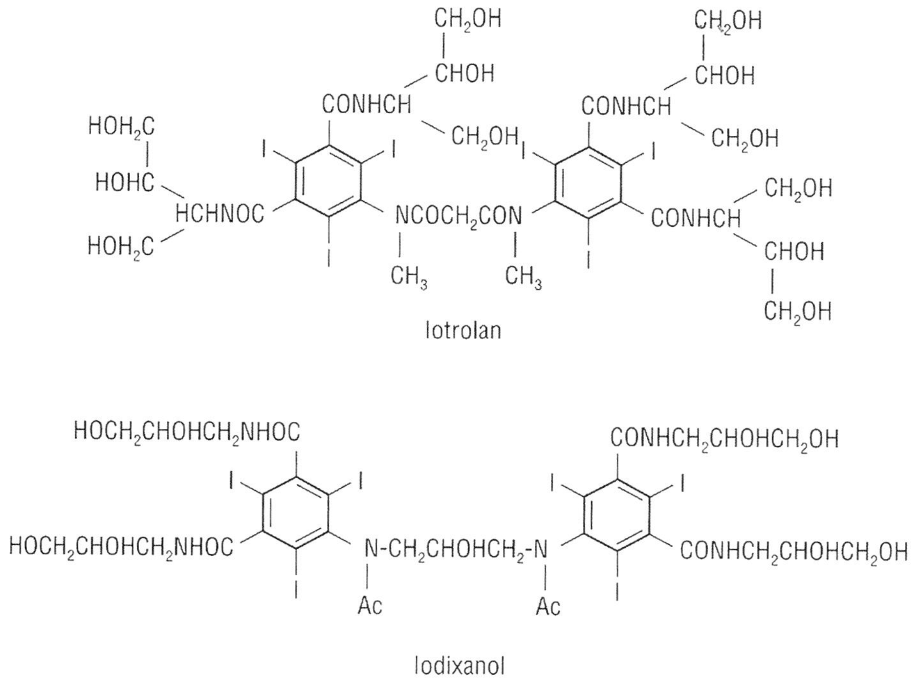

Fig. 38.4 Non-ionic dimmers: iotrolan and iodixanol. Reproduced with permission from Dawson P, Cosgrove DO, Grainger RG. Textbook of contrast media. Oxford: ISIS Medical Media; 1999

multiphasic imaging of the urological system, with adequate organ enhancement in such a short space of time, the same total dose of iodine within the iodinated contrast has to be delivered much more quickly yet still at an even rate. In order that lesions are detected, the scan has to be completed prior to the equilibrium phase of contrast enhancement. The commencement of this phase depends on the flow rate and contrast concentration. Increases in injection rates are limited by the gauge of the venous access cannula and associated delivery systems but are undoubtedly a simple method of increasing contrast flux into the circulation. Given realistic flow rates (4–5 ml/s for arterial phase imaging), modifications of total iodine dose, and hence improved organ enhancement, require an increase in iodine concentration. High concentration contrast (400 mgI/ml) has been shown to improve both aortic and liver enhancement, which may be further raised by a saline bolus "chaser" post-infusion [21, 22]. However, streak artifact can be a limitation if iodine concentrations are too high. High concentration contrast agents, although mainly studied so far in liver imaging, seem likely to have a future role in urological imaging. An additional phase of hepatic imaging has been tested in order to maximize the sensitivity for detection of small hypervascular tumors: arterial and portal venous inflow phases are supplemented by a dedicated "hepatic venous" phase. Due to the speed of the multidetector scanner, the whole liver was imaged in three

separate phases of vascular enhancement [23]. This technique could easily be applied to urological imaging in the assessment of small renal tumors which could be assessed in an additional phase to the standard cortical and medullary phases.

As well as being dependent on the iodine flux (i.e., the rate X concentration of contrast administration), a number of patient factors are recognized as being important in determining vascular concentrations and imaging timing. Various cardiovascular conditions causing a reduced cardiac output delay peak enhancement (aortic and organ) and, counterintuitively, result in increased vessel iodine concentrations; however, there is little effect on organ enhancement since this is a function predominantly of total iodine dose. Patient body mass may have a significant effect on reducing the magnitude of enhancement and so a higher total dose may be appropriate.

With multidetector CT technology and high concentration contrast media, high contrast concentrations allow higher quality arterial phase imaging. This has application not just in CT angiography but also in the detection of small hypervascular urological parenchymal tumors. With accurate contrast bolus timing, standard CT angiography can be performed with reduced total iodine doses. Although total iodine is reduced, a high flow rate and high concentration of contrast must be maintained for optimal imaging [24]. A reduction in contrast dose may be possible for CT angiography, though this is unlikely to be translated into parenchymal urological imaging, as organ enhancement is determined by total iodine dose.

Nephrotoxicity

In a study of 16,248 patients receiving iodinated contrast media the incidence of acute renal failure was 1% [25]. The most important risk factor for contrast-induced acute renal failure was the presence of chronic renal impairment. Other risk factors include diabetes mellitus, cardiac failure, dehydration, hypovolemia, multiple myeloma, ventricular dysfunction, and the use of other nephrotoxic agents [26]. The mechanisms of nephrotoxicity may include renal vasoconstriction, decreased vasodilatation (induced by nitric oxide), increased free radical production, increased oxygen consumption observed during ischemia, an increase in intratubular pressure due to diuresis, tubular obstruction, hyperviscosity, and alterations of red blood cells [27]. The outer medullary tubular cells of the kidney are very sensitive to hypoxia. In this region the balance between perfusion and oxygen consumption is easily disrupted leading to cellular hypoxia [27].

In at-risk patients multiple strategies have been used to reduce the incidence of contrast media-induced nephropathy. In such high-risk patients, serum creatinine levels should be measured before and after the administration of contrast media. Contrast media dose and frequency are both known risk factors for nephroxicity. Whenever possible an interval of several days should be allowed between administrations. The osmolality of the contrast agent is also an important consideration. Many studies have shown that "low-osmolality" contrast agents (LOCM) (600–800 mosm/kg) have a lower renal toxicity than do high-osmolality agents ($\geq$1500 mosm/kg) [28, 29]. Therefore LOCM should be used for high-risk patients. There has been considerable debate regarding the use of iso-osmolar contrast agents (osmolality $\sim$ 300 mosm/kg). One study demonstrated that iodixanol has a better renal safety profile compared with a LOCM [9] but other studies contradict this finding [11, 12]. The need for further studies to clarify the situation, the high cost of iodixanol, and the claimed prothrombotic actions of this agent [30] precludes its widespread use.

In low-risk patients oral hydration and salt intake is sufficient precaution prior to iodinated contrast media. In high-risk patients intravenous water and sodium should be administered in the form of isotonic saline 12 h prior to contrast. In addition, a recent study showed that intravenous sodium bicarbonate may be more effective at preventing acute renal failure than sodium chloride [31].

A number of pharmacological agents have been evaluated in the prevention of contrast media-induced nephropathy. These have proved disappointing. One study showed that mannitol was no more effective in preventing contrast agent-induced nephropathy than was saline [32]. This study also showed that furosemide was ineffective and may increase the risk of nephrotoxicity. Weisberg et al. [33] showed that dopamine and atrial natriuetic peptide (ANP) may significantly increase the risk of acute renal failure in the presence of severe renal impairment. Acetylcysteine, a free radical scavenger, initially seemed to demonstrate efficacy in the prevention of contrast media-induced nephropathy, but subsequent studies have shown that it does not significantly reduce the risk of nephropathy [34–36]. Nevertheless it is still frequently used in high-risk patients.

In patients at risk of contrast agent-associated nephrotoxicity, carbon dioxide (CO_2) gas may have a role as an alternative to iodinated contrast media. CO_2 is an established effective angiographic contrast agent that can be delivered by pump or hand injection. In a recent study in a rat model, although injection of CO_2 markedly affected regional renal blood flow and oxygenation, there were qualitatively different effects in the cortex and outer medulla compared with those seen after injection of ioxaglate. The pronounced decrease in medullary blood flow and oxygenation observed after injection of ioxaglate was absent in the animals injected with CO_2. This might suggest beneficial effects of the use of CO_2 instead of iodinated contrast media in patients with increased risk of developing renal failure [37]. Another study has shown that the risk of impairment of renal function is lower after injection of CO_2 with small amounts of added ioxaglate compared with injection of a larger amount of ioxaglate alone. The amount of injected CO_2 did not correlate with an increase in serum creatinine level, though the amount of injected iodine did significantly correlate with an increase in serum creatinine level and a decrease in estimated creatinine clearance after 2 days [38]. However its efficacy in vascular mapping prior to partial nephrectomy for presumed renal cell carcinoma was shown to be inferior to that achieved with iodinated contrast agents, albeit only in one small study [39].

Gadolinium-based contrast agents have also been used in patients at risk of acute renal failure, but mainly in the setting of conventional angiography. In the largest study to date, gadolinium-based contrast agents did – rarely – cause acute renal failure in patients with underlying chronic renal insufficiency, despite reports of negligible nephrotoxicity in many other studies [40]. A study assessing gadolinium-enhanced CT angiograms suggested the use of at least 16-detector row CT technology for high-quality angiography; the doses administered did not alter the renal function except transiently in one patient [41].

MR Contrast Agents

The first-generation MR contrast agents are "non-specific" small molecular weight gadolinium chelates that distribute into the intravascular and interstitial (extracellular) spaces (Fig. 38.5) [42]. This still allows for physiological evaluation of renal function, and kidney-specific anatomy, in an approach referred to as MR renography [43]. Gadolinium diethylenetriamine pentaacetic acid (Gd-DTPA) is most commonly used for this purpose. The kidney is a target organ for such extracellular fluid space marker agents due to their virtually exclusive excretion by glomerular filtration. Current improvements in functional renal imaging relate to improved spatial and temporal resolution of current MR systems rather than advances in contrast agents.

More recently tissue-specific contrast agents have been developed, most notably liver-specific agents, which are classified as hepatocyte or reticuloendothelial system (RES) specific. Some of these agents have shown considerable promise in the characterization of focal liver lesions [44, 45], such as metastases from urological cancer. Gadobenate dimeglumine (Gd-BOPTA, multihance, Bracco) distributes to the extracellular space but is selectively taken up by functioning hepatocytes and biliary excreted [46]. Hepatobiliary contrast enhancement is prominent at 1–2 h and when compared to gadopentate dimeglumine images were equivalent in the dynamic phase but showed additional information in the delayed phase of imaging [47]. Another hepatocyte-specific agent is Mangafodipir (teslascan, Amersham Health). The manganese ion is a powerful T1 relaxation agent, and this has been shown to be an effective positive liver enhancer, and only a very small amount of agent (5 μmol/kg) can significantly improve contrast between focal liver lesions and healthy parenchyma [48].

RES-specific compounds are largely superparamagnetic iron oxide (SPIO) particles that induce dramatic magnetic field disturbances, which translate into strong T2 and T2* effects. These nanoparticles rapidly target the Kuppfer cells of the liver causing a decrease in T2 signal in healthy parenchyma, but not in metastases.

Smaller SPIOs or ultrasmall SPIO nanoparticles (USPIO) generally circulate longer in the blood space, before passing

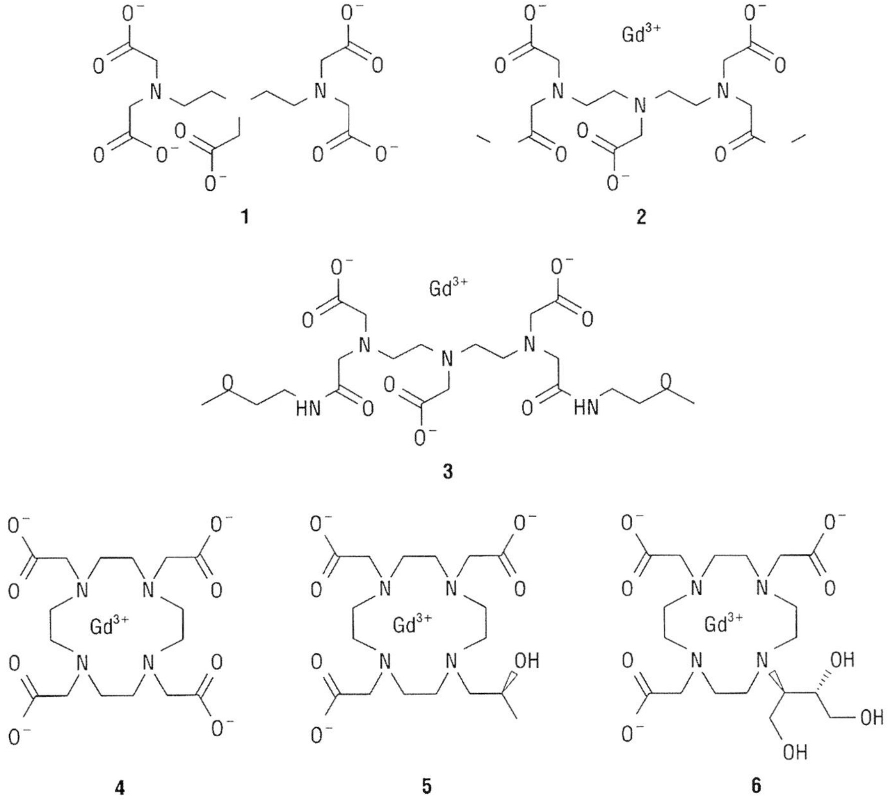

Fig. 38.5 Chemical structures of some common clinically used extracellular gadolinium chelates: 1. gadopentate (Magnevist); 2. gadodiamide (Omniscan); 3. gadoversetamide (Optimark); 4. gadoterate (Dotarem); 5. gadoteriol (Prohance); 6. gadobutrol (Gadovist). Reproduced with permission from Dawson P, Cosgrove DO, Grainger RG. Textbook of contrast media. Oxford: ISIS Medical Media; 1999

into the interstitial space and finally accumulating in the macrophages of lymph nodes, liver, and spleen. They have found increasing application as intravenous MR lymphographic agents, as they homogeneously reduce the signal intensity of normal nodal tissue due to their $T2^*$ susceptibility effect. In lymph nodes containing metastases, there is less USPIO uptake, leading to relative hyperintensity (i.e., no enhancement). A focal area of relative signal hyperintensity may represent an area of segmental malignant infiltration within the node. This has led to an improved detection of metastatic tissue in normal-sized nodes in a number of cancers [49]. High-resolution, GRE, $T2^*$-weighted sequences (pre- and post-contrast) are essential for evaluation of USPIO uptake, and thus for the detection of small metastases. The optimal time for evaluation post-contrast is 24–36 h, allowing sufficient USPIO to accumulate within the nodes (early imaging would result in a significant false negative rate [49]). This has been evaluated to good effect in prostate cancer, with the sensitivity of detection of nodal metastases vastly superior to conventional MR imaging [50]. A prospective study evaluating 216 nodes in 36 patients with genitourinary malignancy resulted in an accuracy level of 98.6% in distinguishing normal and metastatic lymphadenopathy [51]. This technique is unique in its ability to non-invasively detect nodal metastases without the use of multimodality fusion imaging.

MR angiography (MRA) has increasing application, particularly in surgical planning for urological cancer. However, the extracellular agents rapidly pass out of the intravascular space, and so require rapid dynamic imaging in order to provide a sufficient contrast to noise ratio (vessel to background on MR). Gadobutrol is a newer extracellular agent currently licensed in Europe but not the USA and has double the concentration of gadolinium as conventional extracellular agents [52]. This has been shown to be efficacious in pulmonary imaging [53]. Due to the reduced volume required for the same dose of gadolinium, it has been proposed as an agent for MRA. It may certainly be of use in patients with poor vascular access or in pediatric patients.

However, there has been a drive for "blood-pool" compounds that remain in the intravascular space for longer, rather than rapidly passing into the interstitial space, allowing a greater window of opportunity for MRA. This does not just allow for high-resolution MRA but also enables evaluation of multiple selective vascular regions during the same examination, without the need for additional injections of contrast agent or concerns about timing. This also allows for quantification of organ and tumor blood volume and perfusion, which can be assessed pre- and post-therapy to assess tumor response to treatment. A number of agents are in clinical development, such as gadolinium bound to serum albumen (gadofosveset, EPIX Medical), which has so far shown efficacy in enhancing the blood in both first-pass and steady-state MRA [54]. Another type of blood-pool agent is the macromolecule, which because of its size remains for longer in the intravascular compartment. Gadolinium, manganese, and iron-based compounds are being developed. Gadomer-17 (Schering AG) is one of the most advanced compounds, and is small enough to undergo glomerular filtration within 24 h, but remains for long enough intravascularly to produce excellent angiograms and perfusion studies [55]. USPIOs such as ferumoxtran-10 (Sinerem, Guerbet) are also likely to be of use in MRA as well as in MR lymphography. As mentioned previously, they remain in the intravascular space for a considerable time before passing into the interstitium and then ultimately the lymphatics and lymph nodes. Further research into the $T2^*$ effects on first-pass imaging are needed prior to USPIOs being used clinically as an agent for MRA. SPIOs may also be used but are engulfed faster by macrophages and hence remain in the blood pool for less time [56].

A potential limitation of these agents is in the equilibrium phase, in certain anatomical locations, where differentiating arteries from intimately associated veins may be difficult. Another concern is the biological half-life of these agents, as they should be designed not just for efficacy but also for timely elimination as potential toxicity is an anxiety [57]. Hybrid compounds will no doubt be produced in the future that are a combination of polymeric compounds and small agents, providing all the imaging advantages without the concerns regarding slow biological clearance.

Molecular imaging can be defined as the imaging of targeted molecules and will undoubtedly play an increasing role in urological cancer imaging in the future. This can broadly be separated into imaging a labeled molecule or the target (receptor) of that molecule. Currently USPIO nanoparticles are preferred to gadolinium chelates, as the latter have relatively low relaxivity and a rather uncertain toxicity profile. USPIOs are well suited in this regard due to their favorable recycling properties, their ability to produce significant signal change per unit of iron, their ease of chemical linkage due to their dextran coating, and the demonstration of variable magnetic properties with particle size [58]. MR lymphography using USPIOs is an example of molecular imaging, with the nanoparticles targeting the macrophages of the lymph nodes. However, the remit of USPIOs has extended much further; they have been used to label stem cells and T cells and can be conjugated to a range of enzymes, antibodies, and peptides for a variety of advanced imaging applications [59, 60]. Stem cell imaging is particularly interesting, especially with the increased interest and success of stem cell transplantation. This success depends on the ability of stem cells to migrate from the site of injection to the target. MR tracking of magnetically labeled cells following transplantation is an excellent, non-invasive method of determining the distribution of these cells, and hence evaluating the success of the procedure.

The new generation of highly specific MR contrast agents is not just limited to defining anatomy and pathology, but can quantify physiology and metabolic activity of cells. The new agents are synthesized by labeling cells with magnetic particulate agents. This can be achieved by linking the magnetic particles to a peptide, by creating a macromolecule such as magnetodendrimer, or by internalizing a magnetic particle within a cell [61]. In broad terms these new agents can be classified as non-specific, targeted, or activated (or smart) agents [62]. The non-specific agents can quantify many physiological processes such as perfusion and blood volume, but provide no information on cellular processes. Targeted agents combine an imaging agent with a molecule such as an antibody or protein that specifically targets tumor cell surface receptors. For example, magnetically labeled (USPIO) monoclonal antibodies have already been used in vivo for imaging lung cancer [63]. Once the appropriate monoclonal antibodies are labeled, these agents are likely to have a future role in the imaging of urological cancers. A potential drawback of this technique is that background noise may be high. Activated agents are only detectable after interaction with the target receptor; they are not detectable in their native state. Compared with targeted agents, this results in a significant reduction in background noise and an increase in signal and contrast to noise ratio. Examples of these agents include magnetic nanosensors that interact with DNA or RNA sequences [64].

The perfect contrast agent for the urologist and urological oncologist is the tumor-specific agent that allows specific detection of urological tumors at an early stage of disease. This agent is still far from development. The ultimate agents are likely to be monoclonal antibodies labeled with paramagnetic atoms or superparamagnetic nanoparticles, with current studies in small animals achieving an appropriate concentration of magnetic label at the target [65–67]. So far this concentration is nowhere near translatable into humans; biotechnology has much further to advance for this to be used clinically. Specifically the low expression of receptors and the limited sensitivity of the relaxation time enhancers are factors. However current and future advances in contrast media, particularly in biotechnology, are likely to extend the role of MR imaging in urological oncology beyond recognition over the next decade.

The gadolinium-based agents have long been held to be much less nephrotoxic than iodinated contrast agents. However, in higher doses this may not be true and recently nephrogenic systemic fibrosis, a rare multi-system disorder, has come to light [68, 69]. This disorder principally affects the skin in patients with renal insufficiency and occurs most frequently, but not exclusively, following the administration of gadodiamide.

The Food and Drug Administration (FDA) recommend checking for renal impairment by history or laboratory tests. The FDA recommends avoidance of all gadolinium contrast media in patients with renal insufficiency grades 4 and 5 (glomerular filtration rate <30 mL/min per 1.73 m^2) or any grade of acute renal failure in liver transplantation patients or candidates. The European Medicines Agency (EMEA) differentiates between agents and advises avoidance of only gadodiamide and gadopentetate in the same patient categories. Other gadolinium contrast media should only be used after careful consideration of risks versus benefits. Postprocedural haemodialysis is only indicated in patients on regular dialysis. All published cases to date received gadodiamide, gadopentetate or gadoversetamide, which are considered to be less stable due to a linear molecular structure. The aetiological significance of stability differences between the non-ionic linear, ionic linear and macrocyclic agents remains to be shown but the EMEA have classified the gadolinium-containing contrast agents into three groups on the basis of their likelihood of releasing free gadolinium ions. The least likely (safest) to release free gadolinium ions Gd^{3+} in the body have a cyclical structure and include gadoterate *(Dotarem)*, gadobutrol *(Gadovist)* and gadoteriol *(Prohance)*. The intermediate group have an ionic linear structure and include gadopentate *(Magnevist)*, gadobenate *(MultiHance)*, Primovist and Vasovist. The most likely to release Gd^{3+} have a linear non-ionic structure; gadodiamide *(Omniscan)* and gadoversetamide *(OptiMARK)*.

Ultrasound Microbubble Contrast Agents

Ultrasound, unlike all other imaging modalities, has lacked effective contrast agents until comparatively recently. This was rectified with the introduction of microbubbles in the 1990s. These have revolutionized clinical and research applications in this field [70–72]. Microbubbles are less than 10 µm in diameter so they can cross capillary beds and are safe, effective echo enhancers (Fig. 38.6). When administered intravenously, microbubbles remain within the vascular compartment, unlike CT and MR contrast agents (Table 38.1). To be effective as clinical tools, microbubbles must after intravenous injection survive passage through the cardiopulmonary circulation to produce useful systemic enhancement. An ingenious range of methods are employed to achieve stability and provide a clinically useful enhancement period. Microbubbles consist of a gas (air or a perfluorocarbon) which is stabilized by a shell (denatured albumin, phospholipid or surfactant or cyanoacrylate) (Table 38.1). Microbubbles produce marked augmentation of the ultrasound signal for several minutes after an intravenous bolus or for 15–20 min after an infusion with enhancement in gray-scale and Doppler signals of up to 25 dB (greater than 300-fold increase). The most widely used is Sonovue (Bracco, Italy) which is licensed in Europe and Asia and consists of sulfur hexafluoride gas surrounded by a phospholipid shell (Fig. 38.7).

Interactions of Microbubbles with Ultrasound Waves

The interactions of microbubbles with an ultrasound beam are complex [73, 74]. Since a microbubble is more compressible than soft tissue, when it is exposed to an oscillating acoustic signal, alternate expansion and contraction occur. At low acoustic power (< 100 kPa) these oscillations are equal and symmetrical (linear behavior) and the frequency of the scattered signal is unaltered, with the scattering intensity linearly related to that of the incident beam. As the acoustic power increases (100 kPa to 1 MPa), more complex non-linear interactions occur as the expansion and contraction phases become unequal because the microbubbles resist compression more strongly than expansion. Microbubbles resonate (in the diagnostic range (1–20 MHz)) and behave like a musical instrument emitting harmonic signals at multiples (or fractions) of the insonating frequency. These harmonic signals are microbubble specific and may be regarded as a signature or fingerprint unique to that agent. At still higher powers (although within accepted limits for diagnostic imaging) highly non-linear behavior occurs with disruption or scintillation that may be imaged with a number of bubble-specific modes which allow differentiation of contrast signal from background tissue.

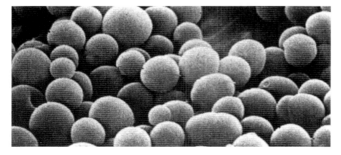

Fig. 38.6 Quantison microbubbles under electron microscopy. Reproduced with permission from Dawson P, Cosgrove DO, Grainger RG. Textbook of contrast media. Oxford: ISIS Medical Media; 1999

Real-Time Imaging

When US contrast agents were initially introduced they were imaged using conventional available B-mode and Doppler mode techniques. While the acoustic powers were in the diagnostic range, these were largely destructive modes. Following the development of non-destructive, low-mechanical-index (MI) contrast-specific modes and the availability of more stable microbubbles (e.g., SonoVue), real-time imaging can be performed allowing clear visualization of contrast-containing vessels, microvessels, and tissue vascularization. In the kidneys, the peripheral vasculature of the renal cortex can be seen up to the renal cortex.

An added opportunity offered by the latest contrast-specific modes is the use of a destructive (high MI) pulse to destroy the bubbles in the particular scan plane and to observe reperfusion of the lesion. The rate of replenishment in the field allows calculation of indices such as microcirculatory flow rate, a measure of tissue perfusion, and this idea has been applied to the myocardium and kidney [75]. These techniques which can demonstrate flow in vessels down to 100 μm in diameter also permit characterization of tumor vascularity and differentiation of benign and malignant lesions [76]. Three-dimensional displays can be constructed demonstrating anatomical vascular structure which may prove important in defining tumor grade and response to therapy. These methods have great potential, especially with the recent interest in monitoring response to angiogenesis inhibitors [77].

Clinical Applications of Ultrasound Microbubbles in Urological Oncology

In kidneys microbubbles are useful in differentiating renal tumors from pseudotumors such as a column of Bertin. In pseudotumors the vasculature exhibits regular and smooth branching compared to the chaotic pattern seen in malignancy [78]. Microbubbles are also useful in the assessment of renal cysts and can reliably distinguish hemorrhagic and inflammatory cysts from solid renal tumors [79, 80]. The presence of septal or mural nodular enhancement is suggestive of malignancy. Microbubbles have not been shown to significantly improve detection of renal cell carcinoma but may be useful to assess tumor vascularity and extent of necrosis and to identify enhancement in tumor thrombus.

In carcinoma of the prostate US contrast has shown promising results but its role in detection, staging, and treatment is still under evaluation [81].

Halpern et al. [82] using contrast-enhanced real-time and intermittent harmonic imaging in addition to power Doppler

Table 38.1 Classification of ultrasound microbubbles

Microbubble	Gas	Stabilization	Company
Blood-pool agents			
Levovist (SHU 508A) **	Air	Palmitic acid	Schering
Echovist*	Air	None	Schering
Albunex**	Air	Sonicated albumin	Tyco
Quantison	Air	Dried albumin	Andaris Ltd
Imavist (Imagent, AFO150)	Perfluorohexane	Surfactant	Schering
Optison* (FS069)	Perfluoropropane	Sonicated albumin	Tyco/Amersham
Echogen (QW3600)	Dodecafluoropentane	Liquid droplet, surfactant	Sonus
SonoVue (BR1) *	Sufhur hexafluoride	Phospholipids	Bracco
Definity (DMP115)	Perfluoropropane	Phospholipids	Bristol-Myers Squibb
BR14	Perfluorobutane	Phospholipids	Bracco
Liver-specific agents			
Levovist (SHU 508A)*	Air	Palmitic acid	Schering
Sonavist (SHU 563A) **	Air	Cyanoacrylate	Schering
Sonazoid™ (NC100100) **	Perfluorocarbon	Not public information	Amersham

*Licensed for clinical use
**No longer commercially available

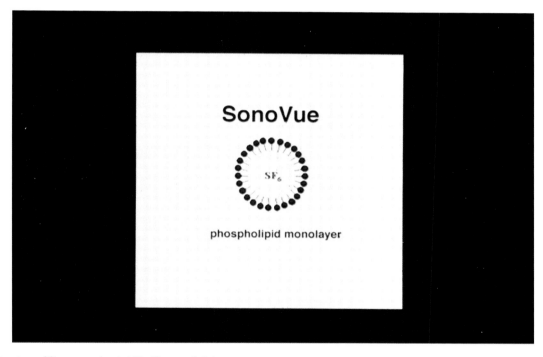

Fig. 38.7 Structure of Sonovue microbubble (Bracco, Italy)

showed a significant increase in sensitivity from 38 to 65% while specificity was maintained at 80%. These results have also been reproduced by other workers [83]. Using Levovist contrast agent and color Doppler-based targeted-biopsy protocol, Frauscher [84] showed positive biopsy rates were significantly improved with targeted cores vs sextant cores (13 vs 4.9%, respectively). In a study of 230 patients comparing contrast-enhanced biopsies to sextant biopsies, targeted biopsies were again found to be superior to systematic biopsy (10.4 vs 5.3%, respectively) [85]. Other studies have confirmed that contrast-enhanced US improves cancer detection, although no advantage of power or color Doppler has been shown [86].

Sedelaar et al. [87] demonstrated a correlation between microvessel density and three-dimensional contrast-enhanced power Doppler imaging. Unal et al. [88] showed that contrast-enhanced power Doppler could be used to discriminate between BPH and cancer with an accuracy of 81%. The association between the increased microvessel density and prostate cancer survival suggest that this line of research may yield valuable indices in the determination of tumor aggressiveness, treatment response, and prognosis.

Enhanced Doppler has also been used to monitor response to treatment. In a study of 68 patients followed up during treatment with enhanced power Doppler, the majority showed a decrease in vascularity within a day or so following commencement of anti-androgen therapy which paralleled falling prostate-specific antigen (PSA) levels [89]. Interestingly in two cases there was a discrepancy in that the vascularity remained high despite a fall in PSA. These patients had escaped from hormonal control at 6-month review. Failure to switch off neovascularity may be an early indicator of relapse which could prompt a treatment adjustment. The emergence of angiogenesis inhibitors is also interesting and enhanced US could provide a quantitative tool to monitor these agents.

Novel Applications of Microbubbles

Quantitation and Functional Studies

Quantitation methods can be divided into "passive" and "active." In the passive approach the passage of a contrast bolus is recorded with minimal microbubble disruption and so low insonating energies are employed. With active approaches, microbubbles are deliberately destroyed so that replenishment of a tissue bed can be measured. Quantification is dependent on the finding that relative microbubble concentration is linearly related to Doppler signal intensity.

Following a bolus injection of microbubbles, their passage through a tissue of interest such as a tumor or organ can be quantified, using low acoustic power, to generate transit time curves, as with nuclear medicine, CT, and MR; from these, functional information can be derived to yield indices such as bolus arrival time, time to peak intensity, area under the curve, wash-in/wash-out characteristics as well as more complex deconvolution indices. Since ultrasound contrast agents are confined to the vascular space (unlike CT and MR agents which diffuse into the interstitial space) they may provide unique functional information not obtainable by other means.

Time intensity curves can be drawn for an area of interest to document microbubble transit through, for example, a tumor bed.

Active quantitation methods are based on the destruction of microbubbles and observation of the effects on contrast enhancement ("reperfusion kinetics"). Intermittent high-power ultrasound pulses are used to destroy microbubbles within the beam and tissue refill observed with nondestructive low MI imaging to demonstrate tissue perfusion in real time. The rate of this refilling can be used to calculate indices such as microcirculatory flow rate, a measure of tissue perfusion, and has been used in the assessment of ischemic myocardium and in renal transplants.

Wei et al. applied the principle to the measurement of myocardial blood flow in dogs [90] by infusing microbubbles while scanning intermittently. They observed an exponential relationship between pulsing interval (PI) and video intensity (VI):

$$VI = VI_{max}(1 - e^{-\beta.PI})$$

where VI_{max} is the maximal video intensity seen at long pulsing intervals (PI) and β is the constant describing the rate of rise of VI. The initial upslope of this curve is proportional to microbubble speed as they refill the slice being insonated. The VI_{max} is proportional to the fractional vascular volume. The product of VI_{max} and β is an indirect measure of tissue perfusion.

This method is time consuming and may be modified by switching the scanner to a low acoustic power mode after the destructive burst and observing the reperfusion in real time. The equation describing the reperfusion is identical to the above.

Future Applications of Microbubbles

Extensive research is also directed toward development of the next generation of microbubbles, which are capable of encapsulating therapeutic agents and releasing them when exposed to high MI or specific US signals. Therapeutic agents could include genes, thrombolytics, and oncological drugs, and this technique has the clinical potential to increasing the therapeutic efficacy while decreasing systemic side effects [91].

References

1. Dawson P, Cosgrove DO, Grainger RG. Textbook of contrast media. Oxford: ISIS Medical Media; 1999.
2. Stacul F. Current iodinated contrast media. Eur Radiol. 2001;11(4):690–7.
3. Dawson P. The non-ionic dimers. Some theoretical and clinical considerations. Eur Radiol. 1995;5:S103–6.
4. Dawson P. The non-ionic dimers. Perspectives and controversies. Eur Radiol. 1996;6:520–4.
5. Adolph JMG, Engelkamp H, Herbig W, Peters PE, Wenzel-Hora BI. Iotrolan in urography: efficacy and tolerance in comparison with iohexol and iopamidol. Eur Radiol. 1995;5 Suppl 2:S63–8.
6. Narimatsu Y, Hiramatsu K. A Japanese multicenter comparison of iotrolan 280 with iopamidol 300 in intravenous urography. Eur Radiol. 1995;5 Suppl 2:S58–62.
7. Pannu HK, Thompson RE, Phelps J, Magee CA, Fishman EK. Optimal contrast agents for vascular imaging on computed

tomography: iodixanol versus iohexol. Acad Radiol. 2005;12(5): 576–84.

8. Rienmuller R, Brekke O, Kampenes VB, Reiter U. Dimeric versus monomeric nonionic contrast agents in visualization of coronary arteries. Eur J Radiol. 2001;38(3):173–8.

9. Aspelin P, Aubry P, Fransson SG, Strasser R, Willenbrock R, Berg KJ. Nephrotoxic effects in high-risk patients undergoing angiography. N Engl J Med. 2003;348(6):491–9.

10. Nicholson T, Downes M. Contrast nephrotoxicity and iso-osmolar contrast agents: implications of NEPHRIC. Clin Radiol. 2003;58(9):659–60.

11. Carraro M, Malalan F, Antonione R, Stacul F, Cova M, Petz S, et al. Effects of a dimeric vs monomeric non-ionic contrast medium on renal failure in patients with mild to moderate renal insufficiency: a double-blind, ramdomised clinical trial. Eur Radiol. 1998;8:144–7.

12. Stone GW, McCullough PA, Tumlin JA, Lepor NE, Madyoon H, Murray P, et al. Fenoldopam mesylate for the prevention of contrast-induced nephropathy: a randomised clinical trial. JAMA. 2003;290:2284–91.

13. Stacul F, Cova M, Assante M, Hougens Grynne B, Haider T. Comparison between the efficacy of dimeric and monomeric non-ionic contrast media (iodixanol vs iopromide) in urography in patients with mild to moderate renal insufficiency. Br J Radiol. 1998;71(849):918–22.

14. Smedby O. Viscosity of some contemporary contrast media before and after mixing with whole blood. Acta Radiol. 1992;33(6): 600–5.

15. Rouviere O, Ecochard R, Berger P, Pangaud C, Fontaine B, Lyonnet D. Low- versus high-osmolality contrast media. Acta Radiol. 2000;41(5):508–13.

16. Justesen P, Downes M, Grynne BH, Lang H, Rasch W, Seim E. Injection-associated pain in femoral arteriography: a European multicenter study comparing safety, tolerability, and efficacy of iodixanol and iopromide. Cardiovasc Interv Radiol. 1997;20(4): 251–6.

17. Tveit K, Bolz KD, Bolstad B, Haugland T, Berg KJ, Skjaerpe T, et al. Iodixanol in cardioangiography. A double-blind parallel comparison between iodixanol 320 mg I/ml and ioxaglate 320 mg I/ml. Acta Radiol. 1994;35(6):614–8.

18. Spencer CM, Goa KL. Iodixanol. A review of its pharmacodynamic and pharmacokinetic properties and diagnostic use as an x-ray contrast medium. Drugs. 1996;52(6):899–927.

19. Morris TW, Dukovic D, Pagani E. Cardiac hemodynamic effects of iodixanol, iopamidol, and ioxaglate following left coronary injections in anesthetized dogs. Acad Radiol. 1995;2(1):33–7.

20. Marten K, Funke M, Engelke C. Flat panel detector-based volumetric CT: prototype evaluation with volumetry of small artificial nodules in a pulmonary phantom. J Thorac Imaging. 2004;19(3): 156–63.

21. Brink JA, Heiken JP, Forman HP, Sagel SS, Molina PL, Brown PC. Hepatic spiral CT: reduction of dose of intravenous contrast material. Radiology. 1995;197(1):83–8.

22. Brink JA. Use of high concentration contrast media (HCCM): principles and rationale–body CT. Eur J Radiol. 2003;45 Suppl 1: S53–8.

23. Foley WD. Dynamic hepatic CT. Radiology. 1989;170(3 Pt 1): 617–22.

24. Herman S. Computed tomography contrast enhancement principles and the use of high-concentration contrast media. J Comput Assist Tomogr. 2004;28 Suppl 1:S7–11.

25. Morcos SK. Prevention of contrast media-induced nephropathy after angiographic procedures. J Vasc Interv Radiol. 2005;16: 13–23.

26. Morcos SK. Contrast media-induced nephropathy. In: Dawson P, Cosgrove DO, Grainger RG, editors. Textbook of contrast media. Oxford: ISIS Medical Media; 1999. 135–48.

27. Heyman SN, Rosen S. Dye-induced nephropathy. Semin Nephrol. 2003;23:477–85.

28. Cigarroa RG, Lange RA, Williams RH, Hillis LD. Dosing of contrast material to prevent contrast nephropathy in patients with renal disease. Am J Med. 1989;86:649–52

29. Moore RD, Steinberg EP, Powe NR, Brinker JA, Fishman EK, et al. Nephrotoxicity of high osmolality versus low-osmolality contrast media: randomised controlled trial. Radiology. 1992;182: 649–55.

30. Jones CI, Goodall AH. Differential effects of the iodinated contrast agents Ioxaglate, Iohexol and Iodixanol on thrombus formation and fibrinolysis. Throm Res. 2003;112:65–71.

31. Merten GJ, Burgess WP, Gray LV, Holleman JH, Roush TS, Kowalchuk GJ, et al. Prevention of contrast induced nephropathy with sodium bicarbonate: a randomised controlled trial. JAMA. 2004;291:2328–34.

32. Solomon R, Werner C. Effects of saline, mannitol and furosemide to prevent acute decreases in renal function induced by radiocontrast agents. N Eng J Med. 1994;331:1416–20.

33. Weisberg LS, Kurnik PB, Kurnik BR. Risk of radiocontrast nephropathy in patients with and without diabetes mellitus. Kidney Int. 1994;45:259–65.

34. Birck R, Krzossok S, Markowetz F, Schnülle P, van der Woude FJ, Braun C. Acetylcysteine for prevention of contrast nephropathy: Meta-analysis. Lancet. 2003;362: 598–603.

35. Alonso A, Lau J, Jaber BL, Weintraub A, Sarnak MJ. Prevention of radiocontrast nephropathy with N-acetylcysteine in patients with chronic kidney disease: a meta-analysis of randomised controlled trials. Am J Kidney Dis. 2004;43:1–9.

36. Fishbane S, Durham JH, Marzo K, Rudnick M. N-acetylcysteine in the prevention of radiocontrast-induced nephropathy. J Am Soc Nephrol. 2004;15:251–60.

37. Palm F, Bergqvist D, Carlsson PO, Hellberg O, Nyman R, Hansell P, et al. The effects of carbon dioxide versus ioxaglate in the rat kidney. J Vasc Interv Radiol. 2005;16(2 Pt 1):269–74.

38. Liss P, Eklöf H, Hellberg O, Hägg A, Boström-Ardin A, Löfberg AM, et al. Renal effects of CO2 and iodinated contrast media in patients undergoing renovascular intervention: a prospective, randomized study. J Vasc Interv Radiol. 2005;16(1):57–65.

39. Sandhu C, Belli AM, Patel U. Demonstration of renal arterial anatomy and tumour neovascularity for vascular mapping of renal cell carcinoma: the value of CO2 angiography. Br J Radiol. 2003;76(902):89–93.

40. Sam AD II, Morasch MD, Collins J, Song G, Chen R, Pereles FS. Safety of gadolinium contrast angiography in patients with chronic renal insufficiency. J Vasc Surg. 2003;38(2):313–8.

41. Remy-Jardin M, Dequiedt P, Ertzbischoff O, Tillie-Leblond I, Bruzzi J, Duhamel A, et al. Safety and effectiveness of gadolinium-enhanced multi-detector row spiral CT angiography of the chest: preliminary results in 37 patients with contraindications to iodinated contrast agents. Radiology. 2005;235(3):819–26.

42. Dawson P, Blomley M. Gadolinium chelate MR contrast agents. Clin Radiol. 1994;49(7):439–42.

43. Huang AJ, Lee VS, Rusinek H. Functional renal MR imaging. Magn Reson Imaging Clin N Am. 2004;12(3):469–86, vi.

44. Hamm B, Thoeni RF, Gould RG, Bernardino ME, Lüning M, Saini S, et al. Focal liver lesions: characterization with nonenhanced and dynamic contrast material-enhanced MR imaging. Radiology. 1994;190(2):417–23.

45. Saini S, Nelson RC. Technique for MR imaging of the liver. Radiology. 1995;197(3):575–7.

46. Spinazzi A, Lorusso V, Pirovano G, Kirchin M. Safety, tolerance, biodistribution, and MR imaging enhancement of the liver with gadobenate dimeglumine: results of clinical pharmacologic and pilot imaging studies in nonpatient and patient volunteers. Acad Radiol. 1999;6(5):282–91.

47. Reimer P, Schneider G, Schima W. Hepatobiliary contrast agents for contrast-enhanced MRI of the liver: properties, clinical development and applications. Eur Radiol. 2004;14(4):559–78.

48. Oudkerk M, Torres CG, Song B, König M, Grimm J, Fernandez-Cuadrado J, et al. Characterization of liver lesions with mangafodipir trisodium-enhanced MR imaging: multicenter study comparing MR and dual-phase spiral CT. Radiology. 2002;223(2):517–24.

49. Kim JY, Harisinghani MG. MR imaging staging of pelvic lymph nodes. Magn Reson Imaging Clin N Am. 2004;12(3):581–6.

50. Harisinghani MG, Barentsz J, Hahn PF, Deserno WM, Tabatabaei S, van de Kaa CH, et al. Noninvasive detection of clinically occult lymph-node metastases in prostate cancer. N Engl J Med. 2003;348(25):2491–9.

51. Harisinghani MG, Weissleder R. Sensitive, noninvasive detection of lymph node metastases. PLoS Med. 2004;1(3):e66.

52. Goyen M, Herborn CU, Vogt FM, Kröger K, Verhagen R, Yang F, et al. Using a 1 M Gd-chelate (gadobutrol) for total-body three-dimensional MR angiography: preliminary experience. J Magn Reson Imaging. 2003;17(5): 565–71.

53. Knopp MV, Giesel FL, von Tengg-Kobligk H, Radeleff J, Requardt M, Kirchin MA, et al. Contrast-enhanced MR angiography of the run-off vasculature: intraindividual comparison of gadobenate dimeglumine with gadopentetate dimeglumine. J Magn Reson Imaging. 2003;17(6):694–702.

54. Grist TM, Korosec FR, Peters DC, Witte S, Walovitch RC, Dolan RP, et al. Steady-state and dynamic MR angiography with MS-325: initial experience in humans. Radiology. 1998;207(2):539–44.

55. Gerber BL, Bluemke DA, Chin BB, Boston RC, Heldman AW, Lima JA, et al. Single-vessel coronary artery stenosis: myocardial perfusion imaging with Gadomer-17 first-pass MR imaging in a swine model of comparison with gadopentetate dimeglumine. Radiology. 2002;225(1):104–12.

56. Frank H, Weissleder R, Brady TJ. Enhancement of MR angiography with iron oxide: preliminary studies in whole-blood phantom and in animals. AJR Am J Roentgenol. 1994;162(1):209–13.

57. Hood MN, Ho VB. Contrast agents: innovations and potential applications for body MR angiography. Magn Reson Imaging Clin N Am. 2005;13(1):189–203, vii.

58. Bogdanov AA Jr, Weissleder R, Frank HW, Bogdanova AV, Nossif N, Schaffer BK, et al. A new macromolecule as a contrast agent for MR angiography: preparation, properties, and animal studies. Radiology. 1993;187(3):701–6.

59. Bulte JW, Zhang S, van Gelderen P, Herynek V, Jordan EK, Duncan ID, et al. Neurotransplantation of magnetically labeled oligodendrocyte progenitors: magnetic resonance tracking of cell migration and myelination. Proc Natl Acad Sci U S A. 1999;96(26):15256–61.

60. Dodd CH, Hsu HC, Chu WJ, Yang P, Zhang HG, Mountz JD Jr, et al. Normal T-cell response and in vivo magnetic resonance imaging of T cells loaded with HIV transactivator-peptide-derived superparamagnetic nanoparticles. J Immunol Methods. 2001;256(1–2):89–105.

61. Hyslop WB, Balci NC, Semelka RC. Future horizons in MR imaging. Magn Reson Imaging Clin N Am. 2005;13(2):211–24.

62. Bradbury M, Hricak H. Molecular MR imaging in oncology. Magn Reson Imaging Clin N Am. 2005;13(2):225–40.

63. Remsen LG, McCormick CI, Roman-Goldstein S, Nilaver G, Weissleder R, Bogdanov A, et al. MR of carcinoma-specific monoclonal antibody conjugated to monocrystalline iron oxide nanoparticles: the potential for noninvasive diagnosis. AJNR Am J Neuroradiol. 1996;17(3):411–8.

64. Lowe MP. Activated MR contrast agents. Curr Pharm Biotechnol. 2004;5(6):519–28.

65. Weinmann HJ, Ebert W, Misselwitz B, Schmitt-Willich H. Tissue-specific MR contrast agents. Eur J Radiol. 2003;46(1):33–44.

66. Gohr-Rosenthal S, Schmitt-Willich H, Ebert W, Conrad J. The demonstration of human tumors on nude mice using gadolinium-labelled monoclonal antibodies for magnetic resonance imaging. Invest Radiol. 1993;28(9):789–95.

67. Shahbazi-Gahrouei D, Williams M, Rizvi S, Allen BJ. In vivo studies of Gd-DTPA-monoclonal antibody and gd-porphyrins: potential magnetic resonance imaging contrast agents for melanoma. J Magn Reson Imaging. 2001;14(2):169–74.

68. Broome DR, Girquis MS, Baron PW, Cottrell AC, Kiellin I, Kirk GA. Gadodiamide-associated nephrogenic systemic fibrosis: why radiologists should be concerned. AJR. 2007;188:586–92

69. Sadowski EA, Bennett LK, Chan MR, Wentland AL, Garrett RW, Diamali A. Nephrogenic systemic fibrosis: risk factors and incidence estimation. Radiology. 2007;243:148–57.

70. Cosgrove DO. Ultrasound contrast agents. In: Dawson P, Cosgrove DO, Grainger RG, editors. Textbook of contrast media, Oxford: ISIS Medical Media; 1999. 451–587.

71. Goldberg BB, Raichlen JS, Forsberg F, editors. Ultrasound contrast agents. 2nd ed. London: Martin Dunitz; 2001.

72. Harvey CJ, Blomley MJK, Eckersley RJ, Cosgrove DO. Developments in ultrasound contrast media. Eur Radiol. 2001;11: 675–89.

73. Harvey CJ, Pilcher J, Eckersley R, Blomley MJK, Cosgrove DO. Advances in ultrasound. Clin Radiol. 2002;57:157–77.

74. Forsberg F, Shi WT. Physics of contrast microbubbles. In: Goldberg BB, Raichen JS, Forsberg F, editors. Ultrasound contrast agents. 2nd ed. London: Martin Dunitz, 2001. pp. 15–24.

75. Harvey CJ, Lynch M, Blomley MJK, Eckersley RJ, Warrens A, Cosgrove DO. Quantitation of real time perfusion with the microbubble optison using power pulse inversion mode in renal transplants. Eur Radiol. 2001;11 Suppl 1;103.

76. Albrecht T, Mattrey RF. Tumor imaging with ultrasound contrast. In: Thomsen HS, Muller RN, Mattrey RF, editors. Trends in contrast media. Medical radiology: diagnostic imaging and radiation oncology series. Berlin: Springer; 1999. pp. 367–82.

77. Folkman J. Angiogenesis. Ann Rev Med. 2006;57:1–18.

78. Correas J, Helenon O, Moreau J. Contrast-enhanced ultrasonography of native and transplanted kidney diseases. Eur Radiol. 1999;9 Suppl 3:S394–400.

79. Quaia E. Characterization and detection of renal tumours. In: Quaia E, editor. Contrast media in ultrasonography. Heidelberg: Springer; 2005. pp. 223–44.

80. Quaia E, Siracusano S, Bertolotto M, Monduzzi M, Mucelli RP. Characterization of renal tumours with pulse inversion harmonic imaging by intermittent high mechanical index technique. Eur Radiol. 2003;13: 1402–12.

81. Padhani AR, Harvey CJ, Cosgrove DO. Angiogenesis imaging in the management of prostate cancer. Clin Pract Urol. 2005;2: 596–607.

82. Halpern EJ, Rosenberg M, Gomella LG. Prostate cancer: contrast enhanced US for detection. Radiology. 2001;219:219–25.

83. Frauscher F, Klauser A, Halpern EJ. Advances in ultrasound for the detection of prostate cancer. Ultrasound Q. 2002;18:135–42.

84. Frauscher F, Klauser A, Halpern EJ. Detection of prostate cancer with a microbubble contrast agent. Lancet. 2001;357:1849–50.

85. Frauscher F, Klauser A, Volgger H, Halpern EJ, Pallwein L, Steiner H, et al. Comparison of contrast-enhanced color Doppler targeted biopsy with conventional systematic biopsy: impact on prostate cancer. J Urol. 2002;167:1648–52.

86. Halpern EJ, Frauscher F, Rosenberg M, Gomella LG. Directed biopsy during contrast enhanced sonography of the prostate. AJR. 2002;178:915–9.

87. Sedelaar JP, van Leenders GJ, Hulsbergen-van de Kaa CA, van der Poel HG, van der Laak JA, Debruyne FM, et al. Microvessel density: correlation between contrast ultrasonography and histology of prostate cancer. Eur Urol. 2001;40:285–93.

88. Unal D, Sedelaar JP, Aarnink RG, van Leenders GJ, Wijkstra H, Debruyne FM, et al. Three-dimensional contrast-enhanced power Doppler ultrasonography and conventional examination methods: the value of diagnostic predictors of prostate cancer. BJU Int. 2000;86:58–64.

89. Eckersley RJ, Butler-Barnes J, Blomley MJ, Cosgrove DO. Quantification microbubble enhanced transrectal ultrasound (TRUS) as a tool for monitoring anti-androgen therapy in prostate carcinoma. Radiology. 1998;209:310.

90. Wei K, Jayaweera AR, Firoozan S, Linka A, Skyba DM, Kaul S. Quantification of myocardial blood flow with ultrasound induced destruction of microbubbles administered as a constant venous infusion. Circulation. 1998;97:473–83.

91. Liang, H, Blomley M, Cosgrove D. Therapeutic application of microbubble-based agents. In: Quaia E, editor. Contrast media in ultrasonography. Heidelberg: Springer; 2005. pp. 393–401.

Chapter 39

Virtual Imaging

M.J. Stone and B.J. Wood

Introduction

Imaging urological pathology does not stop at routine axial techniques. Direct endoscopic visualization of pathology has become a standard tool in urology, and now virtual endoscopy (or virtual reality imaging) and three-dimensional (3D) depictions of pathology may facilitate screening, training, planning interventions, or diagnosis, in addition to the practice and evaluation of clinicians in the performance of procedures for certification. Improvements in radiological imaging techniques facilitate non-invasive diagnosis. Image processing tools may also enhance the planning of urologic interventions.

Virtual imaging of lumens is now easily performed from CT or MRI source data and shows promise for several specific clinical scenarios. Virtual colonoscopy has pioneered endocavitary image processing and is rapidly emerging from the research world to become an accepted screening method to augment standard colonoscopy [1]. Virtual reality imaging has been used to examine many lumens and cavities including the tracheobronchial tree, biliary tree, blood vessels, and the paranasal sinuses [2–4]. Physicians may now fly into just about any anatomic cavity or lumen using CT or MRI and the personal computer. Virtual reality and 3D image processing are tools that have been underutilized in urology and may enhance communication of patient issues in specific settings and may prove useful for screening or planning as well.

Techniques

In virtual reality imaging, 3D images are created from axially acquired source images or 3D source data. Several types of algorithms are available to generate 3D images, including shaded surface display (surface rendering), maximum intensity projection (MIP), and 3D volume rendering. Three-dimensional volume rendering has the advantage of retaining the entire data set; however, it requires much more processing power and time than shaded surface display. The difference in these algorithms may account for increased detection of bladder tumors less than 5 mm in size with volume rendering as compared to shaded surface display [5].

Virtual reality imaging can be employed to create views not otherwise available with the axial source images alone. A surface model can be created to view the pertinent internal anatomy in reference to the skin surface. The surface can be removed to reveal the internal structures. This 3D model can be rotated to allow for different views for improved diagnosis or treatment path planning. The user can use virtual reality to further zoom in on pathology and the user can also employ a "fly through" technique to visualize the inside of a lumen as shown in Fig. 39.1b. The workstation can be designed to show simultaneous virtual reality endoscopic, axial, coronal, and sagittal reformatted views as shown in Fig. 39.2. The virtual reality flight path, viewpoint, and viewing direction are identified on all windows.

Virtual cystoscopy (Figs. 39.3 and 39.4) has shown promise as both a screening technique for bladder neoplasms and a minimally invasive and inexpensive technique to monitor treatment response and follow-up after tumor resection. Positioning during the scan is of importance, as demonstrated by several studies. The patient must be scanned in both the supine and the prone positions for increased sensitivity [5, 6]. Lesions on the anterior wall may be missed on the prone view, while lesions on the posterior wall may be missed on the supine view, due to obscuration by residual urine [5, 6]. A prominent limitation of virtual cystoscopy is in detection of flat tumors or carcinoma in situ. These tumors are seen as submucosal color changes on conventional cystoscopy, but may not be identified on virtual cystoscopy. This actually represents a major weakness of virtual imaging for application to transitional cell carcinoma, which typically grows in thin sheets. However, an advantage of virtual cystoscopy over conventional cystoscopy in screening is the

B.J. Wood (✉)
Diagnostic Radiology Department – Clinical Center, National Institutes of Health, Mailing address: National Institutes of Health; Building 10, Room 1C-660; Bethesda, MD 20892, bwood@nih.gov

J.J.M.C.H. de la Rosette et al. (eds.), *Imaging in Oncological Urology*,
DOI 10.1007/978-1-84628-759-6_39, © Springer-Verlag London Limited 2009

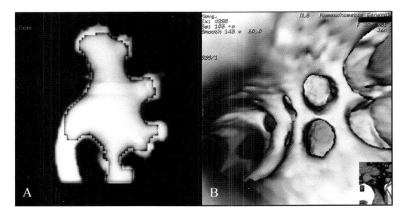

Fig. 39.1 (a) Virtual reality image demonstrating a stone in the collecting system. (b) Virtual reality uroscopic image viewed from within a dilated renal pelvis after virtual electronic stone removal. Endoscopic views can show anatomy with stone or tumor removed prior to actual removal

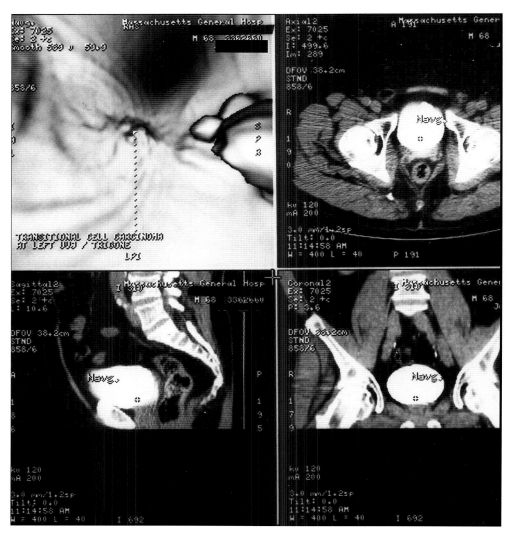

Fig. 39.2 Virtual reality workstation with triplanar and virtual endoscopic views

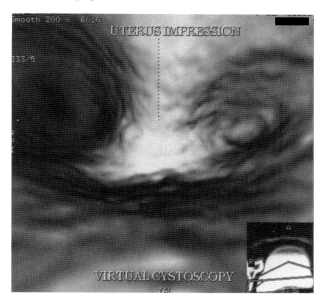

Fig. 39.3 Virtual cystoscopy showing extrinsic impression from an enlarged uterus which could be erroneously interpreted as tumor

visualization of blind spots, namely the bladder neck and in diverticular sacs [5]. Several contrast techniques have been studied in virtual cystoscopy, including insufflation of the bladder with air [5–8] or intravenous contrast administration [8–10], with delayed imaging in the excretory phase. Virtual cystoscopy via intravenous contrast administration may be superior to air virtual cystoscopy because tumors may be

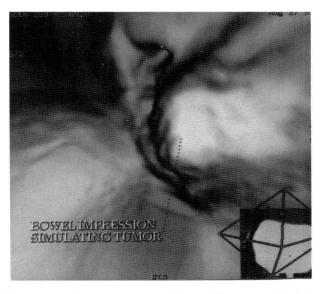

Fig. 39.4 Virtual cystoscopy of extrinsic bowel impression simulating tumor, but easily diagnosed with the addition of the source CT axial images

obscured by residual urine in air contrast studies. Intravenous contrast virtual cystoscopy also allows concomitant intravenous urography study [8] and may prove to be the initial diagnostic study of choice for evaluation of hematuria in the future. Contrast allergy and nephrotoxicity issues should be considered when designing techniques. The exact threshold of detection for tumors is technique dependent and has not been broadly validated. Magnetic resonance (MR) technology is also being examined in virtual cystoscopy (Fig. 39.5) and appears to have similar diagnostic efficacy to CT cystoscopy [11–13]. MR cystoscopy may prove to be favorable over CT given its lack of ionizing radiation and less nephrotoxicity. However, the accuracy of MR has been questioned, and large-scale studies are needed [14].

Virtual reality imaging has also been investigated in both ureteroscopy (Fig. 39.6) and urethroscopy (Fig. 39.7) with promising early results. CT voiding urethrography and virtual urethroscopy may be equivalent to conventional diagnostic methods in evaluating patients with urethral stricture, injury, and hypospadias [15]. Diagnosis of urethral diverticula has also been accomplished with virtual CT urethroscopy and could prove to be superior to conventional urethroscopy [16] and is less invasive. Virtual reality is also valuable for imaging the ureter. In particular, virtual ureteroscopy has been used to effectively evaluate strictured ureteral lumens on follow-up after placement of ureteral metallic stents [17]. Virtual ureteroscopy also shows promise for detecting ureteral tumors as small as 1 mm with currently available techniques [18]. MR can also be used in ureteroscopy (Fig. 39.8).

The upper urinary tract, including the renal calyces, pelvis, and ureteropelvic, junction can also be evaluated using virtual endoscopy (Figs. 39.2, 39.9, and 39.10). Calyceal obstruction has been readily visualized using CT virtual endoscopy, which quickly demonstrates the precise location, morphology, and sometimes the cause of the stenosis [19]. This information can be valuable in diagnosis, as well as pre-procedure planning. MR virtual endoscopy of the upper urinary tract has been shown to be a feasible technique to evaluate neoplasia, stenosis, stricture, and compression of the ureter in patients with urinary tract dilation [20]. Virtual endoscopy has also been investigated as a promising aid in ureteropelvic stenting [21].

Hydronephrosis/CT Urography

IV urography (IVU) has largely been replaced by unenhanced CT in the evaluation of stone disease and enhanced for tumor obstruction. CT urography may provide functional information on renal perfusion, excretion, and urinary system

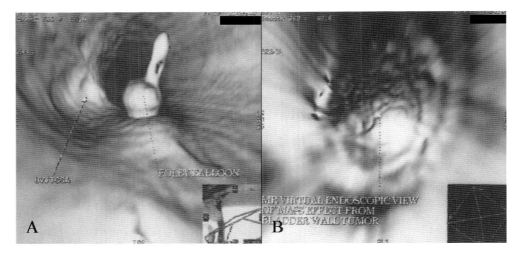

Fig. 39.5 Virtual cystoscopy. (a) CT virtual cystoscopy shows bladder catheter and very subtle, non-specific wall thickening from a flat tumor. (b) MR virtual reality image shows subtle bladder wall mass

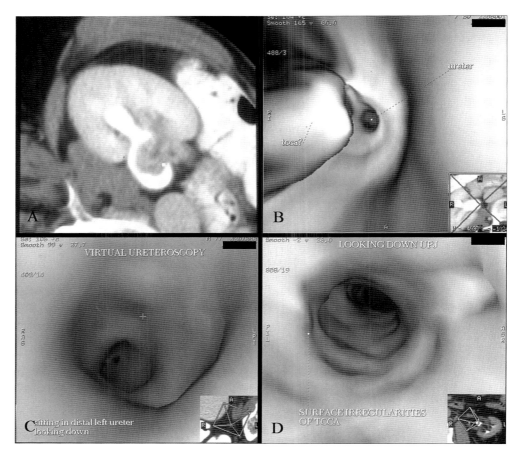

Fig. 39.6 Virtual imaging of the urothelium in the ureter. (a) Axial CT image. (b) Same patient as a, Virtual ureteroscopy demonstrates a bulky finger-like projection of tumor in the same patient. (c) Different patient: representative example of normal smooth urothelium seen in ureteroscopy. (d) Compare to c: Irregular urothelium seen in transitional cell carcinoma (TCC) diagnosed by ureteroscopy. Although no longer smooth, a similar appearance may be seen in normal patients from weeping urothelium or lack of tight contrast/urothelial contact

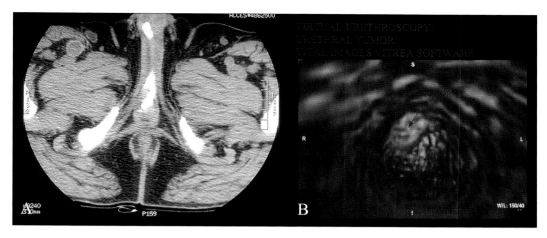

Fig. 39.7 Virtual imaging in the urethra. (a) Standard axial CT image demonstrates a mass in the urethra. (b) Virtual urethroscopy demonstrates a tumor in the urethral lumen

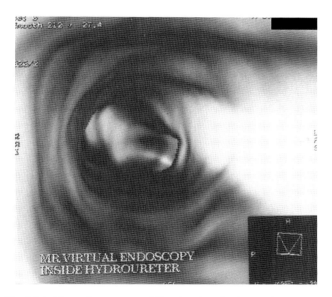

Fig. 39.8 Magnetic resonance (MR) virtual reality image demonstrates hydroureter with the obstructing tumor in the distance

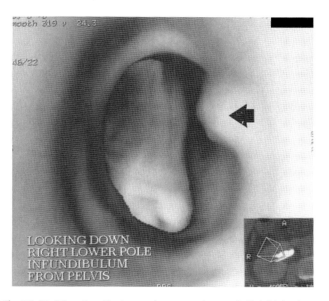

Fig. 39.10 Virtual reality image demonstrating urothelial thickening at the origin of the infundibulum, viewed from within the renal pelvis (virtual perspective demonstrated by inset in lower right corner)

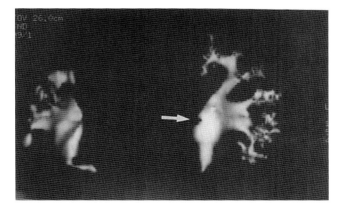

Fig. 39.9 Three-dimensional pyelogram demonstrating a filling defect caused by a tumor

plumbing. The addition of contrast-enhanced 3D models may enhance detection and characterization of hydronephrosis and its underlying cause as well, which may be a weakness of axial imaging, with or without contrast. Excretory phase images may then be processed to allow virtual or 3D models to be built of the urinary lumens or to delineate sites of neoplastic obstruction.

Spatial and 3D relationships as well as mild hydronephrosis are possibly better depicted and easier perceived with 3D models than with axial imaging. The model's similarity to traditional IVU is easier for the urologist and non-radiologist to digest. The distended collecting system is

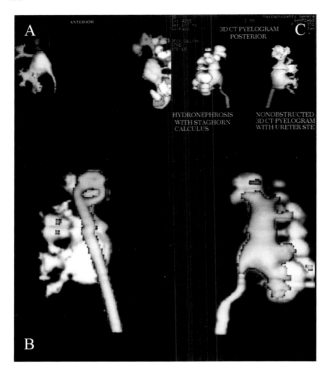

Fig. 39.11 Hydronephrosis. (a) Unilateral hydronephrosis with normal right collecting system. (b) Left hydronephrosis from staghorn stone and small right stones with decompressed right collecting system status post-right ESWL and ureteral stenting. (c) Unilateral hydronephrosis is easily diagnosed with CT urography 3D view

easily flown through with virtual uroscopy, which may depict anatomical detail from within, or even better distinguish obstruction from tumor versus from stone. These models may be more sensitive for unilateral, asymmetric, or segmental hydronephrosis than axial imaging alone (Fig. 39.11).

Case Studies

Bladder and collecting system tumors may be diagnosed and characterized with virtual reality endoscopic models. These models are interactive and the "pilot" may fly into the bladder, ureters, or collecting systems to see tumors, stones, wall thickening, or strictures from up close and inside.

Future cystoscopic or nephroscopic interventions may be practiced and planned from this "simulation endoscopy." Virtual reality methods may assist in the follow-up surveillance of patients with transitional cell carcinoma, in the evaluation of areas difficult to see on cystoscopy, in the analysis of the mucosal and surface detail of bladder tumors, and in the differentiation of blood clot from tumor. This information may be provided without catheterization, and its risks of trauma or infection.

Several cases shown here demonstrate the benefit of 3D CT over axial images alone. Figure 39.12 shows an axial CT slice where a transitional cell bladder tumor was initially missed (a). However, the tumor is easily diagnosed with 3D imaging. Zoomed, narrow angle lens can be employed for close-up view (Fig. 39.4c). The next case compares IVU, axial CT, and 3D imaging. In Fig. 39.13, an IVU shows a filling defect but fails to make the definitive diagnosis. Axial CT of the same patient also shows the filling defect, but fails to distinguish between blood clot and tumor. Three-dimensional CT better depicts the cancer and provides a firm diagnosis.

Virtual imaging can also be used to rule out malignancy (Fig. 39.14). A fluoroscopic spot film shows a dilated ureter and raises the possibility of blockage. Two-dimensional reformat CT shows dilated ureterovesicular junction (UVJ) but does not give the diagnosis. VR cystoscopy depicts edema at the UVJ which is further characterized on the close-up view. This view shows a lack of mucosal irregularity seen in neoplastic growth and fixes the diagnosis as edema as a result of passing a stone.

Figure 39.15 demonstrates another case where axial imaging alone was insufficient to arrive at the correct diagnosis. The question of prostate tissue pressing into the bladder versus a bladder mass cannot be answered on axial imaging (Fig. 39.15a). However, VR cystoscopy (Fig. 39.15b and c) clearly shows polypoid tumor and multiple bladder diverticuli. Three-dimensional imaging must not be used as the only imaging technique, as demonstrated in the case shown in Fig. 39.16. Bladder wall thickening is seen on CT scan (Fig. 39.16a). VR cystoscopy (Fig. 39.16b and c) shaded surface models show irregular mucosa, but viewed alone cannot depict surface depth, demonstrating why axial source images must be simultaneously reviewed. "Perspective volume imaging" can depict tissues behind a surface and may be a better way to examine questionable abnormalities than shaded surface display.

Virtual reality imaging can also be employed to evaluate malignancy in an ileal loop neobladder (Fig. 39.17). Virtual imaging allows the viewer to not only see the tumor in standard axial CT but to "fly through" the ileal loop, to better visualize the tumor.

These cases demonstrate many of the potential future applications of virtual imaging in urologic malignancy.

Teaching/Training/Pre-procedure Planning/Telemedicine

Learning procedures requires repetition for mastery, although the learning curve may be influenced by difficulty of the task, hand–eye coordination, and availability

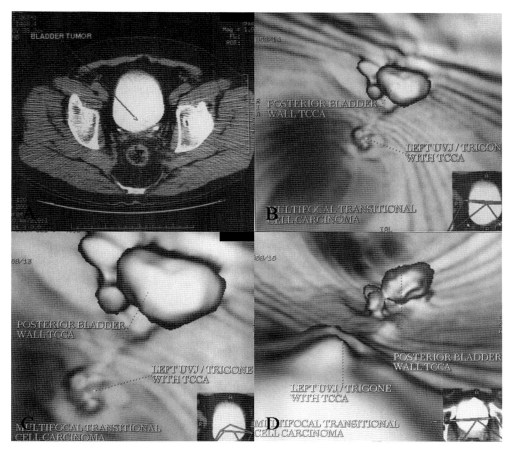

Fig. 39.12 CT versus 3D. (a) Tumor initially missed on review of axial CT alone. (b)Three-dimensional model readily demonstrates the tumor and the extension of growth toward the ureteral orifice. (c) Close-up view of b. (d) Virtual view from the other side of the tumor

of training tools to simulate the task. The OR was once accepted as the main learning environment for surgical trainees' procedural skills. However, concern for patient safety and limitation on resident work hours have caused many to question this system and whether surgical residents can expect to reach clinical competencies under the current system. Use of cadavers has been proposed for surgical training, but they lack realistic conditions and environment of operating on a live subject. Animal surgery for training is limited by differences in anatomy and potential ethical issues. Virtual reality in training may offer an additional tool for procedural training [22, 23]. In the same way, VR could be used to test, certify, or recertify core competencies for surgical procedures [24]. Virtual reality may never fully replicate the experience of performing the procedure, but it may be an ideal bridge in the training cycle for patient safety and physician competence.

Imaging relies upon the recognition of familiar symbols and relationships. Radiologists are repeatedly trained to mentally convert axial or 2D images produced in CT and MR imaging into 3D models associating the anatomy and pathology. However, non-radiology general practiioners without repeated exposure may have difficulty processing or "mental 3D model building" from axial, 2D images when trying to interpret imaging (or plan therapeutic interventions). Three-dimensional models may be rotated, "flown" into and around, and viewed as a fly-through movie for better understanding of the pertinent anatomical relationships. These 3D depictions of the same data are acquired non-invasively, enhance spatial awareness, and give a life-like representation which may be more easily communicated to or among physicians. Utilizing these 3D models may allow planning of the treatment. This may produce a "patient-specific medicine" approach to therapeutic procedures where each patient's anatomy may be mapped and even practiced prior to the actual procedure. However, 3D imaging will not obviate the need for radiologists to examine the source axial images as some pathology is best depicted in conventional 2D images, and derived images (such as 3D or virtual reality) may introduce false findings, and inaccuracies, since there is always the risk that processed images will have less integrity. In actuality, even the axial source

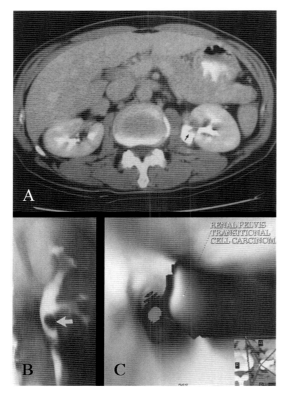

Fig. 39.13 IVU versus CT versus 3D imaging. (a) Axial CT demonstrating a non-specific filling defect. (b) IVU demonstrating filling defect. (c) Three-dimensional image clearly depicts the tumor, which has a more suspicious geometry than expected from a stone, blood clot, or fungus ball

images are "derived" images with volume averaging and borrowing data from adjacent slices (broadening of the slice sensitivity profile). False positive findings may be created in the derived 3D models, such as indentation of the lumen by abutting bowel or uterus, or layering of mucous along a lumen wall, which may simulate tumor. Finally, virtual reality shows initial promise for use in the burgeoning field of telemedicine [25].

Limitations

Obstacles to the full implementation of this technology include further development of the proper software, overcoming the learning curve for image interpretation, as well as dissemination of software and hardware into standard practice.

Conclusion

Three-dimensional and virtual reality models are exciting new tools with which to evaluate the urinary tract. However, their exact role is yet to be clarified, and many potential urological applications need further clinical investigation. Virtual reality and 3D models may be applied to urology training, evaluation, treatment planning, practicing invasive procedures, and complementing communication or diagnosis. The life-like models provide a depiction that is readily digested by physicians and patients alike, who may find spatial relationships easier to conceptualize than from axial images alone.

Whether these models can facilitate identification of mild hydronephrosis, screening for recurrent transitional cell carcinoma, better evaluate the patient with urological malignancy, or provide "one-stop shopping" imaging is yet to be seen.

Acknowledgments

The authors wish to thank the Massachusetts General Hospital for case material and Peter Mueller, M.D., for feeling the fire, buying the mission, and irrigating territory.

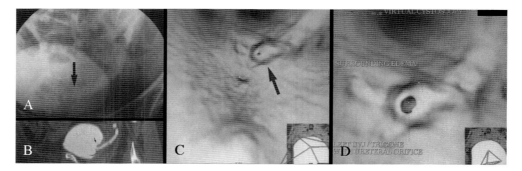

Fig. 39.14 Edema versus neoplasm. (a) Fluoroscopic spot film depicting a dilated ureter. (b) Two-dimensional reformat CT image depicting dilated ureterovesicular junction without extra soft tissue. (c) Virtual cystoscopy with smooth edges gives the likely diagnosis of edema, not malignancy. (d) Close-up view. Recent passage of a stone caused swelling that could have been mistaken for malignancy

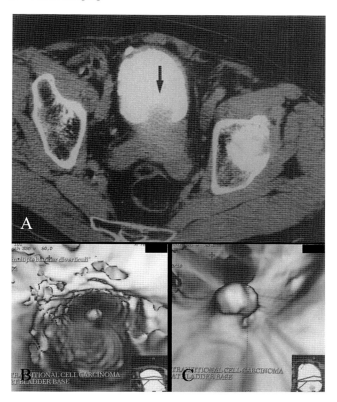

Fig. 39.15 Prostate tissue versus bladder mass. (a) Axial CT image demonstrating apparent filling defect in the bladder (arrow). (b) Virtual cystoscopy depicts polypoid tumor and multiple bladder diverticuli. (c) Close-up of b to better appreciate the polypoid shape of the mass. A median lobe of Alberans can also have this appearance

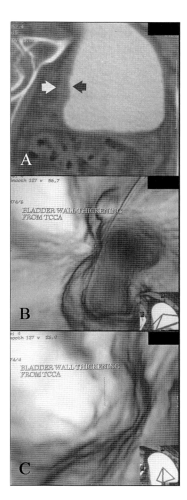

Fig. 39.16 CT versus 3D in bladder wall thickening. (a) Bladder wall thickening seen on CT scan. (b) Virtual reality-shaded surface display model fails to demonstrate wall thickening depth, demonstrating the value of viewing axial images in conjunction with the virtual studies. (c) Close-up view of b to see possibly irregular mucosal detail

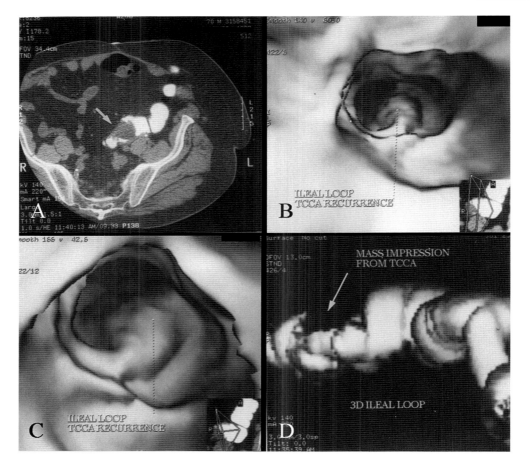

Fig. 39.17 Ileal loop neobladder tumor. (a) CT shows soft tissue filling defect within the ileal loop neobladder, consistent with tumor. (b) Virtual looposcopy shows view from within loop facing tumor. (c) Close- up view of b. (d) Three-dimensional CT loopogram model of loop lumen shows defect from tumor

References

1. Pickhardt PJ, Choi JR, Hwang I, et al. Computed tomographic virtual colonoscopy to screen colorectal neoplasia in asymptomatic adults. N Engl J Med. 2003;349:2191–200.
2. Wood BJ, Razavi P. Virtual endoscopy: a promising new technology. Am Fam Physician. 2002;66:107–12.
3. Simone M, Mutter D, Rubino F, et al. Three-dimensional virtual cholangioscopy: A reliable tool for the diagnosis of common bile duct stones. Ann Surg. 2004;240:82–8.
4. Kim HJ, Yoon HR, Kim KD, et al. Personal-computer-based three-dimensional reconstruction and simulation of maxillary sinus. Surg Radiol Anat. 2003;24:393–9.
5. Tsili AC, Tsampoulas C, Chatziparaskevas N, et al. Computed tomographic virtual cystoscopy for the detection of urinary bladder neoplasms. Eur Urol. 2004;46:579–85.
6. Song JH, Francis IR, Platt JF, et al. Bladder tumor detection at virtual cystoscopy. Radiology. 2001;218:95–100.
7. Browne RFJ, Murphy SM, Grainger R, Hamilton S. CT cystography and virtual cystoscopy in assessment of new and recurrent bladder neoplasms. Eur J Radiol. 2005;53:147–53.
8. Kawai N, Mimura T, Nagata D, Tozawa K, Kohri K. Intravenous urography-virtual cystoscopy is a better preliminary examination than air virtual cystoscopy. BJU Int. 2004;94:832–6.

9. Nambirajan T, Sohaib SA, Muller-Pollard C, Reznek R, Chinegwundoh FI. Virtual cystocscopy from computed tomography: a pilot study. BJU Int. 2004;94:828–1.
10. Kim JK, Ahn HJ, Park T, et al. Virtual cystoscopy of the contrast material-filled bladder in patients with gross hematuria. AJR. 2002;179:763–8.
11. Lammle M, Beer A, Settles M, et al. Reliability of MR imaging-based virtual cystoscopy in the diagnosis of cancer of the urinary bladder. AJR. 2002;178:1483–8.
12. Beer A, Saar B, Zantl N, et al. MR cystography for bladder tumor detection. Eur Radiol. 2004;14:2311–9.
13. Bernhardt TM, Rapp-Bernhardt U. Virtual cystoscopy of the bladder based on CT and MRI data. Abdom Imaging. 2001;26:325–32.
14. Bernhardt TM, Schmidl H, Philipp C, Allhoff EP, Rapp-Bernhardt U. Diagnostic potential of virtual cystoscopy of the bladder: MRI vs CT. Preliminary report. Eur Radiol. 2003;13:305–12.
15. Chou C-P, Huang J-S, Wu M-T, et al. CT voiding urethrography and virtual urethroscopy: preliminary study with 16-MDCT. AJR. 2005;184:1882–8.
16. Chou C-P, Huang J-S, Yu C-C, Pan H-B, Huang F-D. Urethral diverticulum: diagnosis with virtual CT urethroscopy. AJR. 2005;184:1889–90.
17. Siabilis D, Kagadis GC, Liatsikos EN, et al. Ureteral metallic stents: application of virtual endoscopy for ureteral patency control. Int Urol Nephrol. 2003;35:327–30.

18. Russel ST, Kawashima A, Vrtiska TJ, et al. Three-dimensional CT virtual endoscopy in the detection of simulated tumors in a phantom bladder and ureter model. J Endourol. 2005;19:188–92.

19. Liatsikos EN, Siablis D, Kagadis GC, et al. Virtual endoscopy: navigation within pelvicaliceal system. J Endourol. 2005;19:37–40.

20. Neri E, Boraschi P, Caramella D, et al. MR virtual endoscopy of the upper urinary tract. AJR. 2000;175:1697–702.

21. Barbalias GA, Liatsikos EN, Kagadis GC, et al. Ureteropelvic junction obstruction: an innovative approach combining metallic stenting and virtual endoscopy. J Urol. 2002;168:2383–6.

22. Wilhelm DM, Ogan K, Roehrborn CG, Cadeddu JA, Pearle MS. Assessment of basic endoscopic performance using a virtual reality simulator. J Am Coll Surg. 2002;195:675–81.

23. Watterson JD, Beiko DT, Kuan JK, Denstedt JD. Randomized prospective blinded study validating acquisition of ureteroscopy skills using computer based virtual reality endourological simulator. J Urol. 2002;168:1928–32.

24. Ogan K, Jacomides L, Shulman MJ, et al. Virtual ureteroscopy predicts ureteroscopic proficiency of medical students on a cadaver. J Urol. 2004;172:667–71.

25. Mutter D, Bouras G, Marescaux J. Digital technologies and quality improvement in cancer surgery. Eur J Surg Oncol. 2005;31:689–94.

Chapter 40

Optical Imaging and Diagnosis in Bladder Cancer

M. Grimbergen, M.C. Aalders, and T.G. van Leeuwen

Introduction

In this chapter we will review currently used and new optical imaging techniques that have been applied in bladder cancer diagnosis. While some of these techniques are still experimental and some are advancing toward in vivo use, others are commercially available to the urologist. The working mechanisms of these techniques will be discussed along with their potential to solve specific clinical questions that face the practicing urologist. Future prospects of biomedical optics applied to the field of urology are discussed according to the latest technical advances in optical engineering.

Optical Diagnosis

The challenge in optical diagnosis of tissue (in oncology) is threefold: detection, i.e., finding the location of interest; staging, i.e., assessing the state of tumor progression through the layers of the bladder wall; and grading, i.e., obtaining the state of differentiation of the cancer cells. Optical diagnostic techniques have the potential to improve on traditional methods in various ways. Some techniques increase sensitivity and specificity of endoscopic imaging and therefore increase their diagnostic value. Other techniques objectively quantitatively analyze the acquired data and therefore show potential in reducing the variation in tissue classification reporting. However, the challenge for optical diagnostics is to develop a technique capable of reliably discerning non-normal and malignant change at an early stage to minimize recurrence and prevent progression of tumor invasion. Optical diagnosis in general relies on detecting a change in the nature of light induced by the interaction with the subject of interest. Changes in the nature of light that can occur or can be induced by incident light are as follows:

- Spatial: the distribution of light is altered by local absorption, reflection, and/or scattering (white light imaging, confocal imaging, diffuse reflectance spectroscopy, optical coherence tomography, etc.)
- Spectral: the spectrum of detected light is altered by absorption, with or without subsequent emission of fluorescence or by inelastic (Raman) scattering; (autofluorescence, fluorescence, Raman spectroscopy)
- Temporal: the propagation time of light through tissue is altered by reflection, absorption, and/or elastic scattering or by delayed emission of fluorescence. (Fluorescence lifetime imaging)

Tissue Optical Properties

Light can be described as a large number of packages of energy that are known as photons. When light is directed at tissue, some photons are absorbed by individual molecules within the tissue. Absorption can provide a clue as to the chemical composition of a tissue and serve as a mechanism of optical contrast during imaging. Absorption depends on the wavelength of light and the type of molecules present.

Scattering of light occurs in media which contain fluctuations in the refractive index (n). Scattering depends on the structural components of tissue and whether fluctuations in refractive index are discrete steps or more continuous variations. Tissue scattering mainly depends on the size of nuclei, the presence of collagen fibers, and the status of hydration in the tissue and density of lipid membranes in the cells.

The bladder wall consists of several layers of tissue each containing different constituents with particular optical properties. Tissue optical properties are dependent on tissue constituents like oxy and deoxyhemoglobin, nicotinamide adenine dinucleotide hydride (NADH), flavins, collagen, and water.

M. Grimbergen (✉)
University Medical Center Utrecht, Utrecht, The Netherlands

J.J.M.C.H. de la Rosette et al. (eds.), *Imaging in Oncological Urology*,
DOI 10.1007/978-1-84628-759-6_40, © Springer-Verlag London Limited 2009

White Light Endoscopy

White light endoscopy (WLE) of the bladder remains the modality of choice for confirmation of the diagnosis of bladder cancer. The technique is based on spatial variations in reflection and absorption of incident light, which are perceived by the observer as color differences. Variations in the optical properties and structural changes of the bladder wall are related to biochemical and morphological changes of neoplastic bladder wall tissue.

Illumination

In standard endoscopy the incident light is produced by an illumination source, with a broad optical bandwidth emitting a smooth optical intensity spectrum. The deep UV and near-infrared (NIR) parts of the spectrum are usually rejected in order to prevent carcinogenic and heating effects, respectively. The color temperature of the light, determined by the type of source, xenon, halogen, or tungsten filaments, causes a particular reflection spectrum, resulting in different visual perception of an object by the observer (Fig. 40.1).

Imaging

Both color and structural information is used in tissue diagnosis. The level of structural information that can be

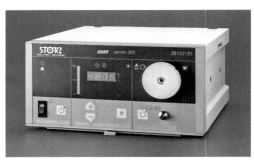

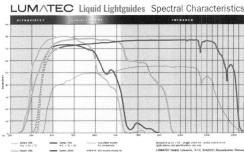

Fig. 40.1 White light source for cystoscopy (from Karl Storz website). Transmission curves for various liquid lightguides (from Lumatec website)

observed with an optical instrument is determined by its image quality. A number of factors determine the image quality as presented to the observer. Contrast and resolution are two optical parameters, which are closely related and form a more distinctive description of the optical performance of an imaging system. Because of the relation between contrast and resolution, the contrast level is often defined at a specific resolution. A graphical presentation of the contrast level for a range of frequencies is the modulation transfer function (MTF) curve. Generally, the contrast will decrease as the frequency increases. The contrast (as a function of frequency) and the smallest detectable object are the main characteristics of an optical system.

Endoscopic Imaging Systems

In white light endoscopic imaging the observer's eye may serve as the image detector. In today's urology, however, video recording and intermediate monitor display have become common practice. Both the charge coupled device (CCD) and the image representation techniques become part of the chain of optical components. A typical endoscopic imaging system consists of an endoscope, a digital image sensor, video processor, and a display. Each of these components has a characteristic frequency response. The image quality of the total system is a multiplication of the MTF's of the individual components.

Flexible Versus Rigid Cystoscopes

The level of detail that can be observed by flexible fiberscopes and rigid Hopkins endoscopes greatly differs due to the difference in image transfer to the camera or eye.

Typical fiber bundles for use in cystoscopy exhibit a diameter of 4–6 mm containing over 30.000 individual fibers. The spatial resolution of these devices is determined by the number of fibers as the number of pixels in the image corresponds to the number of fibers. Individual fibers are made as small as possible with a physical limit of the transmitted wavelength. The rigid endoscopes usually give brighter images with higher contrast (Fig. 40.2).

Chip-on-the-Tip Technology

Distal video sensor chips have recently been introduced into clinical endoscopy. A number of flexible cystoscopes with this "chip-on-the-tip" technology have since emerged.

The optical performance of these devices is solely dependent on the size of the image sensor and image processing.

(a)

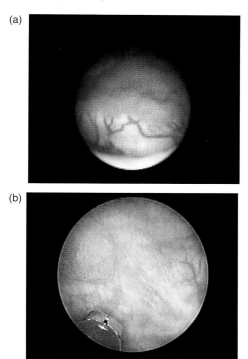

(b)

Fig. 40.2 White light endoscopy images of urologic features (UMCU Department of Urology) (a) flexible scope, (b) Karl Storz 24F rigid cystoscope

A recent study described a single blinded in vitro comparison of fiber-equipped cystoscopes of four major manufacturers with two digital cystoscopes. The image quality was assessed by determining correct interpretation of text at a fixed distance from the cystoscope through dyes with different concentrations [1]. Significant improvement of the digital scopes over the fiber scopes was observed at higher concentrations.

Confocal Imaging

Confocal imaging has emerged in microscopy and has rapidly gained interest because of its relatively easy incorporation in optical systems. Confocal microscopy allows optical cross-sectional imaging of tissue with μm resolution. This optical sectioning is obtained by placing small apertures at the focal plane of both the illumination and the detection pathways. The illumination pinhole limits the illumination of the sample to a single spot. The aperture in the detection path is used to block light from objects out of the focal volume, i.e., above or below the spot of interest. By scanning the focal volume through the tissue, two- or three-dimensional images of a slice/volume within the sample can be obtained (Fig. 40.3).

Targeting specific anatomical structures with fluorescent dyes is used to image subsurface cellular structures in vivo, such as subcutaneous melanoma, subcutaneous vessels and nerves, or microvascular changes in colitis (Fig. 40.4).

D'Hallewin reported the feasibility of performing endoscopic fiber-optic confocal microscopy imaging of the bladder in the rat. This study showed that in vivo assessment of different types of cells is feasible by means of contrast dyes [2]. This technique can also provide depth assessment in case of cancer invasion.

Diffuse Reflectance Spectroscopy

Diffuse reflectance spectroscopy (DRS), also known as elastic scattering spectroscopy, is a non-invasive optical technique based on wavelength-dependent absorption and elastic scattering of photons, to produce a characteristic reflectance spectrum, providing information about the structure and composition of the medium. In biological tissues, scattering depends on the ultra-structure of a tissue, the density of lipid membranes in the cells, the size of nuclei, the presence of collagen fibers, the status of hydration in the tissue, and other factors. An important parameter for diagnosis is the size of the nucleus, which is often enlarged in neoplastic tissue. These enlarged nuclei cause a relatively lower scattering intensity at longer wavelengths. In addition, other parameters like the change in polarization or angular dependence of the scattering may be assessed to obtain diagnostic information.

Mourant et al. developed an optical biopsy system (OBS) for patients with suspected bladder cancer. Elastic-scatter spectra over the wavelength range 250–800 nm were obtained using a fiber-optic probe through one of the lumen of a urological cystoscope. Measurements were done and biopsies were taken from apparently normal areas and areas of uncertain abnormality, as well as those suspected to be cancerous. A diagnostic algorithm for distinguishing malignant from nonmalignant tissue based on the values of the slopes over the wavelength range 330–370 nm has a sensitivity of 100% and a specificity of 97% for the limited number of patients in this study [3].

In a similar investigation, the potential of diffuse reflectance spectroscopy for the detection of neoplasma of the bladder was performed by Koenig et al. This method was based on the difference in blood absorption brought about by the presence of neovasculature in neoplastic tissue. Only the total amount of blood proved to be a useful parameter for the differentiation between neoplastic and benign bladder areas. The sensitivity and specificity for the detection of neoplastic tissue was 91 and 60%, respectively. The relatively low specificity is a result of inflammatory areas also exhibiting an increased blood concentration [4].

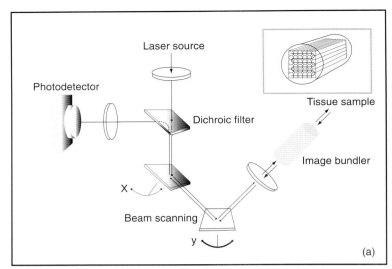
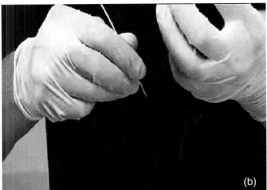

Fig. 40.3 (a) Schematic of a Fibered Confocal Microscopy setup (from J Vasc Res. 2004;41:400–411) and (b) Insertion of a confocal mini-probe through a flexible endoscope (from Mauna Kea Technologies)

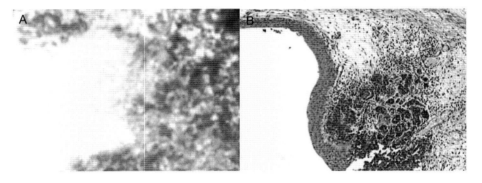

Fig. 40.4 Rat bladder. (a), transurethral Cell-vizio™ images show intensely fluorescing spot corresponding to AY-27 tumor, where small inflammatory cells surrounding tumor were less fluorescent. Field of view $600 \times 500 \, \mu$m. (b) Frozen section from same spot. H & E, reduced from $\times 10$

More recently Demos et al. showed that near-infrared (NIR) polarized elastic light scattering can be used to differentiate between benign and malignant tissue in vitro. Cross-polarized light-scattering images of the samples were recorded under near-infrared polarized illumination at 700, 850, and 1000 nm. They found significant differences in intensity between normal and cancer tissue in 700 nm cross-polarized light-scattering images of in vitro tissue samples [5]. The combination of this technique with autofluorescence (see below) under different excitation wavelengths further enhanced these differences (Fig. 40.5).

Fluorescence-Guided Endoscopy

Fluorescence diagnostics or photodetection (PD) is widely used in various clinical disciplines for localization and identification of neoplastic tissue. The technique is based on concentration differences of fluorescent molecules (the

fluorophore) in normal versus neoplastic tissue. When illuminated by light of a specific wavelength (excitation light), the fluorophores will be promoted to a higher energy (excited) state. Relaxation of the excited molecules to the ground state is accompanied by emission of fluorescence. The distribution of the fluorescence can then be used to demarcate the area of pathologic cells. The emitted "fluorescence" photon is less energetic than the incident photon originally absorbed by the molecule. As the energy of light is inversely proportional to its wavelength, the fluorescent light will have a longer wavelength than the excitation light. Fluorescent and excitation light can easily be distinguished by this change in wavelength.

For optimal detection, the amount of excitation light which is scattered back to the detector, e.g., a CCD camera, is decreased by optical filtering to a level where fluorescence becomes visible. Variations in fluorescence intensity are, besides on the differences in concentration of fluorophores, also influenced by the tissue optical properties.

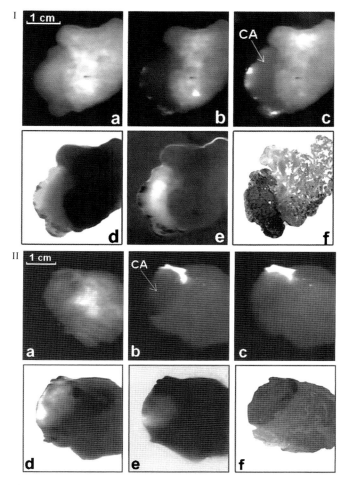

Fig. 40.5 Images of two human bladder tissue specimen I & II. (a) Crosspolarized light scattering under 700-nm illumination. (b) NIR fluorescence images under 532-nm and (c) 632.8-nm laser excitation. (d) Ratio of the autofluorescence image under 632.8-nm excitation over that under 532-nm excitation. e) Interimage ratio of a cross-polarized scattering image recorded under illumination at 700 nm over the fluorescence image under 532-nm excitation. (f) H&E, stained section of the same specimen. (from Demos et al.)

In order to exploit fluorescence as a modality for tissue diagnosis, a difference in fluorescent properties between normal and pathological tissue is required. In cells and the ultrastructure of tissue there are a number of constituents that have natural fluorescent characteristics. Endogenous fluorescence relies on discerning local variations in the presence of these naturally occurring fluorescent molecules. Another strategy is to exogenously apply a fluorescent dye, which is predominantly absorbed by tumor cells to attain the desired contrast.

Autofluorescence

When intrinsic tissue fluorescence is used (autofluorescence), fluorescence is emitted by naturally occurring tissue elements like NADH, porphyrins, flavins, and collagen. Variations in concentration of these elements may be used to characterize tissue. Autofluorescence is usually induced with wavelengths in the UV part of the spectrum (<400 nm). Unfortunately, information is only obtained from a very superficial tissue layer, as the penetration of UV/blue light in most tissue types is limited to the upper 500 μm. Autofluorescence imaging requires sensitive equipment, which was only recently developed. Commercial devices are currently available for the detection of early stage cancer of the GI tract, ENT, and lung (e.g., the Xillix Life™ systems). Interpretation of the autofluorescence images is difficult because of the large influence of tissue optical properties, particularly scattering, and the imaging geometry. Currently, autofluorescence is still an experimental technique.

In a comprehensive study of laser-induced fluorescence spectroscopy in the urinary bladder, Anidjar et al. [6] used excitation wavelengths of 308, 337, and 480 nm. They stated that by using 308 nm, one could obtain more information to discriminate cancer from normal tissue than with the longer excitation wavelengths (480, 337 nm). They calculated a ratio of the obtained fluorescence maxima at 360 and 440 nm and found higher mean fluorescence ratios ($I_{360}:I_{440}$) for tumors (3.04) than for normal (0.87) and/or inflammatory (1.28) bladder lesions. Using a threshold value to differentiate between cancer and normal tissue, they were able to discriminate all malignant lesions from the corresponding benign sites correctly without any false-negative results, suggesting a 100% sensitivity and specificity for the detection of bladder cancer. However, the investigation was based on a limited number (n = 66) of biopsies, which were mainly taken from visible carcinomas (n = 31), normal tissue (n = 22), and only few inflammatory areas (n = 13).

A recent publication by Zheng et al. [7] determined the optimal excitation and emission wavelengths for autofluorescence diagnosis of bladder cancer in 52 tissue samples. Fluorescence excitation wavelengths varying from 220 to 500 nm were used to induce tissue autofluorescence, and emission spectra were measured in the 280–700 nm range. Significant changes in fluorescence intensity were found at the excitation wavelengths of 280 and 330 nm. A diagnostic algorithm based on the combination of the fluorescence peak intensity ratios of I_{350}/I_{470} at 280 nm excitation and I_{390}/I_{470} at 330 nm excitation yielded a sensitivity of 100% [95% confidence interval (CI) 0.95–1.0] and a specificity of 100% (95% CI 0.90–1.0). However, excitation of tissue with UVB light always bears a problem associated with UV irradiation: the carcinogenic risk. The UV radiation exposure limit for continuous wave radiation at 308 nm on skin has been determined as 120 mJ/cm^2 for 8 h of exposure on the skin [8]. Kochevar [9] showed that the photobiologic effects on epithelial cells using continuous wave radiation and pulsed excimer laser irradiation are the same. Therefore, the same exposure limit was assumed reasonable. If fluorescence imaging is to be performed similar to video endoscopy, larger surfaces will have to be irradiated for longer times. This might result in undesirable high dose exposure to UV light.

Exogenous Fluorescence

To increase the fluorescent signals, administration of a fluorescent dye to the patient that will accumulate preferentially in neoplastic tissue can be performed. The success of photodetection with exogenously administered photosensitizers depends on the differential gradient of the concentration of the dye in tumor versus host tissue. The dye should be tumor selective, with a rapid clearance from the body after the diagnostic procedure and minimal side effects, like photosensitization of the skin. The first photosensitizers applied in PD were hematoporphyrin derivatives (HPD) and its more purified form photofrin. These dyes have relatively low tumor specificity and cause a prolonged skin photosensitization in the patient. Despite these disadvantages, photofrin is still widely used in clinical PDT. Second-generation photosensitizers are now also available, of which the most commonly used is aminolevulinic acid.

Aminolevulinic Acid

Aminolevulinic acid (ALA) is a precursor of protoporphyrin IX (PpIX) in the heme synthesis, and it is naturally available in the human body in small concentrations. Adding excess amounts of (exogenous) ALA leads to much higher concentrations of PpIX, which selectively accumulates in neoplastic tissue. This selective accumulation of PpIX is thought to be due to an altered activity of heme biosynthetic pathway enzymes in neoplastic tissue. Excess PpIX production after administration of ALA also occurs in normal tissue, with a preference for mucosa, e.g., in stomach, intestines, skin, and bladder. Despite the concurrent accumulation of PpIX in normal tissue, useful tumor to normal concentration ratios are obtained with most investigated tissue types (e.g., bladder, skin, cervix, esophagus, brain). The tumor selectivity, short half-life (< 24 h), and mild photosensitization at lower dosages make ALA an attractive fluorescent dye for PD applications [10–14].

Kriegmair et al. were the first to describe intravesical ALA application in humans. A total of 68 patients with bladder cancer were instilled with a 3% ALA solution for 1–3 h, followed by blue light examination of the bladder [15]. A sensitivity and specificity of 100% and 68.5%, respectively, were obtained. In a larger series (106 patients), these results

were further confirmed [16]. The largest published series to date was presented by Zaak et al. and included 1012 cystoscopies and 552 biopsies containing dysplasia, CIS, and/or papillary tumors [17]. The sensitivity (92.4%) and specificity (65%) were comparable to prior published data. Furthermore, approximately one third of the false-negative results consisted in GII dysplasia, and about 50% small Ta tumors.

Other studies later also reported similar results [18, 19]. None of the earlier mentioned authors observed skin photosensitization, and Filbeck et al. could not observe any changes in minimal phototoxic dose after UVA light exposure before or after ALA administration [20]. A mixture of ALA and lubricant was found to induce PpIX fluorescence in urethral tumors [21].

All reports on ALA-induced PpIX-guided fluorescence detection confirm the high sensitivity to detect bladder cancer ($>90\%$), including carcinoma in situ. Minor discrepancies can be attributed to different factors such as instillation time, the interval between instillation and blue light excitation, different levels of experience and skill in white light endoscopy (e.g., suspicious versus inflammatory) or blue light endoscopy. Photobleaching is dependent on the concentration of photosensitizer, fluence and fluence rate [23, 24]. In the conditions applied during fluorescence cystoscopy, photobleaching results in the absence of fluorescence after 30 min illumination [24, 25]. Finally, the sensitivity will be dependent on the number of biopsies performed and the number of patients included in the study.

The specificity however varies greatly from study to study, ranging from 71% [16], 57% [26] to 33% [27]. In the most ideal conditions, however, still one third of positive results must be considered false. This is partly due to inexperience in blue light endoscopy. PpIX can be detected in normal mucosa, although at a five- to tenfold lesser concentration [28]. When normal mucosa is excited by a parallel beam, a high amount of red fluorescence will result from the excitation of a large amount of normal cells, containing a minimal dose of PpIX but resulting in a strong fluorescence, comparable to tumoral fluorescence when excited with a perpendicular beam. This results in false-positive fluorescence, which can be observed in bladder neck, trigone, diverticular under "experienced" observation, but also whenever the excitation is not strictly perpendicular to the inspected tissue. The presence of an inflammatory reaction, due to transurethral manipulation, bacterial, chemical, or radiocystitis or scar tissue, induces false-positive results [16, 27, 29].

On the other hand, in case of hyperplasia, a benign condition sometimes resulting in false-positive fluorescence, monosomies, or partial deletions of chromosome 9 could be detected in 70% of the cases, together with p53 alterations [30, 31]. Those alterations are believed to be an early event in the development of bladder cancer [32], since they can be detected in papillary and flat bladder carcinoma in situ [24, 25]. Longer follow-up of the patients and bladder sites presenting false-positive results should provide more information.

Although the mechanisms of selective fluorescence are not fully understood, the clinical relevance of the technique of fluorescence is now generally accepted. Blue light endoscopy has been proven to give more information as compared to white light cystoscopy [33]. The best sensitivity estimate for white light endoscopy is 46.7% (95% confidence intervals 39.4–54.3) as compared to 93.4% (95% confidence intervals 90–97.3) for fluorescence endoscopy. Not only the detection rate is increased but also a significant reduction in recurrence rate of 20% is observed at control cystoscopy [22].

Hexyl esters of ALA reduce the incidence of false-positive results but without significantly improving the specificity [28]. The results from the first European multicenter study conducted in 19 centers in 286 patients confirmed the advantages of hexaminolevulinate fluorescence cystoscopy over standard white light cystoscopy in the detection of bladder cancer. The second multicenter phase III study at ten centers in Germany and the Netherlands in 146 patients with known or suspected bladder cancer was successfully completed in March 2003. The independent blind reviewer acknowledged that imaging with hexyl aminolevulinate would result in better treatment options in every fifth patient compared with standard cystoscopy [44].

Hexyl-aminolevulinic Acid

Recent studies have shown that only limited amounts of ALA enter the target cells or penetrate through the tissue when topically instilled, which consequently limits the amount of PpIX in the targeted tissue [34]. Almost all of the possible disadvantages accompanying the use of ALA can be ascribed to the physical–chemical properties of the molecule itself. Applied under physiological conditions, ALA is a zwitterion [35]. Because the lipid bilayer of biological membranes is relatively impermeable to charged molecules, the cellular uptake of ALA is shallow. Consequently, in order to increase the transport across cellular membranes, fairly high drug doses and long administration times have to be used. This deficiency results in a low penetration depth [36–38] and an ALA-induced PpIX distribution that is not optimized for the PDT of the deep layers of, e.g., nodular lesions in the urothelium [39, 40] after topical ALA application. Systematic studies have shown that the modification of a drug to an ester, an amide, or a urethane by the addition of a long-chain hydrocarbon improves penetration through biological barriers [41–43].

Hypericin

Hypericin is a hydroxylated phenantroperylene quinone which emits red fluorescence at 594 and 642 nm when illuminated with blue light. Hypericin-induced fluorescence is limited to the epithelium and the specificity for malignant cells was 95% in the study of D'Hallewin et al. (Fig. 40.6).

Eighty-seven patients with known TCC/CIS or positive urine cytology were studied, using hypericin-induced fluorescence cystoscopy [45]. An instillation time of 2 h was used and no photobleaching occurred. In this population the sensitivity and specificity for detecting CIS was 94% and 95%, respectively. Numerous investigators assessing the potential clinical efficacy of hypericin as a method for PDT showed, in vitro and in vivo, potent photocytotoxic activity for hypericin. Recent data from an in vitro study also detailed the type of cell death (apoptosis versus necrosis) and the biochemical background of the phototoxicity induced by photo-activated hypericin. These aspects suggest a promising clinical potential for hypericin in whole bladder wall PDT.

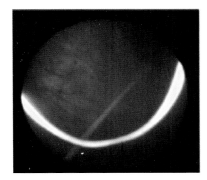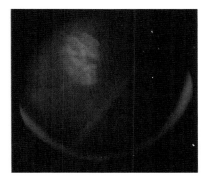

Fig. 40.6 Bladder with resection loop under white light inspection (left) and fluorescence inspection (right) [44]

Raman Spectroscopy

Inelastic scattering is a fundamental interaction in which energy is exchanged between light and matter. In Raman scattering, photons can lose or gain energy, which corresponds to the difference in the initial and final vibrational energy levels of the scattering molecule. The probability for a photon to be subject to inelastic scattering is rare, affecting roughly one in every million elastically scattered photons. A Raman spectrum is an intensity plot of scattered photons as a function of the energy difference between the incoming and scattered photons, also known as the Raman shift. Typically Raman peaks are spectrally narrow and in many cases can be associated with the vibration of a particular chemical bond in a molecule. Therefore, Raman spectroscopy provides chemical information of the tissue.

Biological tissue structures consist of many Raman active molecules. A tissue Raman spectrum therefore is a summation of the intensity at each shift of the biological tissue structures probed by the technique. In recent years, the diagnostic value of this technique [46] is being explored, because the molecular specific information can provide information to differentiate between tissue types. Several biological molecules such as nucleic acids, proteins, and lipids have distinctive Raman features that yield molecular-specific structural and environmental information. Thus the transitional changes in tissues that occur with disease progression yield characteristic Raman features that allow differentiation, e.g., between precancers and cancers. One of the more prominent changes that occur with cancer and precancer is increased cellular nucleic acid content that can be sampled by Raman spectroscopy. Based on these biochemical differences, several groups have studied the potential of vibrational spectroscopy for cancer diagnosis in various organ sites. These groups have shown that features of the vibrational spectrum can be related to molecular and structural changes associated with neoplastic transformation.

Raman spectroscopy has been applied to in vitro detection of cancers of epithelial and mesenchymal origin such as breast, colon, esophagus, and gynaecologic tissues. A recent study of Raman spectroscopy in diagnoses of bladder disease pertains to the in vitro assessment of the bladder wall composition in relation to bladder outlet obstruction [47]. Bladder outlet obstruction leads to loss of bladder function as a result of structural damage. The authors present the first results of Raman spectroscopy, applied for the detection of changes in molecular composition of the bladder wall to asses the diagnostic value. Raman spectroscopic mapping of unfixed sections of damaged and undamaged bladder wall from a guinea pig model of bladder obstruction was used to detect changes in composition of bladder muscle tissue. Collagen infiltra-

tion in muscle fibers was clearly visualized. Other compositional changes that are revealed include the accumulation of glycogen in obstructed bladder wall as well as an apparent but as-yet unknown change in protein composition. These initial findings show that Raman spectroscopy can be a valuable diagnostic tool for evaluation of the extent of bladder structure loss.

An in vitro sample study was performed by Crow et al. [48] to determine the sensitivity and specificity of Raman spectroscopy in a confocal microscopy setup. Bladder samples collected during cystoscopic procedures were snap-frozen and a section was taken for histological examination. Samples were classified as normal, cystitis, carcinoma in situ (CIS), TCC, and squamous cell carcinoma (SCC). Scanning was carried out on an optimized Raman system, using an acquisition time of 10 s. In all, 1685 spectra were recorded from 76 patients (590 benign and 1095 malignant spectra). These spectra were analyzed using principal-component-fed linear-discriminant analysis to construct a diagnostic algorithm. The algorithm was tested for its accuracy in predicting the histological diagnosis. The accuracy achieved by the algorithm for normal, cystitis, CIS, TCC, and SCC were, respectively (sensitivity), 91%, 79%, 86%, 84%, and 98% and (specificity) 96%, 92%, 97%, 96%, and 100%.

Combined Fluorescence and Raman Spectroscopy

To improve the low specificity of fluorescence imaging and to provide in vivo pathology, optical biopsy by means of Raman spectroscopy after region selection by fluorescence imaging was proposed. Raman spectra were recorded and evaluated from bladder wall biopsy samples obtained from both: white light endoscopy (WLE) and 5-ALA fluorescence-guided endoscopy. The spectral features in NIR Raman spectra of biopsies with and without ALA were evaluated and have not been shown to be significantly different. Principal-component-fed linear-discriminant analysis was used to construct a diagnostic algorithm based on the WLE data. To determine the influence of the fluorescent marker on the performance of the diagnostic algorithm it was used to predict pathology class of the 5-ALA FGE biopsies. A similar algorithm developed from the FGE group showed a training performance of 82%. The combination of NIR Raman spectroscopy after region selection by 5-ALA-induced fluorescence diagnosis in bladder cancer diagnosis proves to be feasible in vitro. Future research is concentrated on applying this technique in vivo.

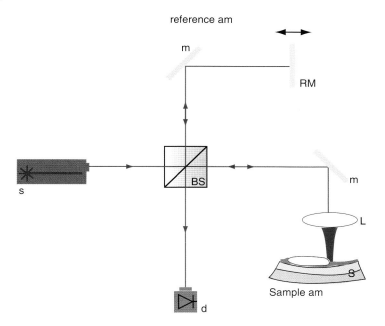

Fig. 40.7 A schematic drawing of an OCT setup. Light emitted by a light source (ls) is split by a beam splitter (BS) into two beams, traveling through the reference arm or the sample arm. Via mirror (m), the light in the sample arm is focused into a sample (S) using a lens (L). In the reference arm, the light is directed to a translating reference mirror (RM). Backreflected light from both arms is recombined by the beam splitter (BS) and the interference signal is monitored by the detector (d)

Optical Coherence Tomography

Since its introduction in the early 1990s, OCT has become a powerful method for imaging the internal structure of biological systems and materials [49]. OCT is analogous to B-mode ultrasound, except that it uses light rather than sound. Whereas in ultrasound the location of reflecting object is determined by measuring echo delay times, in OCT depth resolved measurement of the backscattered light is achieved through low-coherence interferometry. The heart of the OCT setup is a Michelson interferometer (Fig. 40.7); light emitted by a light source is split by a beam splitter in two beams. One is directed into the reference arm and is reflected by a translating reference mirror. The other beam is directed into the sample arm and is reflected by a tissue sample. The backreflected beams recombine at the beam splitter and are guided to a detector. It is important to note that interference between the two light beams will only be detected when the difference in optical path lengths traveled by the light in both arms is less than the so-called coherence length of the light source. This phenomenon is used to determine the optical path length the light has traveled in the sample arm: if interference is observed while scanning the path length in the reference arm (i.e., moving the reference mirror), the backscattered light from different positions within the sample (i.e., in depth) can be measured ("coherence gating"). Conse-

quently, the axial resolution is directly related to the coherence length of the light source, which is inversely related to the bandwidth of the light source. The transverse resolution for OCT imaging is determined by the focused spot size, as in microscopy [50]. In contrast to conventional confocal microscopy, the lateral resolution is decoupled from the axial resolution. Furthermore, OCT provides cross-sectional images of structures below the tissue surface in analogy to histopathology. Standard-resolution OCT can achieve axial resolutions of 10 μm.

In accordance with the terminology of ultrasound imaging, a measurement of reflectivity versus depth is called an A-scan. The OCT image, or B-scan, is constructed from adjacent A-scans, with the reflectivity now plotted as a gray or color scale. The contrast of an OCT image is determined by differences in the optical properties (e.g., scattering and absorption) [51] of different tissue layers and their components (Fig. 40.8). The imaging depth is also determined by the optical properties of the tissue [52]. Using wavelengths in the near-infrared, where hemoglobin and melanin absorption are low and scattering is reduced, permits imaging depths of up to 2 mm in tissues [53, 54]. Although this depth is shallow compared with other clinical imaging techniques like ultrasound, the image resolution of OCT is 1–2 orders of magnitude better than conventional ultrasound imaging, magnetic resonance imaging, or computed tomography. Recently, using state-of-the-art lasers as light sources,

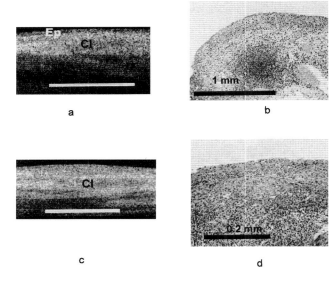

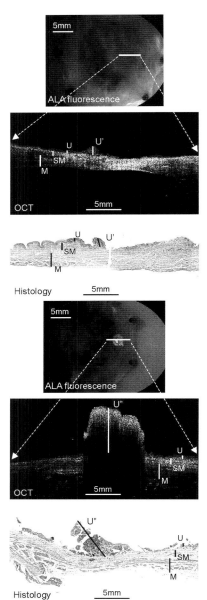

Fig. 40.8 Optical coherence tomography of chronic nonproliferative cystitis (a and c) with corresponding histological findings (b and d). Diffuse cellular infiltration (CI) of submucosa is indicated by inhomogeneous and spotted pattern. Boundary between mucosa and submucosa is blurred due to diffuse infiltration of transitional epithelium (Ep) and submucosa (c)

ultrahigh-resolution imaging with axial resolutions as fine as 1–2 μm has been demonstrated (Table 40.1) [55].

Table 40.1 Overview of light sources and their specifications. The center wavelength (λ) is proportional to the imaging depth (d_i). The bandwidth of the light source ($\Delta\lambda$) is inversely proportional to the coherence length (l_c). The maximal power (P_{max}) is also given. SLD: super luminescent diode; AF: autofluorescent fiber; Ti:Al$_2$O$_3$: titanium sapphire laser

Light source	λ (nm)	$\Delta\lambda$ (nm)	P_{max} (mW)	l_c (μm)	d_i (mm)
SLD	825	~ 25	~ 5	~ 12	0.5–1.0
SLD	1300	~ 50	~ 5	~ 15	1.0–2.0
AF	1300	~ 60	~ 20	~ 12	1.0–2.0
Ti:Al$_2$O$_3$	800	~ 100–250	~ 1000	~ 1–3	0.5–1.5

Most OCT systems for biomedical applications use single-mode fiber, which allows the use of OCT catheters and endoscopes.

Fig. 40.9 Combined ALA fluorescence imaging and OCT

Fluorescence and Confocal or OCT

Xie et al. have demonstrated a combined endoscopic imaging technique that allows for simultaneous front-view surface fluorescence imaging and high-resolution cross-sectional OCT of the tissue (e.g., urinary bladder) under examination [56]. A two-dimensional OCT image (at 5 frames/s) and an ALA fluorescence image (at 8 frames/s) were simultaneously displayed on a computer monitor for instant compar-

ison and guidance. Preliminary results based on rat bladder carcinogenesis studies demonstrate that ALA fluorescence imaging is highly effective and sensitive and covers a large area (diameter 30 mm) of the bladder surface, whereas OCT provides only a cross-sectional scan of, in this case, 5 mm × 32.8 mm. However, because of the superior resolution and the ability to delineate bladder micromorphology (e.g., the normal uroepithelium, submucosa, and upper muscularis layer), OCT can detect both neoplastic lesions (Fig. 40.9b) and precancerous lesions (Fig. 40.9a). In addition, the technique can differentiate inflammatory lesions that may be wrongly positively classified by fluorescence. This suggests that a new cystoscope with ALA fluorescence imaging to guide OCT may substantially enhance the efficiency and sensitivity for rapid diagnosis of early bladder cancers. Because of the complex nature of bladder carcinogenesis, further, more detailed studies are needed to carefully compare the difference between the biochemical and the morphological characteristics provided by fluorescence and OCT imaging.

New Imaging Modalities

Two state-of-the-art imaging techniques, which currently are under development for clinical application, are described with their potential to overcome difficulties posed by currently available imaging and optical diagnostic techniques.

Nano-particles and Quantum Dots

Optical imaging has strong potential for sensitive cancer diagnosis; however it greatly relies upon the use of sensitive and stable optical probes. Recent advances in nanomaterials have produced a new class of fluorescent labels by conjugating semiconductor quantum dots with bio-recognition molecules. These nanometer-sized conjugates are water soluble and biocompatible and provide important advantages over organic dyes and lanthanide probes. In particular, the emission wavelength of quantum-dot nanocrystals can be continuously tuned by changing the particle size, and a single light source can be used for simultaneous excitation of all different-sized dots. Unlike the traditional organic fluorescent probes, high-quality dots are also highly stable with respect to photobleaching and have narrow, symmetric emission spectra [57]. These novel optical properties render quantum dots ideal fluorophores for ultrasensitive diagnostic imaging [58].

Nanoparticles bearing tissue-targeting ligands can moreover improve the focused delivery of a photosensitizer payload to malignant cells, making photodynamic diagnosis or treatment more effective for both imaging and treating of, e.g., infiltrating cancers or those growing near sensitive normal structures. Recent attempts to deliver photosensitizers to cells using nanoparticles have produced limited photodynamic efficacy; e.g., in one case, sequestering of the photosensitizer within a stable nanoparticle kept it from the most sensitive cellular targets. The technology is based on the mechanisms of photodynamic action and identification of the relevant anti-apoptotic proteins as immediate molecular targets of nanoparticle photosensitizer.

Life-Time Fluorescence Imaging

Spectrally resolved fluorescence imaging has a reasonable sensitivity for the detection of cancer but lacks the required specificity for tissue diagnosis. Emission spectra of many tissue fluorophores overlap which limits the obtainable contrast. Life-time fluorescence imaging allows distinction of intrinsic tissue fluorophores by their particular rate of fluorescence intensity decay, which can be used to differentiate between normal and neoplastic tissue in several organs. The FLIM technique is based on gated optical image intensifier technology. The sample is excited with a very short laser pulse and a gated optical intensifier coupled to a CCD camera is used to record the intensity of the fluorescence at some chosen time after the excitation pulse. In the past high-speed wide-field FLIM setups did not comply with clinical demands of resolution and frame rate. Real-time FLIM endoscopy with rigid and flexible scopes was recently shown to be feasible [59, 60]. Technical improvements of the current FLIM systems should allow clinical applications in the near future.

Diagnostic Value of Optical Techniques

In this chapter, an overview of presented techniques and their specific (optical) characteristics and capabilities with respect to the clinical task at hand in bladder cancer diagnosis has been discussed.

The diagnostic value of any modality is determined with respect to histopathology, the gold standard. In table 40.2, the specific information of imaging and optical biopsy systems is presented. However, the presented calculated diagnostic values should not be compared between the imaging and biopsy techniques because of their intrinsic different subjective and objective nature, respectively. In imaging, sensitivity and specificity expresses the contrast between normal and pre-malignant tissue as perceived by the observer in the locations that are biopsied, as the imaging prediction is compared to histopathology.

Combination of wide-field imaging techniques and either or both optical diagnosis and microscopic imaging will likely provide the necessary diagnostic detail to enable in vivo tissue diagnosis.

Table 40.2 Overview of optical charateristics and diagnostic value of imaging and optical biopsy modalities

	Aim	Field of view	Time domain	Sensitivity[1]	Specificity[1]
White light endoscopy	Imaging	Optics related	Video rate	40	60
Autofluorescence imaging	Imaging	Optics related	Video rate		
Exogenous fluorescence imaging	Imaging	Optics related	Video rate	80–90	40–60
Fiber-optic confocal microscopic imaging	Microscopic imaging	Max 500*600 μm	Max 12 fr/s	nca	nca
Diffuse reflectance spectroscopy	Imaging	Optics related	Video rate	nca	nca
Raman spectroscopy	Diagnosis	Single point	1–5 s	>95%	>90%
Optical coherence tomography	Microscopic imaging[2]	5 × 30 mm	5–15 fr/s	nca	nca
Fluorescence life-time imaging	Imaging and diagnosis	Optics related	5–15 fr/s	nca	nca
Nano-particle fluorescence imaging	Imaging	Optics related	Video rate	nca	nca

nca = no clinical assessment
[1] Sensitivity and specificity average of published papers
[2] Cross-section

References

1. Quayle SS, Ames CD, Lieber D, Yan Y, Landman J. Comparison of optical resolution with digital and standard fiberoptic cystoscopes in an in vitro model. Urology 2005;66:489–93.
2. D'Hallewin MA, El Khatib S, Leroux A, Bezdetnaya L, Guillemin F. Endoscopic confocal fluorescence microscopy of normal and tumor bearing rat bladder. J Urol 2005;174:736–40.
3. Mourant JR, et al. Mechanisms of light scattering from biological cells relevant to noninvasive optical-tissue diagnostics. Appl Optics 1998;37:3586–93.
4. Koenig F, et al. Spectroscopic measurement of diffuse reflectance for enhanced detection of bladder carcinoma. Urology 1998;51:342–5.
5. Demos SG, Gandour-Edwards R, Ramsamooj R, White RD. Spectroscopic detection of bladder cancer using near-infrared imaging techniques. J Biomed Optics 2004;9:767–71.
6. Anidjar M, et al. Argon laser induced autofluorescence may distinguish between normal and tumor human urothelial cells: a microspectrofluorimetric study. J Urol 1996;155:1771–4.
7. Zheng W, Lau W, Cheng C, Soo KC, Olivo M. Optimal excitation-emission wavelengths for autofluorescence diagnosis of bladder tumors. Int. J. Cancer 2003;104:477–81.
8. Guidelines on limits of exposure to ultraviolet radiation of wavelengths between 180 nm and 400 nm (incoherent optical radiation). The International Non-Ionizing Radiation Committee of the International Radiation Protection Association. Health Phys. 1985;49:331–40.
9. Kochevar IE. Cytotoxicity and mutagenicity of excimer laser radiation. Lasers Surg Med. 1989;9:440–5.
10. Chang SC, Buonaccorsi G, MacRobert AJ, Bown SG. 5-Aminolevulinic acid (ALA)-induced protoporphyrin IX fluorescence and photodynamic effects in the rat bladder: an in vivo study comparing oral and intravesical ALA administration. Lasers Surg Med 1997;20:254–64.
11. Divaris DX, Kennedy JC, Pottier RH. Phototoxic damage to sebaceous glands and hair follicles of mice after systemic administration of 5-aminolevulinic acid correlates with localized protoporphyrin IX fluorescence. Am J Pathol. 1990;136:891–7.
12. Leveckis J, Burn JL, Brown NJ, Reed MW. Kinetics of endogenous protoporphyrin IX induction by aminolevulinic acid: preliminary studies in the bladder. J Urol 1994;152:550–3.

13. Pottier RH, et al. Non-invasive technique for obtaining fluorescence excitation and emission spectra in vivo. Photochem Photobiol. 1986;44:679–87.
14. Xiao Z, et al. Biodistribution of Photofrin II and 5-aminolevulinic acid-induced protoporphyrin IX in normal rat bladder and bladder tumor models: implications for photodynamic therapy. Photochem Photobiol. 1998;67:573–83.
15. Kriegmair M, et al. Fluorescence photodetection of neoplastic urothelial lesions following intravesical instillation of 5-aminolevulinic acid. Urology 1994;44:836–41.
16. Kriegmair M, et al. Detection of early bladder cancer by 5-aminolevulinic acid induced porphyrin fluorescence. J Urol. 1996;155:105–9.
17. Zaak D, et al. Endoscopic detection of transitional cell carcinoma with 5-aminolevulinic acid: results of 1012 fluorescence endoscopies. Urology. 2001;57:690–4.
18. Ehsan A, Sommer F, Haupt G, Engelmann U. Significance of fluorescence cystoscopy for diagnosis of superficial bladder cancer after intravesical instillation of delta aminolevulinic acid. Urol Int. 2001;67:298–304.
19. Kriegmair M, et al. Transurethral resection and surveillance of bladder cancer supported by 5-aminolevulinic acid-induced fluorescence endoscopy. Eur Urol. 1999;36:386–92.
20. Filbeck T, et al. No generalized skin phototoxicity after intravesical application of 5-aminolevulinic acid for fluorescence diagnosis of superficial bladder cancer. Urol Int. 2000;64:126–8.
21. Holtl L, et al. Photodynamic diagnosis with 5-aminolevulinic acid in the treatment of secondary urethral tumors: first in vitro and in vivo results. Eur Urol. 2001;39:178–82.
22. Riedl CR, et al. Fluorescence endoscopy with 5-aminolevulinic acid reduces early recurrence rate in superficial bladder cancer. J Urol. 2001;165:1121–3.
23. Juzenas P, Sharfaei S, Moan J, Bissonnette R. Protoporphyrin IX fluorescence kinetics in UV-induced tumours and normal skin of hairless mice after topical application of 5-aminolevulinic acid methyl ester. J Photochem Photobiol. 2002;B 67:11–7.
24. Robinson DJ, de Bruijn HS, de Wolf WJ, Sterenborg HJ, Star WM. Topical 5-aminolevulinic acid-photodynamic therapy of hairless mouse skin using two-fold illumination schemes: PpIX fluorescence kinetics, photobleaching and biological effect. Photochem Photobiol. 2000;72:794–802.
25. Steinbach P, et al. Cellular fluorescence of the endogenous photosensitizer protoporphyrin IX following exposure to 5-aminolevulinic acid. Photochem Photobiol. 1995;62:887–95.

26. Jichlinski P, et al. Clinical evaluation of a method for detecting superficial surgical transitional cell carcinoma of the bladder by light-induced fluorescence of protoporphyrin IX following the topical application of 5-aminolevulinic acid: preliminary results. Lasers Surg Med. 1997;20:402–8.

27. Filbeck T, et al. 5-aminolevulinic acid-induced fluorescence endoscopy applied at secondary transurethral resection after conventional resection of primary superficial bladder tumors. Urology 1999;53:77–81.

28. Lange N, et al. Photodetection of early human bladder cancer based on the fluorescence of 5-aminolaevulinic acid hexylester-induced protoporphyrin IX: a pilot study. Br J Cancer 1999;80:185–93.

29. D'Hallewin MA, Vanherzeele H, Baert L. Fluorescence detection of flat transitional cell carcinoma after intravesical instillation of aminolevulinic acid. Am J Clin Oncol. 1998;21:223–5.

30. Hartmann A, et al. Frequent genetic alterations in simple urothelial hyperplasias of the bladder in patients with papillary urothelial carcinoma. Am J Pathol. 1999;154:721–7.

31. Hartmann A, et al. Occurrence of chromosome 9 and p53 alterations in multifocal dysplasia and carcinoma in situ of human urinary bladder. Cancer Res. 2002;62:809–18.

32. Simoneau AR, et al. Evidence for two tumor suppressor loci associated with proximal chromosome 9p to q and distal chromosome 9q in bladder cancer and the initial screening for GAS1 and PTC mutations. Cancer Res. 1996;56:5039–43.

33. Schneeweiss S, Kriegmair M, Stepp H. Is everything all right if nothing seems wrong? A simple method of assessing the diagnostic value of endoscopic procedures when a gold standard is absent. J Urol. 1999;161:1116–9.

34. Lange N, et al. Routine experimental system for defining conditions used in photodynamic therapy and fluorescence photodetection of (non-) neoplastic epithelia. J Biomed Opt. 2001;6:151–9.

35. Novo M, Huttmann G, Diddens H. Chemical instability of 5-aminolevulinic acid used in the fluorescence diagnosis of bladder tumours. J Photochem Photobiol. B 1996;34:143–8.

36. Loh CS, et al. Oral versus intravenous administration of 5-aminolevulinic acid for photodynamic therapy. Br J Cancer. 1993;68:41–51.

37. Peng Q, Moan J, Warloe T, Nesland JM, Rimington C. Distribution and photosensitizing efficiency of porphyrins induced by application of exogenous 5-aminolevulinic acid in mice bearing mammary-carcinoma. Int J Cancer. 1992;52:433–43.

38. Peng QA, et al. Distribution of 5-aminolevulinic acid-induced porphyrins in noduloulcerative basal-cell carcinoma. Photochem Photobiol. 1995;62:906–13.

39. Chang SC, MacRobert AJ, Bown SG. Biodistribution of protoporphyrin IX in rat urinary bladder after intravesical instillation of 5-aminolevulinic acid. J Urol. 1996;155:1744–48.

40. Iinuma S, Bachor R, Flotte T, Hasan T. Biodistribution and phototoxicity of 5-aminolevulinic acid-induced PpIX in an orthotopic rat bladder tumor model. J Urol. 1995;153:802–6.

41. Bridges JW, Sargent NS, Upshall DG. Rapid absorption from the urinary bladder of a series of n-alkyl carbamates: a route for the recirculation of drugs. Br J Pharmacol. 1979;66:283–9.

42. Jain MK, Vaz WL. Dehydration of the lipid-protein microinterface on binding of phospholipase A2 to lipid bilayers. Biochim Biophys Acta. 1987;905:1–8.

43. Jain MK, Zakim D. The spontaneous incorporation of proteins into preformed bilayers. Biochim Biophys Acta. 1987;906:33–68.

44. Jocham D, et al. Improved detection and treatment of bladder cancer using hexaminolevulinate imaging: a prospective, phase III multicenter study. J Urol. 2005;174:862–6.

45. D'Hallewin MA, Kamuhabwa AR, Roskams T, de Witte PA, Baert L. Hypericin-based fluorescence diagnosis of bladder carcinoma. BJU Int. 2002;89:760–3.

46. Hanlon EB, et al. Prospects for in vivo Raman spectroscopy. Phys Med Biol. 2000;45:R1–59.

47. de Jong BW, et al. Identification of bladder wall layers by Raman spectroscopy. J Urol. 2002;168:1771–8.

48. Crow P, Uff JS, Farmer JA, Wright MP, Stone N. The use of Raman spectroscopy to identify and characterize transitional cell carcinoma in vitro. BJU Int. 2004;93:1232–6.

49. Huang D, et al. Optical coherence tomography. Science 1991;254:1178–81.

50. Van Leeuwen TG, Faber DJ, Aalders MC. Measurement of the axial point spread function in scattering media using single-mode fiber-based optical coherence tomography. IEEE J Selected Topics Quantum Electron. 2003;9:227–33.

51. Faber DJ, et al. Oxygen saturation-dependent absorption and scattering of blood. Phys Rev Lett. 2004;93.

52. van der Meer FJ, et al. Quantitative optical coherence tomography of arterial wall components. Lasers Med Sci. 2005;20:45–51.

53. Fujimoto JG, et al. Optical biopsy and imaging using optical coherence tomography. Nat Med. 1995;1:970–2.

54. Schmitt JM, Knuttel A, Yadlowsky M, Eckhaus MA. Optical-coherence tomography of a dense tissue - statistics of attenuation and backscattering. Phys Med Biol. 1994;39:1705–20.

55. Drexler W, et al. In vivo ultrahigh-resolution optical coherence tomography. Optics Lett. 1999;24:1221–3.

56. Xie TQ, Zeidel ML, Pan YT. Detection of tumorigenesis in urinary bladder with optical coherence tomography: optical characterization of morphological changes. Optics Expr 2002;10:1431–43.

57. Chan WCW, et al. Luminescent quantum dots for multiplexed biological detection and imaging. Curr Opin Biotechnol. 2002;13:40–6.

58. Santra S, Dutta D, Walter GA, Moudgil BM. Fluorescent nanoparticle probes for cancer imaging. Technol Cancer Res Treatment 2005;4:593–602.

59. Munro I, et al. Toward the clinical application of time-domain fluorescence lifetime imaging. J Biomed Opt. 2005;10:051403.

60. Siegel J, et al. Studying biological tissue with fluorescence lifetime imaging: microscopy, endoscopy, and complex decay profiles. Appl Optics 2003;42:2995–3004.

Chapter 41

Elasticity Imaging

R. Souchon

Introduction

It has been noticed since the early days of medicine that a significant number of pathologic conditions are associated with changes in the elastic properties of biological tissues. Nowadays palpation is routinely used in most medical specialties, and many breast or prostate cancers are primarily detected by this means.

Still, palpation remains a highly subjective practice; it is usually limited to organs that are close to the surface of the body and only detects large abnormal masses. Unfortunately none of the many imaging modalities available today (ultrasound B-scans, MRI, CT) provide direct information about the elastic properties of soft tissues. As a consequence research in elasticity imaging has received a growing interest in the scientific community since the late 1980s, and several new elasticity imaging techniques have emerged over the following decade.

In 2005, most of these new techniques were available in specific research laboratories only. However some of them are reaching the stage of clinical evaluation, and the first applications envisioned are often in prostate and breast cancer detection. It is therefore of interest to present them in this book.

In a very simple approximation, the elastic properties of a medium can be characterized by two elastic constants,[1] the bulk modulus and the shear modulus. Two related constants, the Young's modulus and the Poisson's ratio, are also widely used in the literature. Palpation detects contrasts in shear modulus. However none of the new imaging modalities is able to measure an elastic modulus directly. Instead, a mechanical stimulus is applied to the body and the response of the tissues is measured using ultrasound or MRI. There

exist two groups of methods that differ in the type of stimulus. The first group uses a static force and measures the internal strains or displacements generated inside the tissues to create an image. Methods in the second group use a dynamic stimulus, which is often – but not always – a cyclic vibration.

Static Methods

Quasi-static Elastography

Ultrasonic elastography [1] appears as a simple and cost-effective imaging technique because it uses a standard ultrasound scanner and a compression (or expansion) of the organ that can be as simple as manually pushing with the tip of the transducer. The principle is to apply a quasi-static force to the organ being imaged and to form an image of the local internal strains (i.e., percentage deformations) undergone by the tissues (Fig. 41.1). The resulting strain image is called an elastogram. In a first approximation, the local deformation is inversely proportional to tissue stiffness. Stiff masses therefore appear as low strain areas, in contrast to the higher strains visible in softer tissues.

Two radio-frequency (RF) images are acquired, one before the compression is applied (the pre-compression

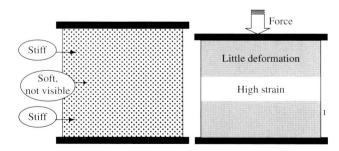

Fig. 41.1 Principle of quasi-static elastography. (Left) A three-layer phantom. (Right) A force is applied onto the phantom; the soft internal layer undergoes higher strain than the stiff surrounding layers

---

[1] In the most general case, mechanical properties are determined by a set of 81 parameters called the elastic constants or elastic moduli.

R. Souchon (✉)
INSERM, U556, Lyon, France

J.J.M.C.H. de la Rosette et al. (eds.), *Imaging in Oncological Urology*,
DOI 10.1007/978-1-84628-759-6_41, © Springer-Verlag London Limited 2009

image) and one after (post-compression). Each RF image is formed by the set of A-lines.[2] The pre-compression RF image is divided into small windows, and a correlation-based algorithm detects where each window has moved during the compression by finding the corresponding pattern in the post-compression image. This process provides an image of tissue displacements. Strain is the ratio of the change in length divided by the initial length; it is directly estimated from the gradient of the displacements, and the resulting strain elastogram is displayed. It is also possible to measure lateral strains. The ratio between the lateral and axial strains has been used to form static and dynamic images of tissue compressibility (Poisson's ratio) which is an intrinsic tissue parameter [1].

The whole process can be accomplished in real time (≥ 10 frames/s). The accuracy of the measurement depends on the direction of the compression, which must be aligned with the direction of propagation of the ultrasonic beam to obtain a high-quality elastogram. Using a large compression surface is preferable to ensure that the elastogram is representative of the underlying elastic properties, but small compressors such as the tip of an end-fire transducer can also be used, provided their influence on the elastogram is compensated for [2].

An advantage of elastography is the immediate availability of the corresponding sonogram, allowing simultaneous display on the scanner. Image registration is perfect because both images are calculated from the same acquisition data. While assessing the potential of elastography to detect prostate cancer, König et al. [3] encountered classification problems during examination directly after acute prostatitis and in patients with chronic prostatitis. They recommended that "real-time elastography should not be interpreted without considering the conventional sonogram at the same time."

Several studies showed the potential of this technique for kidney imaging (Fig. 41.2) [4] and for the detection of prostate cancer (Figs. 41.3–41.5) [2, 3, 5, 6]. In a study conducted in 151 patients with prostate cancer, König et al. [3] concluded that "real-time elastography [...] is a cost-effective and safe new method for detecting prostate cancer, which achieves a high sensitivity rate of 84% in comparison to 64% when using conventional diagnostic modalities." In 2005, at least three major ultrasound companies propose commercial scanners with real-time elastographic capabilities. Clinical evaluation is ongoing and their results will in the near future provide a first insight into the role of elastography in urologic oncology as well as in other medical specialties.

---

[2] A-line: the raw ultrasonic signal received by the scanner after beam-forming.

Acoustic Radiation Force Imaging (ARFI)

Biological tissues, like other composite materials, have a hierarchical structure and the mechanical properties associated with the material depend on the scale used to make the measurements. ARFI is an ultrasound-based technique that images elastic properties of biological tissue on a small scale by exerting a highly localized compression inside the organ [7]. Localized compression is achieved non-invasively using the acoustic radiation force generated by an ultrasonic transducer. The volume of tissue to which significant force is applied is the focal zone of the transmitting transducer, typically $1-8$ mm^3. The same transducer is used in standard A-mode to measure the amplitude of local displacements, typically on the order of 10μm, with a correlation-based technique identical to that used in elastography. The displacement images are correlated to local variations in tissue stiffness and to eventual variations in ultrasonic absorption and/or reflectivity.

When ultrasound propagates through an object, a force is produced. Acoustic radiation force is a unidirectional force that is applied to absorbing or reflecting targets in the propagation path of an acoustic wave. This phenomenon is caused by a transfer of momentum from the acoustic wave to the propagation medium. In a first approximation the radiation force is entirely in the direction of wave propagation, and its amplitude is proportional to the temporal average acoustic intensity of the wave. ARFI interleaves "pushing" beams up to 1 ms in duration with standard A-mode beams to push the tissues and track their displacements. Displacement estimation is performed with a correlation algorithm that compare pre- and post-displacement A-line, as in elastography. An image of the local displacement amplitudes is created by electronically moving the focus of the transducer array. The amplitude of the radiation force depends on the absorption and reflection encountered along the path of the acoustic beam and is therefore uncontrollable and unknown in a clinical situation. If the force is not constant when the focus is moved, the displacement images must be interpreted carefully because the variations in local displacements may not be representative of the underlying elastic properties.

By firing several tracking beams after the initial pushing beam, ARFI can also measure the displacement as a function of time. The excitation and recovery velocities, as well as the peak in displacement amplitude, can be determined from these measurements.

In practice, an advantage of ARFI is its easy implementation using only a standard ultrasound scanner whose firing sequences have been modified to include alternating "pushing" and "tracking" beams. No external compression device is necessary. Because of their high intensity and long duration, the "pushing" beams have a high thermal index

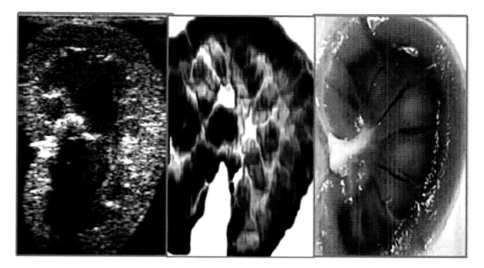

Fig. 41.2 Ovine kidney ex vivo: (a) sonogram, (b) elastogram, and (c) pathology showing the internal structure of the organ ([4], courtesy Pr. Jonathan Ophir)
Reprinted with permission from World Federation of Ultrasound in Medicine and Biology

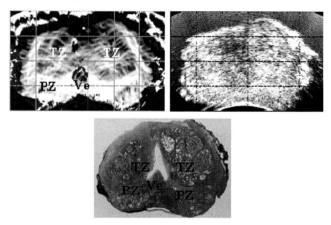

Fig. 41.3 Prostate ex vivo: the zonal anatomy was visible in (a) the strain elastogram (dark is stiff) and (c) gross pathology, but not in (b) the sonogram [5]
Reprinted with permission from World Federation of Ultrasound in Medicine and Biology

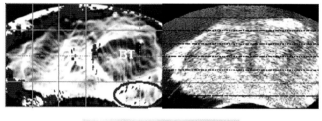

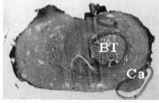

Fig. 41.4 Prostate ex vivo: left posterior cancer (bottom right in the images) and BPH shown in (a) the strain elastogram, (b) the corresponding sonogram, (c) gross pathology [5]
Reprinted with permission from World Federation of Ultrasound in Medicine and Biology

(TI). Nevertheless examination is feasible within the AIUM guidelines. Feasibility of ARFI was recently demonstrated in vivo in the abdomen, bicep, thyroid, and breast [8], but no application has been reported to date in the field of urologic oncology.

Dynamic Methods

Many dynamic methods rely on the transmission of shear waves (also called transverse waves) into the body, i.e., mechanical vibrations wherein particle displacement is perpendicular to the direction of propagation of the wave. It

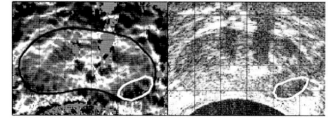

Fig. 41.5 Corresponding (a) elastogram and (b) sonogram of a prostate cancer in vivo [6]
Reprinted with permission from World Federation of Ultrasound in Medicine and Biology

appears therefore of interest to introduce shear waves before the various dynamic imaging modalities are presented. You can get an approximate idea what a shear wave is by dropping a stone into still water and observing the water surface[3]: the wave propagates horizontally, while the oscillating motion is vertical. In biological tissues, low-frequency vibrations mostly propagate as shear waves, whereas high-frequency vibrations (such as MHz-range ultrasonic pulses generated by ultrasound scanners) mostly propagate as compression waves. Shear waves are relatively slow (1–10 m/s) compared to compression waves ($\sim$1500 m/s). The speed of shear waves is approximately proportional to the square root of the shear elastic modulus, which is the parameter of interest in elasticity imaging [9]. The speed of the wave can be estimated using either ultrasound or MR, and the shear elastic modulus is calculated based on the estimated speed. A modulus image is created by measuring the local speed of the wave in each position in the imaging plane. As opposed to strain or displacements that represent the behavior of the tissues, the shear modulus is an intrinsic property of the tissues.

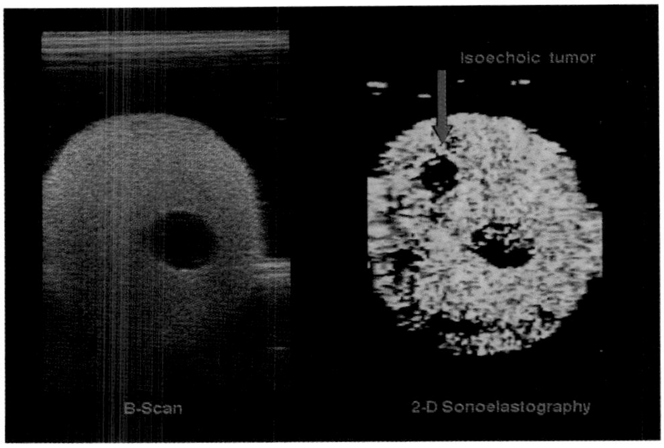

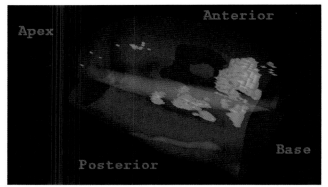

Fig. 41.7 (a) Sonogram and (b) corresponding sono-elasticity image in a prostate phantom with two stiff inclusions, one of which was not visible in the sonogram. Dark corresponds to low-amplitude vibration (i.e., stiff), and highlighted areas to "normal" vibrations (courtesy Pr. Kevin J. Parker)
Reprinted with permission from the Rochester Center for Biomedical Ultrasound at the University of Rochester, Rochester, NY

Sono-elasticity Imaging

In sono-elasticity [9, 10], a low-frequency vibration is applied to the surface of the body using a mechanical vibrator (Fig. 41.6). The vibration is typically 50–500 Hz in frequency and 100 µm in amplitude. The amplitude of the vibration is measured from Doppler signals using a standard ultrasound scanner and is displayed in a vibration ampli-

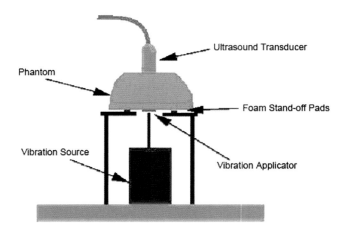

Fig. 41.6 Experimental setup for the acquisition of sono-elasticity images in phantoms (courtesy Pr. Kevin J. Parker)
Reprinted with permission from the Rochester Center for Biomedical Ultrasound at the University of Rochester, Rochester, NY

---

[3] These water waves are in reality surface waves, not shear waves, and serve only here as illustration.

Fig. 41.8 Sono-elasticity image (3D) of the prostate phantom showing the inclusions in pale red (courtesy Pr. Kevin J. Parker)
Reprinted with permission from the Rochester Center for Biomedical Ultrasound at the University of Rochester, Rochester, NY

tude image (Figs. 41.7 and 41.8). Stiff regions undergo low-amplitude vibrations that are easily detected in the image. The Doppler signals can be further processed to estimate the phase of the shear wave, and the speed of the wave can be measured from the resulting phase maps. Finally the shear elastic modulus is directly estimated from the speed of the wave, and a shear modulus image can be displayed. However refraction and reflection of the propagating wave occur at internal tissue boundaries, and can induce a bias in the vibration amplitude image and in the shear modulus estimates.

The first experiments were conducted with the imaging transducer facing the vibrator. Alternatively, the imaging transducer and the vibrator can be positioned side by side, allowing easy clinical implementation. Rubens et al. [11] compared sono-elasticity images to standard ultrasound in 10 prostate cancer specimens in vitro. They displayed "normal" vibration amplitude as a green tag overlay on the sonogram. Stiff non-vibrating regions were displayed as normal B-mode. They reported that "sensitivity and specificity with sono-elasticity imaging were 85% and 84%, respectively, and 30% and 100% with standard ultrasound when compared to pathologic findings." Moreover "64% of pathologically confirmed tumors visible in sono-elasticity imaging were isoechoic on conventional ultrasound images." Initial in vivo experience has been reported in ophthalmology, but so far not in urology.

Transient Elastography

Transient elastography uses a shear wave of short duration to avoid the formation of standing waves, and to remove corresponding measurement artifacts. Transient elastography, or pulsed elastography, was proposed by Catheline et al. [12] in 1999. This technique uses a short-duration shear wave (typically 20 ms), as opposed to sinusoidal shear waves used in sono-elasticity. The propagation of the wave in the imaging plane is tracked using a specific ultrafast ultrasonic imaging system operating at very high frame rate (up to 10,000 frames/s). This frame rate enables to follow the evolution of the pulsed wave on a few centimeters into the tissues with millimetric resolution. The pulsed shear wave induces a transient displacement whose axial component is measured from consecutive A-lines. The shear modulus is calculated from the displacement estimates using the wave propagation equation, and a shear modulus image is displayed. This technique requires sophisticated hardware but it offers significant advantages: The acquisition takes place before unpredictable wave reflections occur, and the elastic modulus can therefore be estimated without a priori knowledge of boundary conditions.

In early experiments, the shear waves were generated at the surface of the body by two electromagnetic vibrators aligned on each side of a linear transducer array. However the success of the imaging technique was very sensitive to the positioning of the imaging probe and penetration depth was limited because shear waves are rapidly attenuated. These early problems were soon eliminated by supersonic shear imaging (SSI), a transient elastography technique that uses the radiation force generated by the imaging transducer to induce the pulsed shear wave deep within the body [13]. Another advantage of supersonic shear imaging is its easy clinical implementation: The examination can be performed with a standard transducer array connected to the ultrafast system.

The first clinical images reported with transient elastography were breast adenocarcinomas. These images were initially acquired with the vibrators [14] and later with SSI [13]. Breast adenocarcinomas were 3–5 times stiffer than normal surrounding tissues and were clearly visible in the modulus images. In 2005 no image has been reported in urology yet.

Magnetic Resonance Elastography (MRE)

MRE is a technique that images propagating mechanical waves using MRI [15]. In the presence of magnetic field gradient, the motion of nuclear spins causes a phase shift in a nuclear magnetic resonance (NMR) signal. The phase shift is proportional to the displacement amplitude. In MRE motion-sensitizing gradient sequences are synchronized with mechanical vibrations (shear waves) of the body, and a "snapshot" of the instantaneous amplitude of tissue displacement is created from the phase shift. Extremely small displacements can be measured using this technique (~100 nm).

The propagating wave can be observed at various points in time by adding a synchronous delay between the gradient sequence and the vibration, thus providing "snapshots" of the wave during one oscillatory cycle. Compiling the displacement images together in time order makes a "movie" of the propagating wave. The displacement "movies" can be processed to estimate and display the shear modulus of the tissues.

The motion-sensitizing gradients can be placed along any axis, so with multiple acquisitions it is possible to acquire all components of the displacements. The use of three-dimensional displacements leads to a mathematical formulation that accounts for eventual reflections or standing waves. MRE has the advantage of sensitive motion detection in all directions with equal sensitivity, but it is slower than ultrasound-based methods.

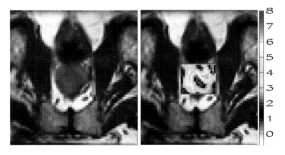

Fig. 41.9 (a) Magnitude MR image and (b) elasticity distribution (in kPa) superimposed inside the prostate gland in vivo. The peripheral portion appears stiffer than the central zone (Kemper et al. [16], courtesy Dr. Ralph Sinkus)

The technical feasibility of in vivo MRE of the prostate gland was shown by Kemper et al. [16] in healthy volunteers. They noted in their study that the modulus images correlated with the zonal anatomy of the prostate: the central portion was 30% softer than the peripheral portion (Fig. 41.9). The existence of a contrast between the two zones of the prostate was previously observed by Souchon et al. [6] using quasi-static elastography, but with an inverse contrast (i.e., softer peripheral zone). This observation suggests that the static properties and the dynamic properties of biological tissues may be different, and thus static and dynamic elasticity imaging methods may provide complementary information.

Ultrasound-Stimulated Vibro-Acoustography

Vibro-acoustography [17] uses a cyclic and highly localized acoustic radiation force[4] to image the acoustic response of a material to a mechanical vibration. Two transducers (or two groups of elements from the same transducer array) are used to transmit two tone bursts (i.e., a few sine cycles) of slightly different frequencies f_1 and $f_1 + \Delta f$. The difference in frequency Δf is small, typically in the range of kHz, whereas the central frequency of the transducers and the frequency f_1 are in the range of MHz. The transducers are positioned so that their beams intersect within an object. The interaction of the two beams produces a beat[5] at the frequency Δf, resulting in a low-frequency radiation force f effectively vibrating the object in the selected region. The vibrated target acts as a local sound source and produces an acoustic field that can be measured some distance away by a sensitive microphone (or a hydrophone in water). An image of the amplitude (or of the phase) of the acoustic field is formed by probing the region of interest point by point by raster scanning. By this means, vibrations of extremely small amplitudes (as low as a few nanometers) can be detected.

The amplitude and phase of the acoustic field are determined by the mechanical properties of the object, but also by its geometry and by the amplitude of the applied force. In most medical applications, the mechanical properties and the amplitude of the radiation force are unknown. Estimating the elastic modulus from the amplitude image is therefore difficult, and a more practical approach is to display and interpret qualitative amplitude images directly.

Vibro-acoustic spectrography is able to detect the resonance frequencies of an object by varying the frequency Δf of the vibration. Detection of the resonance frequencies can be used to distinguish between objects made of identical materials but having different geometries, such as tuning forks [17]. Small objects whose resonance frequencies are known a priori can be detected with high contrast by vibro-acoustography [18].

One of the first applications of vibro-acoustography was the detection of calcifications in human arteries and vessels [17]. The technique was later applied in vivo to detect breast arterial calcifications, but its potential in urologic applications has yet to be investigated.

Conclusion

Pathological conditions are often associated with changes in tissue elasticity. The detection of abnormal masses by palpation is a standard practice, but many nodules elude detection by palpation by virtue of their small size or of their deep location within the body. Elasticity imaging techniques open up new opportunities in medical imaging. Quantitative information about tissue stiffness is now available with high resolution and high penetration depth. Some of the techniques already operate in real time. It is expected that the resulting images convey clinically significant information that is currently unavailable with existing imaging modalities such as MRI, CT scans, or standard B-mode ultrasound.

Elasticity imaging also opens up exciting possibilities that extend beyond strain or modulus imaging: Viscosity, permeability (the ease with which fluids flow within an organ), nonlinear elasticity (elastic properties changing under load), and tissue connectedness (i.e., how a tumor is attached to surrounding tissues) are some of the new parameters that may be explored with elasticity-based techniques.

As of 2005, initial clinical evaluation of most elasticity imaging described in this chapter was already beginning. The next challenges will be to assess their clinical benefits. In the field of urologic oncology, and specifically for prostate cancer detection, clinical evaluation of ultrasonic elastography and MRE is now only beginning.

Acknowledgments

The author would like to acknowledge Prof. Jonathan Ophir, Prof. Kevin J. Parker, and Dr. Ralph Sinkus for their valuable contribution to this section.

---

[4] We refer the reader to the section on acoustic radiation force imaging (ARFI) for details on radiation force.

[5] Similar to the low-frequency oscillation heard when striking two guitar strings that are slightly out of tune with each other.

References

1. Ophir J, et al. Elastography: ultrasonic estimation and imaging of the elastic properties of tissues. J Eng Med. 1999;213(3):203–33.

2. Lorenz A, et al. A new system for the acquisition of ultrasonic multicompression strain images of the human prostate in vivo. IEEE Trans Ultrason Ferroelectr Freq Control. 1999;46(5):1147–53.

3. König K, et al. Initial experiences with real-time elastography guided biopsies of the prostate. J Urol. 2005;174:115–7.

4. Kallel F, et al. Elastographic imaging of low-contrast elastic modulus distributions in tissue. Ultrasound Med Biol. 1998;24(3):409–25.

5. Souchon R, et al. Prostate elastography: in vitro study. Proc. IEEE Ultrasonics Symp. 2003a;2:1251–13.

6. Souchon R, et al. Visualisation of HIFU lesions using elastography of the human prostate in vivo: Preliminary results. Ultrasound Med Biol. 2003b;29(7):1007–15.

7. Nightingale KR, et al. On the feasibility of remote palpation using acoustic radiation force. J Acoust Soc Am. 2001;110(1):625–34.

8. Nightingale K, et al. Acoustic radiation force impulse imaging: in vivo demonstration of clinical feasibility. Ultrasound Med Biol. 2002;28(2):227–35.

9. Yamakoshi Y, et al. Ultrasonic imaging of internal vibration of soft tissue under forced vibration. IEEE Trans Ultrason Ferroelectr Freq Control. 1990;37(2):45–53.

10. Lerner RM, et al. Sono-elasticity: medical elasticity images derived from ultrasound signals in mechanically vibrated targets. Acoustic Imaging. 1988;16:317–27.

11. Rubens DJ, et al. Sonoelasticity imaging of prostate cancer: in vitro results. Radiology. 1995;195:379–83.

12. Catheline S, et al. Diffraction field of a low-frequency vibrator in soft tissues using transient elastography, IEEE Trans Ultrason Ferroelect Freq Contr. 1999;46(4):1013–1020.

13. Bercoff J, et al. Supersonic Shear Imaging: a new technique for soft tissues elasticity mapping. IEEE Trans Ultrason Ferroelec Freq Contr. 2004;51(4):374–409.

14. Bercoff J, et al. In vivo breast tumor detection using transient elastography. Ultrasound Med Biol. 2003;29(10):1387–96.

15. Muthupillai R, et al. Magnetic resonance elastography by direct visualization of propagating acoustic strain waves. Science. 1995;269(5232):1854–7.

16. Kemper J, et al. MR elastography of the prostate: initial in-vivo application. Fortschr Röntgenstr. 2004;176(8);1094–9.

17. Fatemi M, Greenleaf JF. Ultrasound-stimulated vibro-acoustic spectrography. Science. 1998;280:82–5.

18. Mitri FG, et al. Improving the use of vibro-acoustography for brachytherapy metal seed imaging: a feasibility study. IEEE Trans Med Imaging. 2004;23(1):1–6.

19. Fatemi M, et al. Vibro-acoustic tissue mammography. IEEE Trans Med Imaging. 2002;21(1):1–8.

Chapter 42

Future Directions

D. Cosgrove

Remarkable improvements in medical imaging over the past few decades have rendered it an essential component of almost every part of medical practice, none more so than in oncology, including urological oncology. Many hospitals now use multidisciplinary meetings, where clinicians join with diagnosticians such as pathologists and imagers, to discuss the findings of their patients and to formulate the best patient care plans; this represents a significant improvement on the old system where the consultant in charge often took these decisions in isolation.

As well as the major impact that diagnostic imaging has made on oncology, it has also improved several aspects of therapy by providing image guidance for external beam radiotherapy and for minimally invasive procedures such as interstitial ablation. The role of the traditional surgeon and the imager is fusing, a trend that is likely to continue since this approach is kinder to patients and is cost-effective.

Many of these established methods are described in this section as well as new methods both as potential diagnostic tools and as ways to improve treatment.

Improved Imaging: Contrast Agents, Image Fusion, Virtual Imaging, and Robotics

An area where major improvements have been developed is the field of contrast agents (Chapter 38). Non-ionic dimeric iodinated agents have improved the safety of contrast-enhanced CT while at the same time improving image quality by providing denser pyelograms.

New families of agents for MR have opened new fields of application. An important example in urology is the use of nanoparticle superparamagnetic iron oxides (SPIOs) for imaging pelvic lymph nodes: normal lymphoid tissue takes up the particles over a 24–36 h period but metastatic tissue does not. The iron quenches the T2∗ signals so that the metastases show as foci of high signal, allowing the detection of metastases in normal-sized nodes with high accuracy. This may be considered a form of molecular imaging (see below).

Ultrasound contrast agents in the form of microbubbles that resonate in the sound field and produce unique signals that can be separately displayed alongside the reference gray scale image have had a major impact on oncological imaging. They have two special properties that make them useful. Being much larger than the molecular scale agents generally used for CT and MR, they remain in the cavity into which they are administered and so behave as blood pool agents following intravenous injection, and they can be destroyed by ultrasound at the high end of the FDA-permitted power range, thus permitting destruction-reperfusion imaging and quantification. In uro-oncology they have proved useful in characterizing renal and prostatic masses but in general abdominal imaging their main uses are for focal liver lesions where the combination of arterial perfusion hemodynamics and the liver-specific late phase caused by their phagocytosis by Kupffer cells allows both detection of metastases and characterization of masses.

An important trend in modern imaging is the fusion of information from two (or more) modalities with complementary characteristics. The best-known example is positron emission tomography (PET) with CT, in which the functional information on tumor metabolism provided by imaging the distribution of ^{19}F-deoxy glucose (FDG) with PET complements the excellent anatomical imaging of CT. By combining the two in a single hybrid scanner, the color-coded PET images can be superimposed on the CT images and this so improves the detection of metastases that it is rapidly becoming routine, despite its high initial and running costs. PET-MRI systems have also been proposed, though the technical challenges of maintaining adequate image quality for both modalities are formidable. New and promising PET tracers are being developed that will be especially relevant to oncology.

D. Cosgrove (✉)
Imaging Sciences Department, Imperial College, Hammersmith Hospital, Du Cane Road, London W12 0NN, UK

Fusion of CT or MRI with ultrasound is also attractive because the real-time and interactive nature of ultrasound is so useful for interventional procedures such as biopsies and interstitial ablation. Many of these systems are experimental but a commercial device (Virtual Navigator, Esaote, Florence, Italy, http://www.esaote.com/products/brochures/Navigator/Navigator.pdf) makes use of prescanned 3D data sets to provide an updated resliced view of the entire cross-sectional image of the patient in the plane of the real-time ultrasound scan which is superimposed upon it. Fiduciary markers align the two image sets, and the position of the ultrasound transducer is tracked with electromagnetic sensors. The ability to "see" the whole field while observing the needle pathway in real time simplifies and improves the accuracy of the procedure. Anticipated advances will include corrections for movement such as breathing and the effects of the intervention.

Virtual imaging (Chapter 39) in which 3D image sets from CT or MRI are redisplayed so as to emulate the endoscopist's view has been further advanced as a replacement for colonoscopy but can also be used for viewing the bladder and ureters in a way that may be more familiar to the surgeon than tomographic slices. The field is advancing rapidly because of the development of fast computers and elegant display algorithms, many owing their development to the PC games industry. The addition of i.v. contrast for CT and obtaining scans in both supine and prone positions improves the detection of tumors so that virtual cystoscopy might eventually be used instead of conventional cystoscopy. A limitation that seems to be insuperable is the inability to visualize non-raised lesions such as in situ bladder tumors.

Another development that relies on fast computing is robotic surgery (Chapter 36), either to assist the surgeon who controls the position of the surgical instrument remotely with image guidance or to perform the procedure according to a presurgical plan. The original development of such aids was in neurosurgery where the rigid skull facilitates the planning and implementation of the procedure. More recently, robots that can operate inside a CT scanner with guidance that is updated by repeated scanning have been developed. Similarly, MRI-controlled systems have been developed, despite the formidable challenges of devising pneumatic motors and avoiding the use of electronics to ensure MR compatibility.

New Imaging Techniques: Optical Imaging and Elastography

Optical imaging (Chapter 40) makes use of visible light in one of several modes (e.g., reflectance, coherent tomography) or of fluorescence, the best established being fluorescence retinal angiography. A general limitation is the depth of tissue that the light can penetrate, which, for short wavelengths needed to obtain useful spatial resolution, is restricted to around 0.5 mm. Thus, optical imaging in urology is most promising for the urothelium. Using conventional endoscopes, spectral filtering can highlight pathologies that are not as well seen with white light. More detailed information can be obtained by confocal tomography in which both the illuminating and the viewing light beams are passed through a small pinhole. Only a very restricted depth of tissue is imaged; to create an image, the light is scanned across the surface and the image is built up in a raster fashion. Highly detailed images result and the method can be performed through a fiber endoscope to interrogate the superficial layers of the bladder. Many native molecules such as collagen and NADH autofluoresce and this can be exploited to form images of the bladder surface but background signals degrade the contrast. This can be improved by adding fluorescent dyes, of which aminolevulinic acid (ALA) and even better, hexyl ALA, is one of the most promising because the porphyrin it forms accumulates preferentially in malignancies. It can be instilled into the bladder and imaged under ultraviolet illumination with excellent sensitivity but less high specificity. Fluorescence indicates abnormal tissue, including in situ changes and even abnormalities of the protein p53, which induces apoptosis and controls the development of many cancers. Hypericin is another promising fluorochrome.

Inelastic imaging is a method in which incident photons are frequency shifted and so is exquisitely sensitive to the local chemistry. The resulting Raman shifts indicate local chemical composition with great precision, though the process is inefficient and therefore noisy. Chemical changes can be detected and the method has been applied to the bladder wall with high sensitivity to transitional cell carcinomas. Many of these methods can be combined in hybrid imaging techniques that are being explored.

New optical techniques are very exciting. In one, quantum dot imaging, a new class of nanometer fluorochromes is used; they have the key advantage that their emission wavelength can be tuned by changing the particle size. Another potentially important technique is a temporal approach in which the decay of fluorescence is monitored to provide a temporal rather than an intensity indicator of activity. Fluorescence lifetime imaging (FLIM) can distinguish the numerous intrinsic natural fluorescing molecules by measuring the rate of decay of the fluorescence.

In elastography (Chapter 41), an image of the tissue's stiffness is created. The method is promising in oncology and elsewhere simply because palpation for stiffness is a well-tried basic clinical method. The concept is simple: two images are created, one before and one after the tissue is distorted by an applied force, and the difference is used to form an image of the tissue's response to the stress. The resulting elastogram or strain image can use MR or ultrasound but the latter has been the most exploited to date. It has the advantage that, in the simplest systems, the transducer can be used to apply the stress, either manually or via a motor. There are commercialized manual systems, and promising results have been reported for the breast while early work on the prostate is also promising.

More complex systems have also been developed. In one, vibro-elastography, two ultrasonic beams with slightly different frequencies are sent simultaneously. The frequencies are chosen so that the interference frequency is a few kilohertz and this vibrates the tissue. Imaging can use MR or ultrasound, both of which are sensitive to the changes induced by tissue compression to produce elastograms. Another approach, transient elastography, uses an acoustic transducer to send a focussed beam into the tissue to generate a shock wave that travels at right angles away from it. Ultrasfast ultrasound scanning is used to image the tissue compression produced by the shock wave and create an elastogram. Both these methods have the advantage that they generate the tissue compression internally and so can be used in organs that are inaccessible from the skin, such as the brain.

Molecular Imaging and Drug/Gene Delivery

The role of nanoparticle SPIOs as molecular imaging agents for lymph node macrophages has already been mentioned, and similar nanoparticles may be tagged with agents that bind specifically to cell surface receptors. Examples include monoclonal antibodies to cancers, but this application is not straightforward because the targeted receptors are scanty and non-specific binding serves to reduce the signal to background ratio.

Microbubbles can also be targeted for imaging of molecular processes such as with integrins for the activated endothelium of inflammation. Targeting tumors may be more difficult because they may not cross the capillary walls, but two factors are in their favor of this potential application: the increased permeability of the poorly formed neovascularization of tumors and the fact that disruption of microbubbles produces local rupture of the capillary endothelium. An extension of this approach that could prove to be of great clinical value is the possibility of loading targeted microbubbles with anti-tumor drugs or small interfering RNA (siRNA) and then using higher power ultrasound to release them at high local concentration for improved therapeutic ratios.

Conclusions

Recently developed and upcoming imaging methods continue to improve patient care, especially in oncology, which is dependent on them for detection, diagnosis, treatment planning, and follow-up monitoring. Advances promise to improve many of these aspects as well as to improve treatment, both conventional and minimally invasive, as well as working with new treatments such as stem cell therapy and novel anticancer approaches such as antiangiogenesis and targeted gene therapy.

Index

Printed in the United States of America